Toward a Science of
FAMILY NURSING

Toward a Science of
FAMILY NURSING

Edited by

Catherine L. Gilliss, RNC, DNSc

Betty L. Highley, RN, MS, FAAN

Brenda M. Roberts, RN, MS

Ida M. Martinson, RN, PhD, FAAN

Addison-Wesley Publishing Company
Health Sciences Division, Menlo Park, California
Reading, Massachusetts · New York · Don Mills, Ontario
Wokingham, England · Amsterdam · Bonn · Sydney
Singapore · Tokyo · Madrid · San Juan

Sponsoring Editor   Debra S. Hunter

Production Consultant   Wendy Earl

Text and Cover Designer   Gary Head

Copyeditor   Melissa Andrews

Illustrator   Ken Miller

Indexer   Katherine Pitcoff

Compositor   Graphic Typesetting Service

Library of Congress Cataloging-in-Publication Data
Toward a science of family nursing.

 Includes bibliographies and index.
 1. Family nursing.   I. Gilliss, Catherine Lynch,
1949–   . [DNLM: 1. Family.   2. Health Promotion.
3. Nursing Care.   WY 100 T737]
RT120.F34T69 1989   610   88-14470
ISBN 0-201-14238-4

5678910–HA–95 94 93 92 91

Addison-Wesley Publishing Company
Health Sciences Division
2725 Sand Hill Road
Menlo Park, California 94025

FOREWORD

Ann L. Whall, RN, PhD, FAAN

Every few years a comprehensive text is published that through its breadth and depth summarizes the state of knowledge in a field of science. This text by Gilliss, Highley, Roberts, and Martinson represents such an effort. Via text and pictures, with clarity and wisdom, this book identifies the substantive areas in a major nursing subspecialty field. One of the best-kept secrets in nursing is the flourishing subspecialty known as family nursing, which encompasses all the traditional medically based nursing practice areas. The knowledge base in this field has literally blossomed within the last fifteen years. It is now possible to identify with clarity and precision the substantive areas in family nursing. Moreover, the research body in family nursing càn be catalogued, classified, and summarized in an analysis of strengths and weaknesses, and necessary new directions can be identified. The theory that underpins the area of family nursing derives from and contributes to research. A sufficient body of research now exists, making it possible to identify the state of the art and science in each content area in family nursing. This effort has been addressed with intelligence and a good deal of persistence by the editors of this text. As such, they have accomplished what others may have only fleetingly pondered or may have considered too overwhelming to undertake. The editors have identified the needed discussions in the content areas and have appointed a cadre of important contributors to address each area. Moreover, they have classified, through chapter selection, the major spheres of exploration in family nursing. This classification is an important contribution to family nursing. In addition, each chapter leads us to identify future directions and presents insights that may be used in practice.

This text will advance the field in a variety of ways. For example, undergraduate nursing students might selectively use a chapter or several chapters for a particular nursing care problem. Graduate students in masters programs might select the areas of importance to their field of study or they may use the text as a source book to suggest research problems and theory underpinning various interest areas. Professors or instructors in various educational programs similarly will find this text helpful as they identify course content, prepare lecture notes, and examine specific problem areas to address in research. One of the most exciting ways in which this text might be used is at the doctoral level. Nursing has long discussed the need to identify the nature of its knowledge base as well as the way in which it might be subdivided and classified. This text suggests that it is possible to identify the knowledge base with a good deal of intelligence, insight, and creativity. This text could be a springboard for other texts that present new content subdivisions, rather than the old medical categories, in nursing.

Perhaps time must pass before a discipline can identify the major concepts and propositions that constitute a content area and the research strategies that advance knowledge development within it. Once the content is thus identified, it may be analyzed and reclassified. There has been little of this effort in subspecialty areas in nursing. Perhaps hampered by past ideologies and notions, nursing heretofore has not identified family nursing in as comprehensive fashion as is done in this text. I look forward to the future, when other texts that transcend the traditional clinical areas and identify specific areas in nursing are presented. Once we have identified and examined our own knowledge base, we can better prepare for work in an interdisciplinary fashion as we collaborate to produce better health care for the people we serve. Until we understand the content and structure of our knowledge base, our ability to collaborate with other disciplines will be limited. I believe the efforts represented by this text help clarify our knowledge and prepare us to collaborate with professionals from other disciplines. Indeed, it is a brave new world before us.

ANN L. WHALL

Ann Arbor, Michigan
March, 1988

CONTENTS

FOREWORD   v

Ann L. Whall

PREFACE   xiii

THE CAMERA IN NURSING RESEARCH
AND PRACTICE   xxi

Betty L. Highley, Tom Ferentz

SECTION I

ISSUES IN FAMILY NURSING
CARE AND RESEARCH

1 WHY FAMILY HEALTH CARE?   3

Catherine L. Gilliss

2 THEORETICAL PERSPECTIVES ON THE FAMILY   9

Ramona T. Mercer

3 FAMILY RESEARCH IN NURSING   37

Catherine L. Gilliss

4 WHAT IS FAMILY NURSING?   64

Catherine L. Gilliss, Brenda M. Roberts,
Betty L. Highley, Ida M. Martinson

SECTION II

FACTORS INFLUENCING FAMILY HEALTH

5 HEALTHY FAMILIES:
FORMS AND PROCESSES   77
Madeline W. Gershwin, Janet M. Nilsen

6 NUTRITION AND THE FAMILY   92
Yolanda Gutierrez, Katharyn Antle May

7 THE FAMILY AND THE COMMUNITY:
MOBILIZING SOCIAL SUPPORT   113
Hester Y. Kenneth

8 CULTURE AND FAMILY   124
Joan Ablon, Genevieve M. Ames

9 HEALTH CARE FINANCING, POLICY,
AND FAMILY NURSING PRACTICE: NEW
OPPORTUNITIES   146
Susan B. Meister

10 FAMILY LIFE IN THE 21ST CENTURY:
AN ANALYSIS OF OLD FORMS, CURRENT
TRENDS, AND FUTURE SCENARIOS   156
Robert Staples

SECTION III

TRANSITIONS IN THE FAMILY LIFE CYCLE

11 FAMILY TRANSITIONS: EXPECTED
AND UNEXPECTED   173
Sally H. Rankin

12 CHILDBEARING AND ITS EFFECT ON
MARITAL QUALITY   187
Brooke Randell

13 THE PERINATAL FAMILY   199

M. Colleen Stainton

14 THE PROCESS OF GRIEF IN THE
BEREAVED FAMILY   216

Sandra McClowry, Catherine L. Gilliss, Ida M. Martinson

15 CHILD DAY CARE FOR HEALTHY
YOUNGER FAMILIES   226

Roberta S. O'Grady, Meryl Glass

APPENDIX: CHILD CARE RESOURCES   247

PHOTO GALLERY: CHILD DAY CARE

Betty L. Highley

16 THE FAMILY WITH A HOSPITALIZED
CHILD   248

Carol Hardgrove, Brenda M. Roberts

17 TRANSITION TO ILLNESS: THE FAMILY
IN THE HOSPITAL   262

Maribelle B. Leavitt

SECTION IV

PROMOTING FAMILY HEALTH DURING
CHRONIC ILLNESS

18 THE FAMILY AND CHRONIC ILLNESS   287

*Catherine L. Gilliss, Debra Rose,
Jeanne C. Hallburg, Ida M. Martinson*

PHOTO GALLERY: THE STORY OF
BILL HANEY

Tom Ferentz

19 THE FAMILY WITH A CHRONICALLY ILL CHILD:
AN INTERACTIONAL PERSPECTIVE   300
Bonnie Holaday

20 THE FAMILY WITH A CHRONICALLY
ILL ADOLESCENT   322
Marilyn C. Savedra, Suzanne L. Dibble

21 THE FAMILY AND CANCER   332
Kay B. Tiblier

22 THE FAMILY AND CARDIAC ILLNESS   344
Catherine L. Gilliss

23 THE FAMILY AND DIABETES MELLITUS   357
Jeanne C. Hallburg, Marilyn J. Little

PHOTO GALLERY: DIABETES: A TRILOGY
Gail Garvin, Betty L. Highley, Tom Ferentz

24 MENTAL ILLNESS AND THE FAMILY   374
Catherine A. Chesla

25 ABUSIVE BEHAVIOR IN FAMILIES   394
Janice Humphreys, Jacquelyn C. Campbell

26 ALZHEIMER'S DISEASE AND THE FAMILY   418
*Mary Lou Muwaswes, Catherine L. Gilliss, Ida M. Martinson,
Glen Caspers Doyle, Catherine A. Chesla, Joycelyn King*

27 PALLIATIVE CARE NURSING: PROMOTING
FAMILY INTEGRITY   437
Jennifer Lillard, Linda Marietta

28 SUICIDE AND THE ELDERLY   461
Patrick Arbore, Arliss Thompson Willis

29 ALCOHOLISM AND THE FAMILY   472

W. Carole Chenitz, William Granfors

PHOTO GALLERY: EPILOGUE

APPENDIX: VISUAL MEDIA RESEARCH REFERENCES   487

INDEX   489

PREFACE

"Science seeks to understand the real world. Theory is the product of science; research is its tool."

STAINTON, 1982

The 1980's has been an important decade for the evolution of the science of family nursing. In the early part of the decade, Marie Lobo and Suzanne Feetham were tireless in their effort to identify the "community" of people interested in family nursing. They met with special interest groups on the family at national and regional nursing research meetings, collecting names wherever they went, and assembled a long list of doctorally prepared family nurse researchers throughout the United States and Canada. Lobo, Feetham, Barbara Germino, Catherine Gilliss, and Susan Meister organized the first invitational conference for family nurse researchers at the Wingspread Conference site in Racine, Wisconsin, in November 1984. For two and a half days 50 family nurse researchers presented and critiqued their work and discussed strategies for the further development of family research in nursing. This group met again in January of 1986. The significance of these meetings was twofold: First, a powerful network of family nurse researchers was formed; second, the participating nurses shaped the direction of the family nursing research movement by calling for future gatherings to include the many interested others who could not participate in Wingspread. The network spread the word that the next "gathering" would occur in Calgary at the International Conference of Family Nursing in 1988. The Calgary meeting, which will occur concurrently with the release of this volume, will bring together numerous and talented family nurse researchers and clinicians from all over the world.

The meeting activity in family nursing has been paralleled by flourishing writing activities, with contributions from many nurse researchers as well as those in other disciplines in the social and health sciences. Until now, that important work has not been drawn together in one volume. We wrote this book to begin the synthesis of the science of family nursing.

The Audience

This text is intended as a resource for nurse clinicians, graduate students, faculty, and researchers. Preprofessional students with preliminary understanding of family theory and beginning experience in providing care to families will also find it useful. It is not intended as a beginning text or a "how-to" text for family nursing.

Features of the Book

Our book is unique because of its approach, its scope, and its special features. In particular:

A Broad Range of Contributors

While the majority of contributors to this book are nurses, we have also invited professionals in other fields to participate. For example, the perspectives of anthropologists, sociologists, and a nutritionist provide a blend of content appropriate to family nursing. This reflects the interdisciplinary, team-oriented nature of this field.

Divergent Approaches to Family Nursing

The reader will find a variety of divergent approaches to family nursing within this text. Some contributors have focused on the family group and its health and properties, and others have discussed care and study approaches that reflect the nursing of family members. This variation echoes the diversity of our developing knowledge base and the influences of traditional perspectives on the individual as the unit of care. As editors, we find that divergent approaches show a level of scholarship characteristic of graduate education. Had we insisted on a uniform framework or conceptual base, our advocacy for family nursing would have been weakened and the richness of the contributions diminished. Those chapters that do not distinguish clearly between the family viewed as a context and the family viewed as a unit do, however, provide an analysis of current knowledge from which family nursing science and care can emerge.

Use of Photographs as a Research Tool

The use of photographs to advance understanding of family functions and interactions is employed in the photo galleries that appear after chapters 15, 18, 23, and 29 and is further described in the prologue to the photographs, entitled The Camera in Nursing Research and Practice.

Questions for Further Research

In our effort to identify phenomena for study and to promote organization of knowledge, we have ended each chapter with a set of questions intended to identify issues for further investigation. Family nursing science is new, therefore much of the information presented in this volume needs further analysis and refinement. Fresh questions must be asked, new methods employed. Paradigmatic diversity abounds, but the usefulness of those paradigms needs closer examination.

Comprehensive Coverage

Family nursing emerges from and is a part of many traditional areas of nursing practice. This text reflects that diversity, with coverage of families across the life cycle in varying states of health and illness.

Organization of the Book

The book is organized into four sections. In Section I, Issues in Family Nursing Care and Research, the chapters provide a foundation for the book and examine the rationale for and characteristics of family nursing. The research focus of the book is addressed in this unit.

Section II, Factors Influencing Family Health, introduces issues such as alternate family forms, nutrition, the community, and social support. Also included are cultural patterns and governmental health policies that affect family.

Section III, Transitions in the Family Life Cycle, addresses the changes that occur in families as they develop. Changes during the family life cycle are described as transitions or crises, and the nursing care required by families in transition is distinguished from the care needed by families in crisis. Family life cycle events such as childbearing, the integration of an infant into a family, child day care, and hospitalization of a family member are covered in depth.

Section IV discusses Promoting Family Health During Chronic Illness. Chapters cover families with a chronically ill child, a chronically ill adolescent, a member with cancer, a member with cardiac illness, a member with diabetes mellitus, a member with Alzheimer's disease and families with mental illness. Abusive behavior in families, end-stage illness, suicide and the elderly, and the effect of alcohol-

ism on family members are also covered in separate chapters.

Toward a Science of Family Nursing

As we have worked on this book, our enthusiasm for this developing science has grown. Clearly, a major advance in family nursing can be accomplished by building a cumulative science and developing paradigms and theories that adequately address the nurse and the family. In this volume we have collected the important early research in family nursing and we invite the reader to continue the development of this work. We hope to offer a beginning, a departure point, for the long trek *Toward a Science of Family Nursing.*

CATHERINE L. GILLISS

BETTY L. HIGHLEY

BRENDA M. ROBERTS

IDA M. MARTINSON

San Francisco, California
March, 1988

ACKNOWLEDGMENTS

Many people have contributed, in different and special ways, to the development of this manuscript. First, we wish to thank the many patients and caregivers who unselfishly participated in the photographic galleries of this book. In particular, we are grateful to William Haney, whose long and brave struggle with debilitating disease is an inspiration to us all; and to his caregiver Gina, whose commitment to Bill and his care added years and meaning to his life. We also acknowledge Hadley Hall for his administrative role in facilitating entree into care settings and patients' homes.

Our colleagues who contributed chapters to the book provided depth and scope we could not have achieved alone. Ingeborg Mauksch and Ann Whall offered wisdom on the direction and scope of the project. We thank our colleagues in the Department of Family Health Care, particularly Tom Ferentz for his contributions to the photo galleries, and Jacqueline Ventura for her participation in the early discussion of this project. Many associates helped us negotiate the inevitable, unanticipated snafus. Among these we thank Linda Cox, Jeff Longcope, Mitch Allen, and Dudley Kaye. Administrative and technical support were competently provided by Diana Zielinski, Dale Lee, and Marie Elena Sotelo.

The reviewers on the next page offered constructive feedback during the development of this text.

Sister Lucy Callaghan, RN, MSN
Assistant Professor of Nursing
The University of Kansas
School of Nursing

Ann Cain, RN, PhD
Professor of Psychiatric Nursing
University of Maryland
School of Nursing

Marilyn M. Friedman, RN, PhD
Professor
Department of Nursing
California State University, Los Angeles

Ann L. Whall, RN, PhD, FAAN
Professor
School of Nursing
University of Michigan, Ann Arbor

Anonymous Reviewer
Mount St. Mary's College, Los Angeles

We are especially grateful to our sponsoring editor, Debra S. Hunter, who believed in our project; to our production consultant, Wendy Earl, whose equanimity and unstinting support are without equal; and to our designer, Gary Head, who accepted our ideas with respect.

Finally, we have derived inspiration from our families. Following publication of this book, we owe a great debt for their endurance of frozen dinners, lost Sundays at the playground, and missed conversations. We thank them for realizing the importance of this work to us.

ABOUT THE EDITORS

Catherine L. Gilliss, RNC, DNSc, is Assistant Professor in the School of Nursing, Department of Family Health Care, at the University of California at San Francisco.

A background that included graduate study in psychiatric–mental health nursing, preparation as an adult nurse practitioner, and undergraduate teaching experience in community health nursing, led Catherine Gilliss to doctoral study in family health. Her research and teaching contributions since then have focused on the impact of chronic illnesses, notably cardiac illness, on the family. Her research program has included several clinical trials of nursing care designed to improve the health status of the recovering patient and the family. Dr. Gilliss was one of the co-conveners of two national, invitational meetings on family research in nursing known as the Wing-spread Conferences on Family Nursing. She serves on the Board of Directors of the National Council on Family Relations, and as elected Chair of that organization's Family and Health Section. In 1984, Dr. Gilliss was elected to the National Academies of Practice as a Distinguished Practitioner in Nursing.

Betty L. Highley, RN, MS, FAAN, is Professor in the School of Nursing, Department of Family Health Care, at the University of California at San Francisco.

Professor Highley's early career contributions in maternal–child nursing included the development of graduate programs to prepare clinical nurse specialists in that field. As the first chair of the newly formed Department of Family Health Care (1972–80), she provided leadership fundamental to the development of graduate programs in family nursing. Concurrently, Professor Highley attended a number of photographic workshops at the Friends of Photography in Carmel, California and the Eye Gallery in San Francisco. Since 1980, the major focus of her work has been the development of a research and education program using visual data to understand various aspects of the interactions of individuals, families and institutions with health and illness. Her photographs have been exhibited by the University of California and the Eye Gallery in San Francisco. Recently she completed *A Photographic Study of Nursing in Europe* for the European Region of the World Health Organization. The photographs from that book will be exhibited in Bruges, Belgium and Vienna, Austria.

Brenda M. Roberts, RN, MS, is Academic Coordinator and Vice Chairperson in the Department of Family Health Care at the School of Nursing, University of California at San Francisco.

A clinical background in public health nursing and graduate teaching experience in the care of chronically ill neurological patients has provided the stimulus for Brenda Roberts' interest in family nursing. Her teaching responsibilities have included undergraduate instruction in the care of families and nursing leadership. Through her administrative role, she has actively guided faculty in the development of family-centered programs in the Department of Family Health Care since 1978.

Ida M. Martinson, RN, PhD, FAAN, is Professor and Chairperson of the Department of Family Health Care in the School of Nursing at the University of California at San Francisco.

Dr. Martinson is known nationally and internationally for her contributions to the literature on childhood cancer. Her early research on the impact of childhood cancer on the child and family, and home care for the dying child have distinguished her as a truly visionary leader in family nursing care. Her research has included the study of Chinese families caring for childhood cancer victims. She has received numerous honors for these contributions as well as four *American Journal of Nursing* Book of the Year Awards. She was inducted into the Institute of Medicine in 1981. Since 1982, she has held the position of Chair in the Department of Family Health Care.

THE CAMERA IN NURSING
RESEARCH AND PRACTICE

"When I first became interested in photography . . . my idea was to have it recognized as one of the fine arts. Today, I don't give a hoot in hell about that. The mission of photography is to explain man to man and each man to himself. And that is the most complicated thing on earth and also as naive as a tender plant . . .

EDWARD STEICHEN (CAPA, 1972)

This book contains a number of photographs gathered together in galleries, or photoessays, which have evolved out of six years of Visual Media Research activity at UCSF. Selected from our extensive visual data bank, the photographs were taken in conjunction with courses in the use of the camera for research, special documentary projects, a doctoral dissertation, and case studies. The galleries are intended to expand upon concepts and ideas presented in the text, to generate new or different understandings and questions, and to transport the reader beyond the scope of written words.

Using the Camera as a Research Tool

Research relies on collecting, recording, and analyzing information. At a minimum, the camera can serve as a notebook for recording visual content to facilitate more objective recollection by the researcher/observer. Through the analysis of visual recordings, significantly more data can be obtained than through the use of notes, tape recordings, and memory alone. Considering the facility with which photographs lend themselves to communication, it is remarkable that within the health sciences—where there is a decided need for continued exploration of communications—relatively little attention has been focused on visual literacy in the education and preparation of health professionals and researchers.

A primary function of the visual media program is teaching nurses to use cameras in their clinical practice and research. From the time nurses enter into their professional education and throughout their careers, they are involved in fine tuning their skills in observing and listening. Once one has seen and heard, it becomes necessary to reconstruct the information and pass it on to others. This reconstruction is dependent on accuracy of recall.

It is significant to note that often we lack complete confidence in what we hear. We are concerned that we may hear what we want to hear or what we think is being said. We are constantly processing what we hear through our own biases and experiences. Thus, we use a tape recorder to ensure an accurate record.

We are usually more confident about our ability to recall that which has been processed through our eyes. We process what we see through the same veil of life-long experiences and understandings we have grown to mistrust in our ears. There is an old saying: "The eyes believe themselves, the ears believe other people." If we acknowledge this inconsistency in our attitudes toward sensory data, then we can accept the camera as the obvious instrument for recording visual information just as we accept the tape recorder for recording auditory information.

There are numerous examples and anecdotes of clinicians sensing that a patient is going bad or that there is a change in his or her status. This process, which relies on a complex synthesis of subtle nonverbal cues, is difficult to articulate. Through her study of this clinical assessment process, Patricia Benner developed the concept of *perceptual knowledge.* How do we describe perceptual knowledge so that we may teach it to others?

This prologue discusses the use of visual media in research, and includes models from the social sciences and photography. Methodology and design issues are discussed, and suggestions for the use of photography in nursing research are presented.

Background and Historical Perspective

The use of photography is well documented in social science disciplines such as anthropology and sociology. Anthropologist John Collier wrote the first text on visual research. In *Visual Anthropology: Photography As a Research Method,* Collier addresses issues of anthropological fieldwork. Though addressed to anthropologists, Collier's text is the primary model for all the behavioral sciences in which the recording and interpretation of visual data are significant. It is a statement on research procedure and a treatise on observation and interpretation.

While Collier is credited with advancing photography in both academic settings and research, Margaret Mead was the first to use photography in her own research. *The Balinese Character,* although a controversial work, is a classic study done from 1936 to 1939. Her then husband, Gregory Bateson, took photographs while Mead made observations and wrote field notes. The photographs, accompanied by her voluminous notes on each frame, contributed to what is perhaps the most ambitious piece of anthropological fieldwork ever published. Included were 759 photographs arranged on 100 sequential plates and accompanied by Mead's detailed, on-the-spot notes. A methodological issue that evolved from this work is the separation of visual recorder and observer/interviewer.

Within the last decade, a number of sociologists have begun to use photography as a research tool. Howard Becker, a distinguished professor at Northwestern University, has provided the major leadership. In 1981, Becker organized a major travelling exhibition called "Exploring Society Photographically," which surveyed the uses of photography in the social sciences. This exhibit and its accompanying book have had an appreciable impact on documentary photography in the visual arts and the social sciences.

One of the most prominent examples of a photographer whose concerns relate to the health sciences is photojournalist W. Eugene Smith. Originally a war photographer, Smith saw the period after World War II as an opportunity to apply journalism to something other than the sensationalist coverage typical of wartime reportage. Integral to his concept of journalism was an extraordinary conception of a role for photography. It was based on an appreciation for the communicative potential of photographs. Using photographs instead of text as a basis for writing stories, Smith developed the photoessay format while working for *Life* magazine (Johnson, 1981).

Smith's methodology bore striking similarities to anthropological field research. He spent a great deal of time with his subjects, developing close relationships with them to better learn their stories. He broke with journalistic tradition by developing a style that focused on the intent of the activity. In a nonintrusive way, he photographed elements of a scene that defined its content.

Two of Smith's photoessays have particular significance to the health sciences: *The Country Doctor* and *Nurse-Midwife*. These photoessays followed their subjects through daily activities in rural communities. Both stories illustrate many aspects of health care. The nurse-midwife, for example, is shown performing a wide variety of services as the only fulltime caretaker in her area. It is a historical document of a method of health care that is rapidly disappearing. Smith's photographs could serve as a guideline for many specializations in the field of nursing. Furthermore, the photo-essay stimulated donations of sufficient funds to build a clinic for the nurse-midwife.

Visual statements like Smith's teach us about the effects of nurses and doctors working with people. Rather than showing us how to perform a particular skilled function, they speak about how and under what circumstances care is given.

In the mid-1960s, Professor Betty Highley conducted a one-year research study on maternal role identity with a small group of young mothers and their firstborn infants. At the conclusion of the study, Highley photographed some of the subjects. Each mother and infant pair was requested to pose in whatever way was most comfortable without any arranging or suggesting by Highley. When Highley showed the photographs to a group of post-masters students and colleagues, they were able to describe accurately each mother's patterns of response to her infant and to draw conclusions about the mothering style and maternal–infant interactions. In short, they were able to summarize quickly research that had been gleaned over a one-year period. This pointed the way to more directed uses of photography in nursing research.

Methodological and Design Issues

Purpose and Framework

Before undertaking a visual documentation project, the researcher must clearly understand its purpose. To what end are the photographs being taken? What is their intent? The purposes may range from the microscopic analysis of the nonverbal communications of an infant with a tracheotomy to a macroscopic analysis of environmental inventories. Consideration must be given to the visibility of the elements central to the problem.

Secondly, the framework from which visual documentation evolves must be clearly understood. More often than not, the philosophical stance and theoretical underpinnings are more implicit than explicit. The framework from which an individual practitioner or researcher functions will influence the photography. We have discovered that the process of photographing often leads to a self-examination that can result in the peeling away of layers of misconceptions and may lead to a more reality-based understanding.

Design issues are as varied as the problems and purposes being addressed. We emphasize that we are not teaching about a tool that is a panacea for all nonverbal data collection. Rather, it is a tool that, like the tape recorder, can make a significant contribution to our search for knowledge.

Access and Consent

In any photographic study, access and consent become important issues, since some patients or subjects may initially feel invaded by the camera. However, over a period of six years, both in our own work and in students' work, we have encountered a limited number of refusals to participate in a photographic study. In fact, many subjects appear to want to be photographed. There is increasing evidence that in some cases the process of visual recording may have a therapeutic effect (Higgens and Highley, 1986).

No photograph should ever be taken without immediate verbal consent. We usually follow up with a signed consent form. A reasonable approach that is sensitive to the individual(s) being photographed is the most critical factor in gaining access and consent. In some cases it may be necessary to consider the legal implications, especially when photographing the mentally ill, handicapped, disadvantaged and subjects not of legal age.

Fact-Finding and Sampling

Once access and consent are obtained, the fact finding begins. For an agency or service study, the following questions must be considered:

1. What is the philosophy?
2. What are the goals and objectives of the group?
3. What are the nature and range of services offered?
4. What is the client population?
5. Who are the personnel?
6. What are the sociocultural-economic factors concerning services? Clients?
7. What are the legal implications?

Agency Surveys

Once these preliminary stages of research are completed, a systematic protocol for sampling the service can be developed. The photograph represents fragmentary slices of time, so all the cautions of sampling must be respected. In agency surveys, peak leisure and midpoint activities should be sampled. Activities that vis-

ually communicate segments of the service rendered should be sampled. Useful headings for the protocol are time, activity, and days. For example, in a study on child day care centers, to understand better how a day care center functioned as a daytime care facility, we needed to know how activities varied and how they were repeated during the day's care. What times did the activities occur? When were the peak activities and quiet play scheduled, and when was naptime? What time did parents drop off and pick up the children? In short, what was a typical day like and how did the care vary over weeks?

In a survey, the researcher is looking at a superstructure in which services are being given. The focus then, tends to be on the service rather than on the individual. This can be difficult, as there are no individual stories told with the kind of depth that provides the cohesion that is characteristic of case studies.

Case Studies

The case study approach to photographic study involves the study of one situation over an extended period of time. In a study of home care of chronic illness, data may be collected through photographs and interviews of patients, their family support groups, and the providers of their home care services. The purpose of the case study is to document a variety of activities so that the final combination of images presents as fully as possible what life is like for the study group. Photographs must be taken over a number of visits and must include a range of subjects, such as receipt of services to leisure time activities. The timespan covered by the photographs is often a significant factor, particularly when photographing changing conditions such as long-term chronic illness, during which changes might not occur week-to-week, but rather month-to-month or over even longer time periods.

In the case study, the investigator decides what to photograph. This decision requires planning and a certain amount of intuition. Interviews and conversation help identify what is pertinent to document. However, many of the most successful case studies are those in which the subjects of the study are active participants. In the final analysis, a documentary study is a collaboration between the photographer/researcher and the study subject. When this collaborative state is achieved, the documentary process can have a beneficial, therapeutic effect.

In a study of a home care patient with amyotrophic lateral sclerosis (ALS), photographs were taken of his treatment and of visits by the nurse and by the doctor. Photographs of a trip to the hospital revealed the complicated mechanisms the friends who were his caregivers had to undertake to get him there. In fact, what became evident in this project was the importance of the primary caregiver, a woman who had made a major personal commitment to providing his care. It was clear that her role was of the utmost importance to document and we also wanted to investigate what she considered important content. To do this, we left an automatic camera and some film with her for several weeks. She photographed the patient going to the grocery store and the dentist in a wheelchair with a portable respirator. Her images revealed much about the social and physical obstacles they faced. Her portraits of him revealed a lot about her own feelings through her choice of settings and other subjects in the frame (Segments of this study appear following Chapter 18).

Because the case study spans a long period of time, the final visual statement can be valuable in terms of the understanding and documentation of the long-term effects of care upon individuals. There is a fair amount of thematic repetition (the same individuals are seen in a variety of situations), so case studies lend themselves well to public communications outside academia. Case studies are also sometimes components of larger survey projects in which a number of studies are combined to offer an in-depth view of particular aspects of an agency or service.

Another methodological design issue that relates to any photographic project is scripting. When the research is coming out of a knowledge base, it is sometimes possible to chart a project in advance. This advanced planning can be as simple as an outline based on scheduled activities that direct the path of photography through an organization. In some cases, it can be well defined, and scripting can lead to a "shot list", or a list of photographs to be taken that will show a particular care situation or variety of care. This approach is based on advance knowledge of the situation and the method of care. One cautionary note: It is possible for the script to supersede observation with the camera at the setting. This phenomenon can work against, as well as for, the investigatory nature of research.

The Analysis and Function of Photographs

The utilization of photographs in any study must reflect back to the original problem and purpose. The classic form of content analysis, structured by procedures in documentary photography, has worked best for us. We view all the images taken at a site as a visual diary or a raw data bank. These serve as a source for analysis and are edited much like tape recordings. Although any of the standard units of analysis—patterns, themes, numbers of people, time or space—may be used, we find that we search more often for themes and patterns. Once the themes are identified, we look for images that form the clearest visual statement. Images recorded for purposes of practice and research rarely stand alone. Thus, in presentations, it is necessary to combine sequences of images that convey the dimensions of the research.

The photograph freezes images and interactions by recording them on film. This process provides us with recorded visual data that challenges us to search for a language to describe the data. Photographs provide visual evidence of occurrences at a specific time. They recall details and interactions that stimulate and objectify the processes of memory.

The first level of analysis occurs on a contact sheet—a print of all 36 exposures on a roll of film on one piece of paper. This constitutes the raw data, and for some applications it is all that is needed. When images are used only as a visual diary, the contact sheet is adequate. The next level of analysis involves selecting patterns and themes from the contact sheet. These choices are made into 5 × 7 working proof prints used for further editing and content analysis. This step is necessary when sharing the data with others is desirable, since contact sheets are difficult for more than one person to look at and they do not facilitate editing.

If the final presentation is an exhibit, book, or other publication, a final high-quality print is needed. Images selected for final prints meet more rigid criteria of content and aesthetics, with a great deal of emphasis placed on how they will fit into the larger context of a presentable series. In this final stage, selected images are combined in a sequence that conveys the message or messages of the research. As the sequencing begins to take shape, it is often necessary to return to the files or proof sheets to find images that round out an idea that has surfaced in the work. This is also the point at which the demand for content will sometimes sublimate the desire for aesthetic standards, which is a characteristic of research and study photography that would tend to be avoided at all costs in other areas of photography such as the arts. Naturally, it is desirable to compromise aesthetics as little as possible, as they are not separable from content when "reading" photographs. This means that the compositional design scheme, lighting, and other formal qualities of each image have a certain synchronicity, lending themselves to a clarity of reading that is analogous to good grammar, punctuation, and style in writing. An important part of this is to make as high quality photographic prints as possible when using them for presentation.

The Uses of Photographic Nursing Research

1. *Learning more about ourselves and our work.* This reflects the most consistent commentaries from students' course evaluations at the UCSF program.

2. *Sharpening visual senses.* Students consistently say they see more and can articulate more of what they see. The need to be constantly attentive to numerous details in daily life, particularly when working in technologically complex environments such as intensive care units, makes the ability to freeze images and study them a luxury that is often a revelation. It can attune the individual to visual data they unconsciously process all the time, and can increase their awareness of overlooked visual data important to them and their work. Sometimes, the act of photographing alone can do this.

3. *Communicating and educating.* Although this is a function to which much of the photography applies, it specifically refers to the continuum from images as illustration in a text, to slides used in services or in a class, to displays and exhibits.

4. *Evaluating services.* Are we really doing what we say we are doing? In our experience, photographs have revealed inconsistencies in this respect. They have shown contradictions in policy which may range from structure and organization of the physical environment to staff interactions. Because they are detailed recordings, they can be helpful

in fine-tuning an agency and have even been implemental in making changes.

5. *Generating new insights and understandings.* Visual data collection is an investigative process that is constantly focusing attention on what is visible, and what is significant in the visual realm. This activity, and the subsequent analysis of still images, is a continual process of discovery.

6. *Restructuring clinical interactions.* When one begins to talk about a photo, the picture will usually stimulate a wealth of information that goes far beyond the frame of the photograph itself. This is a function most of us identify with snapshots in a family album. It is a reason that visual recording should be considered for many kinds of work and research, even when photographs are not needed in the final product.

7. *Photo interviewing.* This function has many ramifications that range from a personalized tête-a-tête using images to jog the memory, to having subjects take their own pictures, to interviewing with photographs, that is largely untapped (Collier, 1986).

Summary

In our work, we have made a stab at uncovering the potentials for visual data, yet we cannot say that we have a comprehensive formula for its use. We have been encouraged by our colleagues in the fields of nursing and photography. At the same time, we have encountered skepticism from academics. We have also encountered criticism from photographers that we are sacrificing aesthetics for content. We have little doubt that these responses are similar to those experienced by visual researchers in other fields, where the methods for synthesis and analysis are not evolved enough, not "hard" enough, or in some way do not conform with established conventions. We feel it is unfortunate that, with the sophistication of photography and other forms of visual media and their expansion into so many areas of the world, there is not currently a more established tradition in education and research emphasizing visual data.

We are pleased to have this opportunity to share some of our work and our photographs. In our continued and collective search for increased understandings of unlimited and unparalleled complexities of health, illness, families and society, we are suggesting the camera as a valuable research tool.

BETTY L. HIGHLEY

TOM FERENTZ

References

Becker HS (1981): *Exploring Society Photographically.* Chicago: University of Chicago Press.

Capa C (1972): *The Concerned Photographer II* (Introduction). New York: Grossman.

Collier J Jr, Collier M (1986): *Visual Anthropology: Photography as a Research Method,* rev ed. Albuquerque: University of New Mexico Press.

Higgens S, Highley BL (1986): The camera as a study tool: Photo interview of mothers of infants with congestive heart failure. *Children's Health Care,* 15(2): 119–122.

Johnson WS (1981): *Master of Photographic Essay: W. Eugene Smith.* Millerton, NY: Aperture.

Mead M., Bateson G (1942): *The Balinese Character.* New York: New York Academy of Sciences.

Tom Ferentz, BA, MFA, has exhibited his photographs widely in group and one-person exhibits in the United States and Taiwan. He has been a photographer with Visual Media Research since 1981 and is also the founder and Director of the Eye Gallery of photography in San Francisco.

ISSUES IN FAMILY NURSING CARE AND RESEARCH

WHY FAMILY HEALTH CARE?

Catherine L. Gilliss, RNC, DNSc

The modern family unit has a significant role in establishing and maintaining its health. This chapter introduces the distinction between the perspective of the family as a significant context to individual health and the family as a unit of care in its own right. An appreciation of the complex, multivariate relationship between family health and the health of individual members is fundamental to the chapters that follow.

Introduction

For many years, nursing has proposed to deliver *family-centered* service—that is, service directed to individuals in families (ANA, 1975). In clinical areas such as maternity and pediatrics, family-centered services have been relatively easy to deliver. In these settings there is generally more than one family member present. Any family involvement in the assessment, treatment, or discharge planning of a patient has been described as family-centered because the family has been considered a significant context for individual care. More recently, the American Nurses' Association described the family as "the necessary unit of service" (ANA, 1980, p. 5).

Recognizing the family as a significant context for the health of its members is important for understanding the patient and for delivering personalized care; however, when the family is viewed as the necessary unit of service, a new level of understanding is necessary. A complex, multifactorial relationship exists between the family and its members, in which the family can be viewed as a contributor to and context for individual health issues. Likewise, the interactions of family members contribute to family health, which must be viewed within a context of a sociopolitical, cultural community because the family regularly transacts within this larger context. Nursing care can be offered to families and to members of families. In its best sense, it is offered to both.

Campbell (1986a; 1986b) has observed that two models have been predominant in the study of the relationship between the family and individual health: social epidemiology (Cassel, 1976) and systems theory (Brody, 1973; Engel, 1977). He concluded that the linear, disease-oriented, social epidemiologic approach has been popular because of its access to "clean" and highly reliable measures. In contrast, the rich complexities of human relationships, which are the phenomena of systems theory, are difficult to

measure. As a result, family studies have tended to rely heavily on the simplistic and linear social epidemiologic approach and have more often been concerned with the health status of the individual than the health of the family group or the relationships that exist between the two entities.

A growing number of authors have called attention to the interdependent nature of the relationship between the family and the health of its members. Griffin (1980) acknowledged the family system's influence during the course of an illness and the alteration of the family system's structures and functions caused by illness onset. "The interdependence of organizational structures and the nature of family functioning mean that no illness can be seen as an isolated event" (p. 245). In his landmark paper, Mauksch (1974) proposed that we conceptualize family health. He described the components of the family group as "unit members" and "linking processes." Each member functions as an individual, a participant, and a component part of the family. Although these components are interactive, the health of individuals may be distinguished from the health of the family unit. In a classic and comprehensive review of the literature related to the family as a basic unit of health, Litman (1974) highlighted the significance of the family as a unit of care by revealing that the family exhibits characteristic patterns of morbidity, response to symptoms, and use of medical services and facilities. Examples include Widmer and Cadoret's (1980) observations of family visits and complaints prior to the diagnosis of a family member's depression and Huygen's (1978) analysis of family behavior over generations of his own clinical practice. Medalie (1979) has proposed a relationship between life cycle events and family care patterns.

Doherty and McCubbin (1985), recognizing the interdependent nature of the family and the health of its individual members, have proposed a model for organizing health theory, research, and practice. They suggested that the family undergoes a series of six phases in the "family health and illness cycle" as the family responds to the illness of a member. As described by Doherty and McCubbin, these phases include: (1) family health promotion and risk reduction; (2) family vulnerability and illness onset; (3) family illness appraisal; (4) family acute response; (5) family and health care system—the critical choice (whether or not to seek treatment); and (6) family adaptation to illness. According to these authors, a body of knowledge is developing around each of these phases.

The Impact of Individual Illness on the Family

The illness of a family member has been reported to influence the family or other individuals within the family. As a responsive context reacting to illness of child members, the family unit has been studied by many. Kruger et al (1980) described changes in sibling behavior following the diagnosis of cystic fibrosis in a child. Hymovich and Baker (1985) have reported reactive concerns of parents. Davis (1963) documented changes in family functioning associated with the development of polio in a child member. Koch (1985) has described the responses of parents and healthy siblings to cancer in a child member. Barbarin and Chesler (1984) have reported the impact of pediatric cancer on marital quality, perceived stress, and relationships with the medical care staff.

Similarly, adult illness has been reported to affect the family or individuals within the family. Litman (1971) speculated that the perceived severity of a member's illness was directly related to its impact on family relations and observed that the wife or mother's illness had the greatest impact on the family. Klein et al (1968) observed the development of role tensions and multiple somatic symptoms among

"healthy" spouses when the other spouse became ill. Gilliss (1984) has described the spousal stress reported at the time of hospitalization for cardiac surgery and continuing six months thereafter. Clinton (1986) has reported the couvade patterns observed in expectant fathers. Based on the available literature, it appears that the family-as-reactor to illness is easily identified and often studied. The family-as-actor is less often described. Before we examine this perspective, we will try to clarify what is meant by the *healthy family unit*.

The Healthy Family Unit

The attribution of wellness and illness to the family unit is a recent phenomenon in the clinical literature, with the exception of the clinical psychiatric literature wherein the identified patient was viewed as symptomatic of a family problem. Bateson's early work with schizophrenia exemplified this perspective (Bateson et al, 1956).

Barnhill's writing (1979) has stimulated interest in viewing the family unit behaviorally within nursing. His identification of the dimensions of family health is organized into four themes: (1) identity processes; (2) change; (3) information processing; and (4) role structuring. New categories for evaluating family health derived from these themes: clear versus unclear communication; flexibility versus rigidity in response to change; and role reciprocity versus role rigidity or role conflict. A working group of nurse scientists has developed a family assessment tool based on this model (Lasky et al, 1985).

Pratt's description (1976) of the "energized family" characterized the healthy family unit by examining its links to the community, interaction between family members, coping efforts, role structure, and freedom and responsiveness. The healthy family, she concluded, constantly modified its structure to promote more effective functioning. Kantor and Lehr (1975) have contributed *Inside the Family* to facilitate understanding of the family coping with the stresses of everyday life. This naturalistic study of the family resulted in a framework that proposed that the family process may be described by its attempts to adjust space, that is, to maintain closeness or distance between individuals.

Hess and Handel (1959) proposed that separateness and connectedness are "the underlying conditions of a family's life, and its common task is to give form to both" (p. 1). From their naturalistic study of families, they described five essential family processes: (1) establishing a pattern of separateness and connectedness; (2) establishing congruence in meanings and images; (3) evolving modes of interactions into characteristic family patterns/themes; (4) establishing boundaries of the family's world of experiences (limits, intensity, extensity, evaluative abilities); and (5) dealing with the significant biosocial issues of life, such as gender expectations and pacing of expectations.

Other naturalistic studies have contributed to our identification of "normal" family behaviors. Hansen (1981) described the most healthy families as those in which: (1) movement and flow of interaction is smooth and relaxed, and problems are addressed promptly; (2) directives are clear; (3) parents listen to children and hold realistic expectations for them; (4) parental authority is clear without a punitive environment; and (5) there is a high degree of spontaneous agreement in the marital pair.

A more complete discussion of the healthy family will follow in Chapter 5. Let us return to a discussion of the influence of the family on its members.

The Family's Influence on Individual Health

The family has been viewed as a powerful influence to individual compliance with treatment and related clinical status. Mabry (1964) demonstrated a relationship between noncompliance and conflicting behaviors and values within the home. Steidl et al (1980) studied a group of chronic dialysis patients and families and identified a positive relationship between medical condition and family functioning. The correlation between family functioning and adherence to the treatment regimen approached, but did not achieve, statistical significance ($p=.054$). It is not clear whether the health of the family contributes to the improved medical condition of the patient or whether the improved medical condition contributes to the health of the family; however, this question merits further study. The results of a randomized clinical trial of 400 poor, urban hypertensive patients have been reported by Levine et al (1979) at the two-year follow-up and by Morisky et al (1983) at the five-year follow-up. A brief family counseling session was employed as one of the seven treatment conditions in this study. All experimental subjects exhibited a healthier outcome profile (fewer missed appointments, compliance, and lower systolic and diastolic blood pressure) at two and five years than control subjects. Subjects from the family intervention subgroup were the only ones who maintained the statistically significant blood pressure difference at five years. Similarly, good diabetic control has been associated with high levels of family functioning (Edelstein, Linn, 1985).

Shared stressful experiences of family members have been described as correlates of, or contributors to, individual illness. The work of Meyer and Haggerty (1962) demonstrated increased incidence of streptococcal sore throats among children whose families had recently experienced a major change, such as death or unemployment. Roghmann and Haggerty (1972) noted increased use of health care facilities by children whose families were experiencing high levels of stress. Much clustering of illness in families has been reported in the literature (Dingle, 1959; Kellner, 1963). Medalie (1979) related this to the stressful impact of certain family developmental stages on the family members.

Minuchin et al (1978) have contributed their observations on the nature of families with many psychosomatic problems. They contend that children with chronic, severe, relapsing asthma, in spite of competent pediatric management, are candidates for "parentectomy." From their work with diabetic, anorexic, and asthmatic children and their families, they have identified four characteristics of family functioning commonly observed in psychosomatic families who encourage somatization. This cluster includes: (1) enmeshment; (2) overprotectiveness; (3) rigidity; and (4) lack of skill in conflict resolution. As described in case reports (Liebman et al, 1974; Minuchin et al, 1975), family treatment was an effective modality for changing these characteristics and freeing the individual child of symptoms. Barbarin and Tirado (1985) have reported that maintenance of weight loss was accomplished with greater success among women whose family style was enmeshed. This finding suggests that family styles may affect individual health outcomes.

Clearly, evidence is accumulating to support the multifactorial nature of the relationship between patient and family. Although some of this evidence is more than 20 years old, little progress has been made toward systematic organization and refinement of these observations.

Summary

This chapter has attempted to extend the perspective of the reader to consider the family unit as the true recipient of family health care. Within the nursing literature, the role of the family as context for patient health concerns has often been identified. The contextual view is valuable but limited. When the family unit is perceived as a unit of care, new possibilities may be identified for family nursing care and family nursing research.

References

American Nurses' Association (1980): Nursing: A social policy statement. Kansas City, MO: ANA.

American Nurses' Association, Division on Community Health Nursing Practice (1975): Concepts of community health nursing practice, 2nd ed. Kansas City, MO: ANA.

Barbarin O, Chesler M (1984): Coping as interpersonal strategy: Families with childhood cancer. *Fam Syst Med*, 2(3):279–289.

Barbarin O, Tirado M (1985): Enmeshment, family processes and successful treatment of obesity. *Fam Relations*, 34(1):115–121.

Barnhill L (1979): Health family systems. *Fam Coordinator*, 94–100.

Bateson G et al (1956): Toward a theory of schizophrenia. *Behav Sci*, 1:251–264.

Brody H (1973): The systems view of man: Implications for medicine, science and ethics. *Perspect Biol Med*, (Autumn) 71.

Campbell T (1986a): The family's impact on health: A critical review and annotated bibliography. US GPO (DHHS # ADM 86–1461).

Campbell T (1986b): The family's impact on health: A critical review. *Fam Syst Med*, 4(2&3):135–328.

Cassel J (1976): The contribution of the social environment to host resistance. *Am J Epidemiol*, 104:107–123.

Clinton J (1986): Expectant fathers at risk for couvade. *Nurs Res*, 35(5):290–295.

Davis F (1963): *Passage Through Crisis: Polio Victims and Their Families.* Indianapolis: Bobbs-Merrill.

Dingle J (1959): *An Epidemiological Study of Illness in Families.* New York: Academic Press.

Doherty W, McCubbin H (1985): Families and health care: An emerging area of theory, research and clinical intervention. *Family Relations*, 34(1):5–11.

Edelstein J, Linn M (1985): The influence of the family on control of diabetes. *Soc Sci Med*, 21(5):541–544.

Engel G (1977): The need for a new medical model: A challenge for biomedicine. *Science*, 196:129–136.

Gilliss C (1984): Reducing family stress during and after coronary bypass surgery. *Nurs Clin North Am*, 19(1):103–112.

Griffin J (1980): Physical illness in the family. In: *Family-Focused Care.* Miller J, Janosik E (eds.). New York: McGraw-Hill.

Hansen C (1981): Living-in with normal families. *Fam Pract,* 20(1):53–75.

Hess R, Handel T (1959): *Family Worlds: A Psychosocial Approach to Family Life.* Chicago: University of Chicago Press.

Huygen FSA (1978): *Family Medicine: The Medical Life History of Families.* Nijmegen, The Netherlands: Dekker and Van deVegt.

Hymovich D, Baker C (1985): The needs, concerns and coping of parents of children with cystic fibrosis. *Family Relations,* 34(1):91–97.

Kantor D, Lehr W (1975): *Inside the Family.* New York: Harper and Row.

Kellner R (1963): *Family Ill Health.* Springfield, IL: Thomas.

Klein R, Dean A, Bodgonoff M (1968): Impact of illness upon the spouse. *J Chronic Dis,* 20:241.

Koch A (1985): "If only it could be me": The families of pediatric cancer patients. *Family Relations,* 34(1):63–70.

Kruger S, Shawver M, Jones L (1980): Reaction of families to the child with cystic fibrosis. *Image,* 12(3):67–72.

Lasky P et al (1985): Developing an instrument for the assessment of family dynamics. *West J Nurs Res,* 1:40–57.

Levine D et al (1979): Health education for hypertensive patients. *JAMA,* 241:1700–1703.

Liebman R, Minuchin S, Baker L (1974): The use of structural family theory in treatment of intractable asthma. *Am J Psychiatry,* 131:535–540.

Litman T (1971): Health care and the family: A three generational analysis. *Med Care,* 9:67.

Litman T (1974): The family as a basic unit in health and medical care: A social behavioral view. *Soc Sci Med,* 8:495–519.

Mabry J (1964): Medicine and the family. *J Marr Fam,* 26:161.

Mauksch H (1974): A social science basis for conceptualizing family health. *Soc Sci Med,* 8:521–528.

Medalie J (1979): The family cycle and its implications for family practice. *J Fam Pract,* 9(1):47–56.

Meyer R, Haggerty R (1962): Streptococcal infections in families: Factors altering individual susceptibility. *Pediatrics,* 29:539–549.

Minuchin S et al (1975): A conceptual model of psychosomatic illness in children: Family organization and family therapy. *Arch Gen Psychiatry,* 32:1031–1038.

Minuchin S, Rosman B, Baker L (1978): *Psychosomatic Families.* Cambridge: Harvard University Press.

Morisky D et al (1983): Five year blood pressure control and mortality following health education for hypertensive patients. *Am J Public Health,* 73:153–162.

Pratt L (1976): *Family Structure and Effective Health Behavior.* Boston: Houghton-Mifflin.

Roghmann K, Haggerty R (1972): Family stress and use of health services. *Int J Epidemiol,* 1(3):279–286.

Steidl J, Finkelstein F, Wexler J (1980): Medical condition, adherence to treatment regimens, and family functioning: Their interaction in patients receiving long-term dialysis treatment. *Arch Gen Psychiatry,* 37:1025–1027.

Widmer R, Cadoret R (1980): Depression in family practice: Changes in patterns of patient visits and complaints during subsequent developing depression. *J Fam Pract,* 10(1):45–51.

2

THEORETICAL PERSPECTIVES ON THE FAMILY

Ramona T. Mercer, RN, PhD, FAAN

This chapter presents an overview of the theoretical perspectives that have contributed to family practice and research, both for other disciplines and for nursing, and that are judged as promising for considering family relationships into the 21st century. The perspectives addressed include *interactionist, developmental, systems* , and *social exchange.* Major assumptions for each of the frameworks, kinds of problems the theory best addresses, implied methodology, limitations and constraints, and strengths of the theory are discussed.

Ramona Mercer, Professor Emeritus at the University of California at San Francisco School of Nursing (Department of Family Health Care Nursing), has received international recognition for her research on the transition to and attainment of the maternal role, and the effect of postpartum stress on family health and functioning.

Introduction

Historically, health care professionals have focused on individuals or dyads within the family; consequently, the family has been viewed as the environmental context in which the treatment or study occurred. The lack of a theoretical approach that permits viewing the family as an aggregate or as a unit with interacting parts has contributed to this practice. Feetham (1984) identified that a major limitation of family research in nursing has been the lack of a complete conceptual framework guiding data collection and interpretation. In this chapter, four major theoretical perspectives that offer promise either for family practice or for family research are discussed. This author agrees with Feetham (1984) that a single definition of family is not essential; however, therapists and researchers need to be explicit about their definition of family in each report or study.

Over a quarter of a century has passed since Hill and Hansen (1960) identified five conceptual frameworks for study of the family: interactional, structural-functional, situational, institutional, and developmental. Christensen (1964) included these same frameworks as "theoretical orientations" in his classic book, *Handbook of Marriage and the Family*, but with the interactional and situational approaches combined by Stryker (1964). Nye and Berardo (1966) added the anthropologic, psychoanalytic, social-psychologic, economic, and western Christian approaches in their important book, *Emerging Conceptual Frameworks in Family Analysis*. In addition, they questioned whether there was a legal conceptual framework for the study of the American family. Of the original five conceptual frameworks, only the interactional, structural-functional, and family developmental were continuing to generate much new inquiry in the early 1970s (Broderick, 1971). During that time, balance, game, exchange, and general systems theories were being revived and applied to the

family. Burr, Hill, Nye, and Reiss (1979) later integrated middle-range family theories with the general sociological theories of exchange, symbolic interaction, general systems, conflict, and phenomenology.

Holman and Burr (1980) suggested major, minor, and peripheral theoretical perspectives for study of the family. The three major theories they identified were interactionist, exchange, and systems. Minor theoretical perspectives included conflict, behaviorism, developmental, ecosystems, and phenomenology. Those theories considered peripheral to the family were game, psychoanalytic, balance, field, learning (other than behaviorism), situational, transactional, institutional, and structural-functional.

The need to develop relevant therapeutic interventions for problems such as intrafamily violence led in the 1970s and 1980s to the examination of multidimensional processes in an attempt to facilitate theory construction about causality. Gelles (1983) proposed an exchange or social control model of family violence. The popular Double ABCX model was adapted by McCubbin and Patterson (1983) for addressing how families cope with and adapt to stress in normative and catastrophic transitions. Talmadge and Ruback (1985) suggested that attribution and social exchange theoretical frameworks contribute to understanding family interactions.

Miller and Sobelman (1985) also emphasized that clinical pressures had created the need for new paradigms or models of the family in psychology. Old reductionist paradigms based on homogeneous systems and objective determinism achieved in the artificial environment of laboratories fail to consider the wide range of potential variables that explain family behavior. The complexity of human and social problems is such that they can no longer be addressed with simplistic views.

Nursing's metatheory, subsumed under the paradigm of person, environment, and health, has much to contribute to both family theory and family practice because of its holistic approach. However, reconsideration of the linear, additive approach to explaining family phenomena must be reevaluated (Feetham, 1984; Whall, 1980).

This chapter presents an overview of theoretical perspectives that have contributed most to family practice and research, both for other disciplines and for nursing, and that are judged as promising for considering family relationships into the 21st century. The perspectives addressed include interactionist, developmental, systems (subsumed within systems are ecological and stress frameworks), and social exchange. Major assumptions for each of the frameworks, kinds of problems the theory best addresses, methodology implied, limitations and constraints, and strengths of the theory are discussed.

The Interactionist Perspective

The interactionist perspective is broad, and when placed on a continuum, phenomenologic, symbolic interaction, and role theories represent differences in schools of thought within this perspective as well as some areas of overlap (Burr et al, 1979; Stryker, 1964). Although the mediating role of self is central for all three, phenomenology is concerned more with qualitative aspects, and role theory at the other end of the continuum focuses on the more objective and quantifiable aspects of self. George Herbert Mead (1934) is credited with synthesizing the works of William James, Charles H. Cooley, and John Dewey to bring together mind, self, and society as major concepts in the interactionist school known as "symbolic interactionism" (Turner, 1978).

Mead (1934) explicated the human mind's capacity to organize and control responses by selecting one option over another (reflection) and to assign and derive meaning from symbols and gestures in interaction with others. Because of these abilities of the human mind, the self emerges from these interactions with others and is a symbolic object in the mind's eye, apart from the body or from other objects or persons. The social group from which a person derives the symbolic self provides the social attitudes and problems that are assimilated as part of the self. From this perspective, the early influence of family and culture on the individual's development is readily evident. Society or institutions represent the organized and patterned interactions among the individuals making up the society; thus, society is dependent on the capacities of the individual selves (Turner, 1978). Changes that are made in the social order mandate earlier changes in self (Mead, 1934). In other words, family problems such as incest or wife and child abuse cannot be abolished until the selves making up society see these practices as criminal acts that violate and damage individuals and families.

Assumptions

The basic assumptions of the interactionist framework summarized from Burr et al (1979) and Mead (1934) include the following:

1. Complex sets of symbols that have common meanings are acquired through living in a symbolic environment.
2. Individuals distinguish, evaluate, and assign meaning to the symbols.
3. Behavior is influenced by the meaning of symbols or ideas rather than by instincts, needs, or drives; therefore, the meaning an individual assigns to symbols is important in understanding behavior.
4. The individual's reflexive, introspective ability gradually leads to a definition of self through the process of social experience and activity. The self continues to change and evolve over time.

5. The evolving self has several dimensions— the physical body and characteristics and a complex social self. The social self is defined by a person's relationships with other persons and social institutions and has an interacting "me" and "I," which depend on the situation. The "me" is a conventional, habitual self that consists of learned, repetitious responses that others can rely on and of the various roles a person performs. The "I" is spontaneous and unique to the individual. Thus, socially determined attitudes that are a part of the "me" may be expressed in a totally new and different way by the "I."

6. Individuals are actors as well as reactors; they select and interpret the environment to which they respond.

7. Individuals are born into a dynamic social context (society).

8. The infant's nature is determined by the environment and responses to the environment rather than by a predisposition to act a certain way. (This is an assumption that reflects the thinking of the early twentieth century and needs to be revised.)

9. Individuals learn from the culture and become the society.

10. An individual's behavior is a product of his or her life history, which is continually modified by integrating newly acquired information.

11. Little can be learned from the study of animals that applies to people because animals lack reflexive, introspective abilities.

Problems Addressed by Symbolic Interactionism

Family phenomena viewed from the symbolic interactionist approach include internal processes within families such as roles/role conflict, statuses, communication, responses to stress, decision-making, and socialization (Schvaneveldt, 1966). *Processes,* rather than end products of social interactions, are the major focus when a symbolic interactionist perspective is used (Turner, 1978). Stern (1982) used a grounded theory approach to determine the processes involved in stepfather family integration. Through this interactionist approach, Stern (1982) relied totally on qualitative data to derive ten affiliating strategies that stepfathers and children used to make friends. At the other end of the continuum in the interactionist approach, Meleis (1975) and Swendsen, Meleis, and Jones (1978) used role theory as a framework for testing whether role supplementation would contribute to role mastery for new parents. Mercer (1981, 1985) also used role theory to study the process of maternal role attainment over the first year of motherhood. Roberts (1983) described the unique dimension contributed by symbolic interactionism to her study of infant behavior and the transition to parenthood as the symbolic meaning of infant behavior to parental perceptions of role competence.

Olshansky (1985) used the interactionist approach to study how infertility affected mates; she identified a process of taking on and managing an identity of self as infertile prior to either overcoming, circumventing, or reconciling the infertility. Using this perspective, Stainton (1985) described a process of parents' assimilation of the fetus as a member of the family through perceptions of the fetus's appearance, communication, gender, temperament, and sleep/wake cycle. The impact of a spouse's chronic illness on family interactions, presented by Corbin and Strauss (1985), is another example of a family problem that may be studied using a symbolic interactionist approach. Ventura and Stevenson (1986) used a family interactional perspective to study parents' psychologic functioning and family characteristics; parents with more symptoms of depression viewed their two- to three-month-old infants as having a more difficult temperament. The family's higher socioeconomic status was associated with parents being more depressed and viewing their infants as less easily soothed and more distressed.

Methodology

Methodology is predicated on the level of question asked, but the philosophic stance of the researcher also influences the methodology. Within the rubric of symbolic interactionism, a range of beliefs exists, as was noted earlier. Mead was at the University of Chicago, and following his death, Blumer (1969) continued his leadership; this interactionist school of thought became known as the Chicago tradition, and it emphasized the indeterminant, unpredictable, and subjective aspects of self that were best studied by a qualitative approach (Burr et al, 1979). Kuhn emphasized the core self as developing into a relatively stable and structured entity, allowing for continuity and predictability; this school of thought, in which the core self is viewed as highly constrained, is known as the Iowa tradition (Turner, 1978). The Kuhn, or Iowa, tradition uses a more deterministic, quantitative approach. However, Turner (1978) cautioned that these positions only represent boundaries within which symbolic interactionists work, and few follow either Blumer's or Kuhn's positions totally. For example, the previously cited study of maternal role attainment used both quantitative measures to measure the core self and qualitative interview data to get at the process that was occurring from the women's perceptions of their situation at the time (Mercer, 1985; 1986). Also, the assumption that the infant's behavior is a function of the environment rather than any predisposition to act a certain way was rejected for the maternal role attainment study because of widely held support for the view that interaction of the environment and innate capacities influence infant behavior.

Limitations and Constraints

The lack of agreement on concepts and assumptions regarding the symbolic interactionist perspective and the wide application of action- or problem-oriented research have made it difficult to refine the theory and come up with new formulations (Schvaneveldt, 1966). Although middle-range theories have been derived using this perspective, no extension of the interactionist theories has occurred over the past decades. As noted above, the assumption that the infant is asocial or has no predisposition to act in certain ways has been disproved both in studies of temperament and in studies of fetal and neonatal activity.

One of the greatest constraints has to do not with the generation of middle-range theories from the interactionist perspective but with the lack of replication of the research and failure to test the middle-range theories that are discovered. The largely qualitative theory is most often presented without adequate testing or comparative analysis needed to reach a stage of formal theory. Theories are meant to be tested, and without this rigorous challenge by the scientific world, they tend to lie fallow rather than to be validated, extended, or otherwise modified.

Although the focus is on process, interactionists have tended to freeze the process or to examine only small segments of a process. For example, in the study by Stainton (1985) of the assimilation of the fetus into the family, the process needs to be extended to earlier in pregnancy and following birth, until the child is fully assimilated into the family unit.

In viewing the interaction process, the symbolic environment is studied, but adequate consideration of the cultural impact on the family or of social expectations is not always allowed. The situation may not be conceptualized in such a way as to permit this analysis. The family is the framework in which social action takes place rather than the determinant of that action, and the organization and changes of the family unit are the products of the activity of the family members rather than of outside forces that do not consider family members (Schvaneveldt, 1966). However, family units are influenced by and must conform to societal constraints (children go to school at age six, state and federal taxes must be paid) as well as to cultural rules and taboos. These outside forces are an important part of understanding the family roles, responses, adaptation, and organization.

In order to evaluate research using the interactionist's approach, these questions need to be answered: How were the data approached? How was the meaning of symbols validated? Was the approach inductive, deductive, or both? What was the situational context of the study? Which tradition or which theories were used? Which interactionist concepts were or were not used?

Strengths

The wide use of the symbolic interactionist framework indicates its greatest strength. Its utilitarian nature includes the ability to focus on the family as a small group. The concept that an individual's definition of the situation affects attitudes toward others, rather than the converse, presents a very different philosophy for treatment and educational purposes.

Another major strength of the symbolic interactionist perspective is the qualitatively derived theory, which is more explanatory. When subjects as well as researchers respond with "aha," the phenomena identified are valid, at least for that particular population. An example of this explanatory power can be found in Stern, Tilden, and Maxwell's (1980) study of the Filipino-American's culturally induced stress during childbearing. Quantitative approaches would have verified a high level of stress among these clients, but through the interactionist approach, the researchers identified differences in customs, cultural beliefs and practices, and in-

terpersonal style, and they noted language barriers created by health care providers' cadence, accent, and use of idioms; these differences *created* the stress. Consequently, more information was available to health care providers, which could then be used to ameliorate or eliminate care-provider-induced stress.

The Developmental Perspective

The developmental perspective draws from many other theories: symbolic interactionist, discussed previously; systems; structural-functional; psychoanalytic; and cognitive. However, the developmental approach has unique philosophic and methodologic perspectives, both of which contribute to holistic views of the person or the family. Despite its being listed as a minor theory by Holman and Burr in 1980, the developmental perspective raises serious questions that need addressing in family research. Kaye (1985) emphasized that families are social systems of physically separate people whose organization and adaptation (development) as a social system must be explained.

Widely accepted individual developmental stages were introduced by Freud and expanded on by Erikson. Erikson's (1959) epigenetic principle of development has strong structural and functional components that were derived from growth of an organism in utero: ". . . anything that grows has a ground plan, and out of this ground plan, parts arise, each part having its time of special ascendancy, until all parts have risen to form a functioning whole" (p. 52). Havighurst's (1972) developmental tasks' definition follows this principle and has remained central to the developmental approach: The task occurs at a specific period; successful achievement leads to happiness and success with later tasks; failure leads to unhappiness, disapproval by the society, and difficulty in achieving later tasks.

Duvall's (1977) classic book, *Family Development*, represented the synthesis of developmental concepts of that period and particularly of work achieved prior to and during the 1948 National Conference on Family Life. Her stages of family development are based on the age of the oldest child. She identified overall family tasks that include establishing and maintaining: the family home; ways of financing the family; division of labor in the family; continuity of satisfying sexual relationships; intellectual and emotional communication; relationships with relatives; relationships with associates and community organizations; competency in childrearing; and a workable philosophy of life. Her work has been influential in family stage and task development.

Rodgers (1964) suggested that family development be viewed as a system with norms (behavioral expectations) with a career trajectory that fulfills role expectations for individuals within the family and the family as a unit, governed by sanctions from society and the family unit. Deviation from norms or ineffective fulfillment of societal expectations by the family would then lead to sanctions when expectations are not met. Howes (1976) applied Erikson's epigenetic principle of development to Duvall's (1977) family stages to illustrate how families' ineffective dealing with adolescent crises led to dysfunction.

The orthogenetic principle of development argues that wherever a developmental progression occurs there is movement from a state of relative lack of differentiation to a state of increasing differentiation, articulation, and hierarchic integration (Werner, 1948). Werner, however, assumed that development as a process of change occurred in a wide variety of circumstances—whether the different circumstances were in a culture or in an individual's cognitive development (Baldwin, 1968). Werner envisioned development to proceed analogous to the broader genetic principle of spirality: Lower levels of functioning remain along with the development of higher levels of functioning, allowing an individual to move back and forth in polar opposites such as diffuse-articulated, rigid-flexible, and labile- stabile. Under the principle of spirality, differentiation or development may occur both horizontally and vertically. The same achievement may be reached by operations that are genetically quite different. Similarly, families could be envisioned to move from relatively undifferentiated systems to more highly organized systems as they deal with internal and environmental challenges. However, in times of stress, a family could regress to a less organized system.

In summary, developmental concepts include movement to a higher level of functioning. This implies continuous, unidirectional progression. However, during transitional periods from one stage or phase to the next, disequilibrium occurs, during which time the individual may revert to an earlier level of developmental responses. Families face normative and unexpected transitions that also create a period of disorganization, during which the family functions at a lower level than usual. Resolution of the disequilibrium or crisis has potential to lead to a higher level of family functioning (Hill, 1965).

Assumptions

Two basic assumptions of the developmental perspective are now open to question. First, the assumption that the family is a nuclear or conjugal unit that will rear children and exist from the wedding until the last spouse is deceased (Rowe, 1966) does not meet all societal situations. Thus, family must be defined for the specific population under treatment or study. In the 1980s families are frequently disrupted by divorce; then individuals with children from two disrupted families marry to recreate or blend into a new family. In addition, with increased longevity, many individuals enter into second or third marriages long past the possibility or desire for procreation.

Second, the assumption made by Hill and Hansen (1960) that the basic focus is on the individual actor within the family setting must be rejected to foster progress in family developmental research. Although individuals and their development are a part of family study, questions must also be directed toward the family as a unit or social system.

Other family developmental assumptions that are viable include the following:

1. Because of differences in internal and environmental stimulation, families change and develop in different ways (Hill, Hansen, 1960; Rowe, 1966).

2. Developmental tasks are goals that are worked toward rather than specific jobs that are completed at once (Rowe, 1966).

3. Each family is unique in its composition and complex of age-role expectations and positions (Hill, Rodgers, 1964; Rowe, 1966). This means that the father may assume the expressive role of being the major caretaker of the children and the mother may assume the instrumental role of being the wage earner; or it may mean that some couples may be married ten years before entering the stage of the birth of the first child.

4. Human conduct (and family conduct) is a function of its historical milieu as well as the current social context (Hill, Hansen, 1960).

5. All families have enough in common despite their uniqueness to make it possible to chart family development over the family life span (Hill, Rodgers, 1964).

6. Families may arrive at similar developmental levels through quite different processes.

Problems Addressed by a Developmental Framework

Kaye (1985) discussed questions for addressing the "how" or process of the family system as a foundation for developmental psychology.

Kaye's questions are summarized for addressing relevant nursing issues such as:

1. How a family retains its identity as it adapts to loss of a family member or to a chronic illness such as Alzheimer's disease

2. How differences evolve, such as using violence or abuse to other family members as a response to stress

3. How development is influenced by health care practices or social policy and culture or vice versa

4. How family development affects individual development and vice versa, such as when the stage of having a first child occurs with individual unreadiness

5. How new members are created, recruited, and socialized, such as in Stern's (1982) study of stepfather families or the birth and socialization of the child

6. How mediation between society and individual members occurs, such as events that are attended, health practices or attitudes that are adopted

7. How individuals facilitate change in other family members or the family as a whole, such as in situations of substance abuse by a family member

8. How individuals internalize the family gestalt, such as family practices, rules, values, and priorities or how this chain can be interrupted when family practices lead to disastrous results

9. How families prepare members for participation in other systems such as hospitals, clinics

The work of Martinson et al (1987), examining how families adapt following the death of a child from cancer, is an example of a longitudinal follow-up study of family adaptation or development. All studies focusing on expanding or shrinking family boundaries or family transitions benefit from a developmental perspective.

Mercer et al (1986) are using a developmental framework to study antepartum stress and its effects through the first eight months postpartum. Their naturalistic study of the family includes both high-risk women (hospitalized during pregnancy) and low-risk women (those attending the general clinic) and their respective mates. Families are studied longitudinally as they move from hospital to home settings and back to the hospital for birth, and then again in home settings. Effects on individuals, dyads, and the family unit are being studied.

Methodology

A longitudinal design is implied if progression over time is to be measured. Both quantitative and qualitative methods may be used in describing or measuring process as it relates to the end product.

An idiographic, or individual, clinical approach may be used in developmental research. A classic example of this approach is Piaget's study of his own children in arriving at his theory of cognitive development. Durand's (1975) clinical nursing study of a child with Down syndrome who had failure to thrive is an excellent example of the idiographic approach.

The nomothetic approach involves the systematic investigation of a large group of subjects who may be of a particular cohort, such as those born during the depression or those who experienced a common catastrophe. The study of large groups can provide greater ranges in developmental phenomena, and the study of individuals can provide greater depth into the interaction of genetics and environment.

A cross-sectional approach is more economical in that larger numbers of subjects may be studied at different facets of a developmental process; and then comparisons may be made (such as in families with an infant, a school-age child, and an adolescent). However, the comparability of families with quite divergent histories may be argued.

Sammons (1985) used a modified cross-sectional sequential design to study maternal anxiety, somatic symptoms, marital adjustment, and family relationships in a second pregnancy. She combined aspects of traditional cross-sectional design with a short-term panel longitudinal study to examine facets of the childbearing year. She conserved resources (time, finances, and personnel) and avoided the problems of self-selection imposed by studying only those willing to participate in a prolonged, repeated testing design.

Hultsch and Hickey (1978) suggested four metatheoretic models for the study of developmental phenomena—mechanistic, organismic, contextual, and dialectical. The *mechanistic* is based on causality as unidirectional and is assumed to be linear; activity is the result of stimulation. The *organismic* model derives its meaning from organic wholeness. Principles of organization are determined rather than a focus being made on component parts; causality is through the overall design in nature. Changes in structures and functions permit comparison. *Contextualism* denies any final cause; change and novelty are fundamental, with the time and duration of an event being central. The focus is to identify and describe transitions and the contexts in which they occur. In the *dialectical* model, homeostatic balance is deemphasized when development is at a plateau, or stage of rest. Causality is reciprocal rather than unidirectional, and inner and outer contradictions lead to change. The dialectical model deals with conflicts resulting from asynchronies between any two of four dimensions of development—inner biologic, individual-psychologic, cultural-sociologic, and outer-physical—representing multiple internal, external, and temporal dimensions. Methodologically, reciprocal interactions that contribute to a continuously changing organism are assessed using the dialectical model. These metatheoretic models, with quite divergent beliefs about causality and direction, emphasize the importance of evaluating the philosophic assumptions underlying any developmental research.

Limitations and Constraints

Testing developmental theories has been problematic. Erikson's epigenetic principle of development suggests a critical period or specific timing for the unfolding of an organism, just as the developmental tasks concepts did later. There are two views of a sensitive or critical period: (1) a critical period beyond which a given phenomenon will not appear; and (2) a discrete period during which environmental input may exert its greatest effect (Caldwell, 1962). The first view is true biologically; however, it is not true psychosocially, and rigid views on this would be constraining. The resilience of the human is such that development continues to occur over the life span. In a study of transitions in the life cycle of women, achievement of independence (an adolescent task) was accomplished in the seventies after a mate's death (Mercer, Nichols, Doyle, 1987).

The research on early mother-infant attachment and interventions to enhance the first hour of maternal–infant interaction following birth was based on the assumption that the first hour following birth was a sensitive period for the attachment process to occur. However, the findings have not been replicated (Curry, 1982; Lamb, 1982), indicating that human mothers have greater resiliency than animals and fowl, whose young imprint following birth. In addition, research such as Stainton's (1985), cited earlier, has shown that attachment begins during pregnancy.

An example of a discrete period during which environmental input may exert its greatest effect on families was seen in the maternal role attainment study (Mercer, 1986). Women who were in their twenties maintained their same peer social structure more than either teenagers or women who entered the family developmental stage of having a first child at 30 to 42 years. Both the younger and older women found less mutuality with previous friends who did not have children. In addition, women in their twenties had obstetrical outcomes that approximated the national norms or expectations more than the other two age groups. They were "in-step" with societal norms and expectations and in that sense had a slight advantage in this first stage of family development. This age group also perceived its initial birth experiences more positively, and they derived greater gratification in the mothering role at one year.

Another weakness of the family developmental framework is the lack of research, or empirical testing. The longitudinal design to study development over a family's life span requires a strong program of research staffed by a multidisciplinary team. Otherwise, an individual researcher might not live to see a project completed (Hill, Rodgers, 1964). Developmental research will prosper best when externally supported and housed within an institution willing to make commitments to long-term goals.

Problems in dealing with and measuring both individual and family stage development confound research outcomes. For example, failure to consider the impact of individual developmental differences on family dynamics will inhibit progress in family development research. Adults operate at different stage levels and as a result may structure their families quite differently (Peterson, Hey, Peterson, 1979).

The stage development approach projected in the 1950s that focuses on family developmental tasks by the age of the oldest child does not equally address the development of the married couple. Couples are opting not to have children. What developmental stages are universal to families exclusive of childrearing? Hudson and Murphy (1980) reviewed all previous research that tested marital satisfaction by stages of the life cycle and concluded that the family life cycle is not a viable theoretical framework for investigating and understanding patterns of change in marital satisfaction or family discord. However, individual differences in self-perception, motivation, and social support were observed through seven stages of the family life cycle (Tamir, Antonucci, 1981). Parents of young children had higher self-perception scores, and parents of adolescents had lower scores with no gender differences observed. Gender differences were observed in motivation for parents of adolescents; men were more affiliative, and women were more achievement oriented. No gender interactions were observed, but significant stage differences were found in social support; adults at earlier stages of the family cycle used social supports more frequently but were less satisfied than adults in later stages. Tamir and Antonucci concluded that the family life stage was an important variable in measuring individual developmental change since the stages of family life were associated with psychologic and social change during adulthood.

Another constraint of the developmental approach is the problem in operationalizing concepts. For example, how can a higher level of integration, adaptation, or functioning be measured for families? Does a particular stage or age set artificial boundaries? It seems that staging family development by the age of the oldest child creates artificial boundaries for studying marital satisfaction (a curvilinear relationship is observed with satisfaction being higher during earlier and later years of marriage) but may be viable for studying individual development.

Lack of measures or methodology to assess family development further inhibits this research. Groups and group processes are difficult to study and require team efforts. Maintaining cohesive, long-term research teams is difficult, not to mention maintaining long-term contact with families for study.

These constraints, along with the cost in time and money for longitudinal research, may be reasons that the developmental approach has been seldom used in research. Although many nursing schools have curricula based on developmental theory, the lack of research using this approach is yet another limitation.

Finally, in any study over time, historical events may affect both process and outcome. Nesselroade and Baltes (1974) found that developmental change in adolescents was influenced more by the cultural moment than by age sequences. They urge that research models focus on the interaction between cultural change and individual development. In addition to historical events, the Hawthorne effect (the stimulus to action that results from being observed) is perhaps unavoidable in any longitudinal study in which close rapport is established between researcher and family.

Strengths

The theoretical base for developmental theory is broad. Thus, the study of the development of the family allows for innovative and creative approaches. For example, the potential for studying the impact of the individual's level of development (such as the moral stage) on family development, as suggested by Peterson et al (1979), is both challenging and promising.

Much can be gained by initial qualitative approaches to help identify the relevant variables for focus. An example is Kreppner, Paulsen, and Schuetze's (1982) interactional analysis of the family system as it changed following the arrival of a second child, using hermeneutic, or interpretive, methodology. They coped with the problem of analyzing continuity and change simultaneously by following families both as individual cases (idiographic approach) and as representatives of generalizable characteristics in a nomothetic approach (study of groups).

The temporal orientation of development allows for consistency in comparisons of families. A combination longitudinal and cross-sectional design, such as that used by Sammons (1985) to study the incorporation of the second child into the family, can make it feasible for individual researchers to study facets of family development. This kind of combination can also help control for cultural change occurring with family development.

Eclectically derived multivariate models for analysis have potential for identifying those variables that are more salient to family development. A family developmental stage theory based on the developmental level of the adults in the family, or other variables yet to be discovered through multivariate models, may yield more fruitful results.

The Systems Approach

The systems approach to study of the family has been influenced by theory derived from physics and biology by Bertalanffy (1950, 1968). Sociologists were describing the family as a semi-closed or open system prior to his influence. General systems theory includes many theories and has been challenged as a formal theory, with some seeing it as a methodology, a strategy, or a way of looking at the world (Hamilton, 1979). Fawcett (1975) integrated systems theories with nursing theorist Roger's framework to propose a conceptual framework for nursing—the family as a living, open system. Rogers (1983), in relating her own theory to the family, noted that the family is an irreducible energy field, different from its parts (members), in which change is continuous and innovative. Because the whole is more than and different from the sum of its parts, family characteristics cannot be predicted from knowledge about individual family members (Rogers, 1983).

A system is composed of a set of interacting elements (Bertalanffy, 1968); each system is identifiable as distinct from the environment in which it exists. A boundary, which separates the system from the environment, should be such that units inside the system have a higher level of interaction with themselves than with units in the environment (Broderick, Smith, 1979).

An open system exchanges energy and matter with the environment to evolve toward greater order and increased complexity, which is known as *negentropy* (Bertalanffy, 1968); thus, an open system is characterized by a major developmental concept (Werner's orthogenetic principle discussed earlier). A closed system is isolated from its environment (Bertalanffy, 1968) and moves toward increasing disorder and disintegration, which is known as *entropy*. The hierarchy of systems may be based on either structure or function. Systems theory includes *developmental* concepts and also embraces *structural-functional* concepts. In a structural-functional approach, the function or role of the family would be studied with the structure of society as the major focus.

An open system is able to maintain a steady state by several different means, which is known as the *principle of equifinality*. The principle of equifinality is congruent with Werner's developmental concept that the same achievement may be reached by quite different genetic operations.

The system depends on feedback, a circular monitoring of information regarding deviations from goals or the state to be achieved. Negative feedback is a system's response to correct or to intervene with stress-producing stimuli to maintain homeostasis or equilibrium. Seeking therapy when the marital relationship is becoming strained is an example of using negative feedback to maintain a steady state in the marriage. An example of positive feedback is that of selecting and maintaining a family member for scapegoating; the greater the family stress from any situation, the more blame and punishment are directed toward the scapegoated individual, leading to increased psychological disequilibrium of the scapegoated person as well as other family members.

Speer (1970) argued that the concept of homeostasis limited both expectations for and approaches to helping families. He proposed that families have *morphostatic* properties (self-correcting processes that permit stability of the system) and *morphogenic* properties (self-directing processes that allow for change, growth, innovation, and viability of the family system).

Olson et al (1979) proposed sixteen types of marital and family systems based on a balance between cohesion and adaptability. Cohesion refers to the emotional bonds between family members. Adaptability refers to the ability of the system to change its power structure, role relationships, and rules in response to stress. A balance must be maintained on the cohesion dimension between too much closeness leading to enmeshed systems and too little closeness leading to disengaged systems. On the adaptability dimension, too much change can lead to chaotic systems, while too little change leads to rigid systems. A third dimension is the communication between family members (Olson et al, 1983).

The Beavers System Model (Beavers, 1977; Beavers, Voeller, 1983) is a cross-sectional model on which the structure, flexibility, and competence of a family and its members are scored on one dimension and family style on another dimension. Centripetal family members derive greater satisfaction from relationships within the family while centrifugal family members derive greater satisfaction from relationships outside the family, and family style of interaction adapts as the family changes.

Assumptions

Assumptions of the systems perspective include the following:

1. The family system is greater than and different from the sum of its parts.

2. There are many hierarchies within the family system. There is a hierarchy in the levels of analysis, for example, subsystems of the family such as mother-child, family as the system with members as the units and the community as environment, family as an undifferentiated unit in a larger social system with individuals viewed as systems, or family as an environment for individuals who are viewed as systems (Broderick, Smith, 1979). In addition, there are temporal or logical sequences of rules and subrules by which a system operates and different complexities of feedback and control that allow the system to monitor its progress, to correct and elaborate responses, and to change goals (Broderick, Smith, 1979).

3. The family system is recognizable from the community; there is a boundary. Kantor and Lehr (1975) described three types of family structure based on the energy expended in maintaining a boundary—open, closed, and random. In open families, individual members regulate the input and output with the environment, and there are numerous guests, visits with friends, free information exchange, and open doors and windows. Closed families maintain discrete family space distinct and apart from the community; there are locked doors, preservation of territoriality, and secretiveness. Closed families tell their members when, where, and how they may acquire energy. In the random family there are as many territorial guidelines as there are family members; the exception is the norm, with very fluid norms and rules.

4. Family systems increase in negentropic complexity over time, evolving to allow greater adaptability, tolerance to change, and growth by differentiation. This is accomplished through the development of a decision maker who communicates with other family members and the outside world to develop the power base necessary to accomplish its goals (Beavers, 1977).

5. Family systems change constantly in response to stresses and strains from within as well as from the outside environment.

6. There are structural similarities in different family systems (isomorphism) (Bertalanffy, 1968).

7. Change in one part of a family system can affect the total system.

8. Causality is always modified by feedback; therefore, causality never exists in the real world.

9. Patterns in a family system are circular as opposed to linear. It is the cycle of interaction (as in mother-child) that is the irreducible unit, and change must be directed toward the cycle (Minuchin, 1985).

10. A family system is an organized whole; thus, the individuals within the family as parts of the system are interdependent (Minuchin, 1985).

11. Family systems have homeostatic features to maintain stabile patterns; although these are usually adaptive, dysfunctional families may adopt maladaptive behavior as functional within the system, resulting in increased rigidity and resistance to change (Minuchin, 1985).

Problems Addressed by Systems Theory

The systems approach may be used to study expanding or contracting families, families facing a crisis, or families that have special problems. Barnes and Olson (1985) tested the hypothesis that balanced families (Circumplex model) would have more positive parent–adolescent communication than extreme families; the hypothesis was supported by parental response but not by adolescent response. Although the individual level of analysis of parents and adolescents was conflicting, when family level analysis was done using discriminant analysis, families with good parent-adolescent communication scored higher on family cohesion, family adaptability, and family satisfaction.

The natural fit between systems and family developmental theory as a conceptual approach to studying families is illustrated in Smith's (1983) study of families incorporating an adoles-

cent mother and her child. Smith viewed the family as a system that progressed and changed through the life cycle, with an inductive, grounded theory approach. Families incorporated the adolescent daughter and her child in one of three ways: role-sharing, role-blocking, and role-binding. The evolvement of the family into any of these patterns illustrated all of the assumptions of the systems perspective discussed earlier. Assumptions that were particularly highlighted were: family change in response to stress; change in one member of the family system affecting the total system; causality being modified by feedback; the circular cycle of interaction; interdependence of family members in the organized whole; and homeostatic features of the family system patterns that were adaptive (role sharing) for the adolescent mother and other features that were dysfunctional for the adolescent mother's ongoing development (role-blocking and role-binding).

Fawcett (1977) used the framework of the family as a living open system to study the relationship and patterns of change in spouses' body images during and after pregnancy. Her theoretical model used the concepts of openness, pattern and organization, and mutual and simultaneous interaction within the family system. She found that husbands' perceived body spaces changed during and after their wives' pregnancy, although the form and appearance of their bodies did not change.

Holaday's (1981) theoretical framework to study maternal response to their chronically ill infants' crying behavior included concepts from systems theory from both Bowlby's (1969) and Johnson's (1980) behavioral system model. Selected concepts were input variables related to the development of the mother's set goals, the conditions that shift set goals, and the individual differences related to the range of set goals. She found that the chronically ill infant's cry elicited different *patterns* of response, and patterns of maternal response provided information about the establishment of the set goal, or behavioral set, which was the degree of proximity and speed of response.

Methodology

The complexity of studying the family system has been formidable because of the requirements for both data collection and data analysis as implied by the assumptions of the theory. Assumptions eight and nine, that causality is always modified by feedback and that patterns of a family system are circular as opposed to linear, mandate that simple regression models cannot be used. Nonrecursive models that consider the circular effects are essential. However, advanced analytic programs, such as those used by Lavee, McCubbin, and Patterson (1985) (LISREL VI), are able to consider nonrecursive causation, measurement errors, and correlated residuals. Such innovations, along with improved technology for recording interactional observations, should contribute to increased research using the systems approach.

Inductive methodologies, such as those used by Kantor and Lehr (1975) and Smith (1983), have proven fruitful. Through observation, these researchers evolved family theory. Kantor and Lehr (1975) described how they proceeded from a study of microlevel acts and sequences of acts to major elements, influencing family process by combining elements of general systems theory with naturalistic study of family life. Kantor and Lehr came up with one way that families function in interfacing with the outside world. Smith described one way that families function within subsystems in affecting individual family members.

Limitations and Constraints

Many of the systems concepts or theories are difficult to operationalize. Part of this may be that systems' terms are not congruent with words used every day (for example, *negative*

feedback and *negentropy* both have negative labels but indicate positive directions).

We know little about the family as a system; its parameters have not been specified and calibrated (Broderick, Smith, 1979). Little is known about control in the family, boundary maintenance, or how family inputs are converted to family outputs (Broderick, Smith, 1979). How are the information processors or determiners of when to use negative feedback selected within the family? More descriptive research, such as Kantor and Lehrs' (1975), is essential.

The complexity of studying several dimensions simultaneously, as Beavers (1977) describes, raises methodologic and analysis problems. How many variables can one research problem or project attend to with accuracy and reliability?

Nurses have used systems theory to study individuals and dyads; however, few have used this theory to study the family as a unit. The problems of operationalizing variables and in measurement have inhibited the extent of this plausible theory's testing.

Strengths

The approach is strong in its broadness and wholeness; the model provides for studying the dimensions of a family in both breadth and depth. The individual as a unit of the family system is not overlooked; seeming dysfunction of a target member who is actually serving to hold the family together might be overlooked using another framework.

A systems approach lends itself readily to model-building, with nonlinear, nonrecursive, and multi-interaction effects. The flexibility allowed by the systems approach lends itself to multicausality with multiple outputs as well as similar outcomes by different inputs (Broderick, Smith, 1979).

The systems language, although not that in everyday usage, is interpreted similarly across disciplines; hence, there is potential for improving communication between disciplines.

Systems theory, with its broad perspective, has influenced two additional perspectives in which systems theory is central. They are the ecologic and stress frameworks.

The Ecological Framework

The ecological framework represents a blend of developmental, systems, and situational perspectives. This blend seems particularly important for problems addressed by the discipline of nursing and has appeared increasingly in nurse researchers' work since Bronfenbrenner (1977) proposed an experimental ecology of human development.

The ecology of human development as proposed by Bronfenbrenner (1977) is an interactive process of progressive accommodation between the human and the changing environment; human development must be understood within the multiperson environmental systems in which the human is enmeshed. The ecological environment is made of the microsystem, mesosystem, exosystem, and macrosystem. Beginning with the microsystem, each system is contained in or nested in the next larger system. The microsystem includes the immediate settings in which the person fulfills his or her roles (family, school, place of employment, and so on). The mesosystem is made up of the interrelationships of the major settings that are salient at the person's particular period in life. The exosystem includes the major institutions of the society, such as the neighborhood, the mass media, and the local, state, and national government agencies, that constrain or affect the person's immediate settings. The macrosystem encompasses the overarching institutional patterns of the culture.

The ecological framework for viewing the family considers the family as nested within these larger systems and as an open system the family is actively influencing and being influenced by the larger systems.

Assumptions

Assumptions for the family ecological framework are derived from Bronfenbrenner's (1977) definitions and propositions for an experimental ecology of human development.

1. An ecological family study is conducted in a naturalistic setting and involves persons and activities from everyday life. This is congruent with the symbolic interactionist perspective.

2. The properties of the environment in which the research is conducted influence the processes that occur within that context, thus affecting the interpretation and generalizability of the research findings. Ecological validity then is the extent that the investigator defines the environment as it is actually experienced by the subjects.

3. An ecological family experiment investigates the adaptation between the growing family and its environment through a systematic contrast between two or more different environmental systems. Controls are done either by what Bronfenbrenner calls "contrived experiment" (random assignment) or by "natural experiment" (matching); he does not like the term *quasi-experimental* because it implies a lesser level of methodologic rigor.

4. In family ecological research, interactions are usually the principal main effects.

5. Environmental structures in which the family system is nested are interdependent and must be analyzed in systems terms. Therefore, reciprocal rather than unidirectional processes are studied.

6. The environment may have indirect influences on processes occurring within the family system, which must be considered.

7. The ecological family approach allows consideration of interdependencies between, or joint impacts of, environments in which the family is nested.

8. An ecological family experiment involving the family in more than one setting should take into account the possible subsystems and higher order effects that may exist across settings.

9. The ecology of family development encompasses the family life span. Ecological transitions provide a rich context for studying family development.

10. Ecological family systems research and developmental research must consider the larger environments that affect the immediate setting. For example, inflation, unemployment, and nuclear weapons have had a profound impact on family units.

11. Ecological family systems research and developmental research should include creative and innovative restructuring of existing ecological systems. An example of a study of this type would be persuading a company to allot paternity leaves as well as maternity leaves to make it possible for families to allot roles by greater expertise and interests of individuals.

Problems Addressed by Family Ecological Systems Perspective

Feetham (1980) has used the ecological systems approach in studying families with children with myelodysplasia. She developed the Feetham Family Functioning Survey (FFFS) (Roberts, Feetham, 1982) to measure three major areas of family relationships: between the family and broader social units such as school and work; between the family and subsystems within the family; and between the family and individuals within the family. Both parents may complete the FFFS so that discrepant views of family life may be identified. Families experiencing a situational crisis may be studied via the natural kind of experiment described by Bronfenbrenner to determine the impact of the crisis on family functioning.

Barnard et al (1983) evolved an ecological paradigm for assessment and intervention with families that included an interaction of the inanimate and animate supporting environment, maternal adaptation style, and the child's adaptation and temperament. They found that measures of the family ecology were strongly related to the child's IQ and language development among mothers with low education but not among mothers with more than a high school education (Bee et al, 1982).

Methodology

The adaptation or developmental approach requires that families are studied in their naturalistic settings. Families are appropriately studied as they seek medical care for treatment in clinics and hospitals, which are naturalistic settings for health problems under study. Barnard and Eyres (1979) studied expanding families from pregnancy through four years. The clinic and the hospital as well as the home environment were naturalistic settings for this period of study.

As in the developmental perspective described earlier, longitudinal designs are employed to study family adaptation. The external environment and internal environment are considered for their interactive effects on family interactions. Feetham's Family Functioning Survey has subscales that permit measurement of the individual family member's perceptions of these interactions.

Sophisticated multivariate models may be tested with systematic ability to control for variables and to study for interactive effects. In the Bee et al (1982) study cited earlier, a cluster of variables was identified as "family ecology"; these variables included level of stress, social support, and maternal education, and the cluster interacted with the child's IQ and language skills in families of mothers with less education.

Limitations and Constraints

When dealing with families in naturalistic settings, any research is invasive to an extent, and those families who are willing to allow the researcher to study them during normal, stressful, or transition periods may differ from the general population. Therefore, the external validity is limited to the population and the environmental context identified in the research.

The researcher is always dealing with a Hawthorne effect, since the interaction of the family with the researcher as part of the ecology will change variables under study somewhat. Kantor and Lehr (1977) suggested that, over time, the researcher may become such a familiar part of the environment that family responses are not affected by the researcher's presence.

In longitudinal research, subject loss is encountered, and severe attrition limits the validity of the findings if an adequate subject-to-variable ratio is not maintained. Often the variable under study, such as stress, may be a reason for a subject's withdrawal from a research project, which presents an additional threat to external validity.

Complex research requires teamwork, which is not easy to accomplish. The development of an instrument by the Family Dynamics Measurement Group, a subunit of the Family Health Section of the Midwest Nursing Research Society, for the assessment of family dynamics and the group process is reported in four articles (King et al, 1985; White, 1985; Speer et al, 1985; and Lasky et al, 1985). Systems theory provided the framework for the instrument's development. The Family Dynamics Measure tests six bipolar dimensions characterizing family relationships: individuation versus enmeshment; mutuality versus isolation; flexibility versus rigidity; stability versus disorganization; clear communication versus unclear or distorted communication; and role compatibility versus role conflict. It is unclear whether the 112 items deal with family–environmental interactions, but when this group releases the measure for others' use, it will be a most welcome addition to family research. This team provides invaluable data for others who are considering such work.

Strengths

The view of a family and the systems within which it is nested gives a holistic perspective that is critical for understanding family adaptation and family development. All of the strengths of both developmental and systems perspectives are applicable.

Stress and Coping Frameworks

Another example of the merged systems and developmental approaches are the stress and coping perspectives. Many paradigms exist in stress and coping research. Arguments abound regarding laboratory versus naturalistic (field) research in stress and traits (anxiety) versus process (Laux, Vossel, 1982). Lazarus and Folkman (1984) emphasize the circular interaction of a stressor and individual, in which three kinds of appraisals occur: primary, secondary, and reappraisal. *Primary* appraisal determines whether an event is irrelevant, benign or positive, or stressful. *Secondary* appraisal involves an evaluation of the options in the event. *Reappraisal* is a changed appraisal based on new information. This represents the information-processing component of a system, and families have either formal or informal members who jointly or hierarchically serve as information processors for the family in appraising whether events are stressful or benign for the family system. Developmental concepts are inherent in coping and stress research, because cognitive appraisals and coping responses are dependent on the level of ego and cognitive development and the individual's sense of mastery in the context.

Appraisal and coping were divided into three domains by Moos and Billings (1984) according to the primary focus when appraising a situation, dealing with the reality of the situation, and handling the emotions that resulted from the situation: appraisal-focused coping, problem-focused coping, and emotion-focused coping. Appraisal-focused coping relates to how the situation is defined or redefined. Problem-focused coping seeks to eliminate the problem. Emotion-focused coping is directed toward management of emotions that have been aroused by stressors.

An example of problem-focused coping with stress is the popular Double ABCX Model. The Double ABCX Model was adapted from the original ABCX Model, which included only pre-crisis variables to account for family differences in adaptation to a crisis; the Double ABCX Model includes postcrisis behavior as well (McCubbin, Patterson, 1983). The Double ABCX Model's postcrisis variables attempt to describe life stressors and changes that affect the family's ability to achieve adaptation, resources that the family calls on to manage the crisis situation, the processes the family engages in, and the outcome of the family's efforts. The Double ABCX Model has in common with the ecological systems model the nesting of microsystems within the larger systems. Three units of analysis include the individuals within the family, the family as a unit, and the community. The central concept is to describe a continuum of outcomes showing family adaptation or balance in functioning following crisis or transitions.

Four major domains of family stress and coping research were identified during the 1970s that used the ABCX crisis model: family response to events such as wars, disaster, illness; family response to normative transitions over the life span, such as parenthood and retirement; the nature and importance of the family's re-sources and perceptions; and the nature and importance of social support (McCubbin et al, 1980). The Double ABCX Model was the theoretical approach used by Gortner et al (1988) in their randomized clinical experiments of a method to facilitate individual and family adaptation following cardiac surgery.

Social Exchange Theory

Homans (1958) argued that "interaction between persons is an exchange of goods, material, and non-material" (p. 597). The argument was based on economics theories and laboratory studies of animal behavioral responses. Homans also used research on group cohesiveness to illustrate his points; the more cohesive a group the more valuable the exchange between individuals in the group and the greater the reinforcement for the exchanged behavior. More cohesive groups maintain equilibrium by choosing not to interact with the deviate. The more closely an individual's behavior conforms to the group's, the more interactions he or she receives from others and the more positive choices he or she receives from group members.

Homans (1958) proposed that distributive justice (rewards proportionate to costs) was one condition for equilibrium within a group; if costs are higher for a group, rewards must be higher. When individuals enter into social relationships, they are rewarded; in deriving benefits or rewards, the rewarded individual must reciprocate. If the individual fails to reciprocate, there is no incentive for others to continue their interactions with him or her. A balance occurs when there is reciprocation; when a person does not reciprocate, an imbalance occurs. With an imbalance, a unilateral dependence develops, and the person who is able to reciprocate has power over the other who has no means to do so (Blau, 1964); collective approval of power legitimates power.

Nye summarized the general principle of what he called choice and exchange theory (1978, 1979): Individuals avoid behaviors with higher costs and seek rewarding statuses and relationships to maximize their profits. Nye (1979) viewed choice as the more significant part of the theory, and noted that rational or irrational choices are made in deciding rewards and costs. Irrational choices may be perceived after the fact as either over- or underestimating costs and rewards of outcome in a particular situation.

The use of exchange theory for family study has evolved since the 1960s. Safilios-Rothschild (1970) reviewed the research focused on family power structure during 1960–1969 and noted many methodologic and conceptual shortcomings in defining power structure or decision-making within the family. She proposed exchange theory as relevant to family dynamics. Osmond (1978) later proposed reciprocity as a dynamic model for the study of family power.

In applying the exchange or social control model to family violence, Gelles (1983) drew on Blau's (1964) concept of balance in relationships; a person who supplies rewards to another obliges that person to reciprocate. In situations in which it is impossible to break off family relationships because the principle of distributive justice is violated, (e.g., a child or an ill family member who cannot reward parents or mates in proportion to services and goods that they receive from these family members) an imbalance is created. Under some circumstances, family members who are not receiving rewards in proportion to their gifts may respond with anger, resentment, conflict, and violence. For equilibrium to be maintained in the family, rewards must be forthcoming from other resources or areas. Characteristics such as inequality (husbands are larger than wives and parents are larger than children), privacy (the extent of social control is reduced in family matters), and the "real man" image in a culture that considers aggressive sexual behavior or violence as proof of masculinity all contribute to family violence.

Assumptions

Assumptions of social exchange theory are adapted largely from Nye (1979).

1. Individuals as rational beings make choices that result in the greatest reward and least cost; therefore, families will, within the limits of their abilities, make choices that lead to the greatest rewards at the least cost.

2. Individuals make decisions and initiate action rather than the culture or milieu determining decisions and actions. Families make choices and respond to the environment rather than the converse.

3. To obtain rewards, a price must be paid.

4. Social behavior that is unrewarded will not continue, unless that behavior is expected to be the least costly of all responses.

5. When no alternative is thought to be profitable, the alternative that is the least unprofitable will be selected or the one in which there will be the smallest loss.

6. When rewards (or received goods) are felt to be deserved (rewards = costs), recipients feel satisfied; if received goods are less than is felt deserved, anger is the outcome (cost > rewards); and if received goods are greater than is felt deserved, guilt is the outcome (rewards > cost).

7. Reciprocity is essential for social life.

8. Revenge is gratifying when a person feels he or she has been wronged (achieving distributive justice).

9. Costs of receiving punishment are usually greater (person receiving punishment may not consider it due) than rewards of inflicting it.

10. Although a particular society usually agrees on whether something is a reward or cost, individuals and families assign different values to the object, experience, relationship, or position. An object viewed as a reward by

one family (such as a new infant) may be viewed as a cost by another.

11. The more of a commodity that an individual or family has, the less additional units of that commodity are worth to the individual or family.

Problems Addressed by Exchange Theory

Social exchange theory is viewed as promising by sociologists, but no family research by nurses was found using the framework. This may be because the framework is less well known (no nurse theorist based a model on this framework) or the assumptions have less philosophic congruence with nursing problems than other frameworks.

Some of the assumptions of exchange theory are culturally biased. For example, assumptions six, eight, and nine suggest anger when rewards do not equal cost and gratification from revenge or inflicting punishment. An Asian student disclosed in a seminar that in her culture, peace was more highly valued over reward; therefore, these assumptions would not be applicable in her culture.

Gelles (1983) derived propositions from exchange theory to apply in research and treatment and social policy issues around family violence. Nye (1979, 1980) also derived numerous propositions around family violence and conflict but included many propositions related to other areas of family behavior as well, such as maternal employment, timing of marriage and parenthood, sexual behavior, and communication. The kinds of problems that may be addressed by this theory are extensive. Nurses interested in fostering family compliance with medical regimens might ask what the costs of compliance versus the rewards for the family are. If costs of compliance outweigh any reward, effort can be made to improve compliance by increasing its attractiveness and reward value.

By using both symbolic interactionist and exchange theory perspectives, Mutran and Reit-

zes (1984) focused on the impact of social structure, the influence of subjective factors on family interaction, and the influence of family exhanges on how the elderly felt about themselves. Elderly parents who had more resources received less help, and elderly parents who were older and in poorer health gave less aid to children. Maximizing profits did not seem to affect self-feelings when the marital relationship was intact among elderly parents. Exchange patterns were more important in influencing the self-feelings of widows than of married parents.

Other researchers used exchange theory to study decision-making in high- and low-conflict tasks among distressed and nondistressed couples (Gottman et al, 1976). Distressed couples did not differ from nondistressed couples in how they intended their verbal messages to their spouses; however, the distressed spouses viewed the messages more negatively than the nondistressed spouses. High-conflict tasks were better discriminators than low-conflict tasks. The couple's own coded behavior discriminated between distressed and nondistressed couples more than observer-coded studies, suggesting that observers do not attend to all cues, such as facial expressions or tone of voice.

Methodology

Social exchange theory converges with symbolic interactionist theory. Both assume that individuals act toward their environment; both imply the process of reflectiveness about self; both view social organization as emerging from individual responses; and in both, social dynamics arise out of contradictions, inconsistency, conflict, and change (Singelmann, 1972). Both perspectives recognize that individuals appraise and assess situations, that rewards derive meaning from the current definition of the situation and past history, and that interactions are constantly open to negotiation and change (Mutran, Reitzes, 1984). Thus, the methodology appropriate for the symbolic interactionist perspective is appropriate for exchange theory. Observations that are process oriented or use time sampling are important.

Limitations and Constraints

Exchange theory does not deal with the underlying psychodynamics, as does systems theory. If social exchange is viewed from an objective stance only, inaccurate assessments will occur. The researcher may focus on choice and the outcome without getting at the real problem in a family or in a relationship. One of the problems with using exchange theory in research on families is that a simple interaction was often observed rather than the total exchange of services (Mutran, Reitzes, 1984).

Leventhal (1980) described three major problems with equity theory (one subcategory of exchange theory). First, it employs a unidimensional concept of fairness. Second, the focus on fair distribution and lack of consideration of the procedures in the distribution may lead to unequal exchange. Third, the exaggeration of the importance of fairness in relationships may reduce exploration of other motivational forces that may influence an individual's perception and behavior.

Talmadge and Ruback (1985) noted that intimate relationships are characterized by a different type of exchange than reciprocity or power models that emphasize the individual's reward over the well-being of the community or the relationship. Partners' commitments may be to the larger unit (marriage or family) rather than to individual goals. Debts (or imbalance in reciprocities) to families are too great to be repaid, yet imbalance is usually accompanied by a negative effect. Talmadge and Ruback suggest that these notions may help explain intense love–hate relationships in conflicted families.

McDonald (1981) proposed a model for testing marital interactions in an attempt to overcome some of the weaknesses in earlier research using exchange theory. He proposed consider-ing structural and temporal dimensions involved in marital exchange along with the need to study the effects of the social structure on the cognitive orientations of the partners and their subsequent exchange relationship. McDonald concluded that social exchange theory had to consider the inability or the unwillingness of partners in special relationships to calculate rewards and costs in their transactions, as well as the possibility that exchanges were for the purpose of maintaining the relationship rather than to maximize individual outcomes.

Nye (1979) cautioned that choice exchange theory required sophisticated theoretical specification and appropriate research to test it. A researcher needs to consider intervening and antecedent variables that might indicate something about the relationship.

Because theory affects an individual's view of the world, ethical considerations are foremost with social exchange theory. Social exchange theory is susceptible to misuse—for example, as a way to explain violence to children, chronically ill individuals, and the elderly who are unable to provide rewards equivalent to their costs within a family.

Strengths

Gergen (1980) argued that exchange theory maintains an intelligibility that cuts across history. As with all theories, social exchange theory has value in providing interpretations of events and sensitizers to events, in organizing experiences into meaningful analytic units, in integrating analyses from disparate domains, and in sustaining value commitments in a society (Gergen, 1980).

Social exchange theory can also contribute to our understanding about the interdependency of individuals, particularly within families in which irrational factors may operate in exchange situations (Talmadge, Ruback, 1985). Gelles (1983) noted that exchange theory provides a perspective that best integrates key elements of diverse theories that explain human violence and can thus explain and answer a range of questions and issues related to family violence. The potential of research from exchange theory to generate additional hypotheses is great and can help set the direction for future research.

Current Level of Family Theory Development and Future Directions

The major theories proposed by the large number of behavioral scientists discussed in this chapter provide overall frameworks from which nursing problems may be easily researched. However, given the lack of testing of many of the theories, it is important that the nurse researcher bear in mind that theories are to be tested and rejected as well as accepted. Theories that apply in industry or in the military may not always apply in family situations or for family health problems. When classical theories do not apply, it is encumbent on the researcher to suggest alternative frameworks and alternative hypotheses for future testing with specific family groups in specific circumstances.

Within the milieu of classical developmental theory, for example, multiple variations of developmental principles exist, as was suggested by Werner (1948). Nursing research has the potential to contribute to middle-range theories concerning individual development in certain health conditions among particular cultures. Symbolic interactionist approaches would be productive to study family development during a variety of situational and developmental transitions to identify major concepts and variables.

We are fortunate that the work of other disciplines may be borrowed in many situations. An example of using classical theory for nursing research may be seen in the study of compliance, an important concern in the health care of fami-

lies. Individual and family interpretations of causation and control influence compliance to any health regimen. Arakelian (1980) outlines considerations for nurses contemplating researching the social behavioral concept of locus of control. Feldman (1984) also shows scholarly borrowing of concepts from several disciplines to study pain.

Nurses providing health care for families have rich data embedded in routine dialogue and examination that can contribute to knowledge. For example, Riddle (1973) observed over time that some families did well during crises, but others fell apart and were unable to cope with their situation. To discover why some families coped better than others, she analyzed case data and found four areas that distinguished the families who were able to cope with crisis and emerge as a stronger unit. Those families who coped best with crises had better communication patterns, economic support, and emotional support from within and without the family and were able to seek and use help more effectively. This rather simple research provides important findings that can be incorporated into clinical practice and can be tested further.

To maximize resources and potential, family research must continue along multiple tracks. Testing borrowed theory that has been assessed for clinical validity, utility, and valid and reliable operationalization is a must. Family theorists have too far to go not to take advantage of the trial and error of other scientists. Studying the extensive family configurations within the current classical theoretical frameworks can produce middle-range theory, which will provide major guidelines for clinical application.

It is important that the clinician–scientist not ignore the intuitiveness that is an unconscious accompaniment of the art of providing health care for families. These hunches may go astray at times, but the richness that lies beneath far outweighs any temporary detour to greater knowledge. When the same concern, fear, response, or question is repetitive, a pattern is indicated. Under what circumstances and in what dimensions does the pattern occur and continue? Only the clinician–scientist (or clinician and scientist in collaboration) can ask and answer these critical questions.

Summary

The overview of four major theoretical perspectives—symbolic interactionist, developmental, systems, and social exchange indicates convergence of major concepts between social exchange and symbolic interactionist theories and between developmental and systems theories. The family ecological systems approach and stress and coping approaches particularly illustrate the combination of developmental and systems concepts.

These theoretical perspectives all beg for increased naturalistic study that focuses on families within the larger community and societal systems. Bronfenbrenner's (1977) definitions of natural and contrived experiments are particularly relevant to nursing science.

Issues for Further Investigation

1. To what extent is nursing or nurse-client interaction addressed in theories of family behavior?

2. What possibilities exist among theories of family behavior for development of prescriptive theorizing about the role of the nurse in influencing family health outcomes?

3. To what extent is the health-related behavior of families explained by theories developed to address nonhealth-related behaviors?

4. Have particular theories of family behavior been more fruitful than others in explaining and predicting family health-related behaviors?

References

Arakelian M (1980): An assessment and nursing application of the concept of locus of control. *ANS,* 3(1):25–42.

Baldwin AL (1968): *Theories of Child Development.* New York: Wiley.

Barnard KE, Eyres SJ (June, 1979): *Child health assessment, Part 2: The first year of life.* Hyattsville, MD.: DHEW Publication No. HRA 79–25.

Barnard K et al (1983): An ecological paradigm for assessment and intervention. In: *New Approaches to Developmental Screening of Infants,* Brazelton TB, Lester BM (eds.). New York: Elsevier, pp. 199–218.

Barnes HL, Olson DH (1985): Parent-adolescent communication and the circumplex mode. *Child Dev,* 56:438–447.

Beavers WR (1977): *Psychotherapy and Growth: A Family Systems Perspective.* New York: Brunner/Mazel.

Beavers WR, Voeller MN (1983): Family models: Comparing and contrasting the Olson circumplex model with the Beavers systems model. *Fam Process,* 22:85–98.

Bee HL et al (1982): Prediction of IQ and language skill from perinatal status, child performance, family characteristics, and mother–infant interaction. *Child Dev,* 53:1134–1156.

Bertalanffy LV (1950): The theory of open systems in physics and biology. *Science, 111*:23–29.

Bertalanffy LV (1968): *General System Theory.* New York: George Braziller.

Blau PM (1964): Justice in social exchange. *Sociological Inquiry* 24:193–206.

Blumer H (1969): *Symbolic Interaction: Perspective and Method.* Englewood Cliffs, New Jersey: Prentice-Hall.

Bowlby J (1969): *Attachment, Vol I; Attachment and Loss*. New York: Basic Books.

Broderick C (1971): Beyond the five conceptual frameworks: A decade of development in family theory. *J Marr Fam, 33*, 139–159.

Broderick C, Smith J (1979): The general systems approach to the family. In: *Contemporary Theories About the Family Vol 2*. Burr WR et al (eds.). New York: Free Press.

Bronfenbrenner U (1977): Toward an experimental ecology of human development. *Am Psychol, 32*:513–531.

Burr WR et al (eds.) (1979): *Contemporary Theories About the Family Vol 2*. New York: Free Press.

Burr WR et al (1979): Symbolic interaction and the family. In: *Contemporary Theories About the Family Vol 2*. Burr WR et al (eds.). New York: Free Press.

Caldwell BM (1962): The usefulness of the critical period hypothesis in the study of filiative behavior. *Merrill-Palmer Quarterly, 8*:229–242.

Christensen HT (1964): *Handbook of Marriage and the Family*. Chicago: Rand McNally.

Corbin JM, Strauss AL (1984): Collaboration: Couples working together to manage chronic illness. *Image, 14*(4):109–115.

Curry MA (1982): Maternal attachment behavior and the mother's self-concept: The effect of early skin-to-skin contact. *Nurs Res, 31*:73–78.

Durand B (1975): A clinical nursing study: Failure to thrive in a child with Down's syndrome. *Nurs Res, 24*:272–286.

Duvall EM (1957): *Family Development*. Philadelphia: Lippincott. (5th Ed 1977).

Erikson EH (1959): Identity and the life cycle. *Psychol Issues, 1*(1):5–171.

Fawcett J (1975): The family as a living open system: An emerging conceptual framework for nursing. *Int Nurs Rev, 22*:113–116.

Fawcett J (1977): The relationship between identification and patterns of change in spouses' body images during and after pregnancy. *Int J Nurs Stud, 14*:199–213.

Feetham SLB (1980): The relationship of family functioning to infant, parent, and family environment outcomes in the first 18 months following the birth of an infant with myelodysplasia. Unpublished doctoral dissertation, Wayne State University.

Feetham SL (1984): Family research: Issues and directions for nursing. *Annu Rev Nurs Res, 3*:3–25.

Feldman HR (1984): Psychological differentiation and the phenomenon of pain. *ANS, 6*(2):50–57.

Gelles RJ (1983): An exchange/social control theory. In: *The Dark Side of Families*. Finkelhor D et al (eds.). Beverly Hills: Sage Publications.

Gergen KJ (1980): Exchange theory: The transient and the enduring. In: *Social Exchange: Advances in Theory and Research*, Gergen KJ et al (eds.). New York: Plenum.

Gortner S et al (1988): Improving recovery from cardiac surgery. *J Adv Nurs, 13* (5): 5, 649–661.

Gottman J et al (1976): Behavior exchange theory and marital decision making. *J Pers Soc Psychol, 34*:14–23.

Hamilton GA (1979): Miller's living systems: A theory critique. *ANS, 1*(2):41–52.

Havighurst RJ (1972): *Developmental Tasks and Education*. New York: McKay.

Hill R (1965): Generic features of families under stress. In: *Crisis Intervention: Selected Readings*, Parad HJ (ed.). New York: Family Service Association.

Hill R, Hansen DA (1960): The identification of conceptual frameworks utilized in family study. *Marr Fam Living, 22*:299–311.

Hill R, Rodgers RH (1964): The developmental approach. In: *Handbook of Marriage and the Family*, Christensen HT (ed.). Chicago: Rand McNally.

Holaday B (1981): Maternal response to their chronically ill infants' attachment behavior of crying. *Nurs Res, 30*:343–348.

Holman TB, Burr WR (1980): Beyond the beyond: The growth of family theories in the 1970s. *J Marr Fam, 42*:729–741.

Homans GC (1958): Social behavior as exchange. *Am J Sociol, 63*:597–606.

Howes K (1976): Epigenesis: The natural development of family crises leading to the hospitalization of adolescents. *Fam Coordinator, 25*:249–254.

Hudson WW, Murphy GJ (1980): The non-linear relationship between marital satisfaction and stages of the family life cycle: An artifact of type I errors? *J Marr Fam, 42*:263–267.

Hultsch DF, Hickey T (1978): External validity in the study of human development: theoretical and methodological issues. *Hum Dev*, 21:76–91.

Johnson DE (1980): The behavioral system model for nursing. In: *Conceptual Models for Nursing Practice, 2nd ed.*, Riehl JP, Roy C (eds.). East Norwalk, CT: Appleton-Lange, pp 207–216.

Kantor D, Lehr W (1975): *Inside the Family*. New York: Harper and Row.

Kaye K (1985): Toward a developmental psychology of the family. In: *Handbook of Family Psychology and Therapy Vol 1*, L'Abate L (ed.). Homewood, IL: Dorsey Press.

King JM et al (1985): A group dynamics view. *West J Nurs Res*, 7:7–19.

Kreppner K, Paulsen S, Schuetze Y (1982): Infant and family development: From triads to tetrads. *Hum Dev*, 25:373–391.

Lamb ME (1982): Early contact and maternal-infant bonding: One decade later. *Pediatrics*, 70:763–768.

Lasky P et al (1985): Developing an instrument for the assessment of family dynamics. *West J Nurs Res*, 7:40–52.

Laux L, Vossel G (1982): Paradigms in stress research: Laboratory versus field and traits versus process. In: *Handbook of Stress*, Goldberger L, Breznitz S (eds.). New York: Free Press.

Lavee Y, McCubbin HI, Patterson JM (1985): The double abcx model of family stress and adaptation: An empirical test by analysis of structural equations with latent variables. *J Marr Fam*, 47:811–825.

Lazarus RS, Folkman S (1984): *Stress, Appraisal, and Coping*. New York: Springer-Verlag.

Leventhal GS (1980): What should be done with equity theory? In: *Social Exchange: Advances in Theory and Research*, Gergen KG, Greenberg MS, Willis RH (eds.). New York: Plenum Press.

Martinson I, Spinetta J (1987): Final report: A longitudinal study of family bereavement after a death from childhood cancer. Report made to the American Cancer Society, California Division.

McCubbin HI et al (1980): Family stress and coping: A decade review. *J Marr Fam*, 42:855–871.

McCubbin HI, Patterson J (1983): Family transitions: Adaptation to stress. In: *Stress and the Family, Vol 1: Coping with Normative Transitions*, McCubbin HI, Figley CR (eds.). New York: Brunner/Mazel.

McDonald GW (1981): Structural exchange and marital interaction. *J Marr Fam*, 43:825–839.

Mead GH (1934): *Mind, Self, and Society*. Chicago: University of Chicago Press.

Meleis AI (1975): Role insufficiency and role supplementation: A conceptual framework. *Nurs Res*, 24:264–271.

Mercer RT (1981): A theoretical framework for studying factors that impact on the maternal role. *Nurs Res*, 30:73–77.

Mercer RT (1985): The process of maternal role attainment over the first year. *Nurs Res*, 34:198–204.

Mercer RT (1986): *First-Time Motherhood: Experiences from Teens to Forties*. New York: Springer-Verlag.

Mercer RT et al (1986): Theoretical models for studying the effect of antepartum stress on the family. *Nurs Res*, 35:339–346.

Mercer RT, Nichols E, Doyle G (1987): Transitions in the life cycle of women. *Commun Nurs Res*, 20:116.

Miller DR, Sobelman G (1985): Models of the family: A critical review of alternatives. In: *Handbook of Family Psychology and Therapy Vol 1*, L'Abate L (ed.). Homewood, IL: Dorsey Press.

Minuchin P (1985): Families and individual development: Provocations from the field of family therapy. *Child Dev*, 56:289–302.

Moos RH, Billings AG (1982): Conceptualizing and measuring coping resources and processes. In: *Handbook of Stress*, Goldberger L, Breznitz S (eds.). New York: Free Press.

Mutran E, Reitzes DC (1984): Intergenerational support activities and well-being among the elderly: A convergence of exchange and symbolic interaction perspectives. *Am Soc Rev*, 49:117–130.

Nesselroade JR, Baltes PB (1974): Adolescent personality development and historical change: 1970-1972. *Monographs of the Society for Research in Child Development*, 39(1):1–79.

Nye FI (1978): Is choice and exchange theory the key? *J Marr Fam*, 40:219–232.

Nye FI (1979): Choice, exchange, and the family. In: *Contemporary Theories About the Family Vol 2*, Burr WR et al (eds.). New York: Free Press.

Nye FI (1980): Family mini theories as special instances of choice and exchange theory. *J Marr Fam,* 42:479–489.

Nye FI, Berardo FM (1966): *Emerging Conceptual Frameworks in Family Analysis.* New York: Macmillan.

Olshansky EF (1985): The work of taking on and managing an identity of self as infertile. Unpublished doctoral dissertation, University of California, San Francisco.

Olson DH, Sprenkle DH, Russell CS (1979): Circumplex model of marital and family systems: I. Cohesion and adaptability dimensions, family types, and clinical applications. *Fam Process, 18:*3–28.

Olson DH, Russell CS, Sprenkle DH (1983): Circumplex models of marital and family systems: VI. Theoretical update. *Fam Process, 22:*69–83.

Osmond MW (1978): Reciprocity: A dynamic model and a method to study family power. *J Marr Fam,* 40:49–61.

Peterson GB, Hey RN, Peterson LR (1979): Intersection of family development and moral stage frameworks: Implications for theory and research. *J Marr Fam,* 41:229–235.

Riddle I (1973): Caring for children and their families. In: *Current Concepts in Clinical Nursing Vol 4,* Anderson E et al (eds.). St Louis: Mosby.

Roberts CS, Feetham SL (1982): Assessing family functioning across three areas of relationships. *Nurs Res, 31:*231–235.

Roberts FB (1983): Infant behavior and the transition to parenthood. *Nurs Res, 32:*213–217.

Rodgers RH (1964): Toward a theory of family development. *J Marr Fam, 26:*262–270.

Rogers ME (1983): Science of unitary human beings: A paradigm for nursing. In: *Family Health: A Theoretical Approach to Nursing Care,* Clements IW, Roberts FB (eds.). New York: Wiley.

Rowe GP (1966): The developmental conceptual framework to the study of the family. In: *Emerging Conceptual Frameworks in Family Analysis,* Nye FI, Berardo FM (eds.). New York: Macmillan.

Safilios-Rothschild C (1970): The study of family power structure: A review 1960–69. *J Marr Fam,* 32:539–552.

Sammons LN (1985): Maternal anxiety, somatic symptoms, marital adjustment, and family relationships in second pregnancy. Unpublished dissertation, University of California, San Francisco.

Schvaneveldt JD (1966): The interactional framework in the study of the family. In: *Emerging Conceptual Frameworks in Family Analysis,* Nye FI, Berardo M (eds.). New York: Macmillan.

Singelmann P (1972): Exchange as symbolic interaction: Convergences between two theoretical perspectives. *Am Soc Rev,* 37:414–424.

Smith L (1983): A conceptual model of families incorporating an adolescent mother and child into the household. *ANS, 6:*45–60.

Speer DC (1970): Family systems: Morphostasis and morphogenesis, or "is homeostasis enough?" *Fam Process, 9:*259–278.

Speer J et al (1985): Collaboration and the research process. *West J Nurs Res, 7:*32–39.

Sroufe LA et al (1985): Generational boundary dissolution between mothers and their preschool children: A relationship systems approach. *Child Dev, 56:*317–325.

Stainton MC (1985): The fetus: A growing member of the family. *Fam Relations, 34:*321–326.

Stern PN (1982): Affiliating in stepfather families: Teachable strategies leading to stepfather–child friendship. *West J Nurs Res, 4:*75–89.

Stern PN, Tilden VP, Maxwell EK (1980): Culturally-induced stress during childbearing: The Filipino–American experience. *Issues in Health Care of Women, 2:*67–81.

Stryker S (1964): The interactional and situational approaches. In: *Handbook of Marriage and the Family,* Christensen HT (ed.). Chicago: Rand McNally.

Swendsen LA, Meleis AI, Jones D (1978): Role supplementation for new parents—A role mastery plan. *Am J Mat Child Nurs, 3:*84–91.

Talmadge LD, Ruback RB (1985): Social and family psychology. In: *Handbook of Family Psychology and Therapy Vol 1,* L'Abate L (ed.). Homewood: IL: Dorsey Press.

Tamir LM, Antonucci TC (1981): Self-perception, motivation, and social support through the family life course. *J Marr Fam, 43:*151–160.

Turner JH (1978): *The Structure of Sociological Theory,* rev. ed. Homewood, IL: Dorsey Press.

Ventura JN, Stevenson MB (1986): Relations of mothers' and fathers' reports of infant temperament, parents' psychological functioning, and family characteristics. *Merrill-Palmer Quarterly, 32*:275–289.

Werner H (1948): *Comparative Psychology of Mental Development.* New York: International Universities Press.

Whall AL (1980): Congruence between existing theories of family functioning and nursing theories. *ANS, 3*(1):59–67.

White MA (1985): A Parsonian view. *West J Nurs Res, 7*:20–31.

3

FAMILY RESEARCH IN NURSING

Catherine L. Gilliss, RNC, DNSc

A review of family nursing research in selected refereed, nonspecialty journals revealed that the designs and methods (observational and correlational) used in family nursing research are typical of those used in general nursing. This chapter offers an updated review of the trends developing in family nursing research.

Introduction

The family is one of the most complex social systems studied by the nurse clinician or researcher. Yet, because of the apparent influence of the family on the identified patient and the growing awareness of the family group in its own right, nurses are studying relationships between family members, and they are studying the family group in increasing numbers (Feetham, 1984). Murphy (1986) has observed that the development of this interest in nursing is a logical outgrowth of ongoing interdisciplinary efforts to comprehend human growth and development and that there are parallels between the development of family science and family science in nursing. Murphy challenges that "the most urgent task for the family nursing research movement is to facilitate the growth of family research in several different directions" (p. 172). She calls for additional interdisciplinary collaboration but neglects to direct our efforts within nursing.

This chapter will attempt to offer some directions for family research in nursing by examining recent research reports. Three areas will be addressed: (1) the nature of questions asked about the family in nursing, particularly the subject matter of investigations into the family; (2) the nature of the designs employed in nursing research on the family; and (3) the methods employed in the study of the family in nursing research.

Several documents serve as important orienting documents to this analysis. First, Brown, Tanner, and Padrick (1984) described the characteristics of contemporary nursing research and the trends occurring over the last three decades. Their review of four refereed nonspecialty journals included research papers with characteristics essential to the development of a practice discipline: (1) the investigator was a nurse; (2) the research was concerned with a clinical problem; (3) the work was anchored in a theoretical framework; and (4) the work was of sound method. More recently, Jacobsen and Meininger (1985) systematically sampled three nonspecialty journals in nursing and described design and methods published in nursing literature between 1956 and 1983. The design criteria used by these authors (Table 3–1) will be used to permit comparison of their findings to reports of family research. Finally, Feetham's landmark review of family nursing research (1984) offers a model and a starting point for this review. Although the

Table 3–1   Taxonomy of Research Designs

Design	Description
Experiments	Prospective studies in which the investigator manipulated at least one intervention.
True Experiments	Randomized controlled trials in which subjects were assigned to concurrent groups at random.
Quasi-Experiments	Trials in which subjects were not assigned randomly to groups or trials in which comparison groups, if any, were not concurrent.
Observational Studies	Studies of naturally occurring events in which no deliberate intervention was made by the investigator.
Cross-Sectional Studies	Studies in which observations related to one point in time.
Longitudinal Studies	Studies in which observations related to at least two points in time, even if all data were collected simultaneously.

specific criteria proposed by Feetham for analysis of family research were not used to critique the reviewed papers, her criteria contributed to this author's recognition of papers to include in this review.

Methods

Sample

Six nonspecialty refereed journals that focus on the publication of nursing research were selected for review: *Nursing Research, Western Journal of Nursing, Research in Nursing and Health, Advances in Nursing Science, Journal of Advanced Nursing,* and *International Journal of Nursing Studies.* Journal issues from the years 1983 through 1986 were reviewed to locate publications addressing the family, as specified by the following criteria.

Criteria for Inclusion

Feetham proposed the use of four criteria to evaluate whether research in nursing should be identified as family research: (1) the family serves as the basis for conceptualization of the research question; (2) knowledge about the family will probably result from the investigation; (3) the family should be operationally defined; and (4) resulting knowledge will be useful to nursing practice. Additionally, Feetham proposed that critiques of such works should include comment on scientific merit and whether a full or partial model had been tested in the study. For this review, the criteria were modified from Feetham (1984) and Brown, Tanner, and Padrick (1984) as follows:

1. One or more authors were identified as members of the discipline.
2. The topic addressed had ultimate relevance

for clinical practice, whether or not the problem was now couched in a clinical setting.

3. The work tested a theoretical framework or attempted to develop new perspectives on the phenomena under study.
4. The method of investigation was sound; the study had scientific merit.
5. The report addressed an aspect of the family group in health or illness, a family role, or a relationship between/among family members or between the family and the larger environs (e.g., social supports or health care system).

Substantive Categorizations

Feetham (1984) also categorized and grouped reviewed papers according to their content focus in one of five areas: (1) family or family characteristics; (2) family as the environment for the individual; (3) external environment and the family; (4) family- related research; and (5) nursing interventions and the family (see Feetham, 1984, for additional detail). Although this schema has, no doubt, influenced the author, it will not be used for this review. Rather, categorizations by clinical practice specialties will be subcategorized as to whether the reports addressed the family, a dyad, or a particular family role enacted by a family member. This approach was employed to facilitate knowledge organization and the development of middle-range theories for nursing the family.

Procedures

Fifty-nine reports were categorized both by the author and a graduate assistant, with respect to substantive focus, design, and methods. For this subset of 59 reports, 90% agreement was achieved. The six disagreements were settled by consensus. The remaining 31 reports were reviewed by the author.

Table 3–2 Citations Referenced by Journal, Year, and Primary Author

	ANS	J Adv Nurs	Int J Nurs Stud	Nurs Res	Res Nurs Health	West J Nurs Res
1983	Gilliss	Chao Green Hentinen Phillips Rose	Hirshfeld	Andrews Edwardson Hurley Hymovich Mercer Mishel Moore Perry Roberts Toney Weaver	Jones	Ellison Magyary
1984	Richter	Hayes Reutter Robinson Salariya		Austin Brandt Broom Gortner Hymovich Riesch Tilden	Riesch	
1985	Boyd Lenz Smith	Harrison Hinds		Blank Censullo Crawford Cronenwett Hilbert Mercer Miles Sund Tulman Woods	Kviz McBride McCance Pridham Saltzer Sexton Silva	Clinton Ellison Foxall Knafl Laskey Tilden
1986	Brunngraber Campbell (a) Campbell (b) Dixon Phillips Uphold	Ekberg Hanson Siebert	Keane Mogan Uyer Williams	Blank Bramwell Brown (a) Brown (b) Byers Clinton Fawcett (a) Fawcett (b) Jones Majewski Mercer et al Tulman Ventura Walker (a) Walker (b)	Bee Collins Duffy Golas Knafl Lenz Martinson Mercer Schroder- Zwelling	Mercer (a)

Results

Sample

One hundred citations met the study criteria and were examined. Table 3–2 displays the source of the referenced citations by journal and year. Nearly twice the number of reports were located in 1986 (38) as in 1983 (21). The 100 reports were then categorized as to their primary purpose: conceptual, or review of literature; methodologic, or instrument development; or substantive report. Table 3–3 displays the referenced citations by major emphasis and year. Of the 100 citations located, 76 were identified as substantive reports of family research in nursing. These 76 reports were then reviewed and categorized. A complete listing of abstracted citations appears in the appendix at the end of this chapter.

Content Focus

With respect to clinical focus, the majority of reports addressed maternal–child issues, and by far the greatest number of reports focused on perinatal events, pregnancy, birthing, and postpartum. A total of 42 of 76 reports, or 55% of the reviewed reports, were dedicated to infants and their parents or the family during birth. The majority of these reports specifically addressed the mother–infant relationship (15 of 42: Andrews, Andrews, 1983; Bee et al, 1986; Blank, 1986; Byers, 1986; Censullo et al, 1985; Chao, 1983; Golas, Parks, 1986; Magyary, 1983; Mogan, 1986; Riesch, 1984; Riesch, Munns, 1984; Schroeder-Zwelling, 1986; Tulman, 1985, 1986; and Williams, 1986). An additional eight focused on mother–infant or father–infant dyads (Clinton, 1986; Jones, Lenz, 1986; Jones, Parks, 1983; Perry, 1983; Roberts, 1983; Toney, 1983; Ventura, 1986; and Weaver, 1983). The maternal role was the subject of seven papers (Majewski, 1986; Mercer, 1985; Mercer, 1986a, 1986b; Mercer, Hackley, Bostrom, 1983; Walker, Crain, Thompson, 1986a,

1986b) and the parenting role was the subject of one (McBride, 1985). The impact of the birth, or transition in the marital relationship, has been examined by nurse investigators (Broom, 1984; Fawcett el al, 1986; Fawcett, York, 1986; Lenz et al, 1985; and Moore, 1983). The social supports received by parents have also been addressed (Brown, 1986a, 1986b; Cronenwett, 1985; Lenz et al, 1986; and Tilden, 1984). Only one report described behavior patterns observed in the family unit following birth (Smith, 1983).

Reports focusing on the parent–young child dyad were frequent. Most were specific to mothers and children (Brandt, 1984; Ellison, 1983; Hayes, Knox, 1984; Kvis et al, 1985; Saltzer, Golden, 1985; and Uyer, 1986), though several reports addressed both sets of dyads (mother–child, father–child) or the parent–child dyad (Austin et al, 1983; Keane et al, 1986; and Miles, 1985). Fathers and daughters were the subject of one report on incest (Brunngraber, 1986). Several reports looked at the parent or family and their relationship with the health care system or nurse (Edwardson, 1986; Martinson, 1986; Siebert et al, 1986).

There were a number of reports (7 of 76, or 9%) that address the marital dyad in mid-life. The majority dealt with the demands of chronic illness (Bramwell, Whall, 1986; Campbell, 1986b; Ekberg et al, 1986; Foxall et al, 1985; Hilbert, 1985; Hurley, 1983; Sexton, Munroe, 1985). Several reports were concerned with the roles performed by women in their families: wife, spouse, mother (Hentinen, 1983; Silva, 1985; and Woods, 1985). Only one study addressed first-degree relatives (parents, offspring, and children) collectively (McCance et al, 1985).

Elders and their family caregivers were the subject of three reports (Hirshfeld, 1983; Phillips, 1983; and Philips, Rempusheski, 1986). Again, the studies looked at the family assisting the frail elder to respond to increasing debilitation or dementia. One of these reports, however, was devoted to an examination of those families that responded effectively and those who did not (Phillips, Rempusheski, 1986).

Table 3–3 Citations Referenced by Major Emphasis, Year, and Primary Author

	1983	1984	1985	1986
Conceptual or Literature Review	Green	Reutter Richter	Boyd Crawford Harrison	Hanson Knafl Mercer et al
Methodologic or Instrument Development	Gilliss Hymovich Mishel	Gortner Hymovich Salariya	Blank Clinton Ellison Laskey Pridham Tilden	Campbell (a) Collins Uphold
Substantive Reports	Andrews Chao Edwardson Ellison Hentinen Hirshfeld Hurley Jones Magyary Mercer Perry Phillips Roberts Rose Smith Toney Weaver	Austin Brandt Broom Hayes Riesch (a) Riesch (b) Robinson Tilden	Censullo Cronenwett Foxall Hilbert Knafl Kviz Lenz McBride McCance Mercer Miles Moore Saltzer Sexton Silva Sund Tulman Woods Hinds	Bee Blank Bramwell Brown (a) Brown (b) Brunngraber Byers Campbell (b) Clinton Dixon Duffy Ekberg Fawcett (a) Fawcett (b) Golas Jones Keane Lenz Majewski Martinson Mercer (a) Mercer (b) Mogan Phillips Schroeder- Zwelling Siebert Tulman Uyer Ventura Walker (a) Walker (b) Williams

Finally, several investigators attempted to study patterns or characteristics of the family group. Dixon (1986) compared the characteristics of the families of black teens using mental health services to those who did not. Duffy (1986) described the health behaviors practiced by female-headed, single-parent families. Hinds (1985) described the resources needed by families caring for cancer patients at home. Knafl (1985) described how families manage pediatric hospitalizations. Robinson and Thorne (1984) reinterpreted family behavior during hospitalization to suggest its function in serving the family. Rose (1983) described the process by which family members develop an understanding of mental illness in a family member. Sund and Ostwald (1985) provided a profile of young working parents and the stresses experienced in dual-career families.

Design

The reports reviewed fell into one of four categories: true experiments, quasi-experiments, observational cross-sectional or observational longitudinal. The greatest number of reports could be described as being based on data from observational cross-sectional designs (39 of 75, or 52%; N.B.: One design was not categorizable). Longitudinal designs were the bases of 28 reports (37%). Five reports were based on true experiments (Andrews, Andrews, 1983; Golas, Parks, 1986; McCance et al, 1985; Perry, 1983; and Toney, 1983) and three on quasi-experiments (Riesch, Munns, 1984; Uyer, 1986; and Williams et al, 1986).

Methods

Most studies reported the use of multiple methods. The most common approach to data collection included standardized self-report forms, often mailed to the investigator without a face-to-face interview. Standardized observations, such as the Brazelton Neonatal Assessment Screen, were used in many of the infant studies.

New, unstandardized instruments for data collection were employed, and often minimally discussed by investigators, providing little information about the usefulness of these data-gathering tools. Those using qualitative methodologies reported the particular method (such as grounded theory or constant comparison) used in data gathering and analysis.

Discussion

Content Focus

The overwhelming representation of maternal–child, parent–child reports in the family literature base probably comes as no surprise. These reports were easily identified as "family" reports in the literature, and their preponderance may reflect sampling biases; however, reports of this content area may exist in greater numbers as a function of our traditional perspectives on the definition of the family. That is, because we have recognized the parent–child dyad as significant to health, we have studied it. More recent is our observation that the family caregiver–frail elder is a social unit significant to health; therefore these reports are fewer in number. It is important to acknowledge that reports of elders and family members in mid-life may appear with greater frequency in specialty journals inside and outside of nursing. Given the number of reports in mother–child/parent–child nursing, one would expect the beginning development of middle-range theories about the family, particularly during birth, childhood illness, and hospitalization.

Almost 90% of the reviewed reports focus on an individual family role or a family dyad. Feetham (1984) noted the importance of testing full and partial models of family behavior, but to appreciate fully the significance of these pieces of information about the family, the pieces must be reviewed as a whole. Recognition that the family is greater than the sum of its parts and careful reanalysis of the pieces may help us better understand the whole of the family.

Design

Several referenced reports were derived from data collected for umbrella projects. As such, the designs that were described in reports were frequently not representative of the parent project (for example, data reported for one time interval in a longitudinal project may appear to be cross-sectional). However, it is important to note that if this is how reporting is accomplished (as with partial model reporting), knowledge development about the full model will be limited unless an integration of the reports is undertaken.

When compared to the Jacobsen and Meininger (1985) report of designs used in nursing from 1956 to 1983, the profile is similar. Whereas 49% of the Jacobsen and Meininger citations were identified as cross-sectional, 52% of the family citations were so identified; 24% of the nursing designs were described as longitudinal, and 37% of the family reports were similarly categorized. Fewer experiments have been reported in the family literature (27% versus 10%). The differences here are noteworthy. Gilliss (1983) and Feetham (1984) have called for the need to view the family over time to understand family processes and behaviors. Apparently this is a trend in family nursing research that distinguishes this area from other nursing research.

Methods

The methods used in the reviewed sample of family nursing research reports are typical of those used generally in nursing. Over 55% of the studies reviewed by Jacobsen and Meininger (1985) employed questionnaires or standardized tests; 15% used observation; and 13% used interviews. Only 19% of their citations employed medical records or apparatus. This profile represented the family nursing sample as well.

Of special note, however, are the unusual strategies used in the studies earlier described to collect data about family unit patterns or behaviors. Duffy (1986) used card sorts, diaries, and an interview to determine patterns of family health behavior. Sund and Ostwald (1985) and Dixon (1986) employed standardized instrumentation aimed at accessing family patterns (Family Environment Scale; Family Inventory of Life Events and Changes). Qualitative methods were used by Hinds (1986), Knafl (1985), Robinson and Thorne (1984), Rose (1983), and Smith (1983). These approaches included intensive interviews of multiple family members, observation, reflection, and analysis of themes.

Summary

Feetham (1984) used a wide number of sources in her review of the growing body of literature in family nursing. No sampling restrictions were placed on sources for the 62 references cited as appearing in the nursing literature; 30 of these were research publications. During the four years reviewed for this chapter, sampling was limited to 6 refereed nonspecialty journals and 100 papers were located, 76 of which were reports of family nursing research. The productivity of family nurse researchers is rapidly increasing. There is potential to dramatically affect nursing with the growing body of knowledge about the family.

There are some startling gaps in the family literature reviewed for this chapter. Very little has been published on nontraditional families or families from nondominant cultures. Little discussion appears in the nursing literature on the health needs of divorced or reconstituted families. Processes between dyads other than parent–child are underrepresented. There are few studies that address the siblings. How are siblings significantly affected by changes in the health of a brother or sister? Does the impact of this effect change over the life cycle? How does social support from a sibling vary from that provided by friends during an illness?

The transactions that occur between the family group and the community are largely overlooked. Currently there is considerable interest in social support. How social support differs from the support of a partner or family member is not clear. Given our concern for the health of families, closer examination is needed for finding ways we might intervene with communities to promote family and individual health.

With respect to designs and methods, work in family nursing appears similar to the work of other nurse scientists, with the exceptions of our use of more longitudinal designs and fewer experiments. These distinctions are important. They typify our interest in the family and underscore the infancy of nursing science. We are not sufficiently prepared to experiment.

Our methodologic similarity is troublesome. It suggests that although we realize that the phenomenon of our interest is different, we do not yet know how to capture that difference with variation in method of analytic technique. The models offered by Smith (1983), Knafl (1985), Rose (1983), Robinson and Thorne (1984), and Duffy (1986) offer some examples for accessing the complex phenomena our theories suggest we are looking for in family study.

References

Andrews C, Andrews E (1983): Nursing, maternal postures, and fetal position. *Nurs Res*, 32(6): 336–341.

Austin J, McBride A, Davis H (1984): Parental attitude and adjustment to childhood epilepsy. *Nurs Res*, 33(2): 92–96.

Bee H et al (1985): The impact of parental life change on early development of children. *Res Nurs Health*, 9: 65–74.

Blank D (1985): Development of the infant tenderness scale. *Nurs Res*, 34(4): 221–216.

Blank D (1986): Relating mother's anxiety and perception to infant satiety, anxiety, and feeding behavior. *Nurs Res*, 35(6): 347–351.

Boyd C (1985): Toward an understanding of mother–daughter identification using concept analysis. *ANS*, 7(3): 78–86.

Bramwell L, Whall A (1986): Effect of role clarity and empathy on support role performance and anxiety. *Nurs Res*, 35(5): 282–287.

Brandt P (1984): Stress-buffering efforts of social support on maternal discipline. *Nurs Res*, 33(4): 229–234.

Broom B (1984): Consensus about the marital relationship during transition to parenthood. *Nurs Res*, 33(4): 223–228.

Brown J, Tanner C, Padrick K (1984): Nursing's search for scientific knowledge. *Nurs Res*, 33(1): 26–32.

Brown M (1986a): Social support during pregnancy: A unidirectional or multidirectional construct? *Nurs Res*, 35(1): 4–9.

Brown M (1986b): Social support, stress and health: A comparison of expectant mothers and fathers. *Nurs Res*, 35(2): 72–76.

Brunngraber L (1986): Father–daughter incest: Immediate and long-term effects of sexual abuse. *ANS*, 8(4): 15–35.

Byers P (1986): Infant crying during aircraft descent. *Nurs Res*, 35(5): 260–262.

Campbell J (1986a): A survivor group for battered women. *ANS*, 8(2): 13–20.

Campbell J (1986b): Nursing assessment for risk of homicide with battered women. *ANS*, 8(4): 36–51.

Censullo M, Lester B, Hoffman J (1985): Rhythmic patterning in mother–newborn interaction. *Nurs Res*, 34(6): 342–346.

Chao Y (1983): Conceptual behavior of Chinese mothers in relation to their newborn infants. *J Adv Nurs*, 8: 303–310.

Clinton J (1985): Couvade: Patterns, predictors, and nursing management: A research proposal submitted to the Division of Nursing. *West J Nurs Res*, 7(2): 221–243.

Clinton J (1986): Expectant fathers at risk for couvade. *Nurs Res*, 35(5): 290–295.

Collins C, Post L (1986): An instrument to measure coping responses in employed mothers: Preliminary results. *Res Nurs Health*, 9: 309–316.

Crawford G (1985): A theoretical model of support network conflict experienced by new mothers. *Nurs Res, 34*(2): 100–102.

Cronenwett L (1985): Parental network structure and perceived support after birth of first child. *Nurs Res, 34*(5): 347–352.

Dixon M (1986): Families of adolescent clients and nonclients: Their environments and help-seeking behaviors. *ANS, 8*(2): 75–88.

Duffy M (1986): Primary prevention behaviors: The female-headed one-parent family. *Res Nurs Health, 9*: 115–122.

Edwardson S (1983): The choice between hospital and home care for terminally ill children. *Nurs Res, 32*(1): 29–34.

Ekberg J, Griffith N, Foxall M (1986): Spouse burnout syndrome. *J Adv Nurs, 11*: 161–165.

Ellison E (1985): A multidimensional dual-perspective index of parental support. *West J Nurs Res, 7*(4): 401–424.

Ellison E (1983): Parental support and school-aged children. *West J Nurs Res, 5*(2): 145–153.

Fawcett J et al (1986a): Spouses' body image changes during and after pregnancy: A replication and extension. *Nurs Res, 35*(4): 220–223.

Fawcett J, York R (1986b): Spouses' physical and psychological symptoms during pregnancy and the postpartum. *Nurs Res, 35*(3): 144–148.

Feetham S (1984): Family research: Issues and directions for nursing. In: *Annual Review of Nursing Research*. New York: Springer-Verlag.

Foxall M, Ekberg J, Griffith N (1985): Adjustment pattern of chronically ill middle-aged persons and spouses. *West J Nurs Res, 7*(4): 425–444.

Gilliss C (1983): The family as a unit of analysis: Strategies for the nurse researcher. *ANS, 5*(3): 50–59.

Golas G, Parks P (1986): Effect of early postpartum teaching on primiparas' knowledge of infant behavior and degree of confidence. *Res Nurs Health, 9*: 209–214.

Gortner S, Hudes M, Zyzanski S (1984): Appraisal of values in the choice of treatment. *Nur Res, 33*(6): 319–324.

Hanson S, Bozett F (1986): The changing nature of fatherhood: The nurse and social policy. *J Adv Nurs, 11*: 719–727.

Harrison M, Morse J, Prowse M (1985): Successful breast feeding: The mother's dilemma. *J Adv Nurs, 10*(3): 261–269.

Hayes V, Knox J (1984): The experience of stress in parents of children hospitalized with long-term disabilities. *J Adv Nurs, 9*(4): 333–341.

Hentinen M (1983): Need for instruction and support of the wives of patients with myocardial infarction. *J Adv Nurs, 8*(6): 519–524.

Hilbert G (1985): Spouse support and myocardial infarction patient compliance. *Nur Res, 34*(4): 217–220.

Hinds C (1985): The needs of families who care for patients with cancer at home: Are we meeting them? *J Adv Nurs, 10*(6): 575–581.

Hirshfeld M (1983): Homecare versus institutionalization: Family caregiving and senile brain disease. *Int J Nurs Stud, 20*(1): 23–32.

Hubbard P, Muhlenkamp A, Brown N (1984): The relationship between social support and self-care practices. *Nurs Res, 33*(5): 266–270.

Hurley P (1983): Communication variables and voice analysis of marital conflict stress. *Nurs Res, 32*(3): 164–169.

Hymovich D (1984): Development of the chronicity impact and coping instrument: Parent questionnaire (CICI:PQ). *Nurs Res, 33*(4): 218–222.

Jacobsen B, Meininger J (1985): The design and methods of published nursing research: 1956–83. *Nurs Res, 34*(5): 306–312.

Jones L, Lenz E (1986): Father–newborn interaction: Effects of social competence and infant state. *Nurs Res, 35*(3): 149–153.

Jones L, Parks P (1983): Mother-, father-, and examiner-reported temperament across the first year of life. *Res Nurs Health, 6*: 183–189.

Keane S, Garralda M, Keen J (1986): Resident parents during paediatric admissions. *Int J Nurs Stud, 23*(3): 247–253.

Knafl K (1985): How families manage a pediatric hospitalization. *West J Nurs Res, 7*(2): 151–176.

Knafl K, Deatrick J (1986): How families manage chronic conditions: An analysis of the concept of normalization. *Res Nurs Health, 9*: 215–222.

Kviz F, Dawkins C, Ervin N (1985): Mothers' health belief and use of well-baby services among a high risk population. *Res Nurs Health, 8*: 381–387.

Lasky P et al (1985): Developing an instrument for the assessment of family dynamics. *West J Nurs Res*, 7(1): 40–57.

Lenz E et al (1986): Life change and instrumental support as predictors of illness in mothers of 6-month-olds. *Res Nurs Health, 9*: 17–24.

Lenz E et al (1985): Sex-role attributes, gender, and postpartal perceptions of the marital relationship. *ANS, 7*(3): 49–62.

Magyary D (1983): Cross-time and cross-situational comparisons of mother–preterm infant interactions. *West J Nurs Res, 5*(3): 15–25.

Majewski J (1986): Conflicts, satisfactions, and attitudes during transition to the maternal role. *Nurs Res, 35*(1): 10–14.

Martinson I et al (1986): Home care for children dying of cancer. *Res Nurs Health, 9*: 11–16.

McBride A (1985): Differences in women's thinking about parent child interactions. *Res Nurs Health, 8*: 389–396.

McCance et al (1985): Preventing coronary heart disease in high-risk families. *Res Nurs Health, 8*: 413–420.

Mercer R (1985): The process of maternal role attainment over the first year. *Nurs Res, 34*(4): 198–204.

Mercer R (1986a): Predictors of maternal role attainment at one year postbirth. *West J Nurs Res, 8*(1): 9–32.

Mercer R (1986b): The relationship of developmental variables to maternal behavior. *Res Nurs Health, 9*: 25–33.

Mercer R et al (1986): Theoretical models for studying the effects of antepartum stress on the family. *Nurs Res, 35*(6): 339–346.

Mercer R, Hackley K, Bostrom A (1983): Relationship of psychosocial and perinatal variables to perception of childbirth. *Nurs Res, 32*(4): 202–207.

Miles M (1985): Emotional symptoms and physical health in bereaved parents. *Nurs Res, 34*(2): 76–81.

Mishel M (1983): Parents' perception of uncertainty concerning their hospitalized child. *Nurs Res, 32*(6): 324–330.

Mogan J (1986): Parental weight and its relation to infant feeding patterns and infant obesity. *Int J Nurs Stud, 23*(3): 255–264.

Murphy S (1986): Family Study and Nursing Research. *Image, 18*(4): 170–174.

Perry S (1983): Parents' perceptions of their newborn following structured interactions. *Nurs Res, 23*(4): 208–212.

Phillips L (1983): Abuse and neglect of the frail elderly at home: An exploration of theoretical relationships. *J Adv Nurs, 8*(5): 379–392.

Phillips L, Rempusheski V (1986): Caring for the frail elderly at home: Toward a theoretical explanation of the dynamics of poor quality family caregiving. *ANS, 8*(4): 62–84.

Pridham K, Chang A (1985): Parent's belief about themselves as parents of a new infant: Instrument development. *Res Nurs Health, 8*: 19–29.

Reutter L (1984): Family health assessment—an integrated approach. *J Adv Nurs, 9*: 391–399.

Richter J (1984): Crisis of mate loss in the elderly. *ANS, 6*(4): 45–54.

Riesch S (1984a): Occupational commitment and the quality of maternal infant interaction. *Res Nurs Health, 7*: 295–303.

Riesch S, Munns S (1984b): Promoting awareness: The mother and her baby. *Nurs Res, 33*(5): 271–276.

Roberts F (1983): Infant behavior and the transition to parenthood. *Nurs Res, 32*(4): 213–217.

Robinson C, Thorne S (1984): Strengthening family "interference." *J Adv Nurs, 9*(6): 597–602.

Rose L (1983): Understanding mental illness: The experience of families of psychiatric patients. *J Adv Nurs, 8*(6): 507–511.

Salariya E, Cater J (1984): Mother–child relationship—FIRST score. *J Adv Nurs, 9*(6): 589–595.

Saltzer E, Golden M (1985): Obesity in lower and middle socioeconomic status mothers and their children. *Res Nurs Health, 8*: 147–153.

Schroeder-Zwelling E, Hock E (1986): Maternal anxiety and sensitive mothering behavior in diabetic and nondiabetic women. *Res Nurs Health, 9*: 249–255.

Sexton D, Munro B (1985): Impact of a husband's chronic illness (COPD) on the spouse's life. *Res Nurs Health, 8*: 83–90.

Siebert K et al (1986): Nursing students' perceptions of a child: Influence of information on family structure. *J Adv Nurs, 11*: 333–337.

Silva M (1985): Comprehension of information for informed consent by spouses of surgical spouses. *Res Nurs Health, 8*: 117–124.

Smith L (1983): A conceptual model of families incorporating an adolescent mother and child into the household. *ANS*, 6(1): 45–60.

Sund K, Ostwald S (1985): Dual-earner families' stress levels and personal and life-style–related variables. *Nurs Res*, 34(6): 357–361.

Tilden V (1984): The relation of selected psychosocial variables to single status of adult women during pregnancy. *Nurs Res*, 33(2): 102–107.

Tilden V, Stewart B (1985): Problems in measuring reciprocity with difference scores. *West J Nurs Res*, 7(3): 381–398.

Toney L (1983): The effects of holding the newborn at delivery on paternal bonding. *Nurs Res*, 32(1): 16–19.

Tulman L (1986): Initial handling of newborn infants by vaginally and cesarean-delivered mothers. *Nurs Res*, 35(5): 296–300.

Tulman L (1985): Mothers' and unrelated persons' initial handling of newborn infants. *Nurs Res*, 34(4): 205–210.

Uphold C, Harper D (1986): Methodological issues in intergenerational family nursing research. *ANS*, 8(3): 38–49.

Uyer G (1986): Effect of nursing approach in understanding of physicians' directions, by the mothers of sick children in an out-patient clinic. *Int J Nurs Stud*, 23(1): 79–85.

Ventura J (1986): Parent coping: A replication. *Nurs Res*, 35(2): 77–80.

Walker L, Crain H, Thompson E (1986a): Maternal role attainment and identity in the postpartum period: Stability and change. *Nurs Res*, 35(2): 68–71.

Walker L, Crain H, Thompson E (1986b): Mothering behavior and maternal role attainment during the postpartum period. *Nurs Res*, 35(6): 352–355.

Weaver R, Cranley M (1983): An exploration of paternal-fetal attachment behavior. *Nurs Res*, 32(2): 68–72.

Williams P, Williams A, Dial M (1986): Children at risk: Perinatal events, developmental delays and the effects of a developmental stimulation program. *Int J Nurs Stud*, 23(1): 21–38.

Woods N (1985): Employment, family roles, and mental ill health in young married women. *Nurs Res*, 34(1): 4–10.

Appendix Breakdown of Substantive Citations

Author(s), Source, and Purpose	Phenomena Under Study/Sample	Design/Methods	Major Findings
Andrews C, Andrews E, *Nurs Res*, 1983. **Purpose:** Determine if maternal posturing would influence fetal position	Dyadic: Mother–Fetus/100 healthy, gravid women	Randomized clinical trial/Observation of clinical data	Four treatment postures effective for increasing anterior fetal rotations
Austin J, McBride A, Davis H, *Nurs Res*, 1983. **Purpose:** Determine the relationship between parental attitudes and adjustment to childhood epilepsy and seizure control	Dyadic: Mother–Child, Father–Child/50 parents: 33 mothers and 17 fathers (includes 16 couples)	Observational, Cross-Sectional/Standardized instrument, New instrument, Independent raters, Medical record	Attitude and adjustment positively related for mothers (p<.001); not significant for fathers. Perception of seizure control and parental attitudes accounts for 60% variance in mothers' adjustment
Bee et al, *Res Nurs Health*, 1986. **Purpose:** Explore effect of parental life change on children's mental and social development	Dyadic: Mother–Infant/193 primiparous mothers and infants	Observational, Longitudinal/Standardized instrument, Standardized observation, Interview	Significant negative correlations between maternal life change in 1st year and infant IQ and receptive language at four years. Subgroup analysis showed strongest correlations for mothers low in personal coping resources and social support.
Blank D, *Nurs Res*, 1986. **Purpose:** Explore early psychophysiologic mother–infant interaction using tenderness and anxiety theorems of HS Sullivan	Dyadic: Mother–Infant/65 healthy, postpartum mothers and their bottle-fed infants	Observational, Cross-Sectional/Standard instrument, New instrument, Clinical data	Maternal state–trait anxiety was related to infant glucose, cortisol, and formula consumption
Bramwell L, Whall A, *Nurs Res*, 1986. **Purpose:** Examine wives' anxiety in response to husband's 1st myocardial infarction, from perspective of perceptions and interpretation of their support roles	Dyadic: Marital/82 wives of patients (Canadian)	Observational, Longitudinal/Standard instrument, Interview, New instrument	Support role performance had direct negative effect on anxiety. Trait anxiety had direct positive effect on anxiety. Uncertainty was source of anxiety post-discharge

Source/Purpose	Focus/Sample	Design/Method	Findings
Brandt P, *Nurs Res*, 1984. **Purpose:** Determine relationship between social support, stress, and maternal discipline of 6 mo—3-yr-old child with developmental delay	Environment on Mother–Child dyad/91 mothers	Observational, Cross-Sectional/ Standardized instrument	Stress and support interaction variable showed trend in predicting restrictive discipline. For high-stress mothers, social support inversely related to restrictive discipline
Broom B, *Nurs Res*, 1984. **Purpose:** Determine anticipated and actual concerns re: marital relationship during period of transition to parenthood	Dyadic: Marital/22 couples expecting first child	Observational, Cross-Sectional/ New instrument	Only moderate levels of agreement on importance of concerns; low accuracy in estimating the importance of concern to spouse
Brown M, *Nurs Res*, 1986a. **Purpose:** Test a conceptually derived multidimensional formula of social support	Social support and pregnant couple/313 expectant couples, varied in age, SES, education	Observational, Cross-Sectional/ Standardized instrument	Data support unidimensional construct of social support
Brown M, *Nurs Res*, 1986b. **Purpose:** Determine relationship of social support and stress on expectant mothers and fathers	Dyadic: Marital, Marital to social support/313 expectant couples (see above)	Observational, Cross-Sectional/ Standardized instrument	Partner support most important variable to understanding expectant father health. Social support for mothers included larger domain and social networks contributed in same way as partner support. Stress and chronic illness explain more about health for expectant mothers than for the partners
Brumngraber L, *ANS*, 1986. **Purpose:** Examine the long-term effects of father-daughter incest	Dyadic: Father–Daughter/21 retrospective female victims of incest	Observational, Cross-Sectional/ Interview, Standardized instrument	Long-term effects described. Relationships with men and sexuality more adversely affected with time
Byers P, *Nurs Res*, 1986. **Purpose:** Describe the phenomenon of infant crying during aircraft descent	Dyadic: Mother–Infant/37 mother–infant pairs (on 16 non-stop flights)	Observational, Cross-Sectional/ Observation, Interview	A significant negative relationship was found between crying on descent and bottlefeeding. Only 18% of mothers attributed crying to ear pain in infant

Author/Source/Purpose	Sample	Method	Findings
Campbell J, *ANS*, 1986b. **Purpose:** Describe themes from survivor group for battered women	Dyadic: Women–Partners/Ongoing, open-group participants over 19 months (8/82–4/84)	Observational, Longitudinal/Content analysis from clinical care	Five themes emerged: feeling controlled by partner; damaged self-esteem; alternatives to end violence in relationship; decision-making process re leaving the batterer; and affirmation by other group members
Censullo M, Lester B, Hoffman J, *Nurs Res*, 1985. **Purpose:** Compare rhythmic patterning in preterm and term mother–infant interactions	Dyadic: Mother–Infant/30 mother–infant pairs: 15 term and 15 preterm	Observational, Cross-Sectional/Standardized observation	Rhythmic patterning found in dyadic interaction from birth in term infants and from 40 gestational weeks in preterms
Chao Y, *J Adv Nurs*, 1983. **Purpose:** Determine cognitive operations used by Chinese mothers in conceptual behavior toward newborns	Dyadic: Mother–Infant/20 mothers (Chinese)	Observational, Longitudinal/Participant observation	Orienting behavior more important than evaluating or delineating behaviors as mothers conceptualized infant body functions and physical state
Clinton J, *Nurs Res*, 1986. **Purpose:** Identify factors that predict health events experienced by expectant fathers	Father health in pregnancy/81 expectant fathers (515 repeated measures)	Observational, Longitudinal/Standardized instrument, New instrument	Six factors predicted expectant father health: affective involvement in pregnancy; number of previous children; income; ethnic identity; perceived stress; recent health
Cronenwett L, *Nurs Res*, 1985. **Purpose:** Determine differences between men and women in social network structure and support after birth of first child	Fathers-Social network; Mothers-Social network/108 subjects (54 couples) expecting first child in phase I; 100 subjects in phase II; 92 subjects in phase III; and 69 subjects in phase IV	Observational, Longitudinal/Standardized instrument, New instrument	More women than men reported an increased need for social support, no difference in satisfaction with available support. For men, network size decreased and qualities changed
Dixon M, *ANS*, 1986. **Purpose:** Describe differences between families of Black adolescents seeking mental health care (AC) and those who do not (ANC)	Family/52 adolescent clients and a parent; 52 adolescent nonclients and a parent	Observational, Cross-Sectional/Standardized instrument, Interview	Subcale comparison from FES revealed significant differences on 5 of 10 subscales: Cohesion, ANC>AC, $p<.05$; achievement orientation, ANC>AC, $p<.05$; intellectual cultural orientation,

Citation/Purpose	Focus/Sample	Design/Method	Results
			ANC>AC, p<.01; active recreational orientation, ANC>AC, p<.05; and conflict, ANC<AC, p<.01. Care-seeking families described themselves as using formal helpers more than non-client families
Duffy M, *Res Nurs Health*, 1986. **Purpose:** Describe the primary prevention behaviors of female-headed, one-parent families and barriers to accomplishment	Family: Alternate structure/59 females heading one-parent families	Observational, Longitudinal/ Card sort, Interview, Diary	Nutrition identified as most important to maintain health. Time greatest barrier. Relationship found between family ability to grow and change and primary prevention practices
Edwardson S, *Nurs Res*, 1983. **Purpose:** Explore decision-making process of MDs and parents in choosing between hospital and home for child dying of cancer	Parents–Health Care System/ Part I: records of 123 deceased patients; Part II 103 parents of 65 dying or deceased children	Longitudinal, Case Control/ Medical record, Interview, New instrument	Four factors were found to discriminate between home and hospital care: technical monitoring of the last week; time hospitalized; MD usual practice; and distance from treatment hospital
Ekberg J, Griffith N, Foxall M, *J Adv Nurs*, 1986. **Purpose:** Describe the features and contributors of spouse burnout in families with a chronically ill member	Dyadic: Marital/Based on earlier study of 30 chronically ill persons and their spouses	Not clear/Interview, Standardized instrument	Manifestations of spouse burnout, similar to those attributed to health care professionals was seen. Stages 1 and 2 symptoms (exhaustion and cynicism) were noted. No stage 3 behaviors seen (disgust and detachment)
Ellison E, *West J Nurs Res*, 1983. **Purpose:** Determine whether mother and child perspectives vary in concept of parental support	Dyadic: Mother–Child/101 mothers and their 7-to-8-year-old children	Observational, Cross-Sectional/ New instrument	Mothers overestimate amount of parent support provided to child. Mothers overestimate equally for sons and daughters
Fawcett J et al, *Nurs Res*, 1986. **Purpose:** Replicate study of relationship between spouses'	Father health in pregnancy; Dyadic: Marital/54 married couples	Observational, Longitudinal/ Standardized instrument, Perceived body space	Results not duplicated. Wives' body space reports changed; husbands' did not. No relation-

Citation / Purpose	Sample	Design / Method	Findings
strength of identification and similarities in pattern of body change components during and after pregnancy			ship between strength of identification and similarities in patterns of body change
Fawcett J, York R, *Nurs Res*, 1986. **Purpose:** Describe health of parents in early pregnancy, late pregnancy and in postpartum	Dyadic: Marital and health of mothers, health of fathers/70 married couples; 23 early pregnancy; 24 late pregnancy; 23 postpartum	Observational, Cross-Sectional/Standardized instrument, New instrument	Parents reported physical and psychological symptoms during pregnancy and postpartum. Women reported more symptoms than men. No differences in psychological symptoms of women across three times
Foxall M, Ekberg J, Griffith N, *West J Nurs Res*, 1985. **Purpose:** Determine adjustment patterns of chronically ill persons and spouses and factors contributing to their adjustment	Dyadic: Marital/30 married couples	Observational, Cross-Sectional/Standardized instrument	No difference between patient and spouse on overall adjustment. Patients and spouses with low adjustment scores were older women, married longer, and low income
Golas G, Parks P, *Res Nurs Health*, 1986. **Purpose:** Determine the effectiveness of teaching primiparous mothers about infant behavior	Dyadic: Mother–Infant/17 experimental mothers; 16 contrast mothers	True Experiment/New instrument	At four-week office visit, experimental mothers were more knowledgeable about infant behavior. No difference regarding maternal confidence in interpreting cues of own infant
Hayes V, Knox J, *J Adv Nurs*, 1984. **Purpose:** Determine parents' perceptions of their stress and parenting role when children are hospitalized with long-term disabilities	Parenting role/40 parents of 35 children (24 with cancer; 11 other long-term illnesses)	Interview and Constant comparative analysis	Parents made changes in role during hospitalization. Much stress attributed to disparity between health professionals understanding of parents' experience and parents' actual experience
Hentinen M, *J Adv Nurs*, 1983. **Purpose:** Determine the need for instruction and support in wives of myocardial infarction patients	Wife role/59 wives of myocardial infarction patients	Observational, Cross-Sectional/New questionnaire	Wives reported physical and emotional symptoms of stress. Wives needed information on home care of patient. Social support came from immediate family

Citation/Purpose	Sample/Design	Method	Findings
Hilbert G, *Nurs Res*, 1985. **Purpose:** Determine relationship between spouse support and compliance of myocardial infarction patients	Dyadic: Marital/60 couples	Observational, Cross-Sectional/ Standardized instrument	No relationship demonstrated
Hinds C, *J Adv Nurs*, 1985. **Purpose:** Determine the perceived needs of families who care for a member with cancer at home; describe how they cope with these needs and identify what resources they used	Family: 83 family members (43 males; 40 females) of cancer patients (Canadian)	Observational, Cross-Sectional/ Interview	Families needed help with physical care or patients. 31% coped poorly with this aspect. Families needed someone with whom they could discuss their fears
Hirshfeld M, *Int J Nurs Stud*, 1983. **Purpose:** Determine factors that contribute to home care versus institutionalization for family caregivers of elderly with senile dementia	Dyadic: Elder and Caregiver/30 demented elderly and 30 family caregivers	Observational, Cross-Sectional/ OARS, Focused interviews, Participant observation	Concept of mutuality emerged as crucial factor distinguishing those who continue home care versus institutionalization
Hurley P, *Nurs Res*, 1983. **Purpose:** Determine relationship of marital conflict stress to communication variables and voice analysis	Dyadic: Marital/68 middle-class couples	Observational, Cross-Sectional/ Simulations (IMC), Voice analysis (PSE)	Communication variables possibly related to stress. Investigator believes concept, as operationalized, represented problem-solving rather than marital conflict
Jones L, Lenz E, *Nurs Res*, 1986. **Purpose:** Identify predictors of paternal interaction behavior	Dyadic: Father–Infant/114 father–newborn pairs, 2 to 4 days after birth	Observational, Cross-Sectional/ Standardized instrument, Standardized observation, Video observation	Infant state was best predictor, especially for affection/comforting behavior. Infant orientation scores predicted touch/stimulating behavior. Parental competence predicted stimulating behavior

Citation/Purpose	Unit/Sample	Design/Method	Findings
Jones L, Parks P, *Res Nurs Health*, 1983. **Purpose:** Determine mother, father, and examiner reports of infant temperament	Dyadic: Mother–Child, Father–Child, Father–Mother, Examiner–Parents/19 mothers and fathers and 1-year-old infants	Observational, Cross-Sectional, Clinical observation, Standardized instrument	Positive relationship between mother and examiner and father and examiner reported scores. Fathers were sensitive to physical dimension of temperament; mothers to adaptive. Little relationship between father scores and mother scores
Keane S, Garralda M, Keen J, *Int J Nurs Stud*, 1986. **Purpose:** Determine how policy of parental admission during child's admission for acute medical illness was implemented, and assess parental response to policy	Dyadic: Parent–Child in hospital/34 resident parents compared to 23 from the visiting group	Observational, Longitudinal/Interview	Resident parents perceived child to be temperamentally vulnerable and in need of special reassurance and explanation
Knafl K, *West J Nurs Res*, 1985. **Purpose:** Determine how parents define and manage their situation during hospitalization of child; describe what parents see as impact of hospitalization on family life	Family/62 couples (parents) of hospitalized children (ages 5 to 12 years)	Observational, Longitudinal/Intensive interviews	Families defined hospitalization differently. Three management styles emerged: Alone style; some help style; and delegation style
Kviz F, Dawkins C, Ervin N, *Res Nurs Health*, 1985. **Purpose:** Determine relationship between mothers' health beliefs and use of well-baby services in poor, minority, high-risk population	Mother–Health Care System/61 Black mothers	Observational, Longitudinal (Cohort)/Medical record, Interview	Health beliefs of mothers not predictive of clinic visits. Health beliefs did account for 30% variance in number of immunizations at 6 months
Lenz E et al, *Res Nurs Health*, 1986. **Purpose:** Determine the extent to which life change after birth of baby and instrumental support of parenting predict occurrence of illness in mothers of 6-month-olds	Maternal health and social support/155 mothers of 6-month-old infants	Observational, Cross-Sectional/Interview, Standard instrument	Life change and intensity of support positively related to illness. Size of network was negatively related to illness. No evidence for buffering effect of support

Citation/Purpose	Sample	Design/Method	Findings
Lenz E et al, *ANS*, 1985, **Purpose:** Determine the relationship of sex-role attributes and gender to changes in intimacy and overall quality of marital relationship after birth of an infant	Dyadic: Marital/146 males and 147 females with healthy full-term infants; marital intimacy analysis based on 44 women and 52 men	Observational, Longitudinal/ Standardized instrument, New instrument	Positive changes in intimacy and overall relationship at delivery related to marital quality at 4 months. Only "femininity" predicted overall change in quality. None of the entered variables predicted intimacy
McBride A, *Res Nurs Health*, 1985. **Purpose:** Determine if young men and women think differently about parenting	Parenting role/136 college women and 136 college men	Observational, Cross-Sectional/ New instrument	Women more often report child as troubled. Men were more inclined to see failure as the child's fault, and see child as mean
McCance K et al, *Res Nurs Health*, 1985. **Purpose:** Test a preventative intervention to reduce coronary heart disease among first degree relatives of sudden death victims	Health behavior of 1st degree relations/58 1st degree relatives of sudden death victims (representing 19 families)	True Experiment/Standardized instrument, Blood pressure screening and/or serum cholesterol	Significant reductions in alcohol intake. No difference in health beliefs, except for sibling subgroup. More screening behaviors practiced in intervention group
Magyary D, *West J Nurs Res*, 1983. **Purpose:** Describe the interactive patterns that occur between mothers and their preterm infants	Dyadic: Mother–Preterm/16 mother–preterm infant dyads	Observational, Longitudinal/ Standardized observation	Mutual gaze was rare. Interaction characterized by social asynchrony. Infant age and social context significantly affect social synchrony, infant adaptation, and infant initiation
Majewski J, *Nurs Res*, 1986. **Purpose:** Determine relationships among employment status, role conflict, marital satisfaction, employment role attitude, and ease of transition to maternal role	Maternal role and Marital satisfaction/86 first-time mothers	Observational, Cross-Sectional/ Interview, Standardized instrument	No differences were seen between employed and unemployed mothers on role conflict. Mothers experiencing more role conflict experienced more difficulty in transition to maternal role. Marital satisfaction positively related to ease in transition to maternal role
Martinson I et al, *Res Nurs Health*, 1986. **Purpose:** Determine feasibility of home care for child dying of cancer	Dyadic: Parent–Child and health care system/Based on a study of 58 dying children cared for at home during a 2-year period	Observational, Longitudinal/ Medical records, New instrument, Interview	Of 58 children in home care, 79% died at home. Physicians would refer for this service. Parents were satisfied with care

Citation/Purpose	Sample	Method/Instruments	Findings
Mercer R, *Nurs Res*, 1985. **Purpose:** Delineate the process of maternal role attainment in three groups, over the first year	Maternal role/294 postpartum women: 66 15–19 years; 138 20–29 years; 90 30–42 years	Observational, Longitudinal/ Standardized instrument, Interview	Role attainment behaviors of feelings of love for baby, gratification in role, observed maternal behavior, self-reported ways of handling irritated child did not progress in linear pattern over year. Behaviors peaked at 4 mo, declined at 8 mo. No difference by maternal age
Mercer R, *West J Nurs Res*, 1986. **Purpose:** Determine whether age group differences influence maternal role attainment at 1 yr; identify major predictors of maternal role attainment at 1 yr postbirth	Maternal role/294 postpartum women; 242 of these were followed to one year (see above)	Observational, Longitudinal/ Standardized instrument, Interview	Mothers 20–29 years derived greater gratification in mothering role than those 30–39. Two older groups had significantly higher observed maternal behavior scores. The 30–39 group demonstrated higher scores on handling irritating child behavior. 38% variance accounted for, with self-concept accounting for 17%
Mercer R, *Res Nurs Health*, 1986. **Purpose:** Determine relationship between developmental differences in self-concept, personality integration, flexibility, empathy, temperament, and maternal behavior	Maternal role/288 mothers in three age groups: 60 15–19 years; 138 20–29 years; 90 30–42 years	Observational, Longitudinal/ Standardized instrument, Standardized rating	Personality integration and flexibility increased significantly and correlated with age, indicating both are developmental constructs. Two older groups' self-concepts decreased significantly in 1st 8 mo of motherhood. Correlates in each age group described
Mercer R,.Hackley K, Bostrom A, *Nurs Res*, 1985. **Purpose:** Determine which variables contribute to perception of birth experience	Maternal role/294 postpartum women: 66 15–19 years; 138 20–29 years; 90 30–42 years	Observational, Cross-Sectional/ Standardized instrument, Medical record, Interview	Mate emotional support contributed 20% of the variance. Early mother–child interaction contributed 9.8%. A total of 39% was accounted for.

Citation/Purpose	Sample	Design/Method	Results
Miles M. *Nurs Res*, 1985. **Purpose:** Compare emotional symptoms and physical health of parents whose child died suddenly to those whose child died following a chronic disease, to a comparison group	Parents/61 bereaved parents (13 fathers and 48 mothers); 31 experienced death of child by accident; 30 experienced death of child by chronic illness; 81 non-bereaved parents	Observational, Cross-Sectional/Standardized instrument	No differences between bereaved groups. Bereaved significantly different from non-bereaved
Mogan J, *Int J Nurs Stud*, 1986. **Purpose:** Determine relationship of mother-infant feeding behavior to development of obesity	Dyadic: Mother–Infant/78 healthy, primiparous couples and their newborns	Observational, Longitudinal/Observation, Medical record, Clinical data	No interaction differences seen between mother-infants in three groups: normal weight, overweight, and mixed. Infants of overweight parents weighed significantly more at 6 mos
Moore D, *Nurs Res*, 1983. **Purpose:** Compare marital satisfaction between couples engaging in two styles of childbirth preparation	Dyadic: Marital/105 couples after normal, vaginal delivery (70 Lamaze; 35 hospital class method)	Observational, Longitudinal Cohort/Standardized instrument	Husbands' satisfaction scores significantly increased after Lamaze classes
Perry S, *Nurs Res*, 1983. **Purpose:** Determine if parents' perception is related to infant behavior and if structured interaction of parent with infant positively influences parents' perception	Dyadic: Mother–Infant, Father–Infant, Parent–Infant/57 married couples and their newborn	True Experiment, Longitudinal/Standardized instrument	No relationship between infant behavior and parental perception. Structured interaction differentially affected mothers' perception at one week. Perceptions of mother and father became more congruent with time
Phillips L, *J Adv Nurs*, 1983. **Purpose:** Identify variables indicative of caregiver abuse of frail elderly, and generate empirical model to explain variance in abusive relationship	Dyadic: Elder–Caregiver/74 elderly: 44 in "good relationship" group; 30 in "abuse" group	Observational, Cross-Sectional/Standardized instrument, New instrument, Interview	Perception of caregiver and other family members in house to help accounted for 54% of variance
Phillips L, Rempusheski V, *ANS*, 1986. **Purpose:** Determine dynamics of good and poor quality caregiving for frail elders at home	Dyadic: Elder–Caregiver/39 family caregivers: 14 with "good" relationships; 25 with abusive relationships to patients	Observational, Cross-Sectional/Interview (Constant comparative analysis)	Five major constructs were identified for a 4-stage model. Proposed model for dynamics of family caregiving

Riesch S, *Res Nurs Health*, 1984. **Purpose:** Determine relationship between mothers' degree of occupational commitment and quality of mother-infant interaction	Dyadic: Mother–Infant and Mother–Work/50 mothers and infants	Observational, Longitudinal/ Standardized instrument	Positive, significant relationship between degree of occupational commitment and interaction at 34 wks gestation, but not at 6 weeks postpartum
Riesch S, Munns S, *Nurs Res*, 1984. **Purpose:** Test effectiveness of intervention to promote mother's awareness of infant behavior and her own behavior	Dyadic: Mother–Infant/108 mothers of term infants and 32 mothers of preterm infants	Quasi-Experiment/Standardized instrument, Standardized observation, Interview	Mothers of term and preterm infants in treatment groups reported more of own behavior than behavior of neonate. Their reports resembled those of trained raters more than did reports of controls
Roberts F, *Nurs Res*, 1983. **Purpose:** Determine effects of infant behavior on transition to parenthood	Dyadic: Mother–Infant, Father–Infant/64 couples pre- and post-delivery of first child	Observational, Longitudinal/ Standardized instrument, New instrument, Interview	Amount of obligatory infant behavior had an effect on ease of transition. Research model better supported with mothers' data than with fathers'. Fathers had easier transition and showed less change
Robinson C, Thorne S, *J Adv Nurs*, 1984. **Purpose:** Examine concept of family "interference" with health care for a sick member	Family/Not specified	Observational, Longitudinal/ Observation, Interview	Described stages of family involvement with health care system. Proposed interference as a characteristic behavior, with a purpose
Rose L, *J Adv Nurs*, 1983. **Purpose:** Determine process by which families develop an understanding of mental illness and treatment in a member	Family/7 families of patients hospitalized for first psychiatric admission	Observational, Longitudinal/ Interview (Constant comparative analysis)	Past experience, beliefs about mental illness and beliefs about own contribution to illness were influences on process
Saltzer E, Golden M, *Res Nurs Health*, 1985. **Purpose:** Determine the relationships between maternal obesity and child obesity, socioeconomic status, maternal knowledge of nutrition and maternal locus of control for weight loss	Dyadic: Mother–Child/144 children and mothers	Observational, Correlational/ Standardized instrument, Clinical observation	Lower socioeconomic status mothers were heavier, had less nutritional knowledge and were more external in locus of weight control. Trend for lower socioeconomic children to weigh more. Maternal-child weight correlated for low socioeconomic group

Citation / Purpose	Sample	Design / Method	Findings
Schroeder-Zwelling E, Hock E, *Res Nurs Health*, 1986. **Purpose:** Evaluate effects of high-risk pregnancy on development of maternal-infant relationship, differences in anxiety, sensitive maternal behavior, and maternal separation anxiety in diabetic and nondiabetic mothers	Dyadic: Mother–Infant/20 diabetic women and 20 nondiabetic women	Observational, Longitudinal/Standardized instrument, New instrument	No differences on anxiety, maternal separation anxiety, or sensitive maternal behavior
Sexton D, Monroe B, *Res Nurs Health*, 1985. **Purpose:** Determine impact of husband's chronic illness on spouse's life	Dyadic: Marital/76 married women: 46 wives of husbands with COPD; 30 wives of husbands with no chronic illness	Observational, Cross-Sectional/Standardized instrument	Wives of COPD patients reported higher subjective stress and lower life satisfaction than wives of men without chronic illness
Siebert K et al, *J Adv Nurs*, 1986. **Purpose:** Determine whether student nurses perceive children differently when given different information about family structure	Dyadic: Nurse–Family/68 undergraduate nursing students	Observational, Cross-Sectional/Standardized instrument, New instrument	Nurses viewed same excerpt of child behavior more favorably when they thought child to be from a two-parent family
Silva M, *Res Nurs Health*, 1985. **Purpose:** Assess adequacy of spouse comprehension of information for informed consent	Role of spouse/75 spouses of surgical patients	Observational, Cross-Sectional/New instrument	72 of 75 spouses had adequate comprehension of informed consent form. As finding was unexpected, investigator proposed explanation
Smith L, *ANS*, 1983. **Purpose:** Explore normative course of family development in families incorporating teen parent and infant into home	Family/18 families with an adolescent mother and child between 4 and 14 months old	Observational, Cross-Sectional/(Grounded theory)	Three behavioral styles seen in these families: Role-sharing, role-binding, and role-blocking
Sund K, Ostwald S, *Nurs Res*, 1985. **Purpose:** Determine relationship between personal and lifestyle related variables and family stress in dual career families	Parents/92 mother–father pairs	Observational, Cross-Sectional/Standardized instrument	The following were significantly related to family stress reports: parental and child age, income, satisfaction with income, satisfaction with child care, and flexibility in vacation scheduling

Reference / Purpose	Sample	Design/Method	Findings
Tilden V, *Nurs Res*, 1984. **Purpose:** Compare partnered to single women for psychosocial variables in pregnancy	Dyadic: Pregnant female–partner/116 partnered and 25 unpartnered pregnant women	Observational, Cross-Sectional/ Standardized instrument	Single women higher in life stress, lower in tangible support, and high in state anxiety. No difference on informational and emotional support, trait anxiety, depression, or self-esteem
Toney L, *Nurs Res*, 1983. **Purpose:** Determine effects of holding newborn at delivery on paternal bonding	Dyadic: Father–Infant/37 first time fathers	True Experiment/Standardized observation	No differences in paternal bonding as result of holding. Factors associated with bonding listed
Tulman L, *Nurs Res*, 1985. **Purpose:** Compare mothers, handling of newborns to handling by nursing students	Dyadic: Mother–Infant/36 newly delivered women and 36 female nursing students	Observational, Cross-Sectional/ Standardized observation	Differences seen in amount of handling, progression, and timing of handling behavior
Tulman L, *Nurs Res*, 1986. **Purpose:** Determine whether differences exist in patterns of newborn handling between vaginally and cesarean-delivered mothers	Dyadic: Mother–Infant/36 vaginally delivered women and 36 cesarean section-delivered women	Observational, Longitudinal/ Observation	Cesarean mothers handled infants less
Uyer G, *Int J Nurs Stud,* 1986. **Purpose:** Determine whether mothers of sick children can be helped to increase understanding of MD recommendations on treatment, care, and follow-up	Dyadic: Mother–Child and health care system/100 experimental and 100 contrast mothers who brought sick children to clinic	Quasi-Experiment/New instrument	Nursing care positively associated with better understanding in the experimental group
Ventura J, *Nurs Res*, 1986. **Purpose:** Determine relationship of father coping behaviors to infant temperament and parent responses: a replication	Dyadic: Father–Infant, Mother–Father/47 couples: mothers and fathers of 2- to 3-month-old infants	Observational, Cross-Sectional/ Standardized instrument	Mothers found more coping behaviors helpful than did fathers, including social support. Fathers report infants as more distressed to approach

Source/Purpose	Focus/Sample	Design/Method	Findings
Walker L, Crain H, Thompson E, *Nurs Res*, 1986a. **Purpose:** Stability and change were examined in maternal identity and maternal role attainment in postpartum	Maternal role/64 medically normal, middle-class primiparas and 58 multiparous women	Observational, Longitudinal/Standardized instrument	Mothers' attitudes of self became more positive over time. Mothers' attitudes toward baby became less positive
Walker L, Crain H, Thompson E, *Nurs Res*, 1986b. **Purpose:** Determine relationships among subjective and behavioral components of maternal role attainment in postpartum	Maternal role/64 primiparous and 68 multiparas	Observational, Longitudinal/Standardized instrument, Video observation	For primiparas, self-confidence was related to maternal feeding behavior, as were age, education, and socio-economic status. For multiparas only initial attitude toward self was related to maternal behavior
Weaver R, Cranley M, *Nurs Res*, 1983. **Purpose:** Examination of relationships between parental-fetal attachment and strength of marital relationship and expectant fathers' physical symptoms during pregnancy	Dyadic: Father–Infant/100 expectant fathers	Observational, Cross-Sectional/Standardized instrument	Paternal attachment positively related to strength of marital relationship. Positive weak relationship between symptoms and paternal attachment
Williams P, Williams A, Dial M, *Int J Nurs Stud*, 1986. **Purpose:** Report performance of children with high perinatal risk on restandardized Denver Development Screen in Philippines; based on findings, also reported results of nursing intervention aimed at preterm infants and mothers	Dyadic: Mother–Infant/ Part 1; 911 children in Philippines; Part 2: 34 preterm infants divided into experimental group (n = 19) and a control (n = 15)	Quasi-Experiment/Standardized observation, Clinical data	Perinatal events were risk factors for influencing development of Filipino children 2 weeks–6.5 years. Psychosocial performance of children significantly improved after nursing intervention. No differences seen in growth of child or maternal attachment between groups

Woods N, *Nurs Res*, 1985. **Purpose:** Determine relationship between employment, family roles, and mental health in young married women	Women's family roles/140 randomly selected married women	Observational, Cross-Sectional/ Standardized instrument, Interview	Complement of women's roles not associated with mental ill health. Mental health not related to employment or parenting. Poorer mental health seen in women with traditional sex role norms, little task sharing from spouse, and little support from a confidant

4

WHAT IS FAMILY NURSING?

Catherine L. Gilliss, RNC, DNSc

Brenda M. Roberts, RN, MS

Betty L. Highley, RN, MS, FAAN

Ida M. Martinson, RN, PhD, FAAN

Despite a long history of interest in the family, there is a scarcity of literature about the nature of family nursing. There is clinical subspecialty acknowledgment of the family as an important context to personalizing the care of family members, but many nurses consider the process of working with the family group *family therapy*. Unless they are psychiatric mental health specialists, they often feel unprepared to offer what they perceive as family therapy. This chapter explains the distinction between family nursing and family therapy, and reviews assumptions about the nature of interventions in family nursing.

Introduction

In Chapter 1 we presented evidence to support the position that the family group is an appropriate recipient of nursing care services. But what are those services and how are they different from other nursing services? In this chapter, family nursing will be described by reviewing several approaches to the health care of families and by reviewing our assumptions about the nature of interventions in family nursing.

The Family as a Unit of Care

The idea that the family is a unit of care in medicine has been controversial (Carmichael, 1983; Ransom, 1983; Schwenk, Hughes, 1983). The arguments against this position counter that the patient is the object of care. Carmichael (1983) has argued that treatment of the family would result in: (1) organizational problems, as the care offered is inextricably bound to the human body; (2) identification problems, that is, defining *who* is in the family; (3) the need for ethical consent for treatment; (4) support of the fantasy of the mythical nuclear family; (5) medicalization of the family and opposition to viewing the family as a resource to patients under care; and (6) the threat that family therapy would be co-opted as a medical specialty. Others suggest that, although family care is a valid concept, the empirical evidence does not exist to support the position that families would use services that are directed toward the family group (Schwenk, Hughes, 1983).

Those who would try to describe, in practical and operational terms, how the family is served as a client in family medicine fail. In contrast, Ransom (1983) suggests that the "family" in family medicine describes a new way of understanding the problem at hand and the many previously overlooked strategies for intervention. Expanding the perspectives of care providers and researchers to include the family group in the delivery of care may be among the most significant contributions made by advocates of the family as a unit of care.

A recent review of the literature (Whall, 1986) revealed that the family as the recipient of care has been identified as a focus of nursing care, beginning with the teaching of Florence Nightingale. Whall's valuable historical review documents the evolution of recognition of the family as the unit of care and identifies public health or district nursing as the first specialty area that designed its practice to focus on the family unit. A review of the American Nurses' Association Standards of Nursing Practice in other practice areas indicated a growing recognition of the significance of the family in health promotion and maintenance (Whall, 1986).

In describing nursing's scope of practice, the American Nurses' Association identifies the family as "the necessary unit of service" (ANA, 1980, p. 5). Although less controversy exists within nursing about the desirability of delivering nursing care to the family group, confusion exists about what this actually means. As suggested in Chapter 1, family nursing proposes to offer care to family groups and not merely to family members. This is a complex service to describe or operationalize in a health care system that is organized to deliver care to individuals. Family nursing does not eliminate the need to care for the members of a family; however, the family nurse attempts to deliver service to the family group while serving the individual family member. This is accomplished with some ease after the family nurse appreciates the powerful and complex interactions that occur within the family and among its members. The family nurse can then take advantage of influencing the individual member by influencing the family and vice versa.

There are more examples of individuals as recipients of care than there are of families as the unit of care. However, a growing number of examples reflect successful caregiving to a member of a family concurrent with the member's family unit. Early strides in family nursing were made in maternal–child nursing. In the preparation for childbirth, mother, father, and siblings are considered in the assessment, intervention, and evaluation phases of the nursing process. More recently, the father has also been included in "maternal–child" nursing care. Nurses recognize the need to facilitate attachment and are aware of the reorganization that occurs within the family unit with the entry of a new member. At the same time, they are able to focus, if need be, on an immediate individual need, such as neuromotor development of the newborn or mastitis in a nursing mother. However, although individual needs emerge and require attention, facilitating the strength and growth of the family unit remains an ongoing, first-order nursing care goal.

A family member with a terminal illness provides another example of a caregiving situation that is optimally met by family nursing. The increasing number of individuals opting to die at home indicates that this is a health and illness issue best approached on a family level rather than on an individual level. Such an approach recognizes the importance of interchange between and among family members (for completion of unfinished business, caregiving by family members, and so on) in this event. Therefore, not only are nurses competent caregivers to the terminally ill family member, they also direct their interventions to all family members and may, in fact, continue with caregiving activities for family members after the ill member is deceased. Again, the goal is to develop the integrity and strength of the family unit in the event of loss of a member.

Birth and death provide examples that nicely illustrate family nursing. Chronic illness is a health issue that is ongoing, and although more difficult to explicate because of the expanded time frame, it is, nevertheless, a situation in which the family unit needs to be the focus for caregiving. The impact of chronic illness is covered in several subsequent chapters (See Section IV). For now, it is important to point out some of the challenges presented by chronic illness.

First, special attention is required by the nurse in timing interventions. Increased sensitivity is needed by the nurse to know when services need to be provided. Though the family will have needs, their occurrences may not exist throughout the course of a chronic illness. Second, inclusion of family members in caregiving activities may not be as "automatic" as with childbirth or in situations where the identified patient is not as obviously dependent on other family members for care. In chronic illness, the nurse must intentionally and methodically plan for the inclusion of other family members in caregiving activities and permit this involvement to change over time. Designed interventions for spousal support during recovery from cardiac surgery and a program specifically designed for healthy siblings of children with cancer are two examples of caregiving activities targeted at maintaining the integrity of the family unit. Such interventions would not exclude nursing measures directed toward specific needs of the chronically ill family member; however, a family nurse is able to recognize when such services are not sufficient to meet the needs of the family unit.

Settings for Family Care

Settings for family care vary from clinic, to hospital, to home. Although we believe family nursing can be provided in all settings, changes may be needed in the traditional care settings to enable the inclusion of the family in the caregiving process. For example, in the clinic, a member of the family frequently may accompany the patient. In the pediatric clinic, the mother is the family member most commonly present with the child during the visit. This is true even in the pediatric oncology clinic when the disease the child has is life threatening. In contrast to this typical American practice, in one case in a hospital clinic in China, both parents were present for the routine follow-up of a child with a brain tumor. When the parents were asked if they both routinely came, the answer was, "Why of course. This is our only child, and we both are excused from our jobs for any necessary medical checkups." This example illustrates that policy outside the caregiving institution (parental leave policy) as well as within it, is requisite for enabling the inclusion of family members in care. Another consideration for family care in clinic settings is recognizing opportunities for and establishing such services as educational programs and support groups.

The hospital as a setting for family involvement is addressed quite extensively in Chapter 17 on the family in the hospital and in Chapter 16 on children in the hospital setting. Special hospital units where more attention should be given to family needs include the emergency room, where the family is often not acknowledged; the intensive care unit, where family visits are limited to five minutes per hour; and waiting rooms for families who have a member in surgery and recovery. All members of the family unit, not only the member experiencing medical treatment, need to be considered as recipients of care in these acute care settings.

The home would seem the easiest site in which to provide family care because the family members are already present. Research conducted on the feasibility of home care for the dying child (Martinson et al, 1978) revealed that in providing family care, the nurse focused not only on the dying child but also on the parents, siblings, and, frequently, other family members such as grandparents and aunts. Assessment of these family members in terms of their roles in provision of care and their influence in family decision-making regarding health care was

found to be a critical variable. Neighbors, too, were involved in family caregiving activities. In one case, the neighbors called the nurse for assistance. They thought the parents were requesting that they make the coffin for the dying child, and the neighbors felt they could not do this. At the nurse's next contact with the parents, discussion of funeral arrangements, including the coffin, took place. The father was, in fact, making the coffin himself. He wished very much to do so and had only shared this news with the neighbors so as to elicit support and understanding in the use of a homemade coffin. The nurse informed the neighbors, which greatly relieved them. They understood the father's desire to make the coffin as his last act of love for his child.

Models of Family Care

Though many have advocated the considerate treatment of the family as a client, few have tried to describe how this might be accomplished and particularly how this is distinct from family therapy. In nursing, the majority of family nursing texts have approached the family theoretically, trying to explain the family as a sociobehavioral unit (Clements, Roberts, 1983; Friedman, 1986; Miller, Janosik, 1980; Hymovich, Barnard, 1979). These texts have been successful in presenting sets of assumptions and models of how to view families (as systems, developmentally, or structurally, for example). Nurses have used assumptions of theoretic models to identify parameters of individual and family behavior. It has logically followed that nurses have directed their activities toward assessment of behaviors identified in theoretic models. Friedman (1986) has included clear examples of family behavior to enable interventionists to recognize the significant behaviors described. Of interest is the observation made by Whall (1986) that nurse theorists have tended to increase the focus on family as they have continued the exposition and development of their models. As described in Chapters 2 and 3, the use of theoretical frameworks and family research instrumentation has provided opportunity for advances in assessment and has enabled nurses to amass considerable data about family members and, to a lesser extent, families. The translation of such assessment into family nursing interventions is the next logical step but is more difficult to explicate. However, *Families at Risk: Primary Prevention in Nursing Practice* (Leavitt, 1982) and *Nurses and Families: A Guide to Family Assessment and Intervention* (Wright, Leahey, 1984) are exceptions. In these texts, the nurse authors have provided specific clinical suggestions for working with the family. All psychiatric nurses, they have clearly detailed care that is not limited to any particular clinical population. Further elucidation of models of care is needed in the nursing literature. Several models are described in this chapter to stimulate and challenge the reader to revise these and describe others.

Family Primary Care

Health professionals in family primary care have struggled publicly to evolve a description of how to care for the family as a unit in the current health system. A popular strategy for collaboration in family care has been to include a behavioral scientist on the health care team. The role of the behavioral scientist includes training others about the family and conducting family therapy sessions when necessary. This collaborative model is described in the writings of Doherty (1985) and of Baird and Doherty (1986), who propose a series of levels of physician involvement when caring for families. Five levels of physician involvement with families are described.

Level 1 (minimal emphasis on the family) involves contacting the families only when necessary for practical or legal reasons. No special skills or knowledge base need be developed for this level of involvement, which is assumed to be the level for which most physicians are prepared.

Level 2 (ongoing medical information and advice) is accomplished through more regular contact with family members for the purpose of answering questions and advising them on care management. Additionally, gross dysfunction is recognized and appropriately referred to a therapist. Knowledge of the triangular relationship* between physician, family, and client prepares the physician, who must also have the personal skill to openly engage the family.

Level 3 (feelings and support) involvement is based on knowledge about normal family development and reactions to stress. The physician engages the family in discussion of their feelings and reactions and encourages them in their coping efforts. Based on an assessment of the family's level of functioning, the medical advice is personalized to the needs and abilities of the family. When dysfunction is recognized, the physician is able to make a referral recommendation.

Level 4 (systematic assessment and planned intervention) involvement is based on an understanding of family systems and an awareness of the physician's own family system as well as on the macrosystems in which the family and physician interact. The skills necessary for such involvement are more sophisticated and include (1) planning and structuring family conferences; (2) assessing the functioning of the family; (3) supporting individual members without forming alliances; (4) redefining situations to pro-

---

*Triangular relationships are those in which a third party has been involved to stabilize tensions that exist within a dyadic relationship. The third person serves as a distraction from the instability and anxiety based in the dyad. This is commonly seen in families, for instance, when unhappy couples present their acting out teenagers. The triangle can exist when two parties are distracted by a loaded issue. Often health care providers find themselves positioned between family members or between the family and an issue.

mote identification of solutions to problems; (5) helping family members work together to generate new solutions acceptable to all; (6) identifying dysfunction that requires referral; and (7) preparing both family and therapist for their work together.

Finally, *Level 5 (family therapy)* involvement requires a knowledge of family systems and patterns of dysfunctional interaction. In an effort to effect change in these families, several key skills must be developed. These abilities include interviewing and engaging difficult family members who make other members anxious or support one member against another; systematically re-evaluating the family's difficulties and patterns; creatively dealing with the family's resistance to change; and collaborating with other professionals who are involved in the family's care, even when these relationships are conflicted.

The levels proposed in this model are organized around the development of the physician-learner. As such, the proposed organization is especially helpful for structuring a curriculum or learning experiences. For use in nursing education, the major adaptation required is the starting point. Based on current recommendations for essential baccalaureate curriculum content (AACN, 1986), the baccalaureate graduate would be expected to systematically assess families; identify their structure, development, communication and decision-making patterns; and recognize and refer dysfunctional families. These skills would prepare a professional nurse for Level 3 involvement (feelings and support) as a point of entry to nursing practice. This is an important distinction between the two professions and may suggest why nurses seem to have even more difficulty in distinguishing the focus on family care from family therapy. Minimum expectation is that the nurse will have family skills at entry level. However, there are advanced nursing skills in family care that are *not* family therapy. Advanced nursing practice with families has been elusive, but its elucidation is one purpose of this text.

Because this model is oriented to the development and skills of the provider, it does not elucidate the nature of the intervention required for families in response to general, predictable types of experiences that all families face.

Levels of Prevention as Applied to Family Care

The levels of application of preventive measures are not new to students of maternal–child or community nursing. Developed in the writings of Leavell et al (1965) on preventive medicine and in the works of Caplan (1964) on individual and community mental health, there are three levels for application of preventive measures: primary, secondary, and tertiary prevention. *Primary prevention* measures are those that promote health by developing well-being and by reducing risk of a problem before that problem occurs. *Secondary prevention* is accomplished by early identification and treatment of problems. Additionally, further disability is prevented. Finally, *tertiary prevention* involves rehabilitation by educating the affected client(s) to learn new ways to maximize use of their capacities.

Though usually discussed as strategies for delivering care to individuals or communities, the levels of prevention framework can easily be applied to families in the delivery of nursing care. However, sometimes when family nurses use this approach, they slip into descriptions of the care of family members. When the family is the unit of care, a new description of care emerges.

Primary prevention of family problems occurs through identification of families at risk. These may be families who are undergoing transitions in the family life cycle, such as families adding members or otherwise changing their routines because of the growth of their members. Though families are often less accessible to nurses during these expected transitions, the predictability of risk is known. Therefore, nurses need to try to access these families at times of predictable risk. Much of nursing practice involves educating families in anticipation of the next developmental hurdle. Generally, risk reduction is accomplished through educating families and through raising their awareness of personal and family strengths and community resources.

Secondary prevention techniques are needed after a family problem has developed, and prompt identification and treatment are required. For instance, the astute family clinician will recognize difficulty in decision-making about where to put father after his stroke and will engage the family in discussion about their feelings and fears. The school nurse will note that first-grader Sarah does not want to come to school and will confer with Sarah's parents and determine their level of comfort with her entry into school. The staff nurse on the cardiovascular floor will watch Mrs. Jacobs, who is unwilling to take breaks for rest or nourishment, as she hovers over Mr. Jacobs after his coronary bypass surgery. The nurse will engage Mrs. Jacobs in discussions about her feelings of helplessness and fear, offering support at this difficult time and perspective on how long it will last. Further, the nurse will attempt to include Mrs. Jacobs in her husband's care in ways that allow Mrs. Jacobs to see his gradual improvement and prepare her to care for him at home after discharge. The strategies of secondary prevention often include providing information about an event and how others have responded to it, validating the individual's or family's right to feel as they do, and assisting them to mobilize resources that they have and to obtain those they need.

Tertiary prevention is accomplished by teaching families new ways to behave, so as to maximize their resources after the development of a problem. The intervention is targeted at helping families to change. Depending on the degree of change necessary, the complexity and

dysfunction of the family, and the skill level of the nurse, helping the family to make such changes may require the help of someone with more specialized skills, such as a family therapist.

The family nurse works to strengthen family health and effect change, largely through education and encouragement. A distinction that may be helpful when evaluating whether the family need for change requires family nursing or family therapy is to evaluate whether the family needs to change in order to persist as they are or to evolve to a new level of functioning. Family nursing is helpful with the former; family therapy is helpful with the latter.

Watzlawick, Weakland, and Fisch (1974) described two types of change: first-order and second-order change. *First-order changes* are those that occur within a given system that do not change the system but help it to persist unchanged. In contrast, *second-order changes* do result in change of the system. In family nursing, first-order changes are exemplified by the nurse working with new parents to prepare them for life with a baby. Though the couple had enjoyed a fulfilling relationship prior to the arrival of this wanted first child, they had begun to argue about responsibilities for childcare. By helping them to anticipate the child's needs, locate community childcare resources, and discuss the demands on them to fulfill the new roles of parent, the nurse promotes continuation of the relationship patterns established earlier by the couple. No dramatic change of the system was required; rather, some adjustments within the system were made. Second-order changes are more complex to orchestrate and are best referred to family therapists. When it appears that the family cannot be healthy or even stable without changing complex and dysfunctional behavior patterns, the family nurse should refer the family to a therapist.

Some problems are self-limiting. This is true of both individual and family problems. An individual may suffer from the flu for five days without sequelae, and a family may muddle through a stressful, disorganizing experience after the birth of a first child. However, just as the flu can develop into bronchitis, the familial distress related to childbearing can result in the development of dysfunctional patterns of family interaction that may eventually cause considerable stress or even divorce. Our renewed interest in family nursing is based on our belief that early intervention can make a difference to subsequent family health and that we can strengthen the family through early intervention. However, a word of caution is due here. Just as all individuals and all communities do not always achieve health, neither will all families. Involving the family members or treating a family as a unit is not a guarantee that health will be attained for the family or for its members.

The Nature of Interventions in Family Nursing

Models commonly used in the study and care of the family were reviewed in Chapter 2. Specific interventions are usually directed by the theoretical model in use. For instance, in interaction approaches, communication patterns become important. In developmental approaches, education and resource supplementation are key. In systems intervention, the patterns of reinforcement are significant targets. We believe, however, that there are some characteristic features that continuously reappear in the care and study of families in nursing, regardless of the theoretical model in use. These features are described below.

1. Family care is concerned with the experience of the family over time. In that sense, it is considerate of the history and future of the family group.
2. Family nursing is considerate of the community and cultural context of the family group. To that end, efforts are made to facilitate the transaction between the family and community. Community resources are located for the family's use. The family is, in turn, encouraged to contribute resources back to the community through work, play, and social exchange.
3. Family nursing is considerate of the relationships between and among family members and recognizes that in some instances all individuals and the family group will not achieve maximum health simultaneously.
4. Family nursing is directed at families whose members are both healthy and ill. The degree of individual health or illness is not a reliable index of family health.
5. Family nursing is often offered in settings where individuals present problems of physiologic or psychologic distress. However, although family nurses must be competent in the care and treatment of the health problems of individual family members, they must also recognize the relationship of these problems to the health of the family group.
6. The family system is influenced by any change in its members; therefore, when caring for individuals in health and illness, the nurse must elect whether or not to attend to the family. The nature of families and their members is so intertwined that both will be affected by nursing care. Some nurses may be frightened of what they do not understand about the family and may choose to focus on the individual patient. This may prevent them from seeing the impact of their interventions on the family group.
7. Family nursing requires that the nurse manipulate the environment to increase the likelihood of family interaction; however, the absence of family members does not preclude the nurse from offering family care.

8. The family nurse recognizes that the most symptomatic person in a family may change over time. Accordingly, the obvious focus on the nurse's attention may change over time. Despite this, the family nurse assesses the impact of these symptoms on the family, understanding that they are data about the family.

9. Family nursing focuses on the strengths of individual family members and the family group to promote their mutual support and growth where possible.

10. Family nursing requires the nurse to define family. We define the *family* as a group of two or more individuals usually living in close geographic proximity; having close emotional bonds; and meeting affectional, socioeconomic, sexual, and socialization needs of the family group and/or the wider social systems.

Summary

Nursing care is appropriately directed toward the family group; however, few nurses have been formally prepared to understand the family in this way. Few models of family care have proposed specific ways through which the nurse might influence the family. In addition to proposing one model of family nursing, this chapter has described characteristics that are distinctive to family nursing.

Issues for Further Investigation

1. How do parameters of health behavior differ when nursing care is focused on the family unit versus individual members?

2. What models/systems of care are most effective in facilitating delivery of care to family units?

3. What organizational/administrative changes need to be made to facilitate delivery of family care?

4. Within given patient populations (such as children or adults with heart disease, children or adults with diabetes, or families with critically ill neonates), what are typical first- and second-order changes in family systems?

5. What family nursing strategies are effective in responding to and facilitating change?

References

American Association of Colleges of Nursing (1986): Essentials of college and university education for professional nursing: Final report. Washington, DC: AACN.

American Nurses' Association (1980): Nursing: A social policy statement. Kansas City, MO: ANA.

Baird M, Doherty W (1986): Family resources in coping with serious illness. In: *Family Resources: The Hidden Partner in Family Therapy*. Karpel M (ed.). New York: Guilford, pp. 359–383.

Caplan G (1964): *Principles of Preventive Psychiatry*. New York: Basic Books.

Carmichael L (1983): Forty families—A search for the family in family medicine. *Fam Syst Med, 1*(1): 12–16.

Clements I, Roberts F (eds.) (1983): *Family Health: A Theoretical Approach to Nursing Care*. New York: Wiley.

Doherty W (1985): Family intervention in health care. *Fam Relations, 34:* 129–137.

Friedman M (1986): *Family Nursing*, 2nd ed. East Norwalk, CT: Appleton & Lange.

Hymovich D, Barnard M (eds.) (1979): *Family Health Care: Vol 1, Clinical Perspectives*. New York: McGraw-Hill.

Hymovich D, Barnard M (eds.) (1979): *Family Health Care: Vol 2, Developmental and Situational Crises*. New York: McGraw-Hill.

Leavell H et al (1965): *Preventive Medicine for the Doctor in his Community: An Epidemiological Approach*, 3rd ed. New York: McGraw-Hill.

Leavitt M (1982): *Families at Risk: Primary Prevention in Nursing Practice*. Boston: Little, Brown.

Martinson I et al (1978, February): Facilitating home care for children dying of cancer. *Cancer Nurs*, 41–45.

Miller J, Janosik E (1980): *Family-Focused Care*. New York: McGraw-Hill.

Ransom D (1983): On why it is useful to say that "The family is a unit of care" in family medicine: Comment on Carmichael's essay. *Fam Syst Med*, 1(1): 17–22.

Schwenk T, Hughes C (1983): The family as patient in family medicine: Rhetoric or reality? *Soc Sci Med*, 17: 1–17.

Waltzlawick P, Weakland J, Fisch R (1974): *Change: Principles of Problem Formulation and Problem Resolution*. New York: Norton.

Whall A (1986): The family as the unit of care: A historical review. *Public Health Nurs*, 3(4): 240–249.

Wright L, Leahey M (1984): *Nurses and Families: A Guide to Assessment and Intervention*. Philadelphia: Davis.

FACTORS INFLUENCING FAMILY HEALTH

5

HEALTHY FAMILIES

Forms and Processes

Madeline W. Gershwin, RN, MA, MFCC

Janet M. Nilsen, RN, MHS, MA

The image of the family has changed in recent years; new family structures are commonplace today. Social acceptance of alternative lifestyles as well as integration of ethnic groups has changed our image of the "normal" family. A healthy family must now be recognized by the patterns and processes of its daily life. This chapter describes the variety of family forms and the processes by which we recognize health in families.

Madeline Gershwin is Assistant Clinical Professor at the University of California at San Diego School of Medicine (Department of Community and Family Medicine). A certified Marriage, Family, and Child Counselor, she combines private practice with responsibilities as coordinator of the psychosocial curriculum for the University of California at San Francisco and San Diego Intercampus Graduate Studies program in family primary care and nurse mid-wifery.

Janet Nilsen, Assistant Clinical Professor at the University of California at San Francisco School of Nursing (Department of Family Health Care Nursing), is a Family Nurse Practitioner with masters degrees in both health services and clinical psychology. Her teaching and practice combine her expertise in primary care, psychology, and holistic health.

Introduction

The word *family* is most commonly associated with the idealized image of the traditional nuclear family model consisting of parents and children with the extended array of grandparents, aunts, uncles, and cousins. Further, our notions of normal and healthy have been based in large measure on traditional role orientations of father-breadwinner, mother-housewife. In fact, it is estimated that by 1990 only 14% of American families will fit into these prescribed roles ("On the Home Front," 1986). There are significant social trends affecting the structure and function of the family (see Chapter 10), and it is likely that such trends will continue for years to come.

This chapter will describe some of the current family trends, examine family functions, and review both individual and family developmental cycles as they relate to healthy development. Recent research on family health will be examined, followed by a discussion of alternate family forms. Finally, family nursing assessment will be discussed to aid the nurse in determining family health and family strengths.

Today's Family

Walsh (1982) and Glick (1984) have observed several trends that have significantly altered the more traditional family patterns: (1) an increase in divorce; (2) an increase in mothers working outside the home; (3) a lower birth rate coupled with higher life expectancy; (4) later marriages and childbearing; and (5) an increase in the number of adults choosing to remain single. The statistics that give evidence to these changes in social trends are impressive. Although there seems to be some variation in numbers cited, the overall direction is clear.

- Nearly one-half of all marriages in the 1980s will end in divorce (McCubbin, Dahl, 1985)
- One in every three marriages is a remarriage (McCubbin, Dahl, 1985)
- One in five families with children is maintained by one parent, usually the mother (Norton, Glick, 1986)
- From 1970 to 1984 the number of one-parent families more than doubled (Norton, Glick, 1986)
- 45% of children born in the 1980s will experience the divorce of their parents before they are 18 (Rubin, 1986)
- More than 35 million adults are stepparents (Rubin, 1986)
- More than 50% of all mothers with school-age children work outside the home (Walsh, 1982)
- More than 40% of mothers with younger than school-age children work outside the home (Walsh, 1982)
- The number of couples cohabiting nearly doubled from 1970 to 1980 and represent 2.3% of all couple households (this includes gay and lesbian and elderly couples) (McCubbin, Dahl, 1985, p. 118)
- Adults living alone account for about 25% of all households and are predominantly women age 45 or older (Glick, 1984)
- There will be more than 31 million Americans (16% of the population) over the age of 65 by the year 2000 (McCubbin, Dahl, 1985)

In addition to the trends that reflect shifts in family structure derived from the nuclear family (divorced, single parent, and remarriage or stepfamilies), other alternate family forms are becoming more common. A larger percentage of the population is choosing to remain single, and many of those who remain single choose to raise children (either adopted or biologic). In some communities, gay and lesbian couples are choosing to raise children. Another trend (Glick, 1984) reflects a dramatic increase from one-half million in 1970 to nearly two million in 1983 in households composed of unmarried couples who are delaying marriage. Most of these couples are delaying childbearing as well.

At the other end of the age spectrum, it is speculated that "by 2020 every fourth American could be over 65 years old" (Dychtwald, 1986). An increase in life expectancy makes it likely that multiple generations will have to accommodate shifting role relationships. In fact, the likelihood of having elderly members in any given kinship network is greater today than ever before in history (Dychtwald, 1986). Ironically, parents and children can grow old together.

We are confronted with more options to family life than ever before, and coupled with these structural changes are economic, social, and environmental factors that affect family life. For instance, families today face financial hardship in lower socioeconomic groups and in single parent families, placing the focus of energy on basic survival, thus diminishing the available energy for relational needs. In middle and upper income families, the commitment to a broad spectrum of activities outside the home likewise decreases the amount of time spent in addressing relational and communication issues.

Another consideration in examining the diversity of family forms is the multitude of ethnic and cultural variations observed in the United States. Galvin (1986) reports that a 1984 analysis of voting age Americans revealed 28.6 million Blacks, 6.5 million Mexican-Americans, more than 3 million other Hispanics, 2.5 million Asians, and 1.8 million Native Americans. Naisbitt (1982) notes that, "We have moved from the myth of the melting pot to a celebration of cultural diversity," and he further suggests that, "We will be transformed into a bilingual country before the end of the century." This idea is easily conceived when we consider the influx of Hispanic immigrants, their increasing birthrate, and their considerable cultural pride. Even more recent is the impact on American family life of growing numbers of Asian and Middle Eastern immigrants. These groups bring with them very powerful family traditions and heritages that are maintained across generations and are often quite different than those most familiar to western culture.

Functions of the Family

Historically the family served five major functions (Curren, 1983): (1) achieve economic survival; (2) provide protection; (3) pass on values and religion; (4) educate the young; and (5) confer status. As social institutions have taken on many of these functions, the family of today primarily is expected to provide for the relational needs of its members. Some of these needs include love, intimacy, self-acceptance, nurturing, caring, individuation, to give and be given to, to share the joys of posterity, and to have support through adversity. Satir (1972), eternally optimistic about the role of family life, describes the family unit as a "people-making factory." This simple phrase conveys a depth of meaning and implies that it is within the crucible of the family that the foundation of personhood is laid. Satir's early work with families focused heavily on the meeting of relational needs.

Given the dramatic shifts in family structure and function, what are the characteristics in families of today that address these relational and affective needs? What traits or patterns characterize those families that produce stable, adaptive, and contributing members of society? If healthy families today are expected to produce healthy adults, perhaps it would be useful to review current thinking on what basic essentials are needed in childhood to provide for successful adulthood and then successful family life. From there it will be possible to examine what kinds of family interactional patterns support this development and then to examine the impact of environmental, social, and cultural influences.

Individual and Family Development

Children

From the outset, a child has to accomplish specific developmental tasks in order to succeed in growth and development. Mahler (1973), an object relations theorist, details very specifically the psychologic development in the first three years of life. Her conclusions suggest that this is the critical time for the development of an ability to separate and individuate and identify a sense of self. The parental ability to deal effectively with this key stage of development is crucial for the subsequent healthy development of the child. Mahler believes that it is in these early stages that the seeds for major psychologic dysfunction are sown if the child is unable to individuate or develop a sense of self.

Broader stages of development and the key issues to be mastered have been well described by Erikson (1963). Six major psychologic tasks of childhood are defined, which parallel the child's growing physical and mental mastery. Each child in a family is progressing in his or her development at different stages and rates, and the ability of the parents to understand the process and function as satisfactory parents can greatly enhance or retard a child's development. Characteristics of healthy children shift with the demands for adaptation imposed by new developmental phases. In addition, each ethnic group may respond to these stages with its own interpretations and behaviors.

Parents

Superimposed on the child's developmental needs are the developmental needs of his or her caregivers. Depending on the age of the parent(s), adult life cycle issues are also at play. Several authors (Sheehy, 1974; Gould, 1978; Colarusso, Nemiroff, 1981; Levinson, 1978) have outlined specifically the stages of adult develop-ment. Each primarily addresses decades from the 20's to the 60's and the development of intimacy and love; relationship to one's body; reactions to time and death; relationship to children and parents; work; play; finances; relationship to society; and mentor relationships. Each decade involves a shifting perspective and progression to a new relationship within these key areas of life.

Healthy Couples

To complicate matters further, the marital couple and family as a whole progress through their own developmental stages, with issues that require change and adaptation at each stage.

Because the basic foundational unit of a family begins with the couple, let us examine the attributes of a healthy couple. Beavers (1985) believes that the quality of the couple's relationship is a critical factor in the quality of family functioning. He states that the following beliefs are associated with healthy couples:

1. Truth is relative rather than absolute, and reality is subjective. These couples believe that people are limited and finite, and each never possesses the absolute truth. All human computing is subject to error, and honest differences exist between people. In contrast, dysfunctional partners believe that truth is absolute and knowable.

2. Family members' motives are basically neutral or benign. Healthy couples believe that those close to you are basically good. This allows people in the family to err or disagree without the threat of abandonment. Accompanied with this is a respect for ambivalence, a characteristic that is not tolerated in dysfunctional couples. Unhealthy couples also tend to see willfulness, anger, and sexuality as expressions of malevolence in family members and attempt to use control and discipline to deal with them.

3. Human encounters are rewarding. With a respect for uncertainty and a belief that family members are good comes a healthy climate of trust and cooperation. The couple has a sense of optimism and hope and believes that human encounters are generally rewarding.

4. Four basic assumptions: (a) an individual needs a group; (b) causes and effects are interchangeable; (c) any behavior is the result of many variables rather than a single cause; and (d) a social role of absolute power or helplessness prohibits many of the needed satisfactions found in human encounters. This is a systems point of view.

5. There is meaning to human enterprise. A healthy couple shares a sense of purpose that goes beyond the family unit. This may be provided by religion or involvement in a cause such as protecting the environment or preventing nuclear proliferation. A belief that directs energy and provides a community outside the family is vital to healthy couple functioning.

In Beavers's (1985) observations of healthy couples, the following behavior patterns were found: (1) a modest overt power difference; (2) the capacity for clear boundaries; (3) operating mainly in the present; (4) respect for individual choice; (5) skill in negotiating; and (6) sharing positive feelings (p. 69).

The couples studied by Beavers et al represented a white middle- to upper-class group of people, so these behaviors cannot be assumed to translate to other family groups, structures, or cultures. Further study with non-white, non-Anglo, and nontraditional families is needed.

Stinnett, Carter, and Montgomery (1972) found in their study of 408 older couples that companionship and the ability to express true feelings to each other were the most rewarding aspects of their relationships. Also important were respect, love, and sharing common interests. Problems cited were poor health, housing, and financial difficulties. In any case, successful

establishment of a couple relationship represents the first stage of the family life cycle.

Family Life Cycle

The life cycle of the family, as with the individual, consists of a series of periods characterized by states of movement or change and quiescence or stability. The times of change represent an instability in the structure, no matter what its form. Throughout family life, milestones of individual development serve as normative events for the whole system. Births, deaths, entering school, beginning careers, launching, and retiring are examples of normative events. Different cultures may mark developmental transitions very specifically, thus highlighting their importance to the family (for example, Bar Mitzvah, Quincieniera). Additionally, there are events that occur frequently, though not universally, that affect the family unit. These are generated by conflict, illness, or external circumstances and are called paranormative (Carter, McGoldrick, 1980). Stillbirth, natural disaster, disability, and divorce are examples of paranormative events. Many such illness-related events are discussed in later chapters.

The establishment of a couple relationship represents the first stage of the family life cycle (Carter, McGoldrick, 1980; Duvall, 1977). The addition of children, the stages of growth and development of children, the leaving home of children, retirement, and later years all represent major transitional points in family life. At each stage, various tasks and issues that require negotiation and resolution emerge for the family and the individuals (Table 5–1). This framework has emerged from examination of traditional nuclear white middle-class American families. Whether the theoretic principles of the family life cycle can be applied to the particular and unique experiences of other family structures, as

Table 5–1   The Stages of the Family Life Cycle

Family Life Cycle Stage	Emotional Process of Transition: Key Principles	Second Order Changes in Family Status Required to Proceed Developmentally
1 Between Families: The Unattached Young Adult	Accepting parent off-spring separation	a. Differentiation of self in relation to family of origin b. Development of intimate peer relationships c. Establishment of self in work
2 The Joining of Families Through Marriage: The Newly Married Couple	Commitment to new system	a. Formation of marital system b. Realignment of relationships with extended families and friends to include spouse
3 The Family with Young Children	Accepting new members into the system	a. Adjusting marital system to make space for child(ren) b. Taking on parenting roles c. Realignment of relationships with extended family to include parenting and grandparenting roles
4 The Family With Adolescents	Increasing flexibility of family boundaries to include children's independence	a. Shifting of parent-child relationships to permit adolescent to move in and out of system b. Refocus on mid-life marital and career issues c. Beginning shift toward concerns for older generation
5 Launching Children and Moving On	Accepting a multitude of exits from and entries into the family system	a. Renegotiation of marital system as a dyad b. Development of adult-to-adult relationships between grown children and their parents c. Realignment of relationships to include in-laws and grandchildren
6 The Family in Later Life	Accepting the shifting of generational roles	a. Maintaining own and/or couple functioning and interests in face of physiological decline, exploration of new familial and social role options b. Support for a more central role for middle generation c. Making room in the system for the wisdom and experience of the elderly, supporting the older generation without overfunctioning for them. d. Dealing with loss of spouse, siblings, and other peers and preparation for own death. Life review and integration

Reprinted with permission from Carter E, McGoldrick M: *The Family Life Cycle: A Framework for Family Therapy.* New York: Gardner Press, 1980.

well as to cultural variations in the family norm, is a major area for further study.

The family life cycle can be viewed as a developmental process and likened to an ongoing dance in which movement is constant, sometimes quick and intense, other times slow and mellow. The performance of each dancer affects and is affected by all the others, both individually and collectively, no matter who is center stage at any given point in time. *The goal of this process and the function of the system is to further the evolution of each member, moving toward greater flexibility and coherence* (Lewis et al, 1976). This goal, we believe, is often overlooked or minimized in the study of families, and there is a tendency to get lost in the system, forgetting that the system is composed of individuals.

Further, each individual brings to his or her life experience a genetic and constitutional endowment, which increases the complexity of the relationship with the interactional environment. The impact of such genetic programming on family process is not always predictable. The development and nurturance of the individual with other individuals in the system forms a backdrop for examining family function. Barnhill (1979) has identified eight dimensions to be negotiated for healthy family function:

1. Individuation versus enmeshment
2. Mutuality versus isolation
3. Flexibility versus rigidity
4. Stability versus disorganization
5. Clear versus unclear or distorted perception
6. Clear roles versus unclear roles
7. Role reciprocity versus role conflict
8. Clear versus diffuse or breached generation boundaries

Although successful progress in these dimensions signifies healthy system function, it is apparent that the dimensions can be equally well applied to the adaptive capacities of the individual. As the family serves not only to nurture its members but also as intermediary between the individual and society (Getty, Humphreys, 1981), the nurse who understands both individual and family dynamics is best prepared to facilitate family health.

Given this constant movement, change, and growth that is concurrent in children, adults, and the family as a whole, it is important to determine which characteristics best support the health of each individual and the system itself.

Research on Healthy Families

The study of healthy families is a recent development, and to date the primary work has focused on white middle-class nuclear families. However, even with this limitation, important characteristics have been defined.

Olson and McCubbin (1983) sampled a cross-sectional group of 1140 families at various points in the family life cycle and evaluated the families on the basis of cohesion and adaptability using the Circumplex model of families (Figure 5–1). Communication is seen as the facilitating dimension that influences the level of adaptability and cohesion (Olson, Russell, Sprenkle, 1983). The major theoretical variables examined were (1) types of families; (2) family resources; (3) family stress and changes; (4) family coping strategies; and (5) marital and family satisfaction. Using the Circumplex model, 16 types of marital and family systems were identified. The families that fell closest to the center of the model were considered most healthy. However, families tended to move in and out of various styles on the model, depending on the stage in the life cycle. As a general rule, however, the further a person was from the center of the model, the more likely he or she would not be satisfied with his or her marriage, family, or overall quality of life.

Another major study (Lewis et al, 1976) identified five qualities that facilitate the development of healthy adaptive adults: (1) clear and nurturant leadership in the system

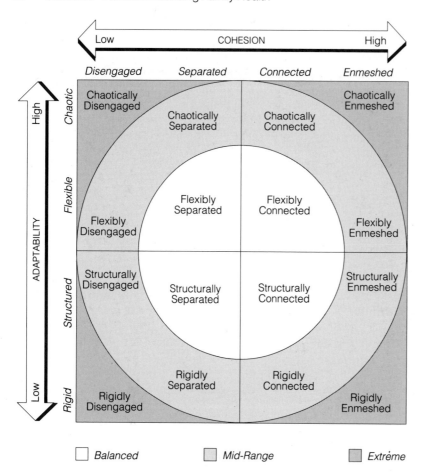

Figure 5–1 Circumplex model: Sixteen types of marital and family systems. Printed with permission from Beavers W, Voeller M: Family models: Comparing and contrasting the Olson circumplex model with the Beavers systems model. *Fam Process* 1983; *22*(3): 71.

with a sense that encounters will be affiliative; (2) a high degree of individuation with respect of each member for each member; (3) the ability to tolerate and work through separation and loss; (4) realistic perceptions both of events and of the passage of time; and (5) open, honest expression of feelings both positive and negative, with awareness and concern for others.

The Beavers and Voeller model (1983) categorizes families as healthy, midrange, and seriously disturbed in relation to these qualities as well as to their style of relating. Family behavioral styles were characterized as centrifugal, mixed, or centripetal (Figure 5–2). Centripetal families receive most relationship satisfaction

from within the family whereas centrifugal families see relationships in the outside world as more satisfying than those in the family. Overall, Beavers found that there was no single quality that optimally functioning families possessed, but that the determinants were a number of variables and the interrelationships of the variables. Healthy families were found to embody the following:

1. An affiliative attitude about human encounters

2. Respect for subjective views

3. A belief in complex motivations

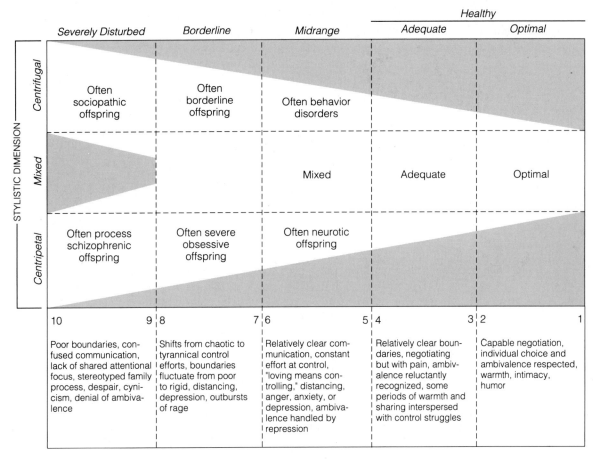

Figure 5–2 Beavers systems model. Printed with permission from Beavers W, Voeller M. Family models: Comparing and contrasting the Olson circumplex model with the Beavers systems model. *Fam Process* 1983; *22*(3): 94.

4. High levels of initiative
5. A flexible family structure with a strong parental coalition
6. Congruent mythology (perceive self as others do)
7. High levels of personal autonomy within the family
8. Open expression of feelings
9. High degree of spontaneity, humor, and wit

The Beavers study suggested the cardinal role of the parental coalition in establishing the level of functioning for the total family.

Curran (1983) notes 15 traits of healthy families, and Stinnett (1979) discusses 6 traits. In both cases, healthy traits suggest good self-esteem, a sense of nurturance, acceptance, encouragement, and support. High on the list are good communication, spending quality time together, commitment to the family, and problem-solving skills. Interestingly, another trait of healthy families is a shared religious orientation or, as Beavers puts it (Lewis et al, 1976), a transcendent value system. The importance of a shared spiritual value system is consistently cited (Curran, 1983; Stinnett al, 1979; Lewis et al, 1976) as a characteristic of the healthy family.

Hanson (1986) investigated the characteristics of healthy single-parent families. In a sample of 42 families (parent and one child), members were given questionnaires that measured various aspects of family health. The study measured characteristics associated with physical and mental health both of parents and of children. Good communication and social support were found to be most correlated with physical and mental health of the two groups. In addition, religiousness was also found to be significant for health in the children. Socioeconomic status and problem-solving were not highly associated with health either in parents or in children.

As the qualities of strong families are reviewed, it becomes clear that they all fall into the category of relational needs. This presumes that more basic survival needs are already met and becomes a basic assumption of the healthy family. The fact that the traits ascribed to healthy families are essentially relational in nature also presupposes a particular value in that the family members are not part of a work unit in the most basic sense. For example, in a more agrarian society, a healthy family quality might be "works together to harvest crops." The family relationships are based on attachment and are affectional in nature (Carter, McGoldrick, 1980).

Alternate Family Forms

If we apply the aforementioned qualities of healthy families to the more common alternative forms (for example, single-parent families and stepfamilies), such structures can be equally healthy or strong. Therefore, we can identify healthy single-parent or stepfamilies if we also recognize the adjustment processes necessary to adapt to these structures. Cooper et al (1983) reported that the particular structure of a family is less significant to a child's development than the level of cohesion in the family. In any given family form, the following qualities can exist: affirming, supporting, and expressing appreciation; good communication; spending quality time together; sharing responsibility; having a high degree of commitment; valuing service to others and respecting others; having a spiritual value system; and possessing an ability to solve problems and seek help appropriately. We might conclude that such traits would characterize family strength whether the family was the traditional nuclear family, a single-parent or stepfamily, or a gay or lesbian family.

Although alternative family structures are becoming the rule rather than the exception, they still represent a deviation from the highly valued, frequently idealized nuclear family norm. Consequently, such family structures experience higher levels of stress and greater than average demands for adaptation. Role definition, always a task requiring subtle shifts, becomes fraught with complexity and confusion. When emotional energy, as well as physical energy and time, is required to address basic psychologic and emotional needs as well as survival needs, there is little left over for enhancement or enrichment. To this extent, single-parent families and stepfamilies may fall short of the healthy family characterization. To echo Abraham Maslow, when basic needs are met, more mature needs arise. Those dealing professionally with families can therefore direct their interventions toward the more basic needs of alternative family forms with the understanding that the real goal is facilitating the development of strength. The same could be said, of course, for the traditional nuclear family that is dysfunctional and therefore deficient in healthy processes. Although we are not specifically addressing the subject, it is important to note that the gay or lesbian family is an alternative family structure with special needs to address. This will continue to be true as more men and women openly acknowledge their homosexuality and choose to raise children in the context of a committed homosexual relationship.

Finally, in relation to the subject of healthy family traits, it must be remembered that these qualities can be expressed in a wide variety of styles. That is, there is not one correct way to show appreciation or express affection; there is no one right way to spend quality time together; there is no mold for religious orientation. Across ethnic and cultural variations and through differences in education, socioeconomic status, geographic locale, interests, and personality style, family strength has the same substance, with different modes of expressions.

Nursing Implications

As nurses move into expanded roles, they encounter families in a wide variety of settings and are concerned with a multiplicity of factors regarding family health. From direct service to consultation and education, nurses have the opportunity to positively affect the health and health care of families. The current approach to nursing practice emphasizes health teaching and health promotion as well as client advocacy. As Reutter (1984) points out, the health care function of the family is not often addressed in the family literature nor is it well defined in the nursing literature. Much of generic nursing education continues to depend primarily on an individual model rather than a systems model, and clinical experience remains hospital-based in the main, although there is no doubt that the paradigm is shifting. Therefore, it becomes necessary for nurses who find themselves working with families or interested in families to conceptualize assessment of the family unit pursuant to the promotion of family health. Orem's (1980; 1983) self-care framework, though individually focused, lends itself to adaptation for developing guidelines to assess family units because of her philosophic appreciation of the role of the family in individual development. Reutter (1984) has developed a Family Assessment Guide that addresses categories consistent with traits of healthy families and considers those aspects of health and self-care not addressed in the family literature. Whall (1981) has employed concepts from Rogers' theory of nursing and has developed a comprehensive family assessment tool based on the systems model (Figure 5–3). Using this assessment tool, it is possible to address all the areas mentioned in research and family literature reviewed in this chapter. Using a systems approach in assessing family health requires nurses to integrate and synthesize knowledge from several disciplines and to use the information in forming nursing interventions. The assessment categories in the Whall model include:

1. Individual subsystem consideration, such as developmental, biologic, psychologic, and social

2. Interactional patterns within the family

3. Unique characteristics of the whole, such as belief systems and group dynamics

4. Environmental interface synchrony, which addresses the family in relation to the environment

This model, derived from Rogers' systems theory, offers a thorough assessment of family emotional and social functioning. Biologic health and behavioral patterns are also addressed. Because Reutter's (1984) work is based on Orem's (1980; 1983) self-care model, she addresses the self-care abilities of the family as well. A skillful family health nurse must determine which approach to understanding a family at a given time will be most useful. These guides, as well as others, will offer avenues to explore family health care needs and to engage families in a commitment for optimum health.

As we continue to shift focus to the family unit and search for ways to strengthen family life and meet relational and affective needs, we will need tools that aid this endeavor. Nurses working with families have the opportunity to contribute to this growing effort by synthesizing what is known about family structure and function with what is currently understood about optimum health.

An Assessment Guideline for Work with Families

The assumption is made that each person and family is characterized by rhythmic developmental sequences which are constantly patterning/re-patterning in mutual simultaneous interaction with the environment. Because these dimensions are essentially boundaryless, there will appear to be some overlap.

I. The Individual Sub-System Considerations
   A. Developmental
      1. Past developmental history of parents and children
         a. Parents' physical and emotional health at time of establishment of the family unit continuing into present time
         b. Developmental landmarks, i.e., age specific tasks, and physical growth for each person.
         c. General psychosexual developmental considerations of members
         d. History of life traumas
         e. Present level of functioning of each member in regard to developmental tasks
   B. Biological
      1. General state of the physical health of each member
      2. Past and present difficulties and care
      3. Past and present physical level of functioning including motor skills, etc.
      4. Genetic factors affecting level of functioning
   C. Psychological
      1. General state of emotional health and psychological growth
      2. Past and present problems including care
      3. General level of functioning with regard to cognitive and affective elements
   D. Social
      1. Class and cultural factors—including types of support systems
      2. General social development of children and adults, i.e., school work and social realms
   E. The nurse as an individual (including development, values, biases, etc.)

II. Interactional Patterns
   A. Executive and sibling system relationships
      1. Clear versus breached generational levels (including inversions and exclusions)
      2. Negotiation patterns and levels
   B. Triadic and dyadic relationships
      1. Positive and negative vectors in relationships (e.g., scapegoating and favoritism)
      2. Cyclical nature of sequencing
   C. Communication patterns
      1. Clarity vs. distortions such as double messages
      2. Usual channels and modes
   D. Role relationships
      1. Role reciprocity and/or role confusion and inconsistency
      2. Complementarity and/or symmetrical patterns
      3. Ways in which intimacy is expressed
   E. Attachment patterns
      1. Commitment and detachment levels
      2. Individuation and enmeshment levels
      3. Mutuality and isolation levels
      4. Implicit and explicit expectations

III. Unique Characteristics of the Whole
   A. Family group psyche
      1. Problem-solving style; i.e., moving toward/against/away
      2. Capacity to validate reality
   B. Family mass
      1. Relative stability and/or disorganization
      2. Capacity for change, i.e., relative rigidity or flexibility

  C. Belief system
      1. Values, myths (including distortions such as sham and pseudomutuality)
      2. Rules regarding expression of beliefs
  D. Group dynamic characteristics
      1. Family power structure
      2. Leadership and problem-solving ability
      3. Cohesiveness and reference groups
      4. "Boundary" characteristics—who is allowed "in" and who is "out"
  E. Family developmental needs
      1. Maturational requirements
      2. Situational requirements
  F. Family typological actions
      1. Centripetal and/or centrifugal
      2. Open, random, or more rigid lifestyle
  G. Economic factors
      1. Distribution of income
      2. Income as related to needs
      3. Style of disbursement

IV. Environmental Interface Synchrony
  A. Developmental needs of family vs. community resources
  B. Family values as compared to community values and beliefs
  C. Requirements of community upon the family
  D. Effect of the family upon the community.

Figure 5–3 An assessment guideline for work with families. From Whall AL: Nursing theory and the assessment of families. *J Psychiatr Nurs*, 1981; *19*:30–36. Reprinted with permission.

Summary

We have begun to recognize that individual development is indeed a dynamic process that continues through the life cycle (Sheehy, 1974; Colarusso, Nemiroff, 1981), and we have noted that family life is described in a developmental cycle (Carter, McGoldrick, 1980; Duvall, 1977). Therefore, when individual members of a family are experiencing developmental transitions, it follows that each will affect one another and the entire family as well. The efforts to explicate these shifts have been focused on the epochs that characterized the traditional white middle-class nuclear American family. This might lead one to conclude that any system that does not progress through the particular epochs associated with this norm is developmentally deficient or irregular. However, study of nontraditionally structured families is showing that the theoretical

principles of the family life cycle can be applied to the alternate family structures. We cling rather tenaciously to the model of the nuclear family as our norm for discussing family life and for understanding family development. Although it is helpful to have some stable parameter from which to assess modifications, there is the danger that, in our attachment to the nuclear family typology, we will be unable to validate the diversity of forms that currently make up the family without resorting to attributions of pathology. Unless social trends reverse dramatically, the number of single-parent families, stepfamilies, aged families, and singles living alone will increase. Family life education and enrichment programs must consider the variety of structures in which individuals grow to personhood.

With some support from available research, we presume that when healthy families reproduce, they produce healthy children. When we encounter dysfunction, we are not surprised to find individual or couple pathology. When we assess maladaptive individual patterns, we expect a dysfunctional family of origin. We are less prepared to find strength in the individual whose family background was severely dysfunctional. And, in fact, when we encounter adaptive, resourceful, reflective individuals from these kinds of families, we are at a loss to explain the source of their abilities. It would seem that other factors or forces are operating that we have not yet begun to comprehend, let alone study. This leads one to develop a healthy skepticism about the absolute nature of any research findings. However, the drive for understanding reflects an evolutionary imperative, and we must continue to investigate not only our environments but ourselves. What are the effects of having children in later life, on parents, children, and the family unit? What is the impact of culture on the identified characteristics of family health (an important question during this wave of new immigration)? What is the impact on gender identity of being raised in a gay or lesbian family? Do healthy families produce healthy individuals or are there other intervening factors? What is the effect on affective family ties of multigenerational relationships? Studies are needed to understand the needs of alternative family forms, to investigate the impact of public policy on family health, and to clarify our understanding of the role that family plays in the development of adaptive, productive human beings.

Issues for Further Investigation

1. What are behaviors that indicate healthy interactional patterns in alternate family forms (as compared with the traditional nuclear family model) and in various cultures?

2. How do transitional points in family life (such as birth, school, career) vary among various cultures and family structures? Are there transitional points in other cultures and family structures that are not operative in traditional nuclear American white middle-class families and are therefore overlooked by health professionals?

3. Do healthy families produce healthy individuals or are there other intervening factors?

4. What are the underlying significant variables when adaptive, resilient individuals emerge from dysfunctional families?

5. How does a family's knowledge of its healthy and dysfunctional family behaviors relate to the effectiveness of family-focused nursing interventions?

6. What are the effects of having children in later life for children, parents, and the family unit?

7. How is gender identity affected when children are raised in a gay or lesbian family?

8. What effects do multigenerational relationships have on the family unit?

References

Barnhill L (1979): Healthy family systems. *Fam Coordinator, 29*:94–100.

Beavers W (1985): *Successful Marriage: A Family Systems Approach to Couples Therapy*. New York: Norton.

Beavers W, Voeller M (1983): Family models: Comparing and contrasting the Olson Circumplex model with the Beavers systems model. *Fam Process, 22*(3):85–98.

Carter E, McGoldrick M (1980): *The Family Life Cycle: A Framework for Family Therapy*. New York: Gardner.

Colarusso CA, Nemiroff RA (1981): *Adult Development*. New York: Plenum.

Cooper J, Holman J, Braithwaite V (1983): Self-esteem and family cohesion: The child's perspective and adjustment. *J Marr Fam, 45*(1):153–159.

Curran D (1983): *Traits of a Healthy Family.* New York: Ballantine.

Duvall E (1977): *Family Development.* Philadelphia: Lippincott.

Dychtwald K (1986): *Wellness and Health Promotion for the Elderly.* Rockville, MD: Aspen.

Erikson E (1963): *Childhood and Society.* New York: Norton.

Galvin KM, Brommel BJ: *Family Communication, Cohesion, and Change.* Glenview, IL: Scott Foresman.

Getty K, Humphreys W (1981): *Understanding the Family: Stress and Change in American Family Life.* East Norwalk, CT: Appleton-Lange.

Glick PC (1984): American household structure in transition. *Fam Plann Perspect, 16*(5):205–211.

Gould RL (1978): *Transformations.* New York: Simon & Schuster.

Hanson SM (1986): Healthy single-parent families: *Fam Process, 35*(1):125–132.

Levinson D (1978): *The Seasons of a Man's Life.* New York: Knopf.

Lewis J et al (1976): *No Single Thread: Psychological Health in Family Systems.* New York: Brunner/Mazel.

Mahler M (1973): Symbiosis and individuation: The psychological birth of the human infant. *Psychoanal Study Child, 29*:89–105.

McCubbin H, Dahl BB (1985): *Marriage and Family: Individuals and Life Cycles.* New York: Wiley.

Naisbitt J (1982): *Megatrends.* New York: Warner.

Norton AJ, Glick PC (1986): One-parent families: A social and economic profile. *Fam Process, 35*(1):9–17.

Olson D, McCubbin A (1983): *Families: What Makes Them Work.* Beverly Hills: Sage.

Olson D, Russell C, Sprenkle D (1983): Circumplex model of marital and family systems. 6. Theoretical update. *Family Press, 22*(3):69–83.

On the home front. (1986, August 28) San Francisco *Chronicle*, p. 24.

Orem DE (1980): *Nursing: Concepts of Practice,* 2nd ed. New York: McGraw-Hill.

Orem DE (1983): The self-care deficit theory of nursing: A general theory. In: *Family Nursing,* Clements I, Roberts F (eds.). New York: Wiley.

Reutter L (1984): Family health assessment—an integrated approach. *J Adv Nurs, 9*:391–399.

Rubin S (1986, August 26): The stepparents's guide to life. San Francisco *Chronicle*, p. 15.

Satir V (1972): *Peoplemaking.* Palo Alto: Science and Behavior Books.

Sheehy G (1974): *Passages.* New York: Dutton.

Stinnett N, Carter N, Montgomery J (1972): Older persons' perceptions of their marriages. *J Marr Fam,* 11:665–670.

Stinnett N, Chesser B, DeFrain J (eds.) (1979): *Building Family Strengths: Blueprints for Action.* Lincoln: University of Nebraska Press.

Walsh F (1982): *Normal Family Processes.* New York: Guilford.

Whall AL (1981): Nursing theory and assessment of families. *J Psychiatr Nurs, 19*:30–39.

6

NUTRITION AND THE FAMILY

Yolanda Gutierrez, MS, RD

Katharyn Antle May, RN, DNSC, FAAN

Because dietary patterns are closely related to levels of health, nurses must understand the nutritional needs of the family populations they care for. This chapter discusses the major factors that influence eating decisions of individuals and families, and it identifies major risk factors in the American diet across the life cycle. It also provides an overview of contemporary dietary issues and identifies family issues that impact dietary patterns.

Yolanda Gutierrez is Associate Clinical Professor at the University of California at San Francisco School of Nursing (Department of Family Health Care). A recognized expert in maternal-infant, childhood, and family nutrition, she has been teaching nutrition content and nutrition counseling to graduate nursing students for over a decade.

Katharyn Antle May is Associate Professor at the Vanderbilt University School of Nursing and Chairperson of its Department of Family and Community Health. Known for her early research of expectant fatherhood, she is also the co-author of Comprehensive Maternity Nursing.

Introduction

The body of knowledge in nutrition and its effect on individual and family health is expanding rapidly with the development of new research techniques. However, despite this new knowledge, many people—even those with a thorough knowledge of basic nutritional principles—do not eat very well. This chapter identifies some of the physiologic and psychologic factors that influence eating decisions and dietary patterns of individuals and families. The relationship between nutrition and lifestyle issues, developmental stages, and adherence and habit formation throughout the life cycle is also discussed. Emphasis is placed on updating nurses' understanding of dietary factors in health promotion to equip them not only to impart information on nutrition in health and disease but also to assist them in the person-centered task of helping to effect desired changes in knowledge, skills, attitudes, and behaviors that may positively influence the nutritional status of family members.

Factors Affecting Family Food Habits

Examining factors that affect food habits provides an understanding of the important effect they have on an individual's nutritional status. In spite of the general view that inadequate income is a major determinant of poor nutritional status, recent research has demonstrated that people who fail to attain an optimum diet can be found at every socioeconomic level. The individual's susceptibility to nutritional problems is affected by his or her behavior as well as by the physical and social environment. Individual food choices and eating patterns are influenced throughout our lives by a complexity of eternal (social, cultural, and economic) factors and by internal (physiologic and psychologic) factors (Figure 6–1). The following section will discuss both internal and external factors as well as developmental factors that influence individual and family dietary patterns.

Family Developmental Stages and Food Decisions

Developmental stages of the family life cycle from inception to dissolution have been found to influence food decisions. Each stage is distinct from the others because of the events and circumstances the family faces at each stage, and these differences are reflected in the diet and food habits of the families, as well as in the information- or assistance-seeking activities of families regarding diet and nutrition.

The life-cycle concept has been used by several nutrition investigators and is useful in providing insight into a wide variety of consumption behavior (Schafer, Keith, 1981). The four life cycle stages of families that have particular importance in relation to dietary patterns are:

Stage 1: *Young families* in which the wife is under 45 years of age and at least one child is under 6 years of age

Stage 2: *Maturing families* in which children, ages 6 to 18, are in school

Stage 3: *Middle-age families* in which the wife is over 45 and there are no children in the home

Stage 4: *Retirement families* in which the wife is over 60 and there are no children in the home

A recent large-scale study used these four life cycle stages to examine factors that influence family food decisions (Schafer, Keith, 1981). Health concerns, cost, and immediate family members were found to be the most important influences on food habits of the 336 married couples randomly selected and interviewed for this study. Other factors affecting food behavior were the influence of mass media, education programs, government information, reference groups, and significant others outside the immediate family.

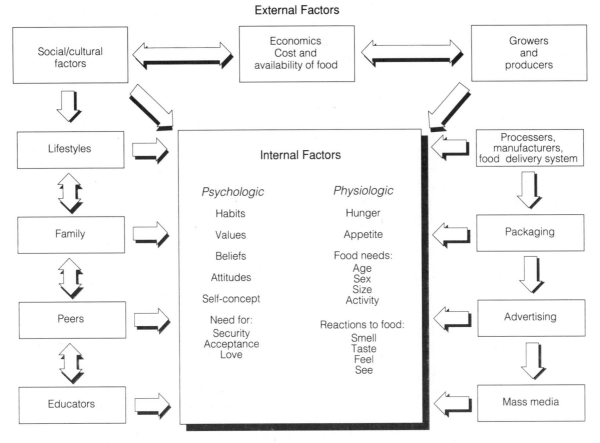

Figure 6-1　Factors affecting food habits. Adapted from: Wenck DA, Boren M, Dewan SP: *Nutrition: The Challenge of Being Well-Nourished*, 2d ed, p. 4. Reston, 1983. Adapted by permission of Prentice-Hall, Inc., Englewood Cliffs, NJ.

Parents in Stage 1 families were, in general, more strongly influenced by external factors than were couples at any other stage: This was probably because these families were in the process of establishing food and diet routines and were more open to new information provided by classes, government sources, parents, relatives, and friends.

Parents in Stage 2 families were more established, with more fixed ideas and attitudes concerning diet, nutrition, and menu preferences. There was a reduction of information-seeking among these families, as well as reduced openness to influence from outside. Strongest influ-

ences on dietary patterns were reported to be concerns about weight among husbands and spousal preferences among wives.

Couples in Stage 3 families, because of the departure of the children, reported changes in marital adjustment and in family role definitions. However, there were only moderate changes in the importance of outside influences on food decisions. There was a pronounced decrease in reported influence of parents and relatives, which is to be expected in this age group.

Couples in Stage 4 families, entering the retirement years, reported a slight increase in the influence of information from the media. This raises the possibility that the elderly may be less likely to seek information from health professionals regarding nutrition.

Thus, it is evident that as families move through the life cycle, their food patterns, how they process information about food, and what factors influence their food decisions change as the unique events at each life cycle stage change. The stage of the family's life cycle is just one of many factors the nurse must consider when providing nutritional care to family members. The following section will consider other important internal and external factors that are likely to affect dietary patterns.

External Influences

Individuals have little control over many external influences on food habits. Food consumption patterns have changed profoundly in recent years because of vast improvements in food production methods, food preservation, food storage, and food transportation. The American public, it seems, has an insatiable desire for new, different, convenient foods that provide instant gratification. Food industry research and development efforts are motivated by the desire to produce food that people will purchase. Unfortunately, the profit motive often places the nutritive value of food last in importance. In addition, consumers generally are unaware of the enormous costs involved in the process of developing and promoting new convenience food products—costs that are inevitably paid by the consumers themselves but that fail to buy improved nutritional health.

Advertising Food advertisers appear to be more successful in changing eating habits than health professionals or educators. This is largely because food has an emotional rather than an intellectual value to most people, a fact well known to manufacturers who use emotional appeals rather than factual information to sell their products. Advertisements emphasize flavor, fun, enjoyment, and psychologic satisfaction

rather than health or nutritional factors. Advertising of food products is particularly effective in families with small children. Research has found that the youngest children paid the most attention to television commercials and that commercials were most often focused on products known as "impulse" purchases. Mothers usually yielded to the child's purchase influence attempts; mothers with 5–7-year-olds yielded 88% of the time in buying breakfast cereals, 55% of the time in buying snack foods, 40% of the time in buying candy, and 38% of the time in buying soft drinks (Ward, Wackman, 1972).

Family Food Cost Another external influence on family dietary patterns is the family food cost. In spite of increased costs and inflation, the food budget of most American families is still

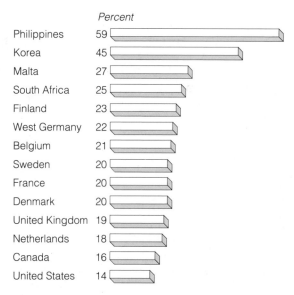

Percent

	Percent
Philippines	59
Korea	45
Malta	27
South Africa	25
Finland	23
West Germany	22
Belgium	21
Sweden	20
France	20
Denmark	20
United Kingdom	19
Netherlands	18
Canada	16
United States	14

1978 data. Canada and United States include non-alcoholic beverages. *Source: U.N. National Accounts of Statistics and National Sources.*

Figure 6–2 Share of income spent on food. Source: *1981 Handbook of Agricultural Charts*, Agriculture Handbook No. 592, U.S. Dept. of Agriculture, Washington, D.C., 1981, Chart 82.

only a relatively small part of their income: About 17% for the average family, compared to higher proportions of income spent on food in many other countries (Figure 6–2). However, this average figure may be somewhat misleading because low-income families in this country may spend up to 40% of their income on food.

Because it is impossible to tell how much foods will cost at any given time, discussion of food costs as an external factor influencing dietary patterns must be on a relative cost basis because certain kinds or classes of food are always less expensive than others, regardless of increasing or decreasing overall food prices. For example, some low-cost but nutritious foods are organ meats, potatoes, dry beans, poultry, eggs, and enriched cereals and flours. More expensive and less nutritious foods include "gourmet" or convenience items, which tend to be higher in sodium, fat, and calories (such as frozen vegetables with sauces), and high-calorie snack foods, including soft drinks, potato and corn chips, candy, pastries, and alcoholic beverages. These foods are often low in nutrient density and typically high in fats, sugars, or salt.

A number of factors can influence how the family divides its food dollar:

• Family income
• Whether the family produces food (gardening, preserving)
• Characteristics of family members (age, sex, activity level, special dietary needs)
• Family time; transportation and energy available for shopping, storing, and preparing food; and storage and cooking facilities in the home
• Number of meals eaten away from home
• Amount and kind of entertaining with food
• Food preferences and the value placed on food and eating

Sociocultural Factors   In every society, food plays a central part in beliefs about life and health. The culture of a given society will greatly determine the food habits of its people. Food is always defined culturally; however, the geographic characteristics of the land, climate, and general social environment will modify food habits as well. Food habits in the United States reflect the economic and cultural diversity of this society, as well as the special nutritional contributions and problems of minority families, especially those in immigrant groups. The story of immigration to the United States is hardly a new one; many subcultural groups have become assimilated to varying degrees. In this process, immigrant groups have contributed dietary patterns to the dominant culture, and, in turn, American food patterns have been adopted.

Individual differences exist in the degree of participation or adaptation of the immigrant family to the dominant culture. Anthropologists recognize that what actually occurs between two cultures in close contact is selective acculturation based on patterns of interaction and conflict. For example, migrant farm workers from Mexico experience two levels of acculturation: one at the level of the Mexican-American culture and the other at the level of the Anglo or dominant culture. Some families will experience more contact with fellow Mexicans, others with Mexican-Americans, and a few with Anglos. The degree of selective acculturation of the individual or family depends on housing, work, and school situations (Melville, 1980) and will be reflected in small or marked shifts from traditional food patterns to those more like the dominant culture.

The pattern of immigration will also determine adaptation and changes in food practices. For example, seasonal immigrants such as farm workers experience different patterns in adaptation to new foods, depending on whether they stay for brief or extended periods, whether they can obtain traditional foods easily, and whether they have adequate income and cooking facilities. Immigrant families intending to stay indefinitely are likely to experience more significant shifts in dietary patterns.

Cultural influences on nutritional status are often most apparent in recently immigrated families, for several reasons. First, a great obstacle faced by many recently immigrated families is poverty. Many are less able to purchase health care, adequate food, and housing and services and may not have legal documentation to enable them to participate in public programs that might assist them with food and health benefits. Second, attention to nutrition is likely not to be a high priority compared to other adjustment problems such as language barriers, lack of employment skills, unfamiliarity with the American lifestyle, housing and transportation problems, and an unstable support network. Finally, immigrant families often have problems in obtaining high-quality foods. These problems include:

- Lack of knowledge or skills necessary to purchase foods in American supermarkets
- Difficulty in finding familiar foods and spices
- Difficulty adjusting to purchasing foods in large quantities for several days, if past practice was to purchase food daily
- Lack of knowledge about supplemental nutrition programs
- Inability to identify nutritive food value
- Lack of knowledge about food preparation and storage
- The strong, often misleading influence of advertising of food products
- Lack of appetite due to stress or other health problems

The shifts in eating habits currently seen among immigrant families are also due in large part to changes in the family structure that affect meal preparation. Traditionally, older family members—the grandmother, for instance—would participate in food preparation. However, new immigrant families often do not have older members, and the mothers are often working outside the home. There has generally been a decline in family togetherness at meals, except for dinner. The influence of school is reflected by children's demands for snack foods and fast foods they may see their friends eat. In addition,

new immigrants frequently experience problems associated with shopping, such as unfamiliarity with American food choices and preparation.

Cultural factors in dietary patterns are also apparent in food habits of families who are well-acculturated, such as second-generation families. Traditional types of foods and food preparation are likely to be used at family events or special occasions. However, with increasing time spent in the dominant culture, dietary patterns become less characteristic of the cultural group and more like modal dietary patterns in the wider culture.

Family Lifestyle   Fast-paced living has become the American way of life, and it probably has a negative impact on nutritional status. Many lifestyle characteristics are linked with food-related behaviors. Individuals may be constantly on the go but largely from a sitting position; many are plagued with problems of overweight and obesity because of an essentially sedentary lifestyle in combination with high caloric intake. These problems are readily seen in specific food choices. Many individuals are often too busy to eat regular meals. Many hurry off in the morning without breakfast and then have a coffee and doughnut snack. Others may skip lunch or grab a hamburger at a fast-food restaurant. At home, worn out from all the day's hurrying, families may relax before dinner with some snack food, a soft drink, or a cocktail.

Snacking and the use of convenience foods has become a trademark of contemporary dietary patterns in the United States. Eating between meals and use of convenience foods are not necessarily poor nutritional practices. The more crucial question relates to the nutritive value of these food choices, which often is quite limited. If a family relies heavily on these foods, members may in fact be at high nutritional risk.

Because these types of foods are quick and easy to serve, they are often the choice of people who live alone, who are not motivated to cook, or who do not have the skills to do so. In addition, the increasingly commonplace single parent family may be especially vulnerable to this poor nutritional practice. If the parent is employed, there may be limited time and energy for food shopping and cooking; the single parent may rely heavily on convenience foods. If the parent is unemployed and dependent on welfare, the food budget may be quite limited. Both situations may place the family members at high risk for nutritional problems.

Internal Influences

The physiologic and psychologic factors that affect individual food choices are so intertwined that it is often impossible to separate them. Many physiologic functions are involved in our appetite and in our enjoyment of food: sight, smell, taste, touch, and, of course, the feeling of satiety and well-being that follows a good meal.

Color and Smell Color and smell of food are usually the most observable and immediate cues that influence food choices. We are conditioned through our early experiences to relate certain colors with certain flavors and with desirable foods. If the food appears in an unfamiliar color, such as green eggs or pink potatoes, we would be likely to reject it on the basis of color alone. Food manufacturers are well aware of the importance of color and use a variety of food-coloring materials to add eye and sales appeal to their foods.

Individuals often judge a food's flavor by its color rather than by its taste. For example, taste testers were given sherbet of three colors—orange, green, and yellow—and were asked to identify the flavor of each. All of the sherbet, regardless of the color, was the same flavor—orange. The taste testers were fooled by the color and identified the flavor of each sherbet based on its color: The orange-colored sherbet had an "orange" flavor; the yellow tasted like "lemon"; and the green had a "lime" flavor (Pangborn, 1964).

Smell also has a powerful effect on food choices. A good-smelling food, such as bread as it is baking, can set up favorable conditions for digestion by stimulating the secretion of saliva and stomach acid. Even before we start eating that freshly baked bread, we are ready to start digesting it. These reactions to color and smell are largely learned responses and reflect early experiences with food, usually within the family environment. However, there are even more complex ways in which physiologic and psychologic responses to food interact.

Psychophysiologic Responses to Food In satisfying physiologic needs, food also fulfills important psychologic needs; thus for most people, food has emotional value as well. For an infant, food means comfort, love, and the security of being cared for. Throughout life, having food available to us when we need it satisfies a basic security need. Early conditioning in the family appears to be an important factor in the development of food habits.

Certain patterns set up during childhood, however, are associated with later nutritional problems such as food intolerance, overeating, and obesity. A common pattern is for parents to offer sweets or desserts as a reward or use food as a substitute for attention or affection. Some individuals learn to hate certain nutritious foods because they were nagged frequently to eat them by overanxious parents or because a parent had a dislike for the food. Others may always eat everything put in front of them because they were taught to do so. Obviously, these are only a few of the family dietary patterns that later affect individual and family food decisions.

It is also important to recognize that there are other influences on an individual's food choices besides the family. Children are imitative, and, as they grow older, they learn food habits from peers. The pressure to conform to certain behavior norms becomes greater as children grow; teenagers are especially known for their need not to be different, and food choices are affected not only by this characteristic but also by the teenager's typical concerns about body size and shape. Advertising is also heavily targeted to this group, and rarely are foods of high nutritive value presented.

It is well known that individuals are strongly affected in their choices of type and amount of food by the sight and smell of good food, by the thought of savory items, and by the sight of other people eating (Rodin, 1981; Schachter, 1968). In addition to these psychologic influences on food choice, there is new evidence that a complex of unique genetic, constitutional, and environmental factors determine the effects of food intake.

It has been shown that elevations in insulin levels produce increased hunger, heightened perceived pleasantness of sweet taste, and increased food intake (Rodin, 1985). However, perhaps even more important, recent research suggests that insulin levels produced by certain types of food intake influence subsequent food intake. Experimental subjects were assigned to one of four groups in which they were asked to ingest liquids before partaking at a large buffet (Spitzer, 1983). These liquids were various mixtures designed to act as preloading doses of nutrients prior to the actual food ingestion. The mixtures included (1) a fructose preload; (2) a glucose preload; (3) a glucose preload made to taste as sweet as the fructose preload with a noncaloric sweetener; and (4) a water preload. All of these mixtures were equicaloric with equal amounts of carbohydrate.

Two hours after the preload ingestion, each subject was presented with the buffet, which contained a large variety of foods. Subjects were instructed to eat whatever they liked until comfortably full. The results were striking: On the average, subjects given glucose preloads ate almost 500 calories more than those given fructose preloads. This suggests that the type of food an individual eats does affect the amount of food subsequently consumed, most likely as a consequence of food effects on insulin-mediated glucose metabolism.

Typically, glucose ingestion produces a sharp increase in both plasma glucose and insulin levels for about an hour after consumption. However, this is followed by a steep decline; two to three hours after ingestion of glucose, plasma glucose levels actually fall below fasting levels for a time, but insulin levels remain elevated. On the other hand, fructose levels produce a gradual increase in plasma glucose and insulin. In addition, the plasma glucose curve does not fall below fasting levels two to three hours after ingestion of fructose, and insulin levels are less elevated. Table sugar, or sucrose, typically accounts for a larger percentage of daily caloric intake than glucose or fructose. Although the sucrose molecule contains equal amounts of glucose and fructose, the effects of sucrose ingestion on plasma insulin levels appear to be similar to those of glucose (Crapo, Kolterman, Olefsky, 1980).

This research on effects of certain types of ingested foods on subsequent caloric intake has implications for individual and family food choices. If the family's food choices include many foods high in sucrose, later choices by the individual away from home may result in higher caloric intake than needed, thus promoting overeating and overweight. Overeating and overweight have become important issues in nutritional health in the last 20 years; the implications of overweight and obesity for individual and family health promotion are discussed in the following section.

Dietary Factors in Promotion of Individual and Family Health

The role of nutrition in health across the life cycle is much like a continuum in that adequacy of nutrition at any stage determines how current physiologic needs are met as well as influencing the body at later stages in development. Food provides the human organism with the raw materials needed for energy to sustain life, promote growth, and replace loss. Each stage of life imposes changing demands on the body; however, basic human nutrient requirements are the same, varying only in the amounts needed for optimum health for a given age and gender.

It is realistic to hope that good nutrition, in combination with other sound lifestyle habits, will prevent or minimize health threats and improve the overall quality of life. However, it is important not to expect more of nutritional practices than they can deliver in terms of individual and family health. In order to maximize the effectiveness of individual and family dietary patterns in promoting health and preventing disease, the nurse must have a clear understanding of what dietary risk factors are present for large numbers of American families and what the most current recommendations are for nutritional practices in health promotion.

Dietary Risk Factors: Problem Areas in the Diets of American Families

Risk factors in the American diet have been shown to contribute directly or indirectly to a variety of health problems. The nutritional problems present in American diets are often many and complex. The simple fact is that our diets have changed radically in the last 50 years; the modern American diet is too high in fat, cholesterol, sugar, and salt and has too little fiber and complex carbohydrate.

These dietary changes are contributing to morbidity and mortality in direct and indirect ways. Of the ten leading causes of death in the United States, six have been linked to dietary patterns: heart disease, cancer, obesity, stroke, diabetes, and cirrhosis of the liver. In response to these findings, dietary goals have been set forth by a number of public and private sources. Overall, these dietary goals (Figure 6–3) are intended to reduce dietary risk factors in American diets.

This section will first examine how typical American diets compare with these current recommendations about nutrient intake. The last part of this section will focus on particular risk factors and how they affect individuals across the life cycle. Overall guidelines for counseling dietary habits across the life cycle are summarized in Table 6–1 on page 102.

Problem Nutrients in the American Diet

Although dietary factors have been implicated in the pathogenesis of certain chronic diseases, establishing a clear relationship between low or high intakes of particular nutrients and subsequent health problems is difficult. One reason for this is that there is disagreement about what level of deficiency in nutrient intake will lead to health problems.

Recommended Dietary Allowances (RDAs), a common standard used to evaluate nutritional adequacy of diets, are set high enough to meet the nutritional needs of "practically all healthy persons" (National Academy of Science, National Research Council, 1980), However, it is important to remember that RDAs are daily amounts of nutrients recommended for populations grouped by sex and age over a period of time; that is, they are not intended to be interpreted as requirements for specific individuals on a day-to-day basis. Current RDAs for energy intake are an exception to this, in that they are calculated not to exceed requirements for healthy individuals.

Research to date has used 80%, 70%, and 66.7% of the RDA for nutrients as the level below which diets may need improvement; other large scale nutritional studies have used other standards for evaluation of dietary intakes. It is also difficult to compare dietary intakes of certain known essential nutrients with current RDAs because composition values of many foods (documentation of the amount of essential nutrients found in food) are not known.

For these reasons, findings of nutritional research on dietary deficiencies and their relation-

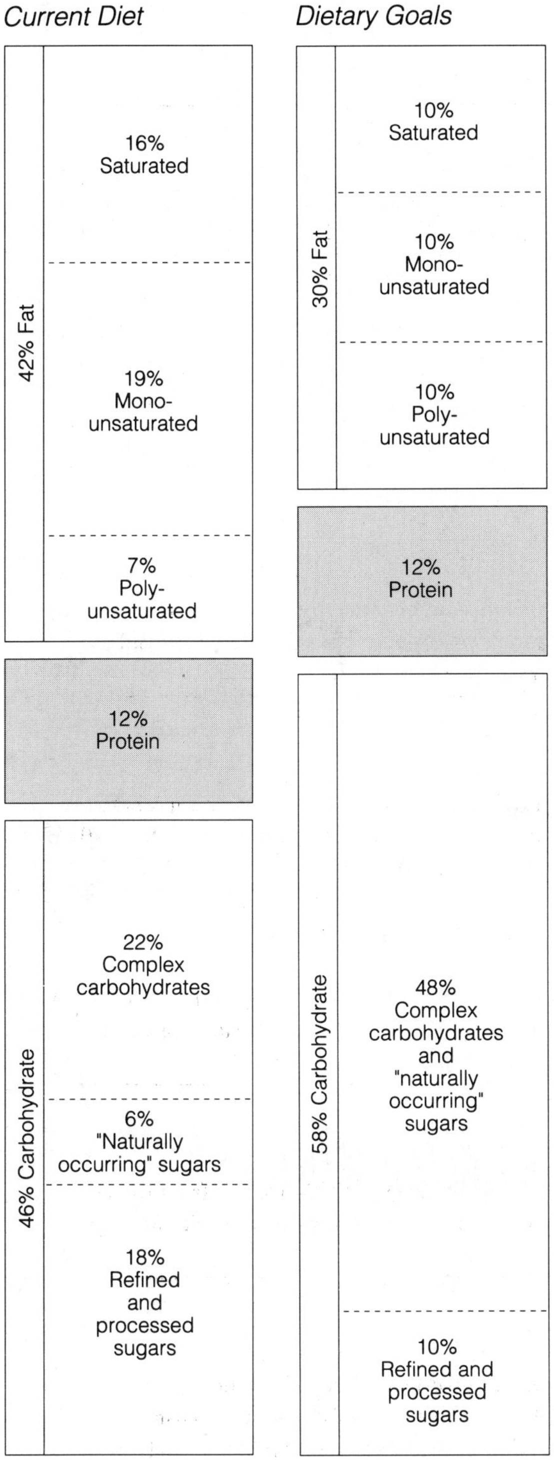

Current Diet

42% Fat
- 16% Saturated
- 19% Mono-unsaturated
- 7% Poly-unsaturated

12% Protein

46% Carbohydrate
- 22% Complex carbohydrates
- 6% "Naturally occurring" sugars
- 18% Refined and processed sugars

Dietary Goals

30% Fat
- 10% Saturated
- 10% Mono-unsaturated
- 10% Poly-unsaturated

12% Protein

58% Carbohydrate
- 48% Complex carbohydrates and "naturally occurring" sugars
- 10% Refined and processed sugars

Goals

1. To avoid overweight, consume only as much energy (calories) as is expended; if overweight, decrease energy intake and increase energy expenditure.

2. Increase the consumption of complex carbohydrates and "naturally occurring" sugars from about 28% of energy intake to about 48% of energy intake.

3. Reduce the consumption of refined and processed sugars by about 45% to account for about 10% of total energy intake.

4. Reduce overall fat consumption from about 42% to about 30% of energy intake.

5. Reduce saturated fat consumption to account for about 10% of total energy intake; and balance that with polyunsaturated and monounsaturated fats, which should account for about 10% of energy intake each.

6. Reduce cholesterol consumption to about 300 milligrams a day.

7. Limit the intake of sodium by reducing the intake of salt to about 5 grams a day.

Suggested Changes in Food Selection and Preparation

1. Increase consumption of fruits and vegetables and whole grains.

2. Decrease consumption of refined and other processed sugars and foods high in such sugars.

3. Decrease consumption of foods high in total fat, and partially replace saturated fats, whether obtained from animal or vegetable sources, with polyunsaturated fats.

4. Decrease consumption of animal fat, and choose meats, poultry and fish, which will reduce saturated fat intake.

5. Except for young children, substitute low-fat and non-fat milk for whole milk, and low-fat dairy products for high-fat dairy products.

6. Decrease consumption of butterfat, eggs and other high cholesterol sources. Some consideration should be given to easing the cholesterol goal for pre-menopausal women, young children and the elderly in order to obtain the nutritional benefits of eggs in the diet.

7. Decrease consumption of salt and foods high in salt content.

Figure 6–3 U.S. dietary goals. Adapted from *Dietary goals for the United States*, Select Committee on Nutrition and Human Needs, U.S. Senate (1977). Washington DC: U.S. GPO.

Table 6–1   Promotion of Good Dietary Habits: Foods for Everyday Use

	Milk and Milk Products	Protein Foods	Breads, Cereals, and Whole Grains	Vitamin C-Rich Fruits/ Vegetables	Dark Green and Yellow Fruits and Vegetables	Other Fruits and Vegetables
First Year of Life						
Number of Servings	24–32 oz	7 mo: 1–3 T	4–6 mo: 4–6 T	4–6 mo: 2–4 T	4–6 mo: 2–4 T	4–6 mo: 2–4 T
	Encourage breast milk or iron-fortified formula, sufficient for the first 4 to 6 months of life. Solid foods by 4 to 6 months. Offer single foods in small amounts. No solids, sugar, or honey in bottles. No Koolaid, sodas, or empty calorie snacks. Always hold your baby when giving bottle. Use iron-fortified cereals.					
Toddler/ Preschool: 1 to 5 years						
Number of Servings	3	2	4	1–2	1–2	1–2
	Use fresh milk, either whole or 2% lowfat. Continue introduction of variety of foods. Regular meals, at least two snacks per day. Be aware of appetite changes. Parents should not be anxious. Don't force-feed. Make snacks part of the food groups.					
Children and Teenagers						
Number of Servings	4–5	3	4	2	1–2	2
	Regular meals. Serve small portions. Offer finger foods frequently. Relax; don't bribe or reward with food. Don't force your child to eat. Keep the TV off when eating. Eat with the rest of the family. Encourage exercise. Avoid fatty foods.					
Young Adults, Men and Women						
Number of Servings	2	2	4	2	1–2	2
	Regular meals. Encourage exercise. Particular attention to calcium and iron-rich foods. Avoid fried foods, salty snacks, sodas, alcohol, cookies, cakes, or other high-sugar snacks. Use cooking methods such as broiling, baking, roasting.					
Pregnant and Lactating Women						
Number of Servings	4–5	4	4	2	2	2
	Small, frequent meals. Use iron and folacin supplements. Avoid alcohol, fried foods, empty calorie snacks. Particular attention to foods from milk group for calcium, vitamin C and A foods. Whole grains for fiber. Protein foods for iron.					
Elderly						
Number of Servings	2	3	4	2	2	2
	Small, frequent meals. Liquids are important even if not thirsty. Use whole grains to avoid constipation. Socializing with groups will help to increase activity and increase motivation to eat with company. May need vitamin and mineral supplements, especially calcium in the order of 1200 mg per day. Avoid alcohol. Nutrient-drug interactions can be minimized by eating a balanced diet and carefully following the instructions for use.					

ship to health problems must be interpreted with caution. However, the findings of one large-scale study, the National Food Consumption Survey of 1977–78 (U.S. Department of Agriculture, 1980), shed some light on the range of potential dietary problems that exist in American diets and helped to highlight certain problem nutrients and the populations most at risk for deficiencies or excess intake.

This study included data representing three-day average dietary intakes of energy (calories) and 12 nutrients in a sample of 37,785 individuals. Intakes were calculated and expressed as a percentage of the 1980 RDA. Subjects were grouped into 22 different sex/age groups; "problem nutrients" were those identified with average intakes below 70% of the RDA in a sizable proportion of any sex/age group. Using this criterion, dietary intakes of calcium, iron, magnesium, and vitamin B6 are problematic for certain groups of Americans.

Calcium Calcium intakes of females 15 to 18 and 34 to 64 years old averaged 66% of the RDA, with other groups of females over 12 years of age averaging 70% to 76%. Men and children had average intakes of 90% or more. Nearly one-half of all females over 12 years of age were in the group showing lowest intake of calcium, as were one-third of males 35 years or older. Those subjects with high intakes of calcium tended to get it from dairy products, and those with low intakes of calcium obtained it largely through grain products.

Iron Intakes of children 1 to 2 years old averaged 55% of their RDA; of this group, 82% had intakes below 70% of the RDA. Females 12 to 50 years old had mean intakes of about 60% of their RDA; about 70% of this group had low intakes (below 70% of the RDA). In infant subjects, those with highest iron intakes received it from milk and fortified grain products. For all other subjects, major sources were meat, eggs and grain products.

Magnesium Females 12 to 22 years of age averaged intakes of 67% of the RDA; up to two-thirds of females over 12 years of age had low intakes (less than 70% of the RDA). Other group average intakes ranged from 77% to 88% of the RDA. About 40% of males 12 to 22 years of age and over 74 years had low intakes of magnesium. Among children and teenagers, milk and milk products and grain products accounted for most magnesium intake. Among adults, the meat/egg group was a far more important source of magnesium.

Vitamin B6 Females over 14 years of age averaged intakes of 61% of the RDA for vitamin B6; about 70% of these had intakes categorized as low. Males over 75 years of age averaged 68% of the RDA. About 40% of young and middle-aged men had intakes in the lowest category. For children and adolescent boys with high intakes, the meat/egg group and grains were the most important sources of vitamin B6. Among teenage girls and women with low intakes (nearly 70%), the meat/egg group was the major source, with grains much less important.

Vitamins A and C Vitamin A intakes were in the low category for about 35% of teenagers and most groups of adults. Among subjects with highest intakes of vitamin A, the most important sources were dark green and deep yellow vegetables. Among children with lowest intakes, the milk group was the most important source. About 25% of preschoolers, 26% of men, and 32% of women had low intakes of vitamin C. Of those with high intakes of vitamin C, the most important sources were from the citrus/tomato group.

Dietary intakes of these essential nutrients were compared according to demographic characteristics as well. A higher proportion of people in the south had low intakes of these nutrients when compared to other regions. Overall, Blacks more frequently had low intakes of these nutrients than did whites. Low-income groups showed intakes most often in the low category on all nutrients except iron.

Nutritional Risk Factors in Young and Middle-Aged Adults

Nutritional risk factors can readily be identified among young and middle-aged adults in the United States, both because of dietary patterns associated with the "American lifestyle" and because of developmental events, such as childbearing. Overall, the following are considered major dietary risk factors affecting many young and middle-aged adults; some of these dietary risk factors will be discussed in more detail.

- Inadequate food intake
- Weight loss diets
- Lack of fruits and vegetables
- Inadequate intake of vitamin C
- Strict vegetarian diets (inadequate vitamin B$_{12}$)
- Inadequate or excess fiber intake
- Excessive intake of sugar, fat, cholesterol, sodium, or alcohol
- Fad dieting
- Lack of variety in food intake
- Inadequate intake of vitamin A
- Inadequate food sources of iron and calcium
- Excessive food intake
- Excessive use of nutritional supplements

Problems with Caloric Intake   The National Food Consumption Survey also examined caloric intakes on the same large sample of Americans that were examined for nutrient problems. One-fourth of all subjects had caloric intakes over the RDA, and one-third had intakes below the RDA. The latter group was heavily represented by women from 19 to 50 years of age. Of all subjects reporting low calorie intake, intakes of 40% to 60% of the RDA for essential nutrients

was not uncommon. This suggests that the long-range implications of low-calorie diets may be seen in disorders related to chronic nutrient deficiencies, especially in adolescent women who adopt low-calorie diets as they are completing their physical growth.

In terms of caloric intake, fat has been of special concern because of possible associations with heart disease and obesity. Findings showed that about one-fourth of this population obtained 45% or more of their food energy from fat (compared to current recommendations of 30%). This trend was especially evident in the population seen to be at high risk for heart disease—men from 35 to 64 years of age; over one-third of this group obtained 45% or more of their food energy from fat.

The Special Problem of Obesity   Obesity is usually defined as body weight in excess of 20% of desirable weight for height and age. Obesity may be described as an American epidemic, affecting one-fourth of the population as a whole. However, it affects certain groups more than others; 60% of black women between 45 and 55 years of age are obese, compared to 30% of white women of the same age. Obesity is six times more prevalent among those in the lowest socioeconomic strata. It may be that social pressures against being overweight among the more affluent may be effective in reducing incidence of obesity.

Morbid or gross obesity (40% or more above desirable weight) has long been related to poor health. It has long been thought that the obese are prone to a variety of diseases, such as hypertension, adult-onset diabetes, hypercholesterolemia, hypertriglyceridemia, heart disease, cancer, cholecystitis, arthritis, and gout. Life spans also tend to be shorter among those with significant obesity. However, in recent years some experts have claimed that even moderate degrees of overweight present a pervasive health hazard and that this threat becomes apparent at 20% or more above ideal weight.

However, other interpretations of the evidence suggest that only two of the leading causes of mortality in the United States have direct relationships to overweight: hypertension and diabetes (Andres, 1980). Further, there is no agreement about the threshold at which ill effects of obesity begin. In fact, investigators have found that health risks are as great, if not greater, in the very thin when compared to obese groups; extremely thin and extremely fat persons do have overall higher mortality rates than those at the middle of the range of body weight (Kannel, Gordon, 1979).

Although risk is increased at the extremes of body weight, it appears that the multitude of health problems attributed to moderate amounts of overweight are unfounded. Further, there is some confusion about the use of weight standards themselves. The most frequently used tables are those compiled by the Metropolitan Life Insurance Company, in which the "desirable" weights by height are based on mortality data. There are two versions of these tables: one published in 1959 and the latest in 1983. In the 1983 tables, desirable weights for the shortest men are 12 pounds heavier than in the 1959 table, and weights for the shortest women are 14 pounds heavier than in the 1959 table.

In February 1984, a 14-member panel of physicians and nutritionists was assembled to evaluate the health risks of overweight and obesity. They concluded that the 1983 tables should be used to evaluate appropriateness of weight for height, except in patients who already have disorders that are aggravated by excess weight, in which case the more stringent 1959 standards should be used. This panel defined obesity as exceeding the desirable weight for height by 20% and concluded that health hazards become significant at this level. By these standards, some 34 million American adults (or one out of five people over 19 years of age) are obese; of those, 11 million qualify as "severely obese," exceeding their desirable weight by 40% or more (Wallis, 1985).

Nutritional Risk Factors in the Elderly

Vitamin deficiencies are common in older people who do not eat a variety of fruits and vegetables and who have inadequate protein and overall calorie intakes. Overuse of laxatives, impaired secretion of bile, and impaired nutrient absorption also contribute to vitamin deficiencies.

Other studies have suggested that the elderly are especially at risk for other nutrient deficiencies. Two studies of low-income elderly showed widespread folacin and zinc deficiencies; in many cases where anemia was present, iron levels in the diet were normal, but folacin was deficient (National Institute on Aging, 1980).

Overall nutritional status of the elderly in the United States is compounded by several risk factors related to socioeconomic status and physical health. Many elderly are at nutritional risk by virtue of low income, solitary living with little available outside support, high stress levels, and relative inactivity. In addition, the elderly are especially likely to experience illness and infection, which negatively affects eating patterns while increasing nutritional needs. Medical therapy also plays a role in nutritional risk among the elderly; the higher the dose and the longer the duration of therapy, the more likely it is that medication will affect nutritional status. Finally, changes associated with aging, such as poor dentition and changes in body weight, place the elderly at particular nutritional risk.

Dietary Patterns and Their Influence in Disease

Finding ways to avoid or postpone the onset of disease is a prominent aspect of the "wellness" trend today. Unfortunately, much misinformation is promulgated under the theme of disease prevention, often motivated by the profit motive in the sale of books, magazines, food products, or special dietary treatments or supplements.

In addition, the picture is further clouded by disagreement, even among well-respected scientific groups. Some suggest that adulthood is too late to begin making dietary changes to prevent disease and that changes must occur earlier, during childhood or even infancy, to be effective. Others point out that considerable research evidence has accumulated that implicates certain dietary practices in adulthood as risk factors in the development of major diseases such as coronary artery disease, cancer, and hypertension.

Dietary Factors and Cancer One approach has been to compile summaries of epidemiologic and animal model research findings on the relationship between diet and disease. On the basis of this type of investigation, there is some evidence that dietary patterns may assist in preventing disease, such as inclusion of certain nutrients or foods that may provide protection from forms of cancer. For instance, the following dietary factors have been found to be associated with level of cancer risk (American Cancer Society, 1984; Ames, 1983; Feinstein et al, 1982; Hodges, 1982; International Collaborative Group, 1982; Mettlin, 1984; Phillips, Snowdon, 1983; Willett, MacMahon, 1984):

- *Factors associated with increased cancer risk*

  High caloric intake
  High intake of fat, protein, or meat
  Alcohol ingestion
  Naturally occurring carcinogens such as aflatoxin, caffeine, and nitrates
  Food mutagens such as flavonoids and cooking products
  Food additives, including colors, nitrates, and artificial sweeteners (cyclamates and saccharin)
  Food contaminants, including packaging materials (polyvinyl chloride), polychlorinated

biphenyls (PCBs), and organochlorine pesticides

- *Factors associated with decreased cancer risk*

  High fiber intake
  High intake of vitamins A, C, and E and selenium, carotene-rich vegetables, cruciferous vegetables (cabbage, broccoli)
  Use of anti-oxidant food additives

These various research findings, many of which are suggesting a relationship between dietary patterns and certain forms of cancer, have been translated into dietary guidelines proposed by the National Academy of Science's Committee on Diet, Nutrition and Cancer (1982) to be "consistent with good nutritional practices and likely to reduce the risk of cancer":

1. Reduce fat intake from the present average of 40% to 30% of caloric intake to reduce the risk of breast and colon cancer associated with high-fat diets.

2. Include fruits, vegetables, and whole grain cereal products; emphasize especially citrus fruits, carotene-rich vegetables, and vegetables of the cruciferous family. Supplements of individual nutrients are not recommended.

3. Minimize consumption of salt-cured, pickled, and smoked foods, including hot dogs, smoked sausages, and smoked fish.

4. Minimize contamination of foods with carcinogens from any source (including intentional food additives).

5. Identify and avoid carcinogenic mutagens in food.

6. Consume alcoholic beverages in moderation because alcohol, especially combined with cigarette smoking, has been associated with increased cancer risk.

However, it must be recognized that the role of nutrition in disease prevention is just now becoming better understood; research in this area is ongoing, and future findings are likely to change or at least refine current concepts. The complexity of research into the relationship of nutrition to disease is shown clearly in current knowledge about dietary factors associated with hypertension.

Dietary Factors and Hypertension   The relationship between dietary intake and development of hypertension in adulthood has been the subject of scientific investigation for many years. Several dietary factors, including sodium intake, obesity, magnesium and calcium intake, alcohol consumption, and polyunsaturated fats in the diet, have been implicated in the pathogenesis of hypertension with varying degrees of certainty.

A large body of evidence suggests that dietary sodium plays a particularly important part in the development of hypertension; yet there is also convincing evidence that some individuals are sodium-sensitive and others are not. The data on the role of these other dietary factors is also suggestive but, at best, preliminary.

It is clear, however, that obesity exacerbates hypertension, and few would disagree that weight loss is an effective treatment for most obese hypertensive individuals. Dietary treatment has become a mainstay of nonpharmacologic therapy for hypertension. Present recommendations include decreasing dietary sodium by reducing processed foods and added salt; losing weight, if obese, by decreasing caloric intake, increasing activity, and improving eating habits; increasing potassium intake through increased intake of fruits, vegetables and juices; increasing dietary fiber with whole grains, fruits, and vegetables; and increasing the proportion of unsaturated fats in the diet by limiting animal fat.

Dietary Factors and Coronary Artery Disease
The difficulty in establishing a clear relationship between dietary factors and disease is also evident in the investigations linking consumption of saturated fats with elevated cholesterol and coronary artery disease. The Select Committee on Nutrition and Human Needs of the U.S. Senate (1977) specified dietary goals for Americans to reduce dietary fat intake because of its association with coronary artery disease (CAD). This was soon followed by similar statements from the Surgeon General, the Department of Health, Education and Welfare, and the Department of Agriculture. Together these reports seemed to establish public health policy on the role of dietary fat intake in coronary heart disease. These conclusions were further confirmed by recent reviews (Epstein, 1977; Lewis, 1980) and by recommendations of noted authorities (Norum, 1978) and professional groups (Blackburn, 1979) throughout the world.

These conclusions, however, are not universally accepted. The most notable dissenting view, that of the National Academy of Science (1980), opposed the universal promotion of fat-controlled diets on the grounds that a causal relationship between dietary fat and CAD had not been conclusively established. Hulley et al (1981) stated that this view is difficult to dismiss since the evidence linking dietary fats to CAD is largely circumstantial. They went on, however, to point out that the evidence is also very extensive, that there is no reason to believe that more convincing findings are likely to be forthcoming, and that some closure on the argument is needed.

It remains the responsibility of the individual clinician to judge whether or not a given patient is likely to benefit from a fat-controlled diet. When dietary intervention is seen as desirable, the following considerations must be kept in mind (Hulley et al, 1981). First, total serum cholesterol, the most widely available test, should continue to be used as a guide. Middle-aged patients with total serum cholesterol levels higher than 210 mg/dL are more likely to benefit from dietary counseling. Other risk factors such as hypertension, cigarette smoking, low levels of high-density lipoprotein, low physical activity, and male gender are relevant because of the multiplicative effects of these risk factors.

Dietary intervention may be particularly important among those who have already had a heart attack because there appears to be a relatively high risk of recurrence, even with lower serum cholesterol levels than were present at the time of the first attack, perhaps because of the presence of advanced coronary arteriosclerosis (Coronary Drug Project Research Group, 1978). Altering serum cholesterol levels among the elderly, who are at particularly high risk for CAD, may not be effective if advanced coronary arteriosclerosis has already developed. Because primary prevention can be started before atherogenesis begins, young people may be prime targets for dietary intervention because good habits learned early may last a lifetime.

Table 6-2 shows the chief points of a fat-controlled diet, giving examples of common high-fat foods, the associated rise in serum cholesterol, and a suitable low-fat substitute, with the resultant drop in serum cholesterol. As noted, foods that raise serum cholesterol levels the most are those with the highest amounts of saturated fat and cholesterol: meats and animal fat, organ meats, butter, and egg yolks.

Future Directions for Nutritional Care of Individuals and Families

Major health problems and the leading causes of death in the United States are diet-related, and their impact could be diminished by improvements in diet. Significant benefits to individual and family well-being could be realized both from new knowledge of nutrient and food needs and from more complete application of existing knowledge.

Early adjustment of diet could prevent the development of conditions such as obesity, hypertension, and coronary artery disease. Minor changes in diet and food habits instituted in the family when children are young might well

avoid the need for major changes that are likely to be more difficult to accept later in life. The most important influence that caregivers can have on a child's nutritional status is to assist him or her in developing sound eating habits. Family circumstances, advertising, and peer influence all contribute to the process of nutritional socialization.

Dietary recommendations for Americans of all ages today stress a wide variety of high-nutrient-density foods. Children may be influenced more by peer pressures and advertising as well as by the dramatic growth demands of adolescence. Adults are likely to be strongly influenced by physiologic factors and by psychologic factors such as a sense of self-responsibility, stress, economic pressures, use of alcohol and tobacco, and nutritional quackery. Although all age and gender groups would benefit from implementation of dietary recommendations, the lower socioeconomic groups would benefit most from this application of current knowledge.

Evaluation of the nutritional status of an individual (that is, the condition of health of the individual as influenced by intake and use of nutrients) permits early intervention both through treatment of established malnutrition and through prevention of nutritional problems in those known to be at high risk. A complete nutritional evaluation of each patient should be obtained by clinical biochemical, anthropometric, and dietary assessment. Nutritional assessment techniques and their use in nutritional support of patients is receiving increasing attention in the scientific literature (Blackburn et al, 1977; Zerfas et al, 1977; Christakis, 1973).

Influences of Economic Conditions on Nutritional Care

Cost pressures in the health care delivery system are endemic, and increases in costs continue to be explosive. Professional nutrition services, which were provided until recently by federal and state funding (Egan, Kaufman, 1985), are

Table 6–2 General Precepts of a Fat-Controlled Diet, with Examples to Indicate the Relative Impact Each Food Change Might Have on Serum Cholesterol Levels

General Precepts	Example of a High-Fat Food*	Approximate Contribution to Serum Cholesterol If Eaten Daily† (mg/dL)	Example of a Fat-Controlled Food	Approximate Contribution to Serum Cholesterol If Eaten Daily† (mg/dL)	Approximate Change in Serum Cholesterol Level (mg/dL)
1. Trim all visible fat	6 oz untrimmed choice porterhouse steak	38	6 oz. trimmed choice porterhouse steak	16	– 22
2. Substitute fish or chicken for beef, pork & lamb	4 oz lamb chop	20	4 oz skinned chicken	7	– 13
3. Eliminate organ meats (liver, kidney, heart, brain, and sweetbreads)	3 oz liver	28	3 oz tuna	5	– 23
4. Substitute polyunsaturated oils for solid cooking fats and monounsaturated oils	1 oz bacon fat or lard	9	1 oz safflower oil	9	– 18
5. Substitute polyunsaturated margarine for butter	1 oz butter	15	1 oz polyunsaturated margarine	2	– 17
6. Substitute egg whites for whole eggs	1 whole egg	19	1 egg white	0	– 19
7. Substitute low-fat desserts for ice cream	4 oz ice cream	8	4 oz skim yogurt	0	– 8
8. Choose lean meats	4 oz hamburger (35% fat)	25	4 oz hamburger (10% fat)	12	– 13
9. Substitute low-fat cheese for regular cheese	2 oz cheddar cheese	12	2 oz low-fat cheese	2	– 10
10. Substitute skim milk for regular milk	½ pint whole milk	5	½ pint skim milk	0	– 5

*The foods listed here were selected because they are common parts of the American diet and because they have a relatively strong influence in raising cholesterol levels. We have not included processed combinations of food (such as hot dogs), whose effects will depend on their ingredients, nor foods that are rare or have little influence on serum cholesterol. Grains, fruits and vegetables are omitted because they do not raise serum cholesterol levels unless eaten in quantities sufficient to induce obesity (exception: coconut).

†The average contribution of each food, if it were eaten daily, is calculated as $2.16S - 1.65P + 0.0677C - 0.5$, where S = % of calories from saturated fat, P = % of calories from polyunsaturated fat, and C = mg of dietary cholesterol per day. This simplified formula is based on metabolic ward studies of the effects of varying dietary composition while calories are kept constant, and it projects averages that do not reflect the possibility of biologic variability among individual persons in their responses to a given food.

Reprinted by permission of the *Western Journal of Medicine*. From Hulley BS et al: Epidemiology as a guide to clinical decisions, II: Diet and coronary heart disease. (July) 1981; 135:25–33.

being cut. Research should now be directed at questions such as the effect of the projected physician surplus on the use of nutritional specialists and on nutritional care; the relative costs and benefits of using other health care providers for nutritional care in the place of physicians, nutritionists, and dietitians; and the implications these changes will have on the quality of nutritional care provided to individuals and families.

Home health care services are on the increase and with them, the need for nutritional services in the community. The need for such services within a home health care agency was demonstrated in one study of 812 patients cared for by a visiting nurse agency, of which 52% had been prescribed therapeutic diets (Gaffney, Singer, 1985). This in itself is not surprising; however, very few such agencies employ registered dietitians, and on examination of this same patient case load, registered dietitians recommended therapeutic diets for 77% of the patient population, based on diagnosis, height, and weight. Further, when the dietitians examined the therapeutic diets as ordered by the referring physician, in 47% of cases the patient might have benefited from a diet different from the one ordered. The results of this study emphasize the need for collaboration between health care providers in order to ensure that the nutritional needs of individuals and families are being met.

Summary

The nutrition specialist is the best-qualified individual to support the family in making adjustments in dietary patterns throughout the life cycle. The importance of nutritional counseling is increasingly recognized in the design of new forms of health care delivery; for example, dietary counseling is specifically included in regulations governing hospice care for the terminally ill patient. In theory, this care should be provided by dietitians and nutritionists; in practice, nurses, aides, and health educators also provide nutritional care.

Issues for Further Investigation

1. What are the changes in family structure and function resulting from immigration that affect family nutrition status?

2. How do family members use food as a mechanism to interact with one another (for example, anorexia, bulimia)?

3. To what extend do social customs influence family traditions regarding eating patterns?

4. How does family nutrition status change throughout each family developmental stage?

5. How are dietary prescriptions as a result of illness or disease adapted to take into consideration family cultural practices and beliefs in daily living?

References

American Cancer Society (1984): Nutrition and cancer—Cause and prevention. *American Cancer Society Special Reports*, 34(2):121.

Ames BN (1983): Dietary carcinogens and anticarcinogens: Oxygen radicals and degenerative diseases. *Science*, 221:1256.

Andres R (1980): Effect of obesity on total mortality. *Int J Obes*, 4:381.

Blackburn GL et al (1977): Nutritional and metabolic assessment of the hospitalized patient. *J Parenter Enteral Nutr*, 1:11.

Blackburn HB (1979): Diet and mass hyperlipidemia: A public health view. In: *Nutrition, Lipids and CHD*, Levy R et al (eds.). New York: Raven.

Christakis G (1973): Nutritional assessment in health programs. *Am J Public Health, 63*:1

Committee on Diet, Nutrition and Cancer, National Research Council (1982): *Diet, Nutrition, and Cancer.* Washington, DC: National Academy Press.

Coronary Drug Project Research Group (1978): Natural history of myocardial infarction in the CDP: Long-term prognostic importance of serum lipid levels. *Am J Cardiol, 42*:489–498.

Crapo PA, Kolterman OG, Olefsky J (1980): Effects of oral fructose in normal, diabetic, and impaired glucose tolerance subjects. *Diabetes Care, 3*:575–581.

Department of Agriculture, Department of Health and Human Services (1985): *Nutrition and Your Health: Dietary Guidelines for Americans.* (2nd ed.). U.S. GPO.

Egan MC, Kaufman M (1985): Financing nutrition services in a competitive market. *J Am Diet Assoc, 85*(2):210–215.

Epstein FH (1977): Preventive trials and the "diet-heart" question: Wait for results or act now? *Atherosclerosis, 26*:515–523.

Feinstein AR et al (1982): Coffee and pancreatic cancer: The problems of etiologic science and epidemiologic case-control research. *JAMA, 246*:957.

Gaffney JT, Singer GR (1985): Diet needs of patients referred to home health. *J Am Diet Assoc, 85*(2):199–202.

Handbook of Agricultural Charts (1981): Food expenditures and income relationship. Agriculture Handbook No. 592, U.S. Department of Agriculture, Washington, DC. Chart 82.

Hodges RE (1982): Vitamin C and cancer. *Nutr Rev, 40*:289.

Hulley SB et al (1981): Epidemiology as a guide to clinical decisions. II: Diet and coronary heart disease. *West J Med, 135* (July):25–33.

International Collaborative Group (1982): Circulating cholesterol level and risk of death from cancer in men ages 40–69 years. *JAMA, 248*:2853.

Kannel WB, Gordon T (1979): Physiological and medical concomitants of obesity: The Framingham study. In: *Obesity in America,* Bray GA (ed.). DHEW (NIH) 79–359. Washington, DC: GPO.

Lewis B (1980): Dietary prevention of ischemic heart disease: A policy for the 80s. *Br Med J, 3*:177–180.

Melville MB (1980): *Twice a Minority: Mexican-American Women.* St. Louis, MO: Mosby.

Mettlin C (1984): Diet and the epidemiology of human breast cancer. *Cancer, 53*:605.

National Academy of Science and the National Research Council (1980): *Recommended Dietary Allowances,* 9th ed. Washington, DC: Food and Nutrition Board, National Academy of Sciences, National Research Council.

National Institute on Aging, U.S. Department of Health and Human Services (1980): Supplemental zinc, taste and health in aging women: Special report on aging, p. 26.

Norum KR (1978): Some present concepts concerning diet and prevention of CHD. *Nutrition and Metabolism, 22*:1–7.

Pangborn RM (1964, November): Speaking of color, from your home advisor. Anaheim: University of California, Cooperative Extension Service.

Phillips RL, Snowdon DA (1983): Association of meat and coffee use with cancers of the large bowel, breast, and prostate among Seventh-Day Adventists: Preliminary results. *Cancer Res, 43* (Suppl.): 2403.

Rodin J (1981): Current status of the internal–external hypothesis for obesity: What went wrong? *Am Psychol, 36*:361–372.

Rodin J (1985): Insulin levels, hunger and food intake: An example of feedback loops in body weight regulation. *Health Psychol, 4*(1):1–24.

Schachter S (1968): Obesity and eating. *Science, 161*:751–756.

Schafer RB, Keith PM (1981): Influences on food decisions across the family life cycle. *J Am Diet Assoc, 78*(2):144–148.

Select Committee on Nutrition and Human Needs, U.S. Senate (1977): Dietary goals for the United States, 2nd ed. Washington, DC: GPO.

Spitzer L (1983): The effects of type of sugar ingested on subsequent eating behavior. Unpublished doctoral dissertation, Yale University.

U.S. Department of Agriculture (1980): Food and nutrient intakes of individuals in 1 day in the United States, Spring 1977. *Nationwide Food Consumption Survey, 1977–78.* Preliminary report no. 2, Hyattsville, MD: U.S. Department of Agriculture, Consumer Nutrition Center.

Wallis C (1985): Gauging the fat of the land: Risks of overweight. *Time, 125* (February 25):72.

Ward S, Wackman O (1972): Television advertising and intrafamily influence. Children's purchase influence attempts and parental yielding. *Television and Social Behavior Vol 4.* Washington, DC: US DHEW.

Willett WC, MacMahon B (1984): Diet and cancer: An overview. *N Engl J Med, 310:*633.

Zerfas AJ, Shorr IJ, Neumarin CG (1977): Office assessment of nutritional status. *Pediatr Clin North Am, 24:*254.

7

THE FAMILY AND THE COMMUNITY
Mobilizing Social Support

Hester Y. Kenneth, RN, DNSc

Social support networks within communities are an important source of resources to families in times of need. Without social support networks, families lack an important aspect of health maintenance. This chapter discusses the power of social support to improve the health of the family, and examines the ways in which family processes and behaviors interact with the social network.

Hester Kenneth, a nurse researcher at Stanford University Hospital, has focused her academic career on community health nursing, with special emphasis on health-promoting behaviors and social support networks.

Introduction

In nursing, the majority of our efforts have been directed to individuals—the clients to whom we provide direct care in institutional settings. As illustrated by the wealth of the theoretical, empirical, and clinical chapters in this volume, nursing interest in the family as a unit of health care has increased geometrically since the early 1970s. This interest has focused primarily on families' internal structures, functions, and processes and only minimally on the family in its social context.

In a recent review of nursing research on the family, Feetham (1984) called attention to the conceptual limitations of much of family research and noted that relatively few family studies are grounded in a theoretical or conceptual model, a factor that has limited the utility of their findings. She further noted that in those studies based on a conceptual model, only partial models with a single or a small number of variables have been examined. There is a need to examine the family in its wider social context in order to determine the range and complexity of factors influencing family health and illness responses and to develop intervention strategies. Exploration of the family in its community context is facilitated by examining it as one component of a social network.

The origins of social network theory lie in anthropology and sociology. Of particular note is Bott's (1955) classic study of 20 urban families in which conjugal role relationships were found to be influenced by the degree of "connectedness" in the network in which the family was imbedded.

Health and social science interest in social network and social support has paralleled the growing attention to the clinical and research interest in the family. Suchman (1964) explored social group influences on health behavior among a probability sample of 2215 urban families and determined that the network aspects of social organization were more closely related to health knowledge, attitudes, and responses than was ethnicity. Comprehensive review articles by Cassel and Cobb (1976) presented cumulative evidence of the relationships between the social environment and a wide variety of disease outcomes. The interest generated was heightened by developing epidemiologic knowledge of the multifactorial causes and the complex processes contributing to health and illness. Research focused on factors mediating disease occurrence, including social network and social support.

Because a number of excellent review articles (Broadhead et al, 1983; Heller, 1979; Mitchell, Trickett, 1980; Norbeck, 1981; Wallston et al, 1983) discuss the development of knowledge about and the controversies related to social support and social network, this chapter describes the current status of knowledge in the field, focuses on its relationship to family research, and discusses the major issues related to integration of theory and research on the family with that on social support and social network.

Definitions

A major dilemma in this evolving interest area is that social support and social network are defined and measured in a number of different ways. Weiss (1974) described six components of social support: attachment or intimacy, social integration, nurturance, worth, alliance, and guidance. Caplan (1974) emphasized the importance of feedback and reciprocity. Cobb (1976) defined social support as "information leading the subject to believe that he is cared for and loved, esteemed, and a member of a network of mutual obligations" (p. 300). Porritt (1979) defined social support as empathic undertanding, respect, and constructive genuineness. Kahn (1979) discussed social support as a multidimensional transactional phenomenon that includes one or more of the following: affect (liking), affirmation (agreement, acknowledgement of rightness), or aid (assistance, monetary or social). Kahn's definition is unique in its focus on the structural aspects of the social network as a whole—size, homogeneity, symmetry, and connectedness. Kahn and Antonucci (1980) described properties of the dyadic links between the individuals such as interaction, frequency, type, magnitude, initiative, range, duration, and capacity. These authors use the term *convoy* to convey the complex construction of the substantive, spatial, and temporal dimensions of social support. The convoy approach is helpful for identifying the way in which different types of social support may operate in different situations at different times in the life cycle.

Social Support

Social support is defined as a dynamic multidimensional construct that is affected by both the person and the situational variables (Norbeck, 1981). Social support refers to the functional and source dimensions of the construct, to the kinds of support available to the focal person, and to the persons who provide the support—partner, family member, neighbor, friend, work associate and so forth. Currently the social support construct is defined as having distinct expressive and instrumental properties. The expressive component—also called emotional, affect, or psychologic support—includes those interactions that provide acceptance and understanding. The instrumental or tangible component of social support includes provision of both material aid, such as financial assistance or a ride to the doctor, and information or guidance, such as childrearing advice.

Social Network

The social network construct is closely related to social support but is seen as distinct from it. *Social network* refers to the structural aspects of the construct: size or range, network diversity, and connectedness. Mitchell and Trickett (1980) summarized the characteristics of the component linkages in social networks as intensity, durability, multidimensionality, directedness or reciprocity, relationship density, dispersion, frequency, and homogeneity. An individual's social network consists of those relatives, friends, neighbors, coworkers, and other acquaintances with whom one interacts. Each member of a family has a personal social network, and collectively these networks make up the family social network (Unger, Powell, 1980).

Conceptual Issues

Several reviews (Heller, 1979; Thoits, 1982; Tilden, 1985; Wallston et al, 1983) have highlighted the conceptual and methodologic issues related to social support and social network. The issues discussed here are those of particular salience to family research and clinical nursing practice.

Although early discussions of the health-related aspects of social support treated it as a global variable, current theoretical emphasis is on determining specific dimensions of the construct and answers to such questions as:

- Is it the quality or quantity of support that influences outcomes?

- What are the effects of different sources of support?

- What types and sources of support are most effective and in what situations?

- How do personal and demographic characteristics influence social support?

- How do the types or sources of support vary over the life span?

- How does social support vary with the family's developmental level?

- What are the costs as well as the benefits of social support?

To achieve conceptual fit between the conceptual–theoretic framework and the operationalization of variables in a study, it is necessary to differentiate between subjective and objective measures of social support and social network. Subjective measures determine the functional dimensions of support perceived by the focal person. Objective measures assess the structure or network dimensions of the construct, and these may be observed.

In the health sciences, research has focused more on the functional, or support, aspects of the network than on its structural, or quantitative, aspects. Determination of the sources as well as types of support has significant health-related implications, and it is necessary for the development of social support interventions in clinical nursing practice. For research on the family in its social context, it is necessary to measure the structural dimensions of the sources of support and their functions in specific situations. In other words, we need to know who does what for whom and under what conditions or circumstances.

Personal variations in the need for social support and the composition of the social network have been identified (Kahn, Antonucci, 1980; Norbeck, 1985; Wallston et al, 1983). Heller (1979) identified individual variations in the need for social affiliation and social competence as potential alternative explanations for the effects of social support. Demographic variables such as age, sex, and marital status also seem to affect access to, development of, and use of social support and the composition of the social network (Heller, 1979; Norbeck, 1985; Wilcox, 1981). Of particular significance for family study, ethnic variations in the need for social support have also been noted (Wallston et al, 1983).

There is evidence that there is a longitudinal dimension to social support and social network, and the term *convoy* is useful for describing the variations in the types and sources of social support at different stages of the life cycle (Kahn, Antonucci, 1980). In addition, there is some indication that there are differences in the social resources that are most helpful during the course of coping and adjustment to life transitions such as parenthood (Richardson, Kagan, 1979; Cronenwett, 1985) and bereavement (Walker, McBride, Vachon, 1977).

Although many writers (Di Matteo, Hays, 1981; Wallston et al, 1983) noted that social relationships have stressful or negative dimensions, the definitions and measures of social support focus only on the positive aspects of the construct. Failure to examine the stressful, enervating, or time-consuming "costs" of social interactions leads to a "theoretical myopia," which prevents development of instruments to measure the negative aspects of support (Tilden, Stewart, 1985).

This issue has particular relevance to nursing research and supports the need to consider the family in its social context. In some situations, individuals' relationships with family ties contribute to their problems (Horwitz, 1978; Liem, Liem, 1978). For example, some kinds of support during rehabilitation or in the long-term management of chronic illness may create dependency (Croog, 1970; Garrity, 1973). Conversely, families may experience stress and exhaustion from their involvement with dependent, aging, or chronically or mentally ill members (Di Matteo, Hays, 1981)

As the health care system in the United States is becoming community rather than institution based, the development of reliable and valid instruments for comprehensive clinical and research assessment of both individual and family social resources becomes a major priority. We need to assess the costs and benefits of all persons in supportive transactions, both receivers and providers (Wallston et al, 1983). To improve the quality of life for the family unit in nursing, we must examine both the negative and the positive dimensions of family relationships and explore community resources to assist families to achieve and maintain equilibrium.

Measurement

As is often true in an evolving field, social support and social network have been operationalized in as many ways as there are investigators. This makes comparability among studies a formidable task. A psychometric review (Rock et al, 1984) of the properties of the social support and social network scales used in 29 behavioral science studies published between 1967 and 1982 found that with only a few exceptions (Lin, Dean, Ensel, 1981; McFarlane et al, 1981; Norbeck, Lindsey, Carrieri, 1983), few data were reported about issues of scaling, reliability, and validity. Theory development and research efficiency in social support and social network require that more emphasis be placed on development of psychometrically sound instruments (Rock et al, 1984).

Published data is available on two instruments developed by nurse researchers. Brandt and Weinert (1981) based the Personal Resource Questionnaire (PRQ) on Weiss's (1974) conceptualization of social relationships. Part one of the PRQ assesses a person's social resources available for specific situations. Part two measures five of Weiss's (1974) relational dimensions: intimacy, social integration, nurturance, worth, and assistance. The authors reported a high level of internal consistency and moderate levels of predictive validity for the tool. Continuing evaluation is in progress (Norbeck, Lindsey, Carrieri, 1983).

The Norbeck Social Support Questionnaire (NSSQ) (Norbeck, Lindsey, Carrieri, 1981; 1983) uses Kahn's convoy construct as its conceptual framework. Designed to be self-administered, it assesses up to 20 network members by asking respondents to "list each significant person in your life" and then to indicate on a Likert scale the level of support from each person listed. The NSSQ measures functional dimensions or types of social support, expressive or instrumental; several properties of network (number, duration of relationship, and frequency of contact); and sources of support in the network (spouse, family member, friend, neighbor, and so forth). Since its introduction in 1980, a series of evaluative studies demonstrated its psychometric properties, high test–retest reliability, internal consistency, and moderate concurrent validity with two other social support measures. The tool's predictive validity has also been established. A distinct advantage of the NSSQ for study of the family in its social or community context is that it measures sources of support from which those most salient at a specific time or in specific situations can be measured.

Sources of Social Support

A classic study by Litwak and Szelenyi (1969) demonstrated that different sources of social support are important in different situations. These authors found that family–kin ties were most useful for long-term commitments such as caring for a member with chronic illness or for shaping values and attitudes. Friendship groups, neighborhood groups, and work groups were found to provide different and supplemental resources to the nuclear family. Friendship groups, based on similarities of age, sex, and stage of the life cycle, were most useful for dealing with changes in social customs and values. Neighbors were most effective for time urgent tasks, such as an emergency ride to the doctor.

Family Support

Several studies found family support to be associated with coping and management of chronic illness (Litman, 1966; De Araujo et al, 1973; Dimond, 1979), adherence to treatment regimen (Oakes et al, 1970; Caplan, Robinson, French, 1976), and adaptations in lifestyle (Heinzelman, Bagley, 1970). For example, family support was associated with the quality of response to rehabilitation among 100 orthopedically disabled patients (Litman, 1966). Perceived family expectation was significantly related to self-reported use of a hand splint by 66 arthritis patients (Oakes et al, 1976). Relatively little is known, however, about the way in which family members influence health behavior or individual adherence to health regimen.

Support from Non-Kin Ties

Other studies demonstrated that support from the network beyond the family may yield other positive outcomes (Granovetter, 1973). In the section that follows, selected studies are discussed to illustrate the contributions of non-kin ties to individual and family health in managing chronic illness and bereavement, in making the transition to parenthood and in childrearing, and in establishing positive health behaviors.

Ties beyond the family serve important informational, normative, and support functions. Finlayson (1976) studied recovery from myocardial infarction in relation to varying levels of social support. Better recovery outcomes were found where support was received from a range of network sources beyond the family of origin. Walker, McBride, and Vachon (1977) examined the role of social networks during the crisis of conjugal bereavement and found that different types of support were needed at different phases of the adaptation process. Intimate ties may be most effective early in the adaptation process, when the bereaved person may need substantial emotional and material assistance. Later, when the bereaved person has worked through acute grief and is ready to renew social contacts, the intimate network, which was helpful earlier in the process, may be less adaptive for resumption of the single role or for introduction to new people.

Both kin and friends contribute in important ways to the transition to the parenthood role. Richardson and Kagan (1979) studied the network properties of size, density, and number of network members providing three kinds of support—encouragement, cognitive guidance, and general socialization—among 40 primi-parous couple pairs with children three to seven months of age. Better psychologic outcomes were found among those couples whose networks were larger and more varied in membership and kinds of support. In contrast, Cronenwett (1985) examined network structure, social support, and psychologic outcomes of pregnancy among 50 married couples and found that relatives predominated in the social networks of both men and women. Women, however, received a greater percentage of emotional support from friends (24%) than did men (15%). Cronenwett noted that relatively few couples described networks in a similar stage of family development.

The variations in the predominant sources of social support found in these studies may be explained by differences in the time the outcomes were measured. Richardson and Kagan (1979) assessed social support three to seven months postpartum, and Cronenwett (1985) measured the outcomes at six weeks postpartum. Support from relatives may be most helpful during the initial transition to parenthood; interaction with network members representing wider and less dense ties may be more helpful during later stages of family development. There is need for systematic exploration of the role that a range of social ties will play in family development over time.

Non-kin ties are also important sources of both expressive and instrumental support during the childrearing years. Cochran and Brassard (1979) found that parents' relationships with friends and neighbors, as well as with kin, influenced performance of the parental role through access to emotional and material assistance, provisions of childrearing controls, and availability of role models. Riley and Cochran (1985) interviewed 96 married and employed fathers of three-year-olds to determine non-spousal sources of childrearing advice and their meanings. Childrearing advice from kin was the most frequent but its content varied less than did the advice from non-kin. The authors suggested that the opportunity to explore different sources of childrearing advice may contribute to the increased involvement of some fathers in childrearing today. "For a man to move beyond the father role modeled by his own father and to join that part of each generation that modifies the social role of the larger society, it may be necessary to seek a wider diversity of social influences and move beyond the domain of kin" (Riley, Cochran, 1985).

In a comparative study of the sources and types of social support in the social networks of 80 Swedish mothers (37 single and 43 married), Tietjen (1985) found that single mothers with the highest levels of support had networks composed largely of friends rather than of relatives, neighbors, and work associates and that it was important to them to maintain a balance of give and take, or "reciprocity," with their network members. In contrast, neighbors were the most important support source for the married mothers, and reciprocity was a less important issue. These findings suggest that nursing assessment of the family in relation to its extended social system of friends, neighbors, and school and work associates holds potential for identifying the means for enhancing family health.

Efforts to foster health promotion behaviors have focused frequently on the individual, sometimes on the family, and less frequently on the community. There is evidence that wider social networks may make an important contribution to participation in positive health behaviors (Coburn, Pope, 1974; Pratt, 1976; Langlie, 1977; Hubbard, Muhlencamp, Brown, 1984). Pratt found that families who coped effectively with health matters had an "energized" pattern of health behavior characterized by extensive and varied ties with the community and its resources. This pattern contributed both to individual members' ability to cope with health matters and to health of the family as a whole (Pratt, 1976). Langlie (1977) found that non-kin interactions contributed to establishment of such risk-reducing behaviors as seat-belt use, exercise par-

ticipation, and positive nutrition behavior. Kenneth (1984) examined the sources of support associated with participation in physical activity among 241 employed subjects ages 25–45 and found that support from peers (friends, neighbors, school and work associates) contributed significantly more to adherence than did family support. Long-term maintenance of positive health behaviors may be enhanced by involvement with friendship ties supportive of the behavior (Kenneth, 1984). This interpretation is consistent with Litwak and Szelenyi's (1969) demonstration that friendship groups provide reference orientation.

For utility in improving the quality of nursing care for families, there is a critical need for nursing research that focuses on the associations among specific family behaviors, their interactions with the social network members, and health and illness responses.

Vignettes from community health nursing (CHN) practice in case management, home care, and hospice situations illustrate some benefits of incorporating the family's social network in their nursing care.

Situation A: Nursing Case Management of a Frail Elderly Couple

Mr. and Mrs. B, a frail elderly couple 92 and 88 years old respectively, lived in a comfortable but modest home in an older section of town. The Bs had spent the majority of their lives in this house and had raised their five children there. Maintaining their independence and living in their own home was extremely important to them. Their children and grandchildren were supportive and visited often, but their efforts to assist their parents in their activities of daily living were rebuffed.

Over the past year, Mr. B had become more and more lethargic and irritable. Mrs. B, his major caretaker, a spritely woman who jealously guarded their independence, refused all outside assistance.

Concerned for Mrs. B's well-being as more and more of her limited energies were consumed by caring for her husband, the private physician referred the family to the local CHN case management program. Critical to effective nursing intervention with this family was comprehensive assessment of family strengths and current needs. These included assessment of the family's current social network and history, as well as their health history and financial status. These revealed that although the couple was presently relatively isolated, they had in the past participated in a number of community activities.

Major needs identified were (1) to provide health supervision, support, and assistance to Mrs. B in her caretaking role; (2) to provide stimulation and health supervision to Mr. B after determining his functional and cognitive abilities; and (3) to assist the couple to take advantage of some of the assistance offers they received from neighbors and friends in their social network while maintaining their independence.

The community health nurse's overall goal with the Bs was to assist them to achieve "supported independence." Only by involvement of members of *their* perceived social network, neighbors, friends, and family members, was this possible. The community health nurse maintained contact with the family through biweekly home visits, timed to alternate with their physician visits. The community health nurse also served as a bridge to other local community agencies, and through her trusting relationship with the Bs was able to assist them to take advantage of services available to help the frail elderly maintain residential independence in the community as long as it was safe for them to do so.

Situation B: Home Care and Hospice Services to a Family with Terminal Illness

The R family was referred to home care *after* Mr. R was diagnosed with metastatic carcinoma of the bowel. The Rs, 78 and 80, married 55 years, had known each other since childhood Sunday School days. Their only child, a son, lived with his wife and his grown family in another city, 500 miles away. They too were fiercely independent and concerned about "needing help," or "taking charity." Their health care was provided by a large Health Maintenance Organization that included a Home Care Program and recently had added hospice care to its range of services.

Although the nursing services of home care were sufficient for providing Mr. R's physical care, the home care nurse encouraged Mrs. R to apply for hospice services so that she could receive much needed respite and support and other hospice services such as equipment use and group and bereavement counseling.

Again Mrs. R was loath to ask for or even to accept help. Neighbors had offered to take her shopping, but she had always refused because she was afraid to leave her husband, believing that his death was imminent.

In her work with the R family, the nurse assisted Mrs. R to identify those people in her network from whom she might consider asking for or receiving assistance. Mrs. R also needed assistance in identifying specific areas in which outside help might be welcome. This was not an easy task. Throughout their marriage, the Rs had been a self-sufficient and independent unit and, except for their strong church affiliation, had few ties to the community in which they had lived for the past 22 years. They maintained close ties to family and friends from the town of their origin on the East Coast.

With the nurse's assistance, Mrs. R identified her need to get to the bank as the major priority, followed by a desire to do a little grocery shopping "to pick out my own things" and get some fresh air.

When a church acquaintance offered to help, Mrs. R was able to respond affirmatively and leave her husband's side for a few hours every week to do some necessary errands and get a brief respite for herself.

At its best, hospice care is organized to provide this kind of respite and support to family members as well as to care for their terminally ill member. Hospice care, however, is still inaccessible in many parts of the United States. Further, current payment mechanisms limit hospice services in time and range of services. Involvement of the family's community support network in their care is often needed both before and after hospice care is formally instituted.

These vignettes illustrate that support from social network members beyond the family is often needed to assist people to manage their care over time. One challenge to nursing is to identify and provide interventions that have sustained impact on family health and well-being.

Summary

There is evidence that different sources of social support are useful in different situations and that ties beyond the family may serve as valuable resources. Integration of family, social support, and social network variables in future studies will provide one means for systematic exploration of the transactions between the social environment and personal and family health. Such research will help provide the necessary foundation for development of nursing intervention strategies to promote family health across the life span.

Issues for Further Investigation

1. Is it the quality or the quantity of support that has the most significant influence on outcomes for the family?

2. What are the differences in the types and sources of support needed during times of crisis as opposed to chronic and long-term situations?

3. What are the effects of different sources of support? For instance, does family as a source of support differ in effect from sources outside the family?

4. How do personal and demographic characteristics influence social support?

5. How do the types and sources of support vary during different stages of family development?

6. What are the costs as well as benefits of social support?

References

Bott E (1955): Urban families: Conjugal roles and social networks. *Human Relations, 8:*345–384.

Brandt PA, Weinert C (1981): The PRQ—a social support measure. *Nurs Res, 32:*4–9.

Broadhead WE et al (1983): The epidemiologic evidence for a relationship between social support and health. *Am J Epidemiol, 117:*521–537.

Caplan G (1974): Support systems. In: *Support Systems and Community Mental Health: Lectures on Concept Development,* Caplan G (ed.). New York: Behavioral Publications, pp. 1–8.

Caplan RD, Robinson EA, French JRP (1976): Adhering to medical regimen: Pilot experiments in patient education and social support. Ann Arbor: Research Center for Group Dynamics, Institute for Social Research, University of Michigan.

Cassel J (1976): The contribution of the social environment to host resistance. *Am J Epidemiol, 104:*107–123.

Cobb SS (1976): Social support as a moderator of life stress. *Psychosom Med, 38:*300–314.

Coburn D, Pope CR (1974): Socio-economic status and preventive health behavior. *J Health Soc Behav, 15:*67–77.

Cochran M, Brassard JA (1979): Child development and personal social networks. *Child Dev, 50:*601–616.

Cronenwett LR (1985): Network structure, social support and psychological outcomes of pregnancy. *Nurs Res, 34:*93–99.

Croog S (1970): The family as a source of stress. In: *Social Stress,* Levine S, Scotch NA (eds.). Chicago: Aldine, pp. 19–53.

DeAraujo G et al (1973): Life change, coping ability, and chronic intrinsic asthma. *J Psychosom Res, 17:*359–363.

Dimond M (1979): Social support and adaptation to chronic illness: The case of maintenance hemodialysis. *Res Nurs Health, 2:*101–108.

Di Matteo MR, Hays R (1981): Social support and serious illness. In: *Social Networks and Social Support,* Gottlieb BH (ed.). Beverly Hills: Sage.

Feetham SL (1984): Family research: Issues and directions for nursing. In: *Annual Review of Nursing Re-*

search Vol 2, Werley HH, Fitzpatrick JJ (eds.). New York: Springer-Verlag.

Finlayson A (1976): Social networks as coping resources. Lay help and consultation patterns used by women in husband's post infarction career. *Soc Sci Med, 10*:97–103.

Garrity TF (1973): Vocational adjustment after first myocardial infarction: Comparative assessment of several variables suggested in the literature. *Soc Sci Med, 7*:705–717.

Granovetter MS (1973): The strength of weak ties. *Am J Soc, 78*:1360–1380.

Heinzelman F, Bagley RW (1970): Response to physical activity programs and their effect on health behavior. *Public Health Rep, 85*:905–911.

Heller K (1979): The effects of social support. Prevention and treatment implications. In: *Maximizing Treatment Gains: Transfer Enhancement in Psychotherapy,* Goldstein A, Kanter FH (eds.). New York: Academic Press.

Horwitz A (1978): Family, kin, and friend networks in psychiatric help-seeking. *Soc Sci Med, 12*: 297–304.

Hubbard P, Muhlencamp AF, Brown N (1984): The relationship between social support and self-care practices. *Nurs Res, 33*:266–270.

Kahn RL (1979): Aging and social support. In: *Aging From Birth to Death: Interdisciplinary Perspectives,* Riley MW (ed.). Boulder, CO: Westview Press for the American Association for the Advancement of Science.

Kahn RL, Antonucci TC (1980): Convoys over the life course: Attachment, roles and social support. In: *Life Span Development and Behavior Vol 3*, Baltes PB, Brim O (eds.). New York: Academic Press.

Kenneth HY (1984a): The benefits, costs and sources of social support associated with establishing and maintaining physical activity among employed adults. Doctoral dissertation, University of California. *Dissertation Abstracts International, 45/09*, 84–25950.

Kenneth HY (1984b): The sources of social support associated with establishing and maintaining physical activity among employed adults: A prospective multivariate study. Abstract, *West J Nurs Res, 6*:81.

Langlie JK (1977): Social networks, health beliefs, and preventive health behavior. *J Health Soc Behav, 18*:244–260.

Liem R, Liem J (1978): Social class and mental illness reconsidered: The role of economic stress and social support. *J Health Soc Behav, 19*:139–156.

Lin N, Dean A, Ensel WM (1981): Social support scales: A methodological note. *Schizophrenia Bulletin, 7*:73–89.

Litman TJ (1966): The family and physical rehabilitation. *J Chronic Dis, 19*:211–217.

Szelenyi T (1969): Primary group structures and their functions: Kin, neighbors, and friends. *Am Soc Rev, 34*:465–481.

McFarlane AH et al (1981): Methodological issues in developing a scale to measure social support. *Schizophrenia Bulletin, 7*:90–100.

Mitchell RE, Trickett EJ (1980): Social networks as mediators of social support. *Community Mental Health J, 16*:27–44.

Norbeck JS (1981): Social support: A model for clinical research and application. *ANS, 3*:43–59.

Norbeck JS (1985): Types and sources of social support for managing job stress in critical care nursing. *Nurs Res, 34*:225–230.

Norbeck JS, Lindsey AM, Carrieri VL (1981): The development of an instrument to measure social support: Phase one. *Nurs Res, 30*:463–469.

Norbeck JS, Lindsey AM, Carrieri VL (1983): Further development of the Norbeck Social Support Questionnaire: Normative data and validity testing. *Nurs Res, 32*:4–9.

Oakes TW et al (1970): Family expectations and arthritis patient compliance to a hand resting splint regimen. *J Chronic Dis, 22*:757–764.

Porritt D (1979): Social support in crisis: Quantity or quality? *Soc Sci Med, 13A*:714–721.

Pratt L (1976): *Family Structure and Effective Health Behavior: The Energized Family.* Boston: Houghton Mifflin.

Richardson MS, Kagan L (1979): Social support and the transition to parenthood. Unpublished paper presented at the American Psychological Association Meeting, New York.

Riley D, Cochran MN (1985): Naturally occurring childrearing advice for fathers: Utilization of the personal social network. *J Marr Fam, 47*:275–286.

Rock DL et al (1984): Social support and social network scales: A psychometric review. *Res Nurs Health, 7*:325–332.

Suchman E (1964): Sociomedical variations among ethnic groups. *Am J Soc, 70*:319–331.

Thoits PA (1982): Conceptual, methodological and theoretical problems in studying social support as a buffer against life stress. *J Health Soc Behav, 23*:145–159.

Tietjen AM (1985): Social network and social support of married and single mothers in Sweden. *J Marr Fam, 47*:489–496.

Tilden VP (1985): Issues of conceptualization and measurement of social support in the construction of nursing theory. *Res Nurs Health, 8*:199–206.

Tilden VP, Stewart BJ (1985): Problems in measuring reciprocity with difference scores. *West J Nurs Res, 7*:381–385.

Unger DG, Powell DR (1980): Supporting families under stress: The role of social networks. *Family Relations, 29*:566.

Walker KN, McBride A, Vachon MLS (1977): Social support networks and the crisis of bereavement. *Soc Sci Med, 11*:35–41.

Wallston BS et al (1983): Social support and physical health. *Health Psychol, 2*:367–391.

Weiss RS (1974): The provision of social relations. In: *Doing Unto Others,* Rubin Z (ed.). Englewood Cliffs, NJ: Prentice-Hall.

Wilcox BL (1981): Social support in adjusting to marital disruption: A network analysis. In: *Social Networks and Social Support Vol 4,* Gottlieb BH (ed.). Beverly Hills: Sage.

8

CULTURE AND FAMILY

Joan Ablon, PhD

Genevieve M. Ames, PhD

Cultural patterns and pressures affect a family's behavioral response to severe health problems. This chapter illustrates this phenomenon by outlining the research findings of a study on Samoan, Irish-American Catholic, and middle-class Protestant families. It also provides a framework encompassing the pluralistic nature of American external society and internal family culture.

Joan Ablon, a Professor in the Medical Anthropology Program at the University of California at San Francisco, shares her expertise with the departments of Epidemiology, International Health, and Psychiatry. She is noted for her anthropological approaches to alcoholism and the impact of dwarfism on the family.

Genevieve Ames, Study Director of the Prevention Research Center at the Pacific Institute for Research and Evaluation in Berkeley, California is known for her qualitative approaches to the study of alcoholism and the family.

Introduction

Family researchers have proposed a distinction between "crisis-proof" and "crisis-prone" families (Hill, Hansen, 1962). We suggest that the cultural patterns of the family play a significant role in determining how families cope with crisis—whether they cope well or poorly. Rarely have researchers or clinicians taken into account the significance of the cultural patterns carried by, developed within, and maintained by individual family units. All families are bearers of the culture of the larger national society within which they live. Likewise, all families develop their own culture, determined by the integration of the roles and personalities of members of an intimate interacting social group. A cognizance of the significance of both external national or ethnic culture and internal family culture is crucial for understanding issues of family health.

All human societies provide cultural blueprints for thought and action for their members. Cultural prescriptions provide the structure for beliefs, values, and normative and expected patterns of behavior for individuals in every society. Anthropologists have concentrated on the concept of culture as central to their studies. Perhaps the most comprehensive concept of culture was proposed by E. B. Tylor in 1871 as "that complex whole which includes knowledge, belief, art, morals, law, custom, and any other capabilities and habits acquired by man as a member of society" (p. 1). More simply, *culture* is composed of the patterns of belief and behavior learned, shared, and transmitted by human beings as members of a social group. Typically, we are not consciously aware of culture as determining or predisposing our thoughts, decisions, or behavior; nonetheless, we are influenced by and through this invisible culture into which we have been socialized and which surrounds us in our daily lives.

Cultural Beliefs and Family Health

The family serves as the first and prototypic mediator of the larger cultural milieu for the individual. American urban life constitutes a highly diversified social setting for most of us. We are exposed daily to widely divergent forms of attitudes and behaviors, and most persons routinely spend parts of their day in several social and cultural worlds. The primary socialization process has typically occurred within the family of orientation (family of birth and childrearing), and the cultural values of this family characteristically form the basis of future value sets. The most meaningful contemporary social field for the individual usually is the household wherein he or she lives, but one may find other significant social fields in the workplace or in social situations with peers. These social fields may expose the individual to different values, some of which may conflict. No one individual incorporates all of these values into his or her personality structure; however, even very divergent cultural elements that are compatible with one's primary value set or that are attractive because of needs or desires may be adopted. The family serves as a basic contextual storehouse of lore, tradition, and values, which influence the course of the actions of its members through time. The impact of the influences of differing families on orientation, procreation, or companionship occurs both serially and cumulatively through time. For our purposes in this chapter, the family serves as a basic context for the imparting of beliefs about health and problem-solving in relation to the challenges of illness, accidents, and stressful situations. In the case of many ethnic groups, the family constitutes a more basic unit for storage of information, problem-solving, and decision-making than it does in many middle-class mainstream American families today.

The contemporary burgeoning of new immigrant populations in America has further increased the cultural diversity that has constituted a continual source of pride for our country. Health care providers are confronted daily by patients from a variety of ethnic backgrounds. To meet the needs of these new populations, health care personnel are paying increasing attention to the fact that communication across cultural boundaries is imperative. Clark (1983a), in the foreword to an excellent collection of articles on cross-cultural medicine in the *Western Journal of Medicine,* discusses a number of potential barriers to clinical care, such as language and communication patterns and divergent expectations for roles and responsibilities. Of particular significance for a consideration of the enormous differences that may exist in cultural beliefs are explanatory models, which have been a subject of considerable analysis by anthropologists (Kleinman, 1980). Clark states:

> Explanatory models in all cultures go far beyond ideas about specific pathogens, dislocations, toxins, traumata, degenerations or biochemical imbalances. They are broadly gauged systems of concepts about the nature of illness and its place in human existence. For example, they explain what disease is, how it comes about, why it exists, what can prevent it or control it or cure it, and why it attacks some people but not others. Human beings seem to have a need to provide explanations for themselves of various kinds of good and ill that befall them. In even the simplest human societies, explanations are advanced and weighed about the reasons for floods, hurricanes, earthquakes, stillbirths, malformations, failed crops, drownings, disease and death. . . .
>
> Explanatory models have many functions; first, they provide criteria for judging whether or not an individual is really sick. Some cultures find it difficult to accept certain "manifestations" of disease that they cannot comprehend. For some, on the one hand, laboratory results may have little meaning in the absence of pain, fear, malaise or other symptoms. . . .
>
> A second function of such models is to deal with multiple levels of causality. In other words,

a disease model not only provides an explanation for how an illness comes to exist; it also affords a reason why a particular patient happened to fall ill. . . .*

Clearly, the pluralistic nature of American society today offers unusual learning opportunities and challenges for health care personnel.†

Family Structure

The nuclear family, widely accepted as the typical American family form, has never been universal in human groups through time (Gough, 1971; Reiss, 1965), nor is it today a universal or even stable form in our own society. In fact, defining the structure of "the contemporary American family" presents a challenge, calling for a comprehensive and realistic assessment of the diverse forms of relationships that exist among us. Although differences in ethnicity account for some degree of this diversity, the core mainstream American nuclear family of the past is also undergoing dramatic changes. Married couples with and without children are still the most frequent family forms as separate households; however, other households forms are becoming increasingly familiar in our metropolitan areas: the single parent household, the single person household, or the household composed of two or more individuals unrelated by blood or legal ties but united by economic need or strong emotional bonds.

For example in 1985, 72% of all households were composed of families. Only 58% of all

---

*Clark M (1983a): Cultural context of medical practice. *West J Med, 139* (6):806–810. Copyright © 1983, California Medical Association. Reprinted with permission.

†For readings on cross-cultural health care and beliefs, the reader is directed to Clark's edited collection in *West J Med* (1983b); Orque et al (1983); Harwood (1981); and Leininger (1978).

households were married couples, with less than one-half of these, or 28% of all households, with their own children under 18. Other forms of family households, those with male householder or no wife present (3%) and those with female householder with no husband present (12%), accounted for 14% of households. Twenty-eight percent of all households were nonfamily households, that is, composed of either a single person or legally unrelated individuals. Significant ethnic differences likewise appear in household composition (U.S. Bureau of the Census, 1986).

We suggest here that *family* be considered as that primary person or group of primary persons that one relates to emotionally or for functional necessities. Thus, family may include persons living in the same household or elsewhere.

Researchers and clinicians are able to determine empirically, in affective, functional terms, who family members are. For example, Bloch (1983) has defined the family in a functional sense for clinicians:

> . . . we will use the term quite broadly to mean that intimate network into which the individual human is born, along with successive representations of that intimate network over a lifetime. *Family* in this sense includes, but is not limited to, either the legal family, or the biological family, or the psychological family. Household members unrelated by blood or marriage may currently be included, or may have been, in the past. Thus, the family has extensions in space—the extended kin network—and in time—the multigenerational and historical family. For each clinical occasion, there is what might be called the "ad hoc" family, defined as those persons immediately involved with the problem, who are assembled to assist with its solution. By the nature of the phenomena involved, there is almost always an intimate psychosocial context that is highly relevant to illness and treatment; experience shows that that context most often coincides with some sector of family as defined above. It is on the foundation of that experience that family therapy builds and that its contribution to medical practice rests. (1983, p. 8)

Stack (1974), in a classic anthropologic study of Black families in the Midwest, described a close networking of individuals involved in interdependent exchanges of goods and services necessary in a context of poverty. From her empirical studies, she presented this functional definition of family members:

> . . . I found extensive networks of kin and friends supporting, reinforcing each other—devising schemes for self-help, strategies for survival in a community of severe economic deprivation. . . . I became poignantly aware of the alliances of individuals trading and exchanging goods, resources, and the care of children, the intensity of their acts of domestic cooperation, and the exchange of goods and services among these persons, both kin and non-kin. (p. 28)

> Ultimately I defined "family" as the smallest, organized, durable network of kin and non-kin who interact daily, providing domestic needs of children and assuring their survival. The family network is diffused over several kin-based households, and fluctuations in household composition do not significantly affect cooperative familial arrangements. . . . An arbitrary imposition of widely accepted definitions of the family, the nuclear family, or the matrifocal family blocks the way to understanding how people in The Flats describe and order the world in which they live. (p. 31)

Although studies in the nursing and health-related literature still tend to focus on nuclear families, it is imperative to be cognizant of the multitude of other family forms that clinicians, particularly those in large metropolitan areas, are seeing in daily practice. In fact, institutions such as hospitals and schools are modifying traditional legal regulations to meet the realities of these varied and increasing new forms.

Family Studies

Lewis, an anthropologist best known for his studies of Mexican and Puerto Rican families (1959; 1961; 1965) has suggested several chief ways in which family studies contribute to our understanding of the individual and culture. The family offers a context in which to bridge the conceptual extremes of the culture of the total population at one pole and the individual at the other. It becomes "the middle-term in the culture–individual equation" (Lewis, 1967, p. 135). Likewise, the descriptions of family members allow for the viewing of real persons living out their lives rather than as stereotypes or abstracted individuals. Further, Lewis observed that for those interested in the relationship between culture and personality, factors in personality development can best be identified and assessed in family contexts. Family studies also provide a perspective for understanding the meaning of institutions such as the family for individuals.

Family studies of interest to health and welfare personnel are the works of Henry (1965); Howell (1973); Stack (1974); Ablon (1980); Ames (1982); and Ablon, Ames, and Cunningham (1984).

Henry, in *Pathways to Madness* (1965), provided a unique group of family studies based on naturalistic observation in homes of families of psychotic and autistic children. Henry argued that by actually living in households where mental illness exists, and presumably was developed, researchers may collect important data to provide an intimate understanding of family life for clinicians. Henry stated:

> For many years it had been my conviction that the etiology of emotional illness required more profound study than had heretofore been possible and that the best way to new discoveries in the field was through study of the disease-bearing vector, the family, in its natural habitat, pursuing its usual life routines—eating, loving, fighting, talking, taking amusements, treating sickness, and so on—in other words, following the usual course of its life. (p. 30)

Henry (1965; 1967) proposed that each family may develop its own "family culture." This culture will be a combination of the values the family carries and transmits from the larger society and the special attitudes and behaviors that result from the systematic interaction of a stable small social unit. Not only will family cultures be idiosyncratic, but similar cultures may well be found in accordance with respective health conditions or chronic illnesses in the family. As researchers we have found Henry's work to be a valuable and unique prototype that has inspired our own research. A case presented below from Ames's research will illustrate the richness of the potential of "interior" family culture research.

Concepts and Methods

Our approach to the study of families uses classical anthropologic theories and methods. The family is seen as a semiclosed system among other systems in society. This approach is compatible with that of other family researchers who have emphasized the nature of the family as an integrated social system with interdependent parts composed of interacting personalities, each having his or her own expected role functions. It follows that the behavior of each part sensitively affects the functioning of the others. A malfunction of one part may lead to a disequilibrium of the total system. The system itself functions to maintain its equilibrium, or homeostasis. This occurs even to maintain conditions perceived as pathologic (Schvaneveldt, 1981; Davis et al, 1974; Steinglass, 1980).

Wedded to the systems orientation is a chief methodologic approach of anthropologic research—that human beings are best studied holistically and in their natural habitats, *in vivo* rather than *in vitro*, to elicit everyday customary and routine behavior. Traditional anthropologic studies of social life attempt to capture the tempo of life and activities naturalistically rather than in laboratory settings or through experimental designs. In the case of families, ideally, naturalistic, in-depth studies involve spending a significant amount of time with families—over at least a year or several years. The holistic perspective can be obtained only through knowledge of a great many aspects of typical behavior. To gain this knowledge, observations are made of family activities, such as mealtime behavior and the carrying out of household tasks, and of leisure activities, including socializing with family members, friends and neighbors. If possible, the researcher accompanies family members to typical events outside of the home. The observation of both normative and unusual household activities is accompanied by the interviewing of all family members, including children where possible. Individual and family life histories are taken in addition to interviews about ongoing family interaction.

Case Studies

The following cases are presented to illustrate the significance of cultural patterns in family health. The first case describes Samoan response to the sequelae of a catastrophic fire. The second describes culturally determined family patterns as they affect drinking behavior in Irish-American families. The third analyzes both external and internal cultural patterns developed in mainstream Protestant families in which there is maternal alcoholism.

American-Samoans in a West Coast Metropolitan Area

Clinicians and behavioral scientists have noted that persons in crisis and postcrisis periods are at high risk for temporary, although frequently disabling, emotional problems. Large bodies of literature describe both the symptomatology of grief and the complicated emotional reactions that accompany severe burn injuries. This case will examine how the cultural values and the form of family system maintained by a Samoan community in a West Coast metropolitan area functioned to alleviate personal and social distress in the wake of a catastrophic fire in which 17 persons died and more than 70 other persons were severely burned. The Samoan family and community have prescribed expectations and actions for caregiving services in times of acute crisis. These services are currently evidenced when the death of a Samoan occurs in this community. The social, religious, and financial security available for Samoans at times of crisis offers a striking contrast to that available for most segments of the larger American society.

The data presented here are from a study conducted by Ablon through (1) interviews and observation of death and crisis situations over a two-year period, 1968 to 1970; and (2) interviews taken during a follow-up study conducted five years after a catastrophic fire that occurred in this Samoan community in 1964 (1971; 1973). A recent restudy of Samoan family life (Janes, Pawson, 1986) confirms the continuation, and even strengthening, of the patterns described in the following paragraphs.

The Evolution of Samoan Population in America

Sizable immigration from American Samoa to Honolulu and the American mainland cities began in the 1950s. Many Samoans on the mainland are naval personnel who retired and settled in California. Many other persons have emigrated to seek wage labor, which will enable them to buy material possessions that they could not afford in Samoa, even though their actual living standard was comfortable. Many come to seek a mainland education for themselves or for their children. Some come simply to investigate the larger world. An estimated 30,000 Samoans now reside in California—chiefly in San Diego, Oceanside, the greater Los Angeles area and the San Francisco Bay area (Janes, Pawson, 1986). A large proportion of men work in shipyards, in warehouses, or in heavy industry, and women often hold jobs as nurses' aides in convalescent homes and hospitals. Samoans lead full and active lives centered about their families, their churches, and their jobs. Many live in a virtually Samoan world. In their homes they are surrounded by extended family members. They speak Samoan, wear brightly colored Samoan dress, and eat traditional Samoan foods. Yet many of their instrumental values could be labeled "middle class." When asked why they seem to adjust rapidly to urban life, Samoans respond: "We work hard and we help one another."

Ablon initially approached a study of this Samoan population in 1968 with a broad focus on the manner in which cultural values and social organization were related to the urban adaptation of this relatively new and exotic ethnic group. In the course of this study, she examined family and community behavior customary at the time of a death and found this information useful in comprehending the complex cultural and social factors operative in times of crisis. She had ample opportunity to observe the extraordinary strength of the extended family. The highly realistic Samoan approach to life, death, and misfortune suggested that as individuals and family groups, Samoans could cope well with disaster. These assumptions were justified by the data collected at the time of the fire.

The Samoan Extended Family

Mead (1930; 1961) provided a functional definition of the Samoan extended family that seems as appropriate to the Samoan family of California today as to that of Samoa in 1925:

> *Aiga* means relative by blood, marriage and adoption, and although no native actually confuses the three ways by which *aiga* status is arrived at, nevertheless, a blanket attitude is implied in the use of the word. An *aiga* is always one's ally against other groups, bound to give one food, shelter and assistance. An *aiga* may ask for any of one's possessions and refuse to take "no" for an answer; usually an *aiga* may take one's possessions without asking. . . . No marriage is per-

mitted with anyone termed *aiga* and all contemporary *aigas* are considered as brothers and sisters. Under the shadow of these far-flung recognized relationships children wander in safety, criminals find a haven, fleeing lovers take shelter, the traveler is housed, fed and his failing resources reinforced. Property is collected for a house building or a marriage; and a whole island is converted into a series of cities of refuge from poverty, embarrassment, or local retribution. (p. 40)

The cohesiveness of the extended family strongly persists in the mainland cities. One example is the prevalence of the extended family household. It is rare to find a household composed of a single nuclear family. The average Samoan household numbers from 6 to 10 persons. Household composition is fluid, and various relatives come and go, the duration of their stays dependent on their reasons for being in the household and in the area. Younger relatives frequently come from Samoa to stay with married siblings, aunts, uncles, cousins, or even close family friends, for the purpose of attending school.

Most Samoans' kin ties can be classified as affective and are relationships that are not only emotionally supportive but also instrumental in that they assist them in practical matters. For instance, the Samoan family and community function as a clearinghouse for information concerning employment and housing. The many small pockets of Samoans working together all over the local area attest to the effectiveness of the family and community as agencies of employment. At the time of this study, the number of Samoan individuals or families receiving any kind of public welfare assistance was negligible. If a person was in financial straits too severe for family assistance to cover the situation, the family would cooperate to send the person back to Samoa, where he always had recourse to ancestral lands and traditional modes of support. Today attitudes toward outside intervention have changed, and increasingly more Samoans seek public welfare assistance.

The mutual aid function of the extended family is extremely important in terms of crisis. The family may serve as an economic cushion while a person is job-hunting or when he or she is temporarily laid off from work. When a family is confronted by the expenses of a funeral or wedding, it expects to receive cash donations as high as $10,000 to $20,000, a sum always adequate to cover expenses, and money usually is left over for redistribution among kin.

Informants categorically state that no matter how infrequently they see any relative, they would feel responsible for helping that relative with money or services at times of crisis or need. Obviously, personal attitudes toward individual relatives, as well as the state of one's personal finances, would enter into the carrying through of this idealized statement. Ablon's observations and interviews at the time of specific crisis situations that arose during the course of her research and Janes' and Pawson's recent study (1986) suggest that most relatives do indeed respond spontaneously with such aid when the need arises.

The Fire of 1964

The fire provided an opportunity to examine the role of social and cultural patterns as they affect individuals, families, and community in a period of acute stress. The fire occurred at a Samoan dance held in a Catholic church social ball. The fire resulted in 17 deaths and 70 moderate to severe burn injuries. Almost all of the dead and injured were Samoans.

The data presented here are based on materials gathered from in-home interviews five years after the fire with 18 families that the fire touched by death or injury and with Red Cross disaster officials, physicians, nurses, and attorneys who were associated with the fire victims over the following days, months, and years. The 18 families contacted numbered less than one-third of those units included in the Red Cross files that comprised the master list of those af-

fected (death to minor injury), and about three-fourths of the families who remained in the area at the time of the interviews. Seven persons in these 18 family units died from burn injuries, and 21 others were hospitalized. Although entire families were interviewed when possible, one person in each family generally acted as a chief informant. The categories of materials chosen for examination were limited to those that one realistically could expect to elicit in significant detail and with some degree of accuracy five years after the event. Although Samoans rarely talked about the fire spontaneously, their memories of it and of subsequent events were quite keen and detailed. Medical personnel were eager to talk about their experiences and likewise retained clear memories of the fire and its aftermath.

Physicians and Red Cross disaster personnel wonderingly described the stoic manner in which Samoans withstood injury and death the night of the fire and during the period immediately following. Medical and disaster personnel had never seen any comparable behavior in times of disaster. The focus in the present account is on the sequelae of this fire and how Samoan families functioned in this crisis period.

Three hundred persons had attended the dance, representing almost every Samoan family in the area. In many families, both father and mother were hospitalized with severe burns. Needs were urgent and all-encompassing: financial, care of children, and general household management. The Samoan extended family household as it has traditionally existed in Samoa proved to be uniquely suited for functioning in time of crisis. Not only did local immediate and distant kin bear the burden of help, but relatives from Samoa and Hawaii came to the assistance of those few who had no close kin in the area.

Interview questions probed the subject of sources of primary assistance at this time. Two-thirds of the 18 families responded that siblings of one or both spouses either moved into their home during their periods of hospitalization and immediate recuperation or took the children of burn victims into their own homes. These siblings managed household affairs and negotiated for the community aid available. Five families stated that parents of one spouse or both spouses took over their responsibilities. In three families, cousins were of primary assistance, and two families reported aunts and uncles were of most help. In several cases there was overlapping of primary assistance by two categories of relatives. Because of the composition of the typical extended family household, these relatives frequently were already living in the household at the time of the fire. Several families stated that their families in Samoa sent them substantial financial aid. Only one widow insisted emphatically that because of her desire to be independent, she refused the aid offered by her relatives here and those who came from Samoa for her husband's funeral.

Some informants reported that they were helping several families, running between the demands of their own crisis period and the demands of babysitting, shopping, or cooking for relatives in other households. The staying power of Samoan family assistance should be noted. In many families varied forms of assistance and childcare were needed for many months as persons remained in burn wards or returned for multiple skin grafts and other procedures. The assistance of family members never flagged.

Informants commented that their days were consumed by attendance at funerals of relatives and friends and related funeral activities. Samoan funeral ritual customarily is elaborate, with several religious services featuring choir singing by all Samoan churches of the area. Even one funeral provides many hours and even days of involvement for a sizable proportion of the Samoan community. The activities and energies entailed by more than a dozen deaths in the weeks following the fire were understandably time-consuming.

Researchers have chronicled a normative grief syndrome with uniform reactions and symptomatology. Many clinicians have stated that "grief work" must be accomplished for bereaved individuals to emancipate themselves from their grief to a new psychologic and social reality (Lindemann, 1944; Silverman, 1967; Committee for the Study of Health Consequences of the Stress of Bereavement, 1984). Interviews with Samoans suggest that this syndrome does not occur in similar form among bereaved Samoans. Likewise, grief work appears to be rapidly and less painfully accomplished by Samoans because of ritualized family and community support and cultural attitudes relating to death.

For example, the widows who were interviewed all reported acute initial shock and distress when confronted by the death of their husbands. Their brief discussions of such distress, however, quickly turned to the amount of assistance they were given by relatives even before the death and extending in the months and years that followed. They immediately were surrounded by their own or their spouse's relatives who took over responsibility for funeral arrangements and household management.

Maddison and Walker (1967) suggested that young widows and those left with dependent children are the widow population at highest risk for emotional problems. Yet Samoan women in these categories appeared to make relatively rapid and satisfactory adjustments. The many functions performed for them by their extended families served to alleviate most of the complicating problems. Silverman (1969), reporting on a study of widows, stated that those she contacted worried about loneliness, financial problems, and raising children alone. The widow "talks about the emptiness of the house, the fact hat thereis no ne to take care of, and no one with whom she can share her evenings and weekends" (p. 335). The nature of the Samoan extended family household precludes many of these specific anxieties. This busy household more than likely existed before the husband's death and normally may be projected into the future, although individual persons may change. In this household there are always many people about; there are one's own or others' children to take care of; and help is forthcoming from other adults and older children.

Immediate funeral expenses are met by the funds collected following the death. Long-term financial support is assured either by family assistance, by the woman's own potential for working, as is the Samoan pattern, or, as a last resort, by a return to Samoa and the ever-available family resources there.

Samoan families responded to burn injuries in a similarly positive fashion. Severe burn injury, long hospitalizations and recuperation periods, and even accompanying permanent disfiguration did not result in the extreme stress and severe emotional disturbances typical of Americans in this situation.

By all accounts, Samoans as individuals and as family groups appeared to have absorbed the disaster amazingly well. In their undemonstrative acceptance of pain, death, and calamities, Samoans present a marked contrast to most Americans. A major factor contributing to the Samoan response was the bulwark of available family and community support. Medical and agency personnel continually commented on the extraordinary emotional, social, and financial support offered by the Samoan extended family and the significance of this for burn victims and the bereaved.

Hill and Hansen (1962) refer to crisis-proof and crisis-prone families. The Samoan family offers an excellent example of a crisis-proof family in that it adapts and successfully can meet unexpected crises. Samoan family and community have their own disaster plan, a complex pattern of expectations and actions that spontaneously becomes activated when a crisis arises. This plan is evident on a small scale at the time of the death of an individual, when all family members—including those so remote in degree that most Americans would have lost all record of relatedness—are expected to donate money and ritual items of goods and food to the bereaved family. This plan was implemented on a large scale at the time of the fire and enabled the Samoan pop-

ulation to absorb an enormously painful disaster with remarkable security and effectiveness.

Irish-Catholic Family Life and Alcohol Use*

Research orientations in the literature dealing with alcoholism and the family have focused primarily on psychologic features of individual family members and, more recently, interactional aspects of the family as a closed system (Ablon, 1976; Paolino, McCrady, 1977). The latter orientation regards the total family unit as the necessary functional context for an understanding of the alcoholic's drinking patterns. Systems and interactional theories posit that the major perpetuator of drinking patterns is the overriding need for the maintenance of the status quo or homeostasis that has developed within the family system (Steinglass, 1980; Davis et al, 1974). Even in the most sophisticated models presented by clinicians, cultural considerations are mentioned as one area that might be reflected through drinking behavior, but no exploration of the implications of sociocultural affiliation is made in any of the published case studies, nor are sociocultural features held constant to allow an analysis of their significance. The extent to which role behavior of family members is the living out of cultural expectations or prescriptions has not been researched.

A cultural case is presented here, wherein the excessive use of alcohol fulfills many specific functions for individual members and for the maintenance of the system as outlined by the systems theorists. A strong and encompassing homeostatic theme or cultural paradigm that perpetuates heavy drinking has been handed down through the generations, and may indeed

*Portions of this section are excerpted from Ablon J (1981): Implications of cultural patterning for the delivery of alcoholism services: Case studies. *J Stud Alcohol*, Suppl 9, 1:185–206. Copyright © 1981, Journal of Studies of Alcohol, Inc. and the Smithsonian Institution. Reprinted with permission.

be more significant than the individual "pathologic needs" typically focused on in treatment.

Drinking Patterns and Family Life

The families in the study were Irish-, German-, and Italian-American Catholic families residing in a metropolitan area of southern California. Survey data rank Catholics nationally and locally the highest among religious groups for the prevalence of alcohol-related problems. Among American ethnic groups, the Irish rank the highest or near highest in terms of heavy intake, loss of control, untoward social consequences, and social support for heavy drinking among associates. Germans and Italians traditionally have a low rate of alcoholism and related problems within their European contexts or as defined ethnic groups in the United States (Cahalan, 1970; Cahalan, Room, 1974; Stivers, 1985).

The Irish in their homeland have ranked internationally among the highest groups for the prevalence of alcohol-related problems. A number of researchers have documented the historical prevalence of heavy drinking among Irish men and the purported relationship of this pattern with characteristics of the family, social, and economic systems (Bales, 1962; Stivers, 1976). Membership in the hard-drinking Irish peer group was suggested to have legitimated the status of landless younger sons who could not inherit land and generally did not marry. In America, heavy drinking became a significant characteristic of the cultural as well as the masculine identity of the Irishman (Stivers, 1976; 1985). However, of particular importance here are the historical and contemporary problematic attitudes and behavior concerning sex and marriage.

Various studies portray marriage among the Irish in Ireland as an uneasy practical alliance providing little affection or intimacy. Sex and procreation were reported to be duties rather than joys or expressive activities. The Irishwoman, in her role as mother and wife, has traditionally been a controlling matriarch on whom sons and husbands were dependent (Messenger, 1969).

Few empirically-based cultural descriptions of the Irish family in America are available. However, Greeley (1972), a sociologist and Irish-American cleric, has presented a discussion of sexual relations and affective characteristics of Irish-Americans in a descriptive study that bears a partial quoting here:

> The Irish are generally not very good at demonstrating tenderness or affection for those whom they love. The Irish male, particularly in his cups, may spin out romantic poetry extolling the beauty of his true love, but he becomes awkward and tongue-tied in their presence and clumsy, if not rough, in his attempts at intimacy. She, on the other hand, finds it hard to resist the temptation to become stiff, if not frigid, in the face of his advance, however much warmth she may feel. For her especially, sexual relationships are a matter of duty, and if she fails in her "duty" to her husband she will have to report it the next time she goes to confession. Some Irishwomen with obvious pride will boast that they have never once refused the "duty" to their husbands, even though in 20 years of marriage they have not got one single bit of pleasure out of it. A sex encounter between a twosome like that is not likely to be pleasurable. (p. 114)

Greeley states that the Irish often tend to drink for reassurance and escape from their "intolerable" psychologic burdens and their need to repress sexuality and aggressiveness. He describes the domination of the Irish-American mother who rules her family by her strong will or by subtly manipulating the sympathies and guilts of her husband and children. Greeley states that, "Many, if not most, of the alcoholic Irishmen I know come from families where the mother rules the roost and have married women who are very much like their mothers (1972, p. 135).

The data presented here from Ablon's study, which explored specific aspects of Irish-American family life, suggest that a combination of restrictive characteristics of lifestyle continue to offer a contemporary variant of the traditional and historical motivations for heavy drinking and alcoholism that have been presented by scholars.

Ablon carried out a study of family dynamics and interaction with 30 families in a middle-class Catholic parish of a West Coast metropolitan area in southern California. Data were gathered over a four-year period through in-home interviewing and extensive participant observation. The wife in every case was the principal informant. The marital unions in 21 of the 30 families represent a mixture of ethnic strains, predominantly Irish and German or Irish and Italian.

Relatively few informants exhibited outward ethnic social indicators such as belonging to national clubs. The most significant elements remaining, although not in the consciousness of informants, appeared to be particular elements of traditional childrearing and role behavior. The Irish and German mothers described were the strong, dominating forces in their families of orientation, and their daughters, the subjects of this study, likewise were strong wives and mothers. Irish, and in fewer cases German, fathers typically were described as nice, quiet men who frequently displayed excessive drinking patterns, as did many of their adult sons.

Ages of subjects ranged from 34 to 64, with a mean of 50 for the men and 47 for the women. The typical level of educational attainment for both men and women was high school graduation. The economic pursuits of two-thirds of the husbands were in city or federal civil service, frequently police or fire departments. Of the remaining one-third, about half worked for large utility companies, and the remainder managed their own small businesses. These occupations tended to be the same as those of their fathers.

A pattern of massive social controls unusual within the context of the contemporary larger society may be quickly identified in the population. This traditional pattern of social control is maintained in large part by the almost unchanging nature of primary relationships constituted by extended kin and friends from high school and even, in many cases, from early childhood. The pattern of tradition constitutes the superstructure that makes for strong, stable families.

Irish-Americans view liberal alcohol use as an expected part of the good life, yet, alcoholism and alcohol-related family problems are common, although hidden from the larger society. Massive denial exists in regard to help-seeking by problem drinkers and, to a lesser degree, by their families.

Social Control and Alcohol Use

Initial surveys of the population pointed up two aspects of family life that appeared to be related: (1) the existence of strong, culturally patterned controls encompassing almost all features of individual and family life, the most significant dealing with marital roles and relationships, and (2) a prevalence of alcohol-related problems.

A correlation between problematic drinking and social control was postulated: Problematic drinking would occur with greatest severity where there were found the highest levels of expressed and accepted family and subgroup societal controls. Thus Irish Catholics, who traditionally have exhibited the greatest amount of control in all features of life, would have more problematic drinking than other Catholics.

The significance of oppressive social controls as they relate to problem drinking lies in the interrelationship of certain specific characteristics and not in the nature of individual elements as they might appear in many populations. For example, perhaps the most important single element that emerged in case histories as problematic—that of religious strictures dealing with sexual behavior—is pervasive, affecting almost all other areas of family life. It is also specific to the Catholic subculture and occurred even more rigidly among Irish Catholics. Other elements of control are commonly found among many groups—for instance among Jews, who have a particularly low rate of alcoholism.

Problem drinking in the sample was found to be linked most closely to the Irish. For example, in 8 cases of the 30, men had an Irish father *and* an Irish mother.

Despite the seeming acculturation and homogenization of the Irish in American society, many characteristics of Irish family life, such as childrearing and marital roles, appear remarkably similar to those common to historical and contemporary Ireland. A number of characteristic patterns emerged from family case materials as features of life and marriage that often appeared—as expressed by the subject or less frequently as defined by the researcher—to preclude or diminish communication and growth of positive, expressive relationships between spouses or between spouses and children. Highly stylized family roles often allow few options for spontaneous or independent action in major areas of the life career.

Patterns of Irish Family Life

A number of patterns emerged with clarity throughout the sample cases:

1. About two-thirds of the subjects had strong domineering mothers and much quieter, passive fathers. The controlling nature of the mothers was much more obvious when the mothers were Irish. In keeping with this, the now adult daughters, the informants in this study, were strong wives and mothers.

2. Strong religious sanctions relating to sex and the negative mystique surrounding premarital sexual experimentation and expression sometimes caused precipitous marriages and were explicitly posited by some informants to have caused young men to drink heavily. Newlyweds encountered the physical and psychologic aspects of marriage with few guidelines. Strictures against birth control and the cultural prescription exhorting procreation in Catholic family life often led quickly to the birth of children before couples could work out their own marital relationship. Newlyweds rarely received any sexual counseling, and the extreme shame and reticence hovering about sex has also worked against such counseling being sought later. It is significant that wives often perceive the biggest family problem to be problem drinking, but husbands perceive the biggest problem to be sexual incompatibility or unwillingness of their wives to have sexual relations. In these cases, almost invariably, women comment on their ignorance of sexual matters when they married and, in fact, to the present day.

3. A significant characteristic of family life was a lack of communication between spouses, despite the great amount of family activity and necessity for conversation about logistical matters. For instance, 18 of the 30 wives brought up their difficulties in communicating their feelings about important issues or even daily events to their spouses.

4. Most men in this population worked for large impersonal bureaucracies as did their fathers. They had little control over their hourly, daily, or weekly work schedules. Many men were in occupations such as the police force, requiring them to work afternoons or night shifts; others were able to meet the economic demands of large families only by working extra jobs. This economic pattern characteristically results in an absentee father. The absentee father essentially relinquishes household and childrearing responsibilities, including the disciplining of children, to his wife. The husband's early dependency on a strong mother appears to feed into an easy capitulation to dependency on the wife, often forced by the issue of occupational time schedules.

5. Many of the legitimizing values and functions of the Irish bachelor group were replaced by the chief peer groups of the husband. The husband's referents for mas-

culine values and behavior tended to be male relatives, workmates, parishmates, and early parochial school friends. One aspect of expected masculine role behavior was heavy drinking.

In summary, both men and women grew up with the model of an energetic, highly capable mother and a father who was remembered as a good quiet man who was rarely at home, or, if so, he was alone in his room silently drinking. Economic demands, now as then, have compounded further the propensity for the mother to be a strong and dominating figure. These strong women have managed and disciplined large families essentially alone, have run the household, and have taken care of aging relatives.

Cultural patterning contributes significantly to shaping the social and economic parameters of a family lifestyle in which alcohol abuse is a common and disturbing element. At a time when American society exhibits seemingly more options for the individual each day, most of these families live locked within cradle-to-grave moral, social, and economic expectations. A careful examination of this family system reveals that in all eight cases in which men had an Irish father and an Irish mother there was excessive drinking. One could posit that the chief progenitors of this situation are an Irish mother, who maintained the Irish tradition and all of the social controls related to that tradition, and a father who provided an alcoholic role model for his son.

One inference from this data could be that many men drink to dull their sexual needs and to blot out the frustration linked to massive personal and social controls that encompass their lives. Through culturally familiar, although only ambivalently condoned, excessive drinking patterns, husbands may register their complaints without actually endangering the fate of their marriage. Wives and mothers in their own appropriate roles have heavily contributed to this

situation and now inherit the many problems attendant to it. Basic intervention techniques that focus on establishing spousal communication and tempering the continuity of culturally inherited role patterns may offer an indirect but effective avenue through which to approach problematic drinking in this population.

Alcoholic Mothers in Middle-class Protestant Families*

Thus far we have focused on external cultural patterns affecting whole-family response to crisis and chronic problems. In demonstrating the need to also conceptualize the family as a cultural system in its own right, we now stress consideration of internal patterns and pressures on the structure and interaction of troubled families. Whereas external pressures are derived from prescribed social and cultural norms, internal pressures are derived from the struggle to maintain a family unit that provides the basic physical and psychologic necessities of human survival (Ames, 1982). The overall impact of these combined pressures on family life forces families to make ongoing adjustments to the factors surrounding the presenting family problem. Such adjustments, often manifested in covert and nonnormative behavior, take on the form of a family culture. Ablon (1979) has suggested that the adjustments a family makes to chronic alcoholism may take on the form of a "peculiar" family culture:

> Because alcoholism affects the total family, in such households all family members may be living within a world of chaos, shame and guilt

*Portions of this section are excerpted from Ames G (1985): Middle-class protestants: Alcohol and the family (chapter 23). In: *The American Experience with Alcohol: Contrasting Cultural Perspectives*, Bennett L, Ames G (eds.). New York, NY: Plenum Press, pp. 435–458. Reprinted with permission from Plenum Press.

often denied and hidden to the extent possible from even close friends and relatives. A peculiar family culture is thus constructed. (p. 199)

An understanding of this culture is critical to effective family treatment.

This study of women alcoholics in middle-class Protestant families (Ames, 1982; 1985) provides a particularly appropriate context for viewing the culture of the family in relation to both external and internal cultural pressures. In spite of recent church-directed efforts to change traditional edicts on the subject, to a large degree, Protestant beliefs and values regarding alcohol use and drinking behavior characterize alcoholism as a moral rather than a medical debility. These external cultural pressures against the mother's alcoholic condition, coupled with internal pressures to maintain individual and unit survival in the face of the disruptive nature of maternal drinking behavior, forced the families described here to make radical changes in role behavior, communication patterns, and family structure and interaction.

In an ongoing struggle to cope with their predicament, the families built boundaries between their private world of adaptive roles and behaviors and their public world of expected or culturally acceptable behavior. Behavioral adjustments to alcoholism, which prior to the onset of the mother's drinking problem would have been considered deviant and which to varying degrees were pathologic, became the norm behind the closed boundaries of the family home. To the degree that these adjustments were learned, shared, and transmitted among all of the family members, they became, in effect, a new kind of family culture. The descriptive materials in the following case profile of Ames's study provide some understanding of how and why alcoholic family culture is developed and maintained.

The data for this study were collected during two years of intermittent but intensive field work in the homes of eight predominantly middle-class Protestant families residing in an affluent suburban area of northern California. Families were visited from 6 to 12 times for periods lasting from 3 to 8 hours. In the course of repeated visits, in-depth life histories and verbal accounts of everyday family routines were taken both from parents and from adult children. Additionally, whole family interaction was observed during mealtime and at different times of the day, week, and seasons of the year. These materials provided a composite picture of each family's perspective on the mother's drinking problem from its inception and on family and community responses to her alcohol-related behavior. Also, these data helped determine whether the family's existing structure and behavioral patterns evolved with the drinking problem or were predispositions to it and whether radical changes in family rules and values had taken place. The mothers in all of the families were seeking treatment from county or private mental health services and in each case, had been identified by such services as alcoholic. Among all the women, the duration of their alcoholism ranged from 4 to 11 years.

Most of the parents referred to their ethno-religious background and present belief system as WASP, the common acronym for White Anglo-Saxon Protestant. All of the families were either actively involved with a church or professed allegiance to the beliefs and guiding principles of an established Protestant denomination. Four of the families were Presbyterian, two were Methodist, and two were Episcopalian. The families were intact in the sense that the parents were living together in the same household with their own or adopted children. Ages of the parents ranged from 35 to 55, and all had attended college. Husbands owned their own businesses or were employed in corporate or professional positions, and in every case were considered the principal provider. All of the women were theoretically positioned in the role of housewife. Although three of the women held part-time jobs, they were often unable to report to work during drinking periods or when suffering from alcohol-related illness.

Alcohol and American Protestantism

The problem of defining alcohol-related beliefs and practices among Protestant populations in the United States is complicated by the differing views held by various churches. The American branches of some large church groups of Europe, such as the Lutherans and the Episcopalians, ordinarily have not opposed *moderate* drinking, but other religious groups, such as the Baptists, Methodists, Presbyterians, Congregationalists, and members of smaller and fundamentalist groups, have a recent history of condemning alcohol use and drunkenness as sinful behavior (Oates, 1966).

When considering the strength behind the molding force of Protestant beliefs about alcohol, it is important to understand the historical roots of such beliefs in the context of religious movements just prior to and during the Temperance Era. It was during the Temperance Era, and with strong sanction, that positions on alcohol taken by several fundamentalist religions transformed frequent, heavy, or moderate drinking from what up to that time had been a normal state of habituation into immoral, depraved, or mentally deranged behavior (Levine, 1978). Methodist and Presbyterian "preachers" in frontier America used alcohol as a central theme in their religious revivalist efforts. The theme of abstinence from alcohol as the road to salvation appealed to the ministry and lay populations alike at a time when millions of Americans were searching for a moral crusade and a revivalistic cause (Rorabaugh, 1979). Ministers of many denominations began preaching the antialcohol theme, and it was out of the strength of this movement that the Methodists, Baptists, fundamentalists, and gospel denominations—and eventually the Salvation Army and the Seventh Day Adventists—arose to become powerful religious institutions in American society (Room, 1982).

In addition to the "loss of grace" theme, temperance reformers declared that those who used alcohol squandered capital; dissipated and destroyed wealth for selfish, nonproductive ends; and deterred opportunities for saving and investing money (Rorabaugh, 1979). This line of argument, coupled with religious proclamations that abstinence was a component for salvation from sin, persuaded the Protestant middle class to accept, and thereafter to maintain, moralistic perceptions of alcohol use, drunkenness, and chronic alcoholism. From the mid-nineteenth century on, abstinence and a religious-oriented lifestyle became the touchstones of middle-class respectability and symbols of elevation to that status level (Gusfield, 1963).

From a similar viewpoint, it has been proposed that the lasting strength of Protestant sanctions against alcohol use or anything other than moderate drinking is related to loss of control. Such symptomatic behavior is not compatible with the dominating middle-class Protestant ethic—that is, cultural prescriptions for behavior—in most regions of American society (Lemert, 1951).

Although in recent years Protestant churches have almost universally recognized the need to plan for future church involvement with alcohol prevention and treatment programs, major churches are still intensely divided over the issue of abstinence. Churches that were historically committed to the tradition of abstinence find it impossible to cooperate in alcohol programs that contradict their own basic edicts (Conley, Sorensen, 1971). Methodist teachings prohibiting alcohol use, historically a strong influence on the position taken by other American Protestant churches (Oates, 1966), have been relaxed to allow for occasional social drinking, although drunkenness is still regarded as sinful behavior and not to be allowed or accepted under any circumstances (Buck et al, 1976). Such edicts of the Methodist Church and similar ones by other Protestant churches have continued to be reinforced by sermons and religious teachings.

Notwithstanding the efforts of churches to moderate the lasting and powerful effects of the Temperance Era, early religious sanctions against alcohol have persisted as a controlling factor for alcohol beliefs and practices among the Protestant middle class even to recent generations. Three surveys over a 20-year period suggest that alcoholism remains a stigmatizing condition in the minds and hearts of many American people. Seventy-five percent of attitude samples from various parts of the United States have persisted in defining alcoholism as a sign of moral weakness (Cumming, Cumming, 1957; Mulford, Miller, 1965; Orcutt, 1976). That this large body of opinion about chronic alcoholism is still significantly prevalent in today's world suggests that it is deeply rooted in the religious and cultural fabric of the dominant middle-class Protestant population. It also suggests that middle-class Protestant Americans share historical commonalities in their alcohol-related beliefs and practices. In the following report on a study of this population, such beliefs are strongly implicated in the way in which families respond to alcoholism and to treatment.

Alcoholism in Protestant Family Environments

In spite of the varying Protestant denominations represented by the present study, families demonstrated pronounced consistencies in their unbending and moralistic responses to alcoholism. These consistencies were in part a reflection of the parents' early life experiences in homes that strongly adhered to Protestant views on alcohol. Parents were socialized to a conceptualization of alcoholism as immoral behavior and beyond that, to a belief that moderate drinking could be tolerated, although for some, abstinence was the preferred norm.

In their early life, and for some in the present, alcohol was rarely or never used for family or church-sponsored parties or at special celebrations such as weddings, holidays, and birthdays. Most of the husbands and virtually all of the wives experienced minimal social pressure to drink as teenagers and, with few exceptions, abstained from alcohol in their high school

years. First experiences with alcohol use and social drinking emerged only after moving out of the more protected family and religious environments of their childhood into the more worldly environments of college, military service, or workplace. After marriage, husbands developed moderate or moderate to heavy drinking practices in response to social and professional pressures to use alcohol. Their wives, most of whom moved directly from college to the housewife role, were occasional social drinkers in their early married years.

The onset of the mother's drinking problems were not related to social peer pressure. In each case it could be traced to a specific precipitating incident related to a traumatic social or health-related problem. The time lapse between choosing to use alcohol for medicinal or relaxation purposes and the development of chronic drinking was relatively short—from one to eight months. Immediately on realizing that they were drinking greater amounts of alcohol than ever before and that their behavior while drinking was causing concern among family and friends, the mothers ceased all drinking in social situations. They drank only in solitude, always out of sight of family, relatives, or friends. As the habitual drinking progressed to chronic alcoholism, the women entered a cyclical pattern of drinking and recovery periods; for years, many cycled between a state of semiconsciousness or total unconsciousness for days at a time, always in the privacy of their room.

Although drinking patterns changed across generations from family of orientation to family of procreation, beliefs and attitudes about alcoholism instilled during childhood did not change. Both the identified women alcoholics and their families accepted more or less on faith that alcoholic behavior was socially and morally deviant behavior. On finally entering treatment (out of desperation and fear of dying), the mothers were introduced to other explanatory models, primarily the disease model; however, family members were generally unimpressed by or uninterested in biomedical or psychosocial explanations for chronic drinking problems. Husbands and children alike were reluctant to describe the erratic behavior of the mother in terms of alcoholic-related language. Her frequent and secluded absences from the family circle during drinking periods and accounts of alcohol-related incidents were explained in relation to an undefined "sickness" or "problem." In turn, her sickness was viewed as a symptom of various nervous and physical ailments or of some recent stressful incident, but never as symptomatic of alcoholism as a sickness. Although family members were often humiliated and angered by the unpredictable nature of the mother's drinking behavior, it was never referred to as "alcoholism." Within their ethnoreligious tradition, alcoholism as a concept was generally equated with drunkenness and lack of willpower. "Weak-willed drunkard" was an unacceptable label for one's own wife or mother.

The resistance to and denial of the mother's alcoholism were continually reinforced by institutional forces in the family's immediate environment. In one case in which both the husband and the wife consulted their minister for counseling about her drinking, the minister announced from the pulpit one Sunday morning that a particular family in the congregation needed prayers to assist them in their struggle to bring a family member "out of darkness into the light." Although he did not mention the family name, the mother, and by association the whole family, was selected out as morally deviant. In another case, the principal of a private religiously oriented school arrived unannounced at one family home to check up on a child who had been absent with sickness for a week. When he confirmed his suspicions that the mother had a drinking problem, he telephoned an alarmed and embarrassed father at his place of business, not to express concern or to offer help, but to suggest that the child be placed in a foster home. Another example of social ostracism was the case in which one mother was dropped from the membership of a community volunteer organization in which prior to her drinking problem she had faithfully participated for 10 years. The president of the group bluntly informed her that they did not accept "alcoholics." Incidents such as these provoked an ever-growing sense of fear and paranoia among all family members.

Given that the families of this particular middle-class Protestant population were socialized to moralistic views of alcoholism and were affected by cultural pressures to conformity, one could assume that the symptomatic behavior of the mother would weaken, if not quickly dissolve, the family unit. In fact, the opposite was true. In their efforts to protect the mother and maintain a pretense of middle-class normality, families created a more cohesive, if unhealthy, family unit. Also, in order to "survive" in both their natural home and their cultural environment, and to appear as productive, participating units within that milieu, the families reinforced certain makeshift behavioral and structural adjustments. Traditional family rules and organization, which at first were tentatively altered, over time became permanently changed to a new and isolated kind of family system.

Because a family system like any social system is made up of interdependent parts—that is, family members—it is logical to assume that a change in the functioning of one member is automatically followed by a compensatory change in the functioning of other family members (Bowen, 1974, p. 115). For example, in families of women alcoholics, if the mother is unable to fulfill her expected role duties in relation to vital necessities of individual and household maintenance such as shopping for food, cooking meals, cleaning the house, and doing the laundry, these duties must be taken over by another family member. Such transference of power and responsibility is more often than not accompanied by hostility on the part of the person or persons forced to take over that role and by fear, shame, and guilt on the part of the mother. Further, the unpredictable nature of role performance of one member often leads to disequilibrium of the whole system.

In the families of this study, when the mother was unable to function in her prescribed role, sometimes for periods as long as two weeks, the family did indeed experience emotional upheavals and a change in family equilibrium. Fathers were especially agitated by the breakdown in cooking and childcare duties. However, as for the question of who stepped into the mother's role and adequately looked to the needs of basic family sustenance, surprisingly, no one did much of anything. The mothers, even in their drinking periods, jealously guarded their claim to maternal role and status. Families, and especially the husbands—either out of concern for the mother's sense of self-esteem or as a path of least resistance or both—made only feeble attempts to take over shopping, cleaning, and other household tasks. In some cases, mothers arranged their daily drinking schedule to accommodate early preparation of the evening meal. Others who drank to prolonged unconsciousness, actually prepared food in advance out of concern for the family's nutritional needs; teenage children coped by buying fast food, and younger children often fended for themselves with cold cuts and canned foods. In one family where the father could not and would not cook, the young children ate canned vegetables from the container when the mother was incapacitated. Ordinarily clean houses became unclean and disorderly, and laundry accumulated until the mother recovered from her drinking period, which sometimes lasted several weeks.

After a time, the periodic malfunction of the maternal role became the normal way of things, and families adjusted by building and maintaining a family system that abandoned normative values of a clean, attractive home and clothing and regular, nutritious, and tasty meals. Mealtime, once an important family ritual, became an irregularly occurring event. It was not unusual for husbands and teenage children to schedule themselves out of the house in the evening, often skipping the evening meals even when the mother was not drinking. This breakdown in family eating patterns was especially agitating

to the mothers and often stimulated them to more drinking. The positive payoff of adaptive change in these and other family behaviors was the mothers' supreme efforts to please and overcompensate during nondrinking periods. Children and husbands seemed to enjoy, and in some cases took advantage of, the compensatory, guilt-ridden periods of "supermomism." As for the mother, these compensatory rewards made the drinking more tolerable and in fact, helped restore the equilibrium of the family system.

In the interests of survival, adaptive measures to alcoholism at the family level do indeed provide a functional, if unhealthy, family system. But in addition to family form, changes have also taken place in traditional family rules, rituals, and values. The adjusted family system becomes what we referred to earlier as a new kind of family culture—that is, an alcoholic family culture. From the perspective of both the family and its immediate cultural environment, the family lifestyle is as culturally deviant as the alcoholism. In order to avoid loss of self-esteem for culturally inappropriate realities of their family life, families organized what Goffman (1963) refers to as a "protective capsule" around their stigmatizing problems, even to the extent of resisting or outright refusing participation in professional treatment. In the process of concealing, denying, and accommodating family behavior, both the chronic alcoholism and the stigma aspects of the situation are reinforced. In sum, the whole family suffers the consequences of culturally derived aspects of alcoholism.

Summary

The aforementioned cases illustrate the power of cultural patterns and pressures in affecting family behavior and response in relation to severe health problems. In the case of Samoans, these patterns contributed toward a very productive and positive reaction to a shared disaster. In the case of Irish-American Catholics, patterns of accustomed behavior fostered severe and painful dysfunctional drinking problems. In the Protestant families, cultural beliefs concerning excessive drinking resulted in massive denial, and internal pressures for the maintenance of the family unit further solidified abusive maternal drinking patterns.

Health care providers rarely have focused on the cultural and social factors that contribute to individual and family health related behavior. A holistic perspective on family life may illuminate the cultural prescriptions regarding attitudes and behavior that relate both directly and indirectly to health maintenance and care. A comprehensive and sensitive understanding of family cultural patterns may provide a more educated basis for effective planning of preventive and intervention programs for families and individual family members.

Issues for Further Investigation

1. The defined individual patient typically engages in a one-to-one relationship with a clinician. The implications and consequences of other family members being included in patient-clinician encounters and in decision-making about therapy and treatment have yet to be explored and systematically studied.

2. Empirically based cross-cultural studies of family responses to health crises, death, and disaster are rare. Such accounts would provide extremely valuable comparative materials for evaluation of the significance of family coping resources.

3. Research has not adequately examined alcohol-related treatment and intervention relevant to specific needs of women.

4. Maternal and paternal alcoholism differentially affect the social and psychologic well-being of young and developing children. These differences need to be more clearly defined in research and treatment.

References

Ablon J (1971): Bereavement in a Samoan community. *Br J Med Psychol*, 44:329–337.

Ablon J (1973): Reactions of Samoan burn patients and families to severe burns. *Soc Sci Med*, 7:167–178.

Ablon J (1976): Family structure and behavior in alcoholism: A review of the literature. In: *The Biology of Alcoholism* Vol 4, Kissin B. Begleiter H (eds.). New York: Plenum.

Ablon J (1979): Research frontiers for anthropologists in family studies. A case in point: Alcoholism and the family. *Human Organization, 38*(2):196–200.

Ablon J (1980): The significance of cultural patterning for the "alcoholic family." *Fam Process, 19*:127–144.

Ablon J, Cunningham W (1981): Implications of cultural patterning for the delivery of alcoholism services. *J Stud Alcohol*, Suppl. 9:185–206.

Ablon J, Ames G, Cunningham W (1984): To all appearances: The ideal American family. In: *Power to Change: Family Case Studies in the Treatment of Alcoholism*, Kaufman E (ed.). New York: Gardner.

Ames G (1982): Maternal alcoholism and family life: A cultural model for research and intervention. PhD dissertation in medical anthropology, University of California, San Francisco.

Ames G (1985): Middle class protestants: Alcoholism and the family. In: *The American Experience with Alcohol: Contrasting Cultural Perspectives*, Bennett L, Ames G (eds.). New York: Plenum.

Bales RF (1962): Attitudes toward drinking in the Irish culture. In: *Society, Culture and Drinking Patterns*, Pittman DJ, Snyder CR (eds.). New York: Wiley.

Bloch DA (1983): Family systems medicine: The field and the journal. *Fam Syst Med, 1*(1):3–11.

Bowen M (1974): Alcoholism as viewed through family systems theory and family psychotherapy. *Ann NY Acad Sci*, 233:111–122.

Bucke ES, Holt JB, Procter JE (eds.) (1976): *The Book of Disciplines of the United Methodist Church*. Nashville: United Methodist Publishing House.

Cahalan D (1970): *Problem Drinkers: A National Survey*. San Francisco: Jossey-Bass.

Cahalan D, Room R (1974): Problem drinking among American men. *Monographs of the Rutgers*

Center of Alcohol Studies 7. New Brunswick, NJ: Publications Center of Alcohol Studies.

Clark MM (1983a): Cultural context of medical practice. *West J Med, 139*(6):806–810.

Clark MM (1983b): Guest editor, special issue on cross-cultural medicine. *West J Med, 139*(6).

Committee for the Study of Health Consequences of the Stress of Bereavement, Institute of Medicine (1984): *Bereavement: Reactions, Consequences and Care.* Washington, DC: National Academy Press.

Conley PC, Sorensen A (1971): *The Staggering Steeple: The Story of Alcoholism and the Churches.* Philadelphia: Pilgrim Press.

Cumming E, Cumming J (1957): *Closed Ranks: An Experiment in Mental Health Education.* Cambridge: Harvard University Press.

Davis DI et al (1963): The adaptive consequences of drinking. *Psychiatry, 37*:209.

Goffman E (1963): *Stigma: Notes on the Management of Spoiled Identity.* Englewood Cliffs, NJ: Prentice-Hall.

Gough K (1971): The origin of the family. *J Marr Fam, 33*:760–771.

Greeley A (1972): *That Most Distressful Nation.* Chicago: Quadrangle.

Gusfield JR (1963): *Symbolic Crusade: Status Politics and the American Temperance Movement.* Urbana: University of Illinois Press.

Harwood A (ed.) (1981): *Ethnicity and Medical Care.* Cambridge: Harvard University Press.

Henry J (1965): *Pathways to Madness.* New York: Random House.

Henry J (1967): My life with the families of psychotic children. In: *The Psychological Interior of the Family,* Handel G (ed.). Chicago: Aldine.

Hill R, Hansen D (1962): Families in disaster. In: *Man and Society in Disaster,* Baker GW, Chapman DW (eds.). New York: Basic Books.

Howell JT (1973): *Hard Living on Clay Street.* Garden City, NY: Anchor Books.

Janes CR, Pawson IG (1986): Migration and biocultural adaptation: Samoans in California. *Soc Sci Med, 22*(8):821–834.

Kleinman A (1980): *Patients and Healers in the Context of Culture: An Exploration of the Borderland Between Anthropology, Medicine, and Psychiatry.* Berkeley: University of California Press.

Leininger M (1978): *Transcultural Nursing: Concepts, Theories and Practices.* New York: Wiley.

Lemert M (1951): *Social pathology: A Systematic Approach to the Theory of Sociopathic Behavior.* New York: McGraw-Hill.

Levine H (1978): The discovery of addiction: Changing conceptions of habitual drunkenness in America. *J Stud Alcohol, 39*:143–174.

Lewis O (1959): *Five Families.* New York: Basic Books.

Lewis O (1961): *The Children of Sanchez.* New York: Random House.

Lewis O (1965): *La Vida.* New York: Random House.

Lewis O (1967): An anthropological approach to family studies. In: *The Psychological Interior of the Family,* Handel G (ed.). Chicago: Aldine.

Lindemann E (1944): Symptomatology and management of acute grief. *Am J Psychiatry, 101*:141–148.

Maddison D, Walker WL (1967): Factors affecting the outcome of conjugal bereavement. *Br J Psychiatry, 113*:1057–1067.

Mead M (1930): *Social Organization of Manu'a.* Honolulu: Bishop Museum Press Reprints, 1969.

Mead M (1961): *Coming of Age in Samoa,* rev. ed. New York: Dell.

Messenger JC (1969): *Inis Beag.* New York: Holt Rinehart Winston.

Mulford H, Miller D (1964): Measuring public acceptance of the alcoholic as a sick person. *Quarterly Journal of Studies on Alcohol, 25*:314–323.

Oates WE (1966): *Alcohol In and Out of the Church.* Nashville: Broadman.

Orcutt JD (1976): Ideological variation in the structure of deviant types: A multivariate comparison of alcoholism and heroin addiction. *Social Forces, 55*:419–437.

Orque M et al (1983): *Ethnic Nursing Care: A Multicultural Approach.* St. Louis: Mosby.

Paolino TJ, McCrady BS (1977): *The Alcoholic Marriage: Alternative Perspectives.* New York: Grune & Stratton.

Reiss I (1965): The universality of the family: A conceptual analysis. *J Marr Fam, 27*:443–453.

Room R (1982): Alcohol as an issue in Papua New Guinea: A view from the outside. In: *Through a Glass Darkly: Beer and Modernization in Papua New Guinea,*

Marshall M (ed.). Boroko, Papua New Guinea: Institute of Applied Social and Economic Research.

Rorabaugh WJ (1979): *The Alcoholic Republic: An American Tradition.* New York: Oxford University Press.

Schvaneveldt JD (1966): The interactional framework in the study of the family. In: *Emerging Conceptual Frameworks in Family Analysis,* Nye Fl, Berardo F (eds.). New York: Macmillan.

Silverman PR (1967): Services to the widowed: First steps in a program of preventive intervention. *Community Ment Health J, 3:*37–44.

Silverman PR (1969): The widow to widow program. *Mental Hygiene, 53:*333–337.

Stack C (1974): *All Our Kin.* New York: Harper & Row.

Steinglass P (1980): A life history model of the alcoholic family. *Fam Process, 19:*211–226.

Stivers R (1976): *The Hair of the Dog.* University Park: Pennsylvania State University Press.

Stivers R (1985): Historical meanings of Irish-American drinking. In: *The American Experience with Alcohol,* Bennett A, Ames G (eds.). New York: Plenum.

Tylor EB (1871): *Primitive Culture.* London: J Murray.

U.S. Bureau of the Census (1986): Household and family characteristics: March, 1985. Series P-20, No. 411. Washington, DC: GPO.

9

HEALTH CARE FINANCING, POLICY, AND FAMILY NURSING PRACTICE

New Opportunities

Susan B. Meister, RN, PhD

The health care services offered to families are often a function of the health policies designed by our governments. Sometimes these policies are proactively developed to serve families; often they are not. This chapter offers a framework for analysis of family data to determine the services necessary to promote family health.

Susan Meister is Director of Health Services Research at Children's Hospital and Health Center in San Diego, California. Also an Associate in Health Policy at the Division of Health Policy Research and Education at Harvard Medical School, she is known for her work with family health policy.

Introduction

The opportunities to be realized by articulating knowledge from family nursing practice with health care financing policy development are the same ones we recognize when a person with a clinical background is appointed to a major health policy position. They are opportunities to join clinical and policy issues.

Making the most of a merger of practice and policy does not require transforming family nurse clinicians into policy analysts or full-time researchers. It requires only that clinicians adapt their perspectives enough to incorporate health care financing policy. In actuality, this will require that family nurse clinicians acquire a new view of families. This view is the focus of this chapter, which proposes that family nurse clinicians systematically examine the relationships between the needs and experiences of families in their caseloads and the health care financing policy.

The Need for a New Perspective on Families

Acquiring a perspective that includes systematic assessment of the relationships between financing policies and family well-being will eventually produce three kinds of benefits: improving the clinician's ability to obtain information about pertinent health policies; potentiating the clinician's ability to use policy information to serve families; and opening new avenues for using clinical knowledge to shape policy development.

This work is justified. Historically, clinical knowledge has sometimes been articulated with health policies, but the current slate of policy issues bears little resemblance to those historical issues. The stakes are higher, implications are more complex, and it is more difficult to antici-

pate the effects of financing policy options. It is especially important to understand those effects in their real context, which is the family. The assumption here is that because family nurse clinicians work with a caseload of families, they have both the commitment and perspective necessary to respond to the new issues in health care financing.

Relationships between Policy and Family

In general, health care financing policies define eligibility, benefits, and payment systems for health services. Because these three factors are critical determinants of access to and use of health services, the policies have direct effects on health status. Changes in any of these factors are defined narrowly, within specific policies. However, the effects of the changes reverberate in a larger system.

Health care financing policy can affect every member of a vulnerable family. These are second-order, interactive effects. For example, when a family "spends down" and meets Medicaid eligibility as medically needy (that is, incurs such large medical bills that their remaining assets fall below the state's Aid to Families with Dependent Children (AFDC) eligibility level), it becomes vulnerable in new ways. Even events unrelated to health, if they create unmanageable demands, can produce health problems for such families. Whether or not such events occur, the results of spending down will require that the family adapt to an unfamiliar and risky financial status.

These effects are a central concern of policy analysis, and they become a major focus of nursing intervention. Commonly, data about probable effects on the family are especially limited. This is a problem because health needs and acquisition of services are family issues. Effective services benefit the family, but the costs (both monetary and nonmonetary) of acquiring those services can range from reasonable to devastating and from expected to unexpected.

The problem is further compounded by the nature of families. Some families are especially vulnerable to financing policies. For example, families with infants, toddlers, and adolescents are more likely to experience catastrophic illness and less likely to have the financial means to cope with the cost of care (McManus, Newacheck, Matlin, 1986). Families with aged members are likely to be faced with costs that exceed the fixed incomes of those members (Harvard Medicare Project, 1986). The most important point, and the one most obvious to clinicians, is that any one family may simultaneously experience multiple vulnerabilities.

Family nurse clinicians, who assist families in managing health and illness, observe the effects of financing policies on families and discover the innovations designed by families to work with (or around) policy problems. Family nurses are, therefore, in an excellent position to reconceptualize family care to include its important relationship with health policy. Reconceptualization calls for:

- Learning to look across a caseload and identify pertinent characteristics
- Relating those characteristics to policy issues
- Identifying current problems, potential risks, early warning signals

Family nurse clinicians appreciate the dynamic states of the family, and this reconceptualization calls for relating families to an equally dynamic entity. Health policy is rarely static and may even appear to be chaotic. The process of policy development may not be orderly but it does possess three discernible elements that bear predictable relationships to each other. These elements should be used to guide efforts at reconceptualization.

Elements of Policy Development

Policy development is usually a recognizable process. The elements of this process have been described by several authors, but one of the clearest descriptions comes from Richmond and Kotelchuck (1983). They describe a tripartite model of social policy development that includes the element of (1) knowledge base, (2) political will, and (3) social strategy.

Briefly, the authors define knowledge base as the set of information that emerges from basic, applied, and clinical sciences. Political will refers to the will of the population, which can become or affect the aims of politicians. These two elements often define the policy agenda. Policy analysis focuses on designing ways to bring knowledge to bear on health issues (social strategy). For example, advances in technology (knowledge base) have produced dilemmas regarding application (political will). In this example, social strategies would be developed and analyzed in an effort to find the best way to apply technology developments.

Richmond and Kotelchuck (1983) emphasize the ebb and flow of this model. Rarely are all three elements equally potent in shaping a policy. More often, an advance in the knowledge base or a change in the political will will precipitate a new focus for policy. However, post hoc analyses of policies will usually reveal that all three elements were active.

Caseload Analysis

A caseload is a naturally occurring group of families, not a group of research subjects or a representative sample. Even so, the concepts embedded in research methods are useful in identifying the characteristics of a caseload. For example, how are age, gender, health status, economic status, and social status distributed in the caseload? Is the group defined by geography or by a common health problem?

This analysis is far from cursory. The clinicians must identify not only obvious characteristics, such as those listed previously, but also the relationships among them. For example, how are these families related to social and health welfare programs? Moynihan (1986) pointed out that in 1984, "every other American household had one or more members participating in one or more government social-welfare or social-insurance programs" (p. 121). The clinician is concerned with identifying relative dependence on these and other programs, such as private health insurance, employment benefits, and community support programs. Together, these dependencies define the kinds of financing policies that could or do affect the families in the caseload.

Financing Policy Issues

A clinician is too busy with the daily demands of practice to perform a continuing analysis of all possible policy issues. Further, the clinician's caseload may not be relevant to some policy issues. In other words, it is most efficient for the clinician to identify relationships between the characteristics of the caseload and the particular financing policy issues.

The analysis of the caseload points out specific financing policies that are directly related to the families. The clinician can identify the direction and magnitude of such effects. Reports of proposals for reform or impending policy decisions would alert the clinician to consider how the proposals could affect the families.

There are also some enduring policy issues that should become part of the clinician's ongoing assessment. These issues are related to comparisons between programmatic goals of health care financing and societal goals for health services delivery. For example, Gornick et al (1985) identify four current concerns about the major public health care financing programs, Medicare and Medicaid. Do these programs provide access for the most needy and vulnerable populations? Do they assure equitable distribution of services? Are the covered services appropriate? Finally, is the system effective and efficient?

These concerns are remarkably close to issues that family nurse clinicians deal with in practice. At a minimum, the nurse assesses the family's health care coverage and, often, becomes involved in making certain that the family receives all possible benefits. Vulnerability, equity, scope of services, and practicality are familiar issues.

Identifying Problems, Risks, and Signals

The caseload analysis enables the clinician to complete an assessment of where the caseload stands in relation to financing policies.

How are current policies affecting the families? The nurse clinician is in the unique position to observe the effects of both federal and state policies, as well as how those policies are implemented in particular institutions. For example, federal and state policies come together to shape the Medicaid program. Focusing on how Medicaid pays for children's hospital services, the nurse can readily identify how the confluence of the federal, state and institutional policies affect quality, equity, access, and effectiveness of care and how the care affects families. It may also be true that families are affecting the institutional policies.

Extant research about the health status of families will help the clinician in making this assessment, but the research is not yet complete. For example, Gilliss (1983) has identified the conceptual, methodologic, measurement, and analytic shortfalls of research that aims to use the family as the unit of analysis. Meister (1984) has addressed a similar issue, describing problems with establishing an empirical measure of family well-being. Feetham (1984) conducted an exhaustive review of nursing research of families and pointed out that although nursing has made progress in identifying some of the behaviors of the family and its members that are related to positive outcomes, research has not yet progressed to the point of identifying actual predictors of family and familial health.

These limitations will have generic effects because it is difficult to describe the relationships between families and policies when research findings have not yet fully defined *family,*

family health, and *family processes.* Even so, the family nurse clinician can identify ways to articulate policy and family effects.

For example, consider the recently proposed Medicare reform of merging Parts A and B of the program (Harvard Medicare Project, 1986). The authors of this proposal suggest that such action would make it easier for beneficiaries of both Parts A and B to understand and use their coverage. Clinicians can determine whether or not this reform would assist the families in their caseloads, even without a sound empirical base for defining *family health.* The nurse would use clinical knowledge and go as far as possible in describing the effects of a given policy on a caseload of families.

The clinician can do more than assess how current policies affect families and estimate how proposed reforms might affect them. It is also possible to watch for early warning signals. Signs of increasing needs for services or emerging inadequacies of health care financing can occur at many levels in the system, and clinicians will see the signs from families. For example, are Diagnostic Related Group (DRG) approaches to reimbursement creating or solving problems for specific kinds of families? What is the net effect on families of the illness-based, improvement-oriented payment system? Are these problems that are, or could be, solved by changes in other financing policies? As noted earlier, health care is delivered in an increasingly complex context, and well-focused surveillance at the point of delivery and by a person capable of detecting effects for individuals as well as their families is exceptionally valuable.

Example: A Hypothetical Caseload

To illustrate the process of reconceptualization, first consider the three hypothetical families described in the following paragraphs. Assume that each family has been seen in a primary care clinic and has become part of the practice of one graduate student in family nursing.

Family A

Mr. A   (father) absent from home, no contact with family for 3 years.

Ms. A   (mother) 22 years old, 8th grade education, unemployed, 7 months pregnant, receives AFDC, lives in a two room apartment in high-crime urban area.

Bobby   (son of Mr. and Ms. A) 4 years old, lives with mother, does not attend formal child day care or school, poorly nourished, recent hospitalization for fractured femur covered by Medicaid.

John   (son of Mr. and Ms. A) 3 years old, lives with mother, growth is at 30th percentile, no regular source of health care, receives episodic care at local emergency room.

Family B

Mr. B   (father) 70 years old, myocardial infarction 6 months ago, receives SSI, no longer able to function independently but able to stay at home with care by his wife. Lives in family home, located in lower-middle-class suburb. Receives monthly Visiting Nurse Association (VNA) visits.

Ms. B   (mother) 68 years old, advanced arthritis, physician visits covered by MediCare, no employment experience, cares for husband full-time, has minimal involvement with financial arrangements for family.

Ms. F   (daughter of Mr. and Ms. B) 35 years old, divorced, employed as a college professor, has health insurance through employer, has two preschool children who attend preschool from 9–4 on weekdays, lives 40 miles from parents and visits them once a month.

Mr. B   (son of Mr. and Ms. B) 33 years old, single, graduate student, works part-time without benefits, lives 500 miles from his parents and visits them once or twice a year.

Family C

Mr. D   16 years old, sporadically employed at minimum wage, has not yet finished high school, lives with his girlfriend in her parents' home.

Ms. E   15 years old, 6 months pregnant, recently dropped out of high school, attends community clinic for pregnant adolescents, brittle diabetic, no employment experience.

Mr. E   (father of Ms. E) 32 years old, in good health, self-employed as a restaurant manager, 2 years of college, has three other children at home: Joan (10 years old, good health), Richard (8 years old, learning disability), Mary (6 years old, unusually gifted and attending private school). His restaurant is not yet financially stable and he does not purchase health insurance for either himself or his family.

Ms. E   (mother of Ms. E) 31 years old, employed as a clerk in a small business, has health insurance through employer, in good health, high school education. Lives with husband, daughter, and daughter's boyfriend in an apartment in a small urban neighborhood.

Caseload Analysis

The analysis begins by using each member of the families to identify the distribution of age, gender, health status, economic status, and social status in the caseload. Table 9-1 shows an abridged version of this assessment.

This caseload includes families at several levels of economic and social status. In most cases, the families have either insufficient resources or resources that are virtually consumed by the needs of the members. No family has much of a buffer, at least in terms of economic or health needs. The families also demonstrate several kinds of intergenerational linkages. These linkages are not casual; in fact, in some cases they are central to the well-being of the members.

This step in the analysis has taken information collected for clinical practice and reordered it. The next step is to integrate the family characteristics and identify relationships among them.

Table 9–1   Caseload Assessment by Family Member

Member	Health	Economic	Social
Absent father 22-year-old woman 4-year-old boy 3-year-old boy	Unknown Pregnant Disrupted Disrupted	Threatened and tentative	Poor, little education
70-year-old man 68-year-old woman	Impaired Impaired	Marginal	Old, fixed income
35-year-old woman 2 preschoolers	Good Unknown	Fairly stable	Middle class
33-year-old man	Normal	Marginal	Student
16-year-old male 15-year-old female	Good Pregnant, diabetic	Poor	Poor education
32-year-old man 10-year-old girl 8-year-old boy 6-year-old girl 31-year-old woman	Good Good Impaired Good Good	Highly stressed and marginal	Middle class

Table 9–2 illustrates the beginning of this step in the analysis.

This kind of summary uses the clinician's information to identify specific needs, dependencies, and vulnerabilities in the families. It is a synopsis of the ways in which a family is or is not coping with enduring and episodic demands. Thus, the analysis yields an outline of the families' current relationships with many policies, including health care financing.

Financing Policy Issues

Each of these families illustrates Moynihan's (1986) points about multiple dependencies on social and health policies. For example, Family A needs both AFDC and Medicaid to manage the basic and health needs of the members. Even with these supports, the family is not doing well. Further, if policies regarding Medicaid eligibility affected either eligibility or access to the children's hospital, every member of the family would be affected.

Family B has marked involvement with several social and health policies. Several members are particularly vulnerable to untoward health events and, should they occur, the intergenerational ties would be pressed into service. This family illustrates the interweaving of social and health policies from several levels of government, as well as the potential for catastrophic effects of small changes in any of those policies.

The third family demonstrates how policies affecting only one or two members can become crucial determinants of the well-being of all members. The economic and health needs of this family are financed through policies affecting one or two members.

This analysis would help the nurse clinician to identify programs and policies that should be part of a working clinical knowledge base. The analysis would also lead the nurse to identify networks related to those programs and assure that the links to those networks were well established. For example, the nurse would develop

Table 9–2   Caseload Analysis by Family Characteristics

	Current Policy Dependencies	Health Services Used	Social Vulnerabilities
Family A	AFDC Medicaid	Children's hospital, Emergency room	Poor Unemployed Limited education Uninsured
Family B	SSI Medicare Tax deduction for childcare Employment benefits Student health	Private MD, University's health services, VNA	Aging on fixed income Intergenerational dependency Uninsured members
Family C	Employment benefits	Community clinic, Employee health services	Needs special education Three generations depend on two incomes Uninsured members

informal ties to the individuals who process paperwork related to benefits, evaluate program effectiveness, and plan new program initiatives. Finally, the clinician's analysis would provide a unique perspective on the relationships among family needs, access to services, equity in use of appropriate services, and viability of the systems' supporting the health of the families.

Identifying Problems, Risks, and Signals

The clinician can then identify how well the families are doing and determine health needs not yet addressed. Obtaining information about policies and programs to meet those needs and designing plans to improve the families' access to such supports may be necessary.

It is also important to identify how well the families are doing in comparison to other families or individuals. Are these families spending more or less, receiving more or less (or different) services than most Americans? Why? Reports on national trends in access to services (Robert Wood Johnson Foundation, 1983), national health care expenditures (Levit et al, 1985), Medicare trends (Harvard Medicare Project, 1986), and Medicaid use (Mauskopf et al, 1985) are useful adjuncts for this comparative analysis.

Over time, the clinician also monitors emerging trends or proposals for policy changes. The caseload analysis helps to sort out the potential impact of proposed changes. It also helps to establish a baseline, from which the clinician can track the status of each family.

For example, capitation is clearly leading the health care financing policy agenda. If the clinician imagines, say, a lump sum payment to the state to cover all health care costs for eligible children during the year, then the caseload analysis can be used to identify what approaches to capitation would help or hinder the families.

In summary, using a caseload of families to systematically examine relationships between families and health care financing policy allows the clinician to see the familial supports in a larger context, to identify problems and respond with policy information or access to the networks involved with programs, and to monitor family status in relation to current or emerging policies.

The method suggested here is a beginning point; each clinician would develop a method specifically tailored to the caseload. The method might also be used by clinicians interested in bringing caseload information to bear on policy decisions.

Caseload Analysis and Policy Development

Much of current policy analysis focuses on identifying methods to achieve cost containment. The optimal method will contain costs and avoid increasing the vulnerabilities of families; perhaps it will even reduce those that exist. However, without data about probable effects on the family, it is difficult to include these concerns in the analysis.

The majority of large, representative databases do not include family data. Those that do, such as the National Medical Care Utilization and Expenditures Survey, are not always used to analyze family implications. Although these databases are certainly valuable, they cannot assure that the analyses supporting policy development will be comprehensive.

There are many well-traveled paths that bring information to policy development; transmission is not the obstacle. The problem is conceptualization. Policy analysis focuses on specific health care financing issues and particular aggregates, and clinicians usually focus on specific health problems and individual families. When the clinician's knowledge is reconceptualized, it becomes more closely related to policy development.

The knowledge of the nurse clinician could apply to any of the three elements of policy development. Meister (1985) used DRGs as an example of the potential for creating links between clinical knowledge and policy development. In that example, health policy for financing children's health services was identified as aiming to increase knowledge about DRGs, respond to the political will, and create a strategy for action. The points of articulation with the clinical perspective were cited as checking the match between DRG research and clinical reality, identifying families' probable needs and reactions to DRGs, and identifying innovations that are both cost-effective and successful.

Translating caseload information for policy development would require another set of analyses to produce information that could be used in macroanalyses such as cost-effectiveness analysis, cost-benefit analysis, decision analysis, or consensus development (Meister, 1986). The requirements are significant, but it is important to remember that data do affect policy decisions. In a recent review, Dobson and Bialeck (1985) demonstrate how data have affected health care financing policies over the past 60 years. The paper points out the increasing reliance on data for policy development, although not always for policy choice. The message that "data matter" refers to macroanalyses of costs, benefits, use, and needs, but it can sometimes refer to research at a less aggregated level.

Clinicians interested in these applications of caseload knowledge might begin by joining forces with a researcher and helping to design studies that include appropriate family variables and analyses. An analysis of providing health care for low-income children (Rosenbaum, Johnson, 1986) would serve well as an example of reconceptualizing data about current health needs and services into an analysis of financing policy issues.

Summary

The important implication of health care financing policy for family nurse clinicians is that each clinician must develop a systematic method for examining the intricate relationships between policies and families. The method could begin with the following questions:

- What are the characteristics of the caseload?
- Which health care financing policies affect these families? How? Which financing policy networks are pertinent to the care of these families?
- What does the well-being of these families suggest regarding the larger goals of policy, such as access, equity, appropriateness of services, effectiveness, and efficiency?
- Are there any early warning signs to be noted in the caseload?
- Are there reasons and resources for bringing the clinical knowledge of this caseload to the policy development arena?

The effects of this work will effect greater contributions to family well-being and it will have the potential to net better health policies as well.

Issues for Further Investigation

1. How does current U.S. government health policy affect specific health problems such as teen pregnancy or alcohol and drug abuse?

2. What constraints do current U.S. health policies impose upon families who are trying to care for their chronically ill members?

3. How can a comparison of countries with disparate morbidity and mortality profiles lead to a better understanding of the influences of health policy on national health?

4. What are the appropriate units of analysis to display family morbidity and mortality in evaluating the impact of health policies?

References

Dobson A, Bialek R (1985): Shaping public policy from the perspective of a data builder. *Health Care Financing Review*, 6:117–134.

Feetham SL (1984): Family research in nursing. In: *Annu Rev Nurs Res Vol 2*, Werley H, Fitzpatrick J (eds.). New York: Springer-Verlag.

Gilliss CL (1983): The family as the unit of analysis: Strategies for the nurse researcher. *ANS, 5*:50–59.

Gornick, M et al (1985): Twenty years of Medicare and Medicaid: Covered populations, use of benefits, and problem expenditures. *Health Care Financing Review*, Annual supplement: 13–59.

Harvard Medicare Project (1986): *Medicare: Coming of Age (A Proposal for Reform)*. Center for Health Policy and Management, John F. Kennedy School of Government, Division of Health Policy Research and Education, Harvard University.

Levit KR et al (1985): National health expenditures. *Health Care Financing Review, 7*:1–35.

Mauskopf J, Rodgers J, Dobson A (1985): State Medicaid program controls and health care services utilization. *Health Care Financing Review, 7*:16–29.

McManus M, Newacheck P, Matlin N (1986): Catastrophic childhood illness. *American Academy of Pediatrics Health Financing Report, 3*:1–2.

Meister SB (1984): Family well-being. In: *Nursing Care of Victims of Family Violence.* Englewood Cliffs, NJ: Prentice-Hall.

Meister SB (1985): Building bridges between practice and health policy. *Am J Mat Child Nurs, 10*:155–157.

Meister SB (1986): Practice and health policy development: Enhancing the health of the nation. In: *Translating Commitment to Reality*, Feetham S, Malasanos L (eds.). Kansas City: American Academy of Nursing.

Moynihan DP (1986): *Family and Nation.* San Diego: HBJ.

Richmond JB, Kotelchuck ML (1983): Political influences: Rethinking national health policy. In: *Handbook on Health Professions Education*, McGuire et al (eds.). San Francisco: Jossey-Bass.

Robert Wood Johnson Foundation (1983): Updated report on access to health care for the American people. Princeton, NJ: Robert Wood Johnson Foundation Special Report.

Rosenbaum S, Johnson– K (1986): Providing health care for low-income children: Reconciling health goals with child health financing realities. *Millbank Memorial Quarterly, 64*:442–478.

10

FAMILY LIFE IN THE 21ST CENTURY

An Analysis of Old Forms, Current Trends, and Future Scenarios

Robert Staples, PhD

The family is a fluid institution that responds to a number of social forces. Throughout history it has been influenced by diverse forces, including the advent of the industrial revolution, changes in technology, and teachings of religious institutions. Today's family faces a challenge to its traditional structure and function. This chapter explores both historical and emerging trends in marriage and the family, with particular emphasis on the Black family in America.

Robert Staples, an internationally known Black sociologist, is a Professor at the University of California at San Francisco School of Nursing (Department of Social and Behavioral Sciences). Considered one of the leading authorities on Black family life, he has written or edited nine books on that subject. He has received distinguished achievement awards from Howard University and the National Council on Family Relations and has lectured at over 400 colleges in the United States, Latin America, Europe, and Asia.

Introduction

Those who are committed to the maintenance of the family in its present form are inclined to view emerging trends in marriage and the family as a deterioration of this social unit. Much of this concern is derived from the enshrinement of myths that surround the American family of the past. It is generally believed that the family was an institution in which one was assured of companionship and socially approved parentage; it was the source of personal warmth, affection, and security. A closer examination of history reveals that the role of the 18th century American family was economic, not emotional. Its basic function was not to provide emotional support for individuals but to preserve and transmit property and to stabilize the working community. Far from being the idyllic unit we believed it to be, it was more easily characterized by the economic and social subjugation of women, numerous cases of infanticide, the selling of wives, and repression of individual needs (Calhoun, 1960).

Changes in the American Family

The changes occurring in American family life need not be viewed as regressive. Moreover, it should be noted that these changes have not occurred in a straight line. Instead, we find periods of sexual freedom followed by sexual conservatism, female equality supplanted by the patriarchal family systems, and so on. Thus, we must be cautious in perceiving the present changes in marriage and the family as irreversible or new. A more realistic approach would view these changes as links in the evolution of the family that are inexorable concomitants in the alteration of extrafamilial institutions that form the infrastructure of human society.

What, exactly, are the changes taking place in the American family constellation? Proceed-

ing from the decade during which these changes began to take place, the decade of the 1960s, we find the family life cycle being modified from the normative expectations that ideal boy and ideal girl fall in love, the marriage is consummated with a sexual union, the husband is expected to make a living while the wife is confined to homemaking, children are brought into the unit as a welcomed asset, and the marriage is expected to last a lifetime.

Today, a more typical emerging pattern is that couples simply get together, premarital sex is a normative expectation for both men and women, heterosexual cohabitation often antedates marriage (if marriage occurs at all), women are becoming more oriented toward careers outside the home, the bearing of children is being shunned by larger numbers of women, and the surety that the majority of marriages established this year will not exist 20 years later.

Although these emergent patterns of family life do not exist to the same extent among all groups, regions, and religions, it is an irrefutable fact that they are the harbinger of new family lifestyles for many Americans. It is merely wishful thinking to believe that such lifestyles are confined to certain sections of the country or a segment of the population we label as socially deviant. Although this author is not personally predisposed toward the conservative, moralistic position about the role of the family, there is much validity in the statement by the noted sociologist Amitai Etzioni (1974) that "the common denominator of all these family substitutes is that they do not last, are highly unstable, and constitute revolving door unions rather than a family." (p. 11) His objection to them is that they are not meeting human needs much better than the traditional family institution.

The Sexual Revolution

Sexologists are not at all in agreement on whether there have been any significant changes in sexual behavior in the past 50 years. Many contend that the changes in sexual behavior really occurred around the turn of the century, after World War II, or in the late 1960s. What is clear is that the public attitude toward sex is much more liberal, and discussion of the subject is more open and candid. A review of research on sexual behavior in the 1970s revealed a sharp increase in liberal premarital sexual behavior over the previous decade. Only a small minority of those surveyed had not engaged in premarital sex by a certain age. Of particular interest was the finding that the standard for sexual behavior before marriage had become similar for males and females (Clayton, Bokemeir, 1980). In the 1980s, according to one survey, the threat of acquired immune deficiency syndrome (AIDS) has caused college students to change their sexual habits. They have become more conservative than the students of the 1970s ("Less But Better Sex for College Students," 1987).

This writer holds the opinion that the trend toward nonmarital sexual relations has been greatest in the last 20 years. One of the most authoritative surveys on premarital sexual behavior (Simenauer, Carroll 1982) reported that 91% of adult single women have had intercourse while single, in contrast to the one-half reported by Kinsey (1953) over 30 years ago. Furthermore, there have been qualitative changes in the kind of nonmarital sexual relations taking place. In the 1970s a number of women ranked love and commitment as secondary in their motives for engaging in nonmarital sexual activity (Shope, 1971). The decline of the double standard is responsible for much of the increase in nonmarital coitus. A few surveys have even uncovered greater nonmarital sexual activity among women than men (Jessor, Jessor, 1977).

Although many would hail these changes as a hallmark of progress, a triumph over our Victorian past, the results of sexual liberation are mixed. In a recent poll of people under age 22, about 50% felt that sex without love is unenjoyable or unacceptable ("The Revolution is Over,"

1984). One might also question the positive values expressed in the findings of Robert and Amy Levin (1975) that the majority of the women they sampled had either engaged in extramarital sexual relations, wanted to, or planned to do so in the future. Although this may give them parity to men, it does nothing to establish trust in a marriage. A basic reason for the misgivings of many Americans, particularly women, about the new sexual freedom is that many have internalized earlier the values of chastity or, at least, sex as a function of love ("The Revolution is Over," 1984). It is not the sexual permissiveness per se that is harmful but the reconciliation of previously established values with their current behavior.

Those who would decry the decline of sexual morals must also acknowledge that American society constantly provides its members with sexual stimuli at every turn—in its advertising, beauty pageants, clothing styles, and so on. Sexual variety is often encouraged, but its exercise is forbidden. People are given numerous opportunities for sexual infidelity, but sexual exclusivity is still the norm for most Americans. Hence, a great amount of our energy is cathected into repression, fantasy, scheming, and guilt. The next stage in the sexual revolution seems to be a pattern of secondary virginity, whereby those disillusioned by a period of premarital sex will choose to remain chaste or at least be very discriminate until marriage. Whether this will be a significant improvement over the present situation remains to be seen.

Signs of a decline in the sexual revolution are evident. *Time* magazine's (1984) cover story proclaimed "The Revolution is Over, in the 80's, Caution and Commitment are the Watchwords." The article cited numerous studies and quotations by sexologists to support its claim that American sexuality had reverted to more traditional expectations. Certainly the increase in sexually transmitted disease and its correlation with the number of sexual partners has brought about a decline in indiscriminate sexual activity. The statistics reveal that 1 in 4 Americans between the ages of 15 and 55 will contract a sexually transmitted disease at some time in their lives. Particularly frightening is the incidence of AIDS, which is usually fatal to its victims and has been found in all segments of the population ("A Nasty New Epidemic," 1985). It should be noted, however, that herpes and AIDS have received an unusual amount of publicity, which has shaped the more conservative attitudes toward nonmarital sexuality. Once the media coverage recedes, it is probable that many Americans will return to their former sexual lifestyles.

Moreover, any proclamation that the sexual revolution is dead may be premature. The liberal sexual values of the 1960s and 1970s still exist but are tempered by other considerations. In addition to the enormous publicity on sexually transmitted diseases, the role of women as traditional gatekeeper of sexual morality was influential in shaping a more conservative sexual attitude in the 1980s. As women age, they become more concerned about their biologic deadline and the prospect of having children before becoming "too old." Consequently, some women have attempted to confine sexual activity to a stable relationship that might culminate in marriage or the birth of children. A survey of college students found female students more determined to have sexual relationships resulting in marriage before age 30 ("Less But Better Sex for College Students," 1987). As always, women have more to lose from permissive sexual activity than men. They are the victims of unwanted pregnancies, abortions, possible damage from unsafe contraceptives, and the risk of cervical cancer associated with having multiple sexual partners.

A contributing factor to the emergence of those attitudes was the economic recession of the 1980s. As men and women became more concerned about their economic security, they retreated into stable relationships and marriage as a form of personal security. Still, sexual attitudes and behavior did not revert back to the 1950s, a period when half of American women married without previous sexual experience.

Studies continue to reveal a minority of women entering marriage as virgins, and there has been only a modest change in male sexual behavior in the 20th century (Clayton, Bokemeir, 1980). Other changes in American dating and marriage patterns make any reversal of changes in sexuality unlikely. For example, the majority of Americans are marrying after the age of 24, and it is unrealistic to expect 6 to 10 years of dating to be asexual. Furthermore, about one-third of Americans over the age of 18 are unmarried and unlikely to lead a celibate existence during their single life. Finally, the increasing psychologic and economic independence of women means that they do not have to adhere to a rigid double standard that favors male permissiveness and female chastity in order to acquire a husband and a reasonable standard of living. Hence, the sexual revolution may have slowed down in favor of a greater selectivity in choosing sexual partners and confining sex to stable relationships, but it is not over.

Singlehood and the Future of Marriage

A decade ago, our society was caught up in debating the validity of traditional marriage and, more especially, in debating the roles of women in marriage. Some even asserted that marriage is an anachronism and childbearing is an oppressive aspect of the female role (Bernard, 1975). During this period in our history, lifestyles alternative to traditional marriage were receiving a great deal of media coverage. "To live a carefree single life, being true to only one's self" seemed the popular philosophy of the day. Whatever we may think about this period and related concerns about the family, there is little question that our views and even theoretical precepts have been altered. Until that time the sociologic explanation of marriage and family life within this society had been a fairly standard and predictable justification of the nuclear family and of its relationship to the larger social order. Furthermore, emphasis was placed on a number of well-defined functions that were attributed to marriage and the resulting nuclear family unit. Murdock (1949) explained that marriage was that structure through which relationships are established and normalized. Others with similar views included Malinowski (1930), who viewed marriage as a universally accepted means through which parenthood was legitimated. Spiro (1954) also followed in this tradition by asserting that the nuclear family is universal— that regardless of the outward structure, the essence of all families is nuclear.

Others viewed marriage and family life as rather fixed in its relationship to the larger social order. Parsons and Bales (1955), for example, have attempted to show that the structure of the nuclear family was the best possible in this highly industrialized, urbanized, and complex society. Furthermore, many of these theorists shared the view that any exception to the perceived norm was not simply considered different, or seen as representing acceptable alternatives, but rather they tended to see exceptions as deviant or unacceptable to the normal functioning of society. The major emphasis from both social scientists and the popular media was that marriage was and should be the goal of most people in our society at some point in their lives. The fact that the American family was faced with a multitude of problems, even at that time, appeared to have little effect on the popular emphasis that marriage and the nuclear family were the best of all possible worlds.

What is most interesting in this area is the widespread discussion and increasing acceptance of alternative lifestyles, and it is within this context that "singlehood" has taken on new dimensions. Singlehood is, of course, not new. Most societies, including this one, have in some form provided for an acceptable state of being single—usually within a religious context. "Natural" periods of being single in our society have also been acceptable: adolescence, early adulthood, and a period of time following the death of a spouse. It seems clear, however, that few, if

any, provisions were made for singlehood outside of some very clearly defined institutional boundaries. Looking at this another way, one could say that being single had little or nothing to do with the wishes and desires of the individual; rather it was a category or status with well-defined parameters. The issue of establishing a lifestyle is a rather recent aspect of American life. Historically, the concept of singlehood, as we are attempting to appraise it, was not nor could have been considered. The issue of individual identity is relevant to this discussion. There was, for most societies in the past, no socially accepted identity outside the context of the family or any other prescribed and accepted group. Marriage was, therefore, not merely a union of two individuals but rather a union of representatives from socially established groups. Again, the issue of free choice was not an option for individuals. It has only been since the transformation of the family from a rural to an urban setting; the combined effects of industrialization and its by-products; the weakening of the economic base of the family and its traditional system of support; and the increasing advent of leisure time that we begin to set the stage for the discussion at hand.

Although times are changing, it is difficult to imagine a society in which large numbers of people reject the concept of marriage. In fact, one cannot envision such a society being able to perpetuate itself. America's forefathers obviously considered singlehood a threat when they imposed a special tax on men who insisted on remaining bachelors. As we look at contemporary America, we see how far we have come from the days when birth, marriage, and death were the three supreme experiences of life. The proportion of never-married adults in the United States continues to increase. In the 1960s, the average American married between the ages of 20 and 24. In 1984, we found 57% of women in that age range still single. In 1960, only 28% were still unmarried. Circa 1984, about 75% of American males were still bachelors at the age of 24 compared to 53% in 1960. It would be easy and comforting to assume that Americans are delaying marriage until a later age. But the proportion of singles has also increased for the age group 25–29. Although many will eventually marry, it is conceivable that a large proportion will remain single throughout their entire lives. Moreover, if we consider the number of individuals divorced, separated, or widowed, over 60 million Americans, or about 40% of all people over the age of 14, are, theoretically, in the state of singleness (U.S. Bureau of the Census, 1984).

One of the most significant factors contributing to singlehood is the fear of an unhappy marriage. There is some evidence that marriage is an unhealthy institution for many who inhabit it, especially women. Bernard (1973) cites studies that reveal that more married women show mental health impairment than single women. However, she notes that more married than single women report themselves as happy. Other studies confirm the stress marriage places on some people. Glenn's (1975) investigation revealed that of all the possible sources of stress, marriage and family problems rank as the primary stress inducer. At the same time, other studies show family life to be the greatest source of satisfaction to Americans. Again, the suicide rates, which traditionally have been lower for married women, were higher than those of single women (Velasco-Rice, Mynko, 1973). Studies continue to show that the higher the income of women in the labor force, the greater the likelihood that they are unmarried (Havens, 1973).

From one point of view, marriage is nothing more than a contract between two consenting adults to work together toward the achievement of mutually defined goals. It was not originally created as an institution designed to provide personal happiness. Until the twentieth century, the family was an economic unit in which the arm of production was lodged. Along with the group production of goods and services came childbearing, sexual access, and socialization. Love and happiness were afterthoughts that came to full expression in the 20th century.

Those qualities must be sought and worked out by a conscious and joint effort. The imperfections of most humans will forever make its achievement a challenging task. Marriage is the most intricate arrangement humans can enter into, particularly because the guidelines of tradition are no longer present. As Stinnett and Birdsong (1978) concluded: "Perhaps many disappointments could be avoided if people only realized that institutions and lifestyles are only as good as the people involved. Happiness and satisfaction are not determined by institutions or lifestyles, but rather they come from within individuals and depend on the quality of relationships between people" (p. 1204).

Although the partisans of singlehood have stressed the negative impact of marriage on mental health, there is another side to the argument. The available data on rates of mental disorder (as measured by admissions to mental institutions or outpatient psychiatric care) show that single people have higher rates of mental illness. This is true for both Blacks and whites, men and women (Brenner, 1973). The National Center for Health Statistics (1976) found that the overall measures of health status indicate that married people had fewer health problems than unmarried people. In one of the most extensive and thorough investigations of the impact of marital status on health, Lynch (1979) discovered that people at every age who live alone have death rates two to three times higher than those of married individuals. In the critical ages between 25 and 50, twice as many people who are divorced or widowed die from hypertensive heart disease than married people of comparable ages. His conclusion is that individuals who live alone are more susceptible to physical and emotional illnesses because they continuously lack the tranquilizing influence of human companionship during life's stresses.

There is an abundance of evidence indicating dissatisfaction with the present form of marriage. It is available in the statistics showing that divorce rates have increased by 109% since 1962. Further evidence emerges from the same set of data, which reveal that since 1960 there has been an increase from 28% to 39% in the number of women who have remained single. Between 1970 and 1981 the number of single parent families has doubled, about triple the growth of two-parent families (U.S. Bureau of the Census, 1982A). Morton Hunt (1972), a noted authority on marriage and the family, states that we can conservatively expect that within another generation, half or more of all persons who marry will be divorced at least once. An even more pessimistic view is that of Etzioni (1974), who predicted that if the proportion of people who choose a nonfamily life continues to increase at the present rate, there will be few families left in the mid-1990s. Although Etzioni was incorrect, based on present trends, Hunt's prediction was quite accurate.

Not only has the divorce rate risen dramatically in the 1970s, but it is a decidedly different kind of divorce pattern. Whereas the general trend in the past has been for the divorce rate to decrease in times of economic hardships, it increased by 5.3 per 1000 population for 1982 during an economic recession, the highest rate in our history and triple the number recorded in 1962 (U.S. Bureau of the Census, 1982). Previously, if a family had strength, it tended to become more cohesive in times of financial stress. Today, however, the fragility of many marriages means that hard times produces an increase in anxiety and irritability among spouses, which ensues in marital dissolution. On the other hand, the impact of a women's liberation ideology was not so strong in previous periods of economic decline. Another changing characteristic of divorce is the number of wives initiating such an action. Although there are not yet national statistics on this phenomenon, it is estimated that whereas in 1960 1 out of 10 divorce requests originated with the wife, 4 out of 10 such actions in 1975 came from the wife's initiative (Pogash, 1975). Even more surprising is the rise in divorce among couples married for 15–20 years. Among such couples, the divorce rate has soared, again

with women initiating the divorce proceedings (Cherlin, 1981).

It is not difficult to understand some of the reasons for the widespread disenchantment with marriage. Studies have long shown that the happiest period of marriage is the first year, and it declines in direct proportion to the length of the marriage (Blood, Wolfe, 1960). This is particularly true of women, for whom marriage has the most negative impact. Although married men are often content with and unharmed by marriage, married women have been found to be in poorer mental health than single women and to have a lower income when they enter the work force (Bernard, 1973). Even the suicide rates are increasing for married women. Many years ago, the sociologist Durkheim (1966) noted that "the wife profits less from family life than the husband. As a result conjugal society is harmful to the woman and aggravates her tendency to suicide."

Nonetheless, marriages are failing for more than the reasons just discussed. In the past era, marriages were not much happier, just more stable. They were not based on the expectations that love, sexual satisfaction, and gratification of emotional needs would be extant. Women were economically dependent on men and hence were subordinate to their wishes and demands. Furthermore, marriage did not bind people for the length of time that it does now. In the past two centuries, couples were often separated by death, whereas contemporary couples can expect half a century or more together. As a result, when people marry early and raise their children by the time they are in their forties, half of their adult lives remain. Boredom with each other is often the main reason for their divorce. In a sense, they are replacing death with divorce.

A continuing rise in divorce will be unabated unless economic forces pressure people to remain married. If American society becomes more homogeneous in its class structure and sex role equality emerges as a reality, individuals will marry more for love and the satisfaction of psychologic needs. Although this sounds good as an ideal, the failure to find or sustain such needs in marriage will make marriages even more vulnerable to dissolution. Hence, what we can expect is a kind of serial monogamy, with the sequences growing even shorter. People will probably continue to marry, if for no other reason than to lead structured lives. And it is quite possible that with the combination of marriage, divorce, and remarriage, they may find greater satisfaction in that pattern than their ancestors found in enforced monogamy.

Childbearing and Childrearing

Changes in attitudes toward the bearing and rearing of children are revealed in a number of ways. An important reason for the current low birth rate is the concern of many citizens about the problems allegedly created by overpopulation. As a result, American society is approaching zero population growth. The year 1982 saw the number of children per household at its lowest point ever, with an average of 1.8 children per family. Moreover, this low rate was partially achieved by the decision of many married couples to remain childless. Lifetime childlessness is now approaching 20%. Alteration of the fertility pattern has been nothing short of revolutionary if we note that the total fertility rate in 1957 was 3.8 children per woman (Glick, 1975; U.S. Bureau of the Census, 1983A).

In addition, parenthood is simply not considered as important a role for many people nowadays. The tragic aspect of this changing attitude is that it is not only confined to people who have no children: It is an ex post facto realization among many parents who have already borne children. It may be reflected most poignantly in the dramatic increase in reported incidents of child abuse. In a national survey, Straus et al (1980) reported an incidence rate of 3.8% of American children abused each year,

meaning that between 1.5 and 2 million children were abused by their parents. Moreover, the child maltreatment was occurring equally among different socioeconomic, religious, and racial groups.

Despite the image of American children as overprotected and permissively reared, they have not always been treated well by society. In earlier centuries, the family provided neither affection nor education. Children were valuable as part of the family labor force but regarded as inherently evil, a tendency which could be exorcised only by stern physical punishment. During that period the child at least had a variety of kinspeople from whom to seek emotional support. Today, they must find affection in either the father or particularly the mother or do without (Mousseau, 1975). This is why the parent's withdrawal of love is such an effective way of controlling children. Up to this point, society has not made a commitment to provide the financial support to make good childcare possible. With only each other to relate to, mother and child may become prisoners in the confined world of the nuclear family.

The decline in extended families is a concomitant of the 20th century. Although fathers are present in 80% of all households with children, their role is still marginal in the socialization of children. Studies continue to show that American men do not associate or interact frequently with their children, spending less than half an hour each day with them (Mackey, Day, 1979). Thus, the child is conditioned early to the realization that survival depends on the relationship with the all-important mothering figure or mothering substitute. Because a majority of children under the age of 16 have mothers in the labor force, other institutions and mediums have become more important in the socialization of the child, such as school, television, and the peer group. The consequences of these multiple socialization figures are a break in generational values and the early entry of children into the world of adults.

Another trend heightening the mother–child relationship has been the rapid growth of female-headed households. Between 1970 and 1981, the number of one parent families doubled, and 80% of them were headed by women. Almost 75% of the men and women maintaining a single parent household were either separated or divorced. About one in five of the nation's families with children are now maintained by one parent (U.S. Bureau of the Census, 1982B). In 1984, one of every four households added since 1980 were families with no husband present. That same year there were 50.1 million family households containing married couples, 9.9 million female-headed households, and 2 million households with only a male parent present (U.S. Bureau of the Census, 1984). It is estimated that nearly 70% of the children born around 1980 will experience a parental death, divorce, or separation and will likely live in a one-parent family at some point during their first 18 years (Espenshade, Braun, 1982).

The sheer weight of those numbers has important implications for the psychosocial development of children. Most of the single-parent households emerge as a result of marital dissolution. Two major studies of the effect of divorce on children show it to be disruptive of parent–child relationships, especially for male children. A couple of years after the divorce, the female's behavior is unaffected by the divorce, but dysfunctional behavior can be expected among boys (Hetherinton et al, 1978; Wallerstein, Kelly, 1979). Presently, 75% of all divorced people remarry, most within the first three years after divorce. However, divorce rates are higher for second marriages than first marriages. When remarriage occurs, the child must adjust to a new set of relationships that result from blending two sets of families (Cherlin, 1981).

Research evidence on the effects on children of living in a one parent home are mixed. One review of the research suggests that (1) father absence in itself is not likely to depress school performance; (2) there is only a small chance of a boy in a father-absent home engaging in delinquent behavior; and (3) no solid research support exists for the thesis that the absence of a father necessarily affects a boy's masculine identity (Herzong, Sudia, 1973). However, it is clear that female-headed households are poorer than two-parent families, possessing less than one-half the median income of married couple households. In 1981, about one-third of all people living within female-headed households had incomes below the poverty line (U.S. Bureau of the Census, 1982B). Many women experience a drop in their family income as a result of a divorce. One group of researchers found that when there is a drop in income of 50% or more, mothers are more likely to experience their children as deviant than when income does not drop (Desimone-Luis et al, 1979).

One can hardly speculate what kind of adults will arise from the childhood experience of children in the 1980s. Because it is a different kind of childhood than adults of an earlier generation experienced does not mean it will have negative consequences. After all, their life as adults may be very different than that experienced by children of the 1940s and 1950s. However, they were reared in a permissive and liberal environment that suggests that the changing values related to marriage and the family will become their own. What we can expect from them as adults in the 21st century is that they will mirror the values under which they were reared and may extend them to even more radical changes in the traditional family.

Changes in Black Family Structure

The family is one of the most fluid institutions in American life. Probably in no other sphere of our society have such rapid and profound changes taken place. Although the changes are most significant for white Americans, Blacks too are influenced to some degree by the same forces. Among the most visible trends are the increase in sexual permissiveness, challenges to the traditional concept of the women's role, the increase in singlehood, the rise in the divorce rate and reductions in the fertility rate. Although Blacks are part and parcel of these dynamics, their different history and socioeconomic status indicates that they will be affected more by economic and sociocultural forces unique to them.

Probably the most significant change in the Black family during the last 30 years has been the proliferative growth of female-headed households. When the Moynihan (1965) report was first issued in 1965, more than three-fourths of all Black families with children were headed by a husband and wife. In 1982 barely one-half of all such families included parents of both sexes. Those households headed by Black women had a median income of $7458 in comparison to the median income of $20,586 for Black married couples and $26,443 for white married couples (U.S. Bureau of the Census, 1983B).

One of the most visible reasons for the dramatic increase in households headed by women has been a corresponding increase in out-of-wedlock births as a proportion of all births to Black women. Approximately 52% of all children born to Black women in 1982 were conceived out of wedlock. This high percentage of out-of-wedlock births is largely attributed to the births to teenage mothers. Among women who turned 20 during the second half of the 1970s, 41% of Blacks but only 19% of whites had already given birth. Within that same group of young Black women, about 75% of all births were out of wedlock, compared with only 25% of births to young white women (U.S. Bureau of the Census, 1984). Although Black women were twice as likely to have had nonmarital sexual intercourse than white women by the age of 19, their rate of sexual activity was remaining constant while such activity was rapidly increasing among white teenagers (Zelnik, Kantner, 1977). In the 1980s, the rate among older teenagers stabilized and that of younger teenagers increased ("Report: More early teens becoming sexually active, 1987").

Not only has the number and proportion of Black female-headed households grown rapidly, but the majority of adult Black women are not married and living with a spouse. In 1982 approximately 56% of all Black women over the age of 14 were never married, separated, divorced, or widowed. Under the age of 30, the majority of them will fall into the never-married category; past age 30, most of them will be listed as divorced and separated, with a small percentage counted among the widowed. The high divorce rate creates a number of female-headed households among Black women over age 30. One out of two white marriages will end in divorce, and two out of three Black marriages will eventually dissolve. Black women who divorce are less likely than their white counterparts to remarry. One in four adult Black women is currently divorced (U.S. Bureau of the Census, 1983B).

The problems Blacks face are essentially the same as for the past century. Those problems are not related to family stability but to the socioeconomic conditions that tear families asunder. In general, the problems are poverty and racism. Although the past decade produced a decline in racial segregation and white stereotypes of Black inferiority, Blacks are still singled out for discriminatory treatment in every sphere of American life. Moreover, any national effort to further remedy these practices has a low priority in the federal government.

A low socioeconomic status continues to plague many Black families. Whereas some Blacks have achieved a higher standard of living as a result of the civil rights movement, large numbers of Blacks continue to live below the poverty level. A disproportionate number of these Blacks will be female heads of families. They will have more responsibilities and less income than any other group in American society. Yet no effective programs are being proposed to meet the needs of one-half of all Black families. Obviously, there is a need for a public policy and program to meet the needs of women who cannot find employment. Even if they could find jobs, the childcare facilities in the Black community are few and inadequate. The persistence of employment and salary discrimination against women will continue to handicap Black women in their struggle to maintain a decent life for their families.

Poverty is not the only reason for the high divorce rate of Blacks. The increase in the Black divorce rate in recent years is due to sociopsychologic factors as well. A primary cause is the economic independence of Black women. Marital stability among whites in the past was based on the subordinate status of women. Once white women were emancipated from the economic domination of men, their divorce rate increased radically. Black women have been independent—economically and psychologically—for a much longer period of time. There is nothing inherently wrong with the equality of sex roles in the family, but when men are socialized to expect unchallenged leadership in family affairs, conflict is an inevitable result.

Many of the methods and goals of the women's liberation movement are of importance to Black women. As a result of women declaring their independence from the domination of men, there will be a greater acceptance of women heading families by themselves. Perhaps the society will then make provisions for eliminating some of the problems endured by female-headed households, for example, childcare facilities. The demand for equal employment opportunities for women and income parity for women in the same jobs as men is very important to Black women. It is Black women who are the most victimized by employment and income discrimination against women. They are most likely to be heads of households who will earn the low salaries paid women on the assumption that they do not have families to support.

Based on present trends, it appears that dichotomy is emerging among Blacks, largely determined by class and gender. College-educated Black males will continue to have a high rate of marriage, and those unions will probably be more egalitarian than in the past. Although middle-class Black women have not affiliated organizationally with mainstream feminist groups, the egalitarian ideology has had an impact. Moreover, it is quite possible that college-educated Black women will reach economic parity with their Black male cohorts by the year 2000. Their income is increasing at twice the rate of Black males with similar education and had reached 90% of the income of Black males in 1978 (Hacker, 1985). One mitigating factor in Black women's push toward sex-role equality is the limited pool of males eligible for marriage in their class level. Middle-class Black males may opt for a mate who does not demand total equality when they are in a position to pick and choose. Whatever the character of their marriage, the excess number of Black female college graduates presages that large numbers of them will remain without a spouse (Staples, 1981).

On the other hand, lower-class families have been attenuated by the pervasive economic forces that plague them. Almost one-third of Black children are born to women under the age of 19, most of them out of wedlock. More than half the Black children born in the United States are born out of wedlock, and a minority of Black children live with two parents. Those lower-income Blacks who do marry have one of the highest rates of marital dissolution in the country. Many of the men cannot afford to marry or find a woman who will take a chance on marrying them. Fortunately, lower-income Blacks have other structures to buttress the effects of those changes in family patterns. Boyfriends, and often the biologic father, play very supportive roles in the financial and emotional support of mother and child. The process of informal adoption means that most Black children will be placed in homes where they receive affection and the appropriate socialization. Although the structure may be different, the functions of the nuclear family are still carried out.

Internal Adaptations

The changes in the interior of the Black family, although ideologically in the direction of nativism, are statistically in the direction of assimilation and acculturation. Examples of this phenomenon are seen in the diffusion of Blacks into predominantely white suburbs, the increase in interracial dating and marriage, the higher incidences of suicide and mental illness, and a decline in the extended family pattern. However, these patterns reflect variations in the Black community. It is surprising, given the pace of racial integration in American society, that more Blacks have not become assimilated into the majority population's mode of behavior. The integration of the school systems, desegregation of suburbia, and greater access to knowledge of majority cultural norms through the mass media have provided, without precedent, opportunities for Black acculturation. Instead, we find Blacks in separate facilities and organizations on white university campuses. Many Blacks who moved to the suburbs continue their social lives in the inner cities. Although the extended family may not live together in the same household, its functions of providing emotional solidarity and other kinds of assistance are still carried out. Moreover, the concept of the extended family is broadened to include all members of the Black community. These internal adaptations are made by the Black community to prevent the trend of racial integration from weakening their cultural unity.

Another most important adaptation under consideration by segments of the Black community is the adoption of polygyny as the Black marriage system. The assumption is that there are not enough Black males to go around and that the sharing of husbands could stabilize Black marriages and provide certain legal benefits to women now deprived of them. In African society, the practice of polygyny is closely related to the economic system, and people are socialized to accept it. At least one study has confirmed the existence of informal polygyny among Blacks in the United States (Scott, 1980). The actual number of Black polygynous marriages is infinitesimal. Such marriages are illegal in this country, and, thus, no legal benefits can accrue to the second wife.

It is difficult to predict the future of Black families because there are several parallel trends occurring at the same time. Many Blacks are entering the middle class as a result of higher education and increased opportunities. At the same time, the future is dim for Blacks in the underclass. The forces of automation and cybernation are rendering obsolete the labor of unskilled Black men, who are in danger of becoming a permanent army of the unemployed. The status of Black women is in a state of flux. Some welcome the liberation from male control, but others urge a regeneration of Black male leadership. Easier and cheaper access to contraceptives and abortions may mean a continued decline in the Black fertility rate. Whatever the future of Black families, it will parallel changes in all American families.

The Future of the Family

Based on present trends, it seems reasonable to expect the family to continue in the same direction as over the last 25 years. Sexual relations will precede marriage; people will have a trial period of cohabitation before entering into marriage, and they will increasingly delay marriage until their late twenties or early thirties; the divorce rate will continue to increase, and remarriage will occur more slowly; couples will limit their families to one or two children; and the dual wage earner family will be the norm for almost all households. However, there will be no radical reconstruction of family forms. Although a multiplicity of options will be available to individuals, most people will continue to marry and bear children. Those marriages will be subject to dissolution, and a majority of American children may spend most of their lives in single parent or blended families.

Whereas the form and function of the future family may be the same as in the 1980s, it will be a qualitatively different kind of family. The greatest changes will manifest in gender roles. Despite the current inequality between the sexes, the available trend data favor increasing parity between men and women. It is estimated that two-thirds of the growth in the labor force between the present and 1995 will be accounted for by women, and males will continue to be a minority of the labor force (Brookes, 1986). Already, women have achieved an educational level superior to men; they currently account for 52% of all undergraduate college enrollments and are gradually approaching equity in graduate and professional schools. Although women currently earn on average only 61% of male salary levels, that differential may be narrowed to 10% by the year 2000. Those changes in the educational and economic levels of women may presage even greater changes in the family (Hacker, 1985).

As women gain true economic parity with men, they will increasingly become independent of marriage as a means to ensure a decent standard of living. Marriages will be created and maintained because they have affectional ties instead of being based on economic or social need. Within those marriages, relationships will be egalitarian, and men will be expected to participate equally in housework and childcare. Because expectations will be higher, the divorce rate will be higher. Single-parent households will continue to increase, and males will be more likely to become the custodial parent. Not only will women have more economic and educational leverage but also greater flexibility in mate selection. They will take more of the initiative in dating and sexual behavior and in marriage proposals. The old adage about men marrying down and women marrying up will be circumvented by the fact that women will have a superior educational level to men and near

parity in income. Moreover, the marriage squeeze for women in the 1980s will be reversed in the 1990s when there will be a shortage of women in the marriageable ages between 25 and 35.

Summary

It would be wise to temper our predictions with the knowledge that changes in the family have been cyclical, not unilineal. The family does not exist in a vacuum, and changes in extrafamiliar institutions can alter radically patterns of family life. Economic changes, in particular, seem capable of redirecting family life in conservative or liberal directions. In times of economic depression or recession, the direction of change is usually conservative. The economic recession of 1980–82 produced more conservative attitudes toward sexuality, marriage, divorce, and the role of women. Liberal attitudes and family arrangements flourished during the 1920s and 1960s. Most of the family trends extant now have been seen in other historical epochs and were subsequently reversed.

Changes in the family during the 1960s were facilitated by a number of factors. The advent of the birth control pill made the sexual revolution possible, and technologic advancements that made housekeeping easier allowed women to enter the labor force. Political legislation made divorce easier to obtain, and court decisions created accessible abortions for many women. Accessible and affordable housing made independent living possible for young people. Given any radical changes in the economy, polity, or technology, the family could undergo changes not possibly foreseen at this point in time. All we can realistically predict is that the family will continue to be an important institution in the lives of most Americans. As long as humans have the need for companionship, its place will be secured, no matter what form it evolves to meet that universal desire for belongingness.

Issues for Further Investigation

1. Given the changes in family structure anticipated in the 21st century, what social institutions and social resources, for example, child day care for well and ill children, will be needed by the families of the future?

2. What factors significantly and differentially affect families of varying socioeconomic status and racial/cultural background?

3. To what extent will anticipated changes in the structure of the American family (blended families, single-sex families, single-parent families, single people) alter the function of the family?

4. What are the economic factors that perpetuate traditional role separation in the American family? Are there social policy changes that could influence these long-standing patterns of family life?

5. What are the effects of procreational technologies on the future structures and functions of the family?

References

Bane MJ (1976): *Here to Stay: American Families in the Twentieth Century.* New York: Basic Books.

Bernard J (1973): *The Future of Marriage.* New York: Bantam Books.

Bernard J (1975): *The Future of Motherhood:* New York: Penguin.

Blood R, Wolfe D (1960): *Husbands and Wives: The Dynamics of Married Living.* Glencoe, IL: Free Press.

Brenner HM (1973): *Mental Illness and the Economy.* Cambridge: Harvard University Press.

Brooks WF (1986): An affirmative action explosion in employment. *The San Francisco Chronicle,* October 7, p. 53.

Calhoun AW (1960): *A Social History of the American Family.* New York: Barnes & Noble.

Cherlin A (1981): *Marriage, Divorce, Remarriage.* Cambridge: Harvard University Press.

Clayton R, Bokemeir J (1980): Premarital sex in the seventies. *J Marr Fam,* 42:759–776.

Desimone-Luis J, O'Mahoney K, Hunt D (1979): Children of separation and divorce: Factors influencing adjustment. *J Divorce,* 3:37–42.

Durkheim E (1966): *Suicide.* Glencoe, IL: Free Press.

Espenshade T, Braun R (1982): Life course analysis and multistate demography: An application to marriage, divorce and remarriage. *J Marr Fam,* 44:1025–1036.

Etzioni A (1974): Marriage and maternity as endangered species seen in perspective. *Hum Behav,* 3:10–11.

Glenn N (1975): The contribution of marriage to the psychological well-being of males and females. *J Marr Fam,* 37:594–599.

Glick P (1975): A demographer looks at American families. *J Marr Fam,* 37:15–27.

Hacker A (1985): Women—Men at work. *San Francisco Sunday Examiner and Chronicle, This World.* January 6, pp. 15–16.

Havens E (1973): Women, work and wedlock: A note on female patterns in the United States. In: *Changing Women in a Changing Society,* Huber J (ed.). Chicago: University of Chicago Press.

Herzog E, Sudia CE (1973): Children in fatherless families. In: *Review of Child Development,* Caldwell BM, Ricciuti HN (eds.), 3.

Hetherington EM, Cox M, Cox R (1978): Family interaction and the social, emotional, and cognitive development of children following divorce. Paper presented at the Symposium on the Family: Setting Priorities. Washington, DC.

Hunt M (1972): The future of marriage. *Playboy,* 19:116–118.

Jessor SL, Jessor R (1977): *Problem Behavior and Psychosocial Development: A Longitudinal Study of Youth.* New York: Academic Press.

Kinsey A, Pomeroy WB, Martin CE (1953): *Sexual Behavior in the Human Female.* Philadelphia: Saunders.

Less-but-better sex for college students. *The San Francisco Examiner,* July 14, 1987, p. A-3.

Levin RJ, Levin A (1975): Sexual pleasure: The surprising preferences of 100,000 women. *Redbook,* *145:* 51–58.

Lynch JJ (1979): *The Broken Heart.* New York: Basic Books.

Mackey WC, Day RO (1979): Some indicators of fathering behaviors in the United States: A cross-cultural examination of adult male–child interaction. *J Marr Fam,* 41:287–298.

Malinowski B (1930): Parenthood: The basis of social structure. In: *The New Generation,* Calveston V, Schmalhaven L (eds.). New York: Macaulay.

Most Americans like marriage. *The San Francisco Chronicle,* June 15, 1987, p. 1.

Mousseau J (1975): The family, prison of love. *Psychology Today,* 9:52–55.

Moynihan D (1965): The Negro family: The case for national action. Washington, DC: GPO.

Murdock G (1949): *Social Structure.* New York: Macmillan.

A nasty new epidemic. *Newsweek,* February 4, 1985, pp. 72–73.

National Center for Health Statistics (1976): quoted in *The San Francisco Examiner,* June 20, 1976.

Parsons T, Bales R (1955): *Family Socialization and Interaction Process.* Glencoe, IL: Free Press.

Pogash C (1975): More runaway wives than ever seek freedom. *The San Francisco Chronicle,* March 2, p. 26.

Report: More early teens becoming sexually active. *The San Francisco Examiner,* June 5, 1987, p. A-11.

The revolution is over, in the 80s, caution and commitment are the watchwords. *Time,* April 19, 1984, pp. 74–83.

Scott J (1980): Black polygamous family formation: Case studies of legal wives and consensual wives. In: *Alternative Lifestyles,* 3:41–64.

Shope DF (1971): Sexual responsiveness in single girls. In: *Studies in the Sociology of Sex,* Henslin JM (ed.). New York: Appleton-Century-Crofts.

Simenauer J, Carroll D (1982): *Singles: The New Americans.* New York: Simon & Schuster.

Spiro M (1954): Is the family universal? *American Anthropologist,* 56:839–846.

Staples R (1981): *The World of Black Singles: Changing Patterns of Male-Female Relations.* Westport, CT: Greenwood.

Stinnett N, Birdsong C (1978): *The Family and Alternate Lifestyles.* Chicago: Nelson-Hall.

Straus M, Gelles RJ, Steinmetz S (1980): *Behind Closed Doors: Violence in the American Family.* Garden City, NY: Doubleday.

U.S. Bureau of the Census (1982): Households, families, marital status and living arrangements. Washington, DC: GPO.

U.S Bureau of the Census (1982): Households and family characteristics. Washington, DC: GPO.

U.S. Bureau of the Census (1982): Fertility of American women. Washington, DC: GPO.

U.S. Bureau of the Census (1983): America's black populations, 1970–1982: A statistical view. Washington, DC: GPO.

U.S. Bureau of the Census (1984): Households, families, marital status and living arrangements. Washington, DC: GPO.

Velasco-Rice, J, Mynko L (1973): Suicide and marital status: A changing relationship. *J Marr Fam,* 35:239–244.

Wallerstein JS, Kelly JB (1979): Divorce and children. In: *Basic Handbook of Child Psychiatry: Vol 4,* Noshpitz J (ed.) New York: Basic Books.

Zelnik J, Kantner JF (1977): Sexual and contraceptive experience of young unmarried women in the United States, 1976 and 1971. *Fam Plann Perspect,* 9: 55–59.

TRANSITIONS IN THE FAMILY LIFE CYCLE

11

FAMILY TRANSITIONS

Expected and Unexpected

Sally H. Rankin, RN, MSN

Throughout the life cycle, changes are experienced by all families. Some changes occur gradually, while others are rapid and may be unexpected. This chapter distinguishes the expected, gradual period of change known as *transition* from the unexpected, rapid change called *crisis*, and explores the nursing care options for both situations. The chapter also introduces a framework for examining family development throughout the life cycle.

Sally Rankin is a doctoral candidate at the University of California at San Francisco School of Nursing (Department of Family Health Care). Her work to date addresses ongoing individual and family adaptation to cardiac surgery and chronic illness.

Though all the changing scenes of life,
In trouble and in joy,

NEW VERSION OF THE PSALMS OF DAVID, PSALM 34

Introduction

The changing scenes of life are indeed reflected in the troubles and joys of families, especially in the transitions that occur in family life over the years. Expected transitions are normative for families just as they are normative for individuals. Viewing expected transitions as normative assists nurses in understanding important aspects of family life. First, this outlook differentiates transitions from crises, which are unexpected transitions not considered normative that frequently imply a negative outcome if the appropriate arsenal of resources and social supports is unavailable. Second, an appraisal of expected transitions as normative assists the nurse in deciding when interventions should be preventive or anticipatory, when they should be supportive, and when they should be therapeutic with the intention of altering the state of the family system (Gorman, 1966). Because expected transitions are viewed as a normal aspect of change confronted by all families, most interventions involved in periods of transition are preventive or supportive. Unexpected transitions require more active involvement in family support. These will be reviewed in Chapter 17.

The concept of psychosocial transitions has been previously developed by Parkes (1971) and used by nurses in their understanding of individuals. His work is also applicable to families and transitions because the family is generally affected by any change occurring within the family boundary, whether initiated by one or more members. Psychosocial transitions are those changes in the personal world of the individual or family that are lasting in their effects, are of short duration, and affect a large part of the family's or individual's "life space" or personal environment in which the family or individual responds to others and initiates and organizes behavior (Parkes, 1971).

A complementary conceptual schema that enlightens our understanding of family transitions exists in the work of family sociologists and developmental psychologists in the area of family development. Among the better-known theorists and writers are Duvall (1977) and Carter and McGoldrick (1980); their work has influenced much of our thinking in work with families. These theorists subscribe to a stage or phase approach to family development, with the stages predicated on the developmental needs and issues pertinent to the oldest child. Typically, they view the family as moving through a series of seven or eight stages throughout the life cycle.

This chapter will meld the two approaches, psychosocial transitions and family development, and will suggest a framework that permits the nurse to comprehend the complexity and plasticity of families. Additionally, this framework will allow health professionals working with families to appreciate the diversity of families and to interpret the definition of *family* in its widest possible perspective—a group of two or more individuals usually living in close geographic proximity, having close emotional bonds and meeting affectional, socioeconomic, sexual, and socialization needs of the family group and the wider social system. This definition allows a vantage point that includes traditional, as well as nontraditional family units, so that our knowledge of family transitions is expanded from conventional ideas. For example, the transition to parenthood may include transitions from a nuclear family unit to a blended family unit, or a transition from productive career to disability may include the homosexual couple in which one member has contracted AIDS. For the purposes of this chapter, a traditional family is one that consists of heterosexual adults who are legally married. Children are not a requirement of traditional marriages. A nontraditional family consists of adults of the same or different sex who maintain a stable relationship without the legitimation of marriage.

The importance of psychosocial transitions in the life of the individual and the family is explicated in the next portion of the chapter. Following this is a brief review of the developmentalists' work on stages in family development. Finally, a framework for understanding family transitions is presented that incorporates a stage and transition approach. Because the family itself is in transition, the framework encompasses many family lifeways and patterns. We obtain a glimpse of the family in this inclusive developmental mirror. Consideration of common psychosocial transitions helps to better reveal the important tasks and characteristics of families during these phases in their history. However, no family system can be understood outside of its own unique context; therefore, the importance of understanding the unique perspective of each family is emphasized. Families may experience transitions in different ways. Even the same family may respond differently as its resources and needs change from one transition to the next.

Psychosocial Transitions and Family Life

Parkes (1971), borrowing Lewin's concept of "life space", illustrates the importance of change within the personal world of the individual or family. Life space is the psychologic "field" that consists of the individual or family and the environment (Deutsch, 1968). The family and the environment are variables that are mutually dependent on each other and together combine to form the life space. When the person or family is confronted with change, the life space must be reorganized. Parkes distinguishes five types of transitions that require major reorganization of life space: (1) changes in personal relationships; (2) changes in roles and status; (3) changes in familiar environment; (4) changes in physical and mental capacities; and (5) changes in loved possessions. Each of these transitions has an impact on the family and will be discussed in turn.

Changes in Personal Relationships

Changes in personal relationships have the greatest potential for creating family disequilibrium. Parkes asserts that changes in personal relationships occur at each stage of the life cycle. The young family, which will later be referred to as the emerging family, experiences changes in personal relationships with marriage and with the birth of each child. Additionally, such important events as going to school, obtaining a job, getting a divorce, and experiencing the death of loved ones are all psychosocial transitions portending changes in personal relationships.

The timing of the change in personal relationships often predicts the family's adaptation to the transition or crisis. Neugarten (1979) notes that individuals develop a concept of a "normal, expectable life cycle." When death occurs later in life, and as such is expected, the family experiences a transition and usually is able to integrate the loss in a way that allows for the continuity of the family. However, when the loss is unexpected or is unusual at that point in the life cycle (such as the loss of a child), the demands are greater and may overwhelm the family. Such changes are the subject of Chapter 14. Loss of an adolescent child through suicide implies dual problems related to issues of timing and stigmatization. Families that must cope with a stress such as adolescent suicide usually require intervention that we have classified earlier as therapeutic—that is, a change in the family system itself is required in order for the family to achieve equilibrium. Additionally, these families need supportive interventions from nurses and other health care professionals as well as referrals to parent and family self-help groups coping with similar problems, all of which may assist families in coping with the change in personal relationships (Hatton, Valente, 1984).

The significance of the change in personal relationships was exemplified in a study comparing the reactions of older (over 70 years) married couples and younger (under 50 years) couples to cardiac surgery. Older couples were unexpectedly resilient to the stressors of surgery (Rankin et al, 1986). Communication patterns between patients and spouses were observed to be well-developed and generally satisfactory. Coping patterns revealed a tendency to avoid rather than to express conflict. The years spent in developing a stable marital relationship seemed to have greater payoffs for the older couples, resulting in a smoother transition to the change in the personal relationship as necessitated by the events of cardiac surgery.

Other changes in personal relationships do not have the same dire implications for the family as the death of a child or adolescent, but they still portend a necessary transition; one such event is a young mother taking a job (Kelly, Voydanoff, 1985). Although the job may provide the family with a better standard of living, issues involving separation and attachment are confronted if it becomes necessary to locate and use suitable child day care (Portner, 1983). These transitions are further developed in Chapter 15. Even the most apparently benign changes in personal relationships often have greater implications for family equilibrium than initially realized.

Changes in Role and Status

A second psychosocial transition having significance for families is that involving a change in role and status. Frequently such a change accompanies an alteration in personal relationships such as the birth of the first child, which not only changes personal relationships but also adds the additional role constellation involving parenthood.

However, alterations in role and status also occur independently of changes in personal relationships, such as those role and status changes that frequently accompany illness. Pearlin (1983) recognizes the social origins of stress and notes that many are embodied in role strains, the "hardships, challenges, and conflicts" that people experience in normal social roles. Realignment of role and status may involve role restructuring. An example of the necessity for role restructuring invoked by this type of psychosocial transition occurs in spousal caregiving situations. Role restructuring involves changes in stable role sets rather than transitions to new roles (Cantor, 1983; Clark, Rakowski, 1983). In the marital dyad where one spouse must assume caregiver duties, the husband–wife role set remains the same but must be restructured around the changed competencies of the patient. For example, wives of cardiac surgery patients frequently complain that they have to do household tasks that previously had been the husband's responsibilities. Husbands of cardiac surgery patients complain about their added duties in meal preparation and housecleaning. In fact, when men are the caregivers, they frequently respond to their added duties by obtaining help from female family members and relinquishing the caregiver role as quickly as possible. It may be the inability of these men to restructure roles that explains why they are less likely to maintain caregiving activities for longer than a couple of weeks. This inability to restructure can result in divorce or desertion, as often occurs when wives who are disabled either from alcoholism or spinal cord injury are divorced or deserted by their husbands (Crewes, as cited in Treischmann, 1978). Interestingly, wives are not as likely to leave their husbands following impairment. This may be illustrative of gender role differences that make role restructuring and psychosocial changes in role and status more easily accomplished by women than men in situations involving caregiving.

Changes in Familiar Environment

A third type of psychosocial transition that families encounter involves changes in familiar environment. One of the most common changes in familiar environment occurs when families move to another home. If changes in schools and occupations as well as alterations in friendships occur, the move may occasion some stressful experiences for the family. Even if the move is desired and signals greater opportunity for the family, the transition required may have stressful consequences (Hull, 1979; Lipson, Meleis, 1983). An example of such consequences may be evident in the families who have left war-torn Central American countries hoping to escape a repressive political situation, but then find it necessary to take work of lesser status, learn a new language, and use their children as emissaries in a land that is frequently cool to their hopes and dreams.

Changes in Physical and Mental Capacities

A fourth psychosocial transition that may affect both individuals and their families is a change in physical and mental capacities. Changes in physical capacities are often accompanied by changes in psychologic function. Therefore, these two will be considered conjointly.

One of the most poignant examples of this dual psychosocial transition involves families coping with Alzheimer's disease (Pratt et al, 1985). Whether the physical change is the most difficult in terms of caregiving that is necessitated or whether the progressive dementia carries a heavier burden seems to depend on the age of the caregiver and the family's developmental stage (Montgomery et al, 1985; Worcester, Quayhagen, 1983). For example, younger families who must confront the progressive deterioration of a 50-year-old woman who was previously an active wife and mother may find the dementia very demoralizing in terms of their interface with the community and health care professionals. When the client is elderly and dependent on an elderly spouse for care, the client's change in physical capacities may necessitate institutionalization, which results in a schism in lifestyle for both the client and the spouse.

Changes in physical capacities in one family member also affect families with middle-aged adults responding to the stresses of cancer. For example, one wife and mother remarked that her teenaged son was taking on many of the maintenance chores previously performed by her husband because her husband was so debilitated by his chemotherapy treatments. Both husband and wife were aware of this role change necessitated by the change in physical capacity, and the husband admitted to resentment of the ease with which his son assumed his old tasks. Another example occurring with middle-aged adults who experience physical changes is the change that frequently occurs with coronary artery bypass graft surgery. The home recovery period is commonly accompanied by depression, so the patient and family must not only contend with the fatigue, anorexia, and discomfort prevalent with this type of surgery, but they may also have to cope with periods of crying and mood swings (Kolitz, Pimm, 1984). The changes in psychologic status have been convincingly documented in such popular books as *Heart Sounds* by Lear (1981). Changes in physical capacities affecting children and adolescents are covered comprehensively in Chapters 19 and 20.

Changes in Loved Possessions

A fifth psychosocial transition that Parkes identifies is changes in loved possessions. Changes in loved possessions may occur in a normative context, as with moves and losses of desired objects, or in a nonnormative context, as with burglaries or other crimes or with natural disasters such as fires, floods, and earthquakes. The literature regarding the high death rates following moves of the elderly from one nursing home to another illustrates the importance of changes in loved possessions for individuals as well as the previously discussed changes in environment (Rowland, 1977; Wolanin, 1978). The propensity for families to rebuild in the same location following fires or to repair following earthquakes or floods indicates the need for constancy and the regard that most families have for their possessions. Although nonpsychiatric nurses are not as likely to be involved in the aftermath of changes necessitated by this psychosocial transition, they should be aware of this transition and its ability to evoke grief and mourning behavior.

Framework for Family Development

The early work completed by Duvall (1977), Duvall and Hill (1948), Carter and McGoldrick (1980), and Hill (1949) has given important direction to our understanding of family developmental stages. Additionally, nurses such as Meister (1977) and Stevenson (1983) have added to the nursing understanding of family's and individual development with work that suggests interventions appropriate to the family's or individual's developmental level. As Mederer and Hill (1983) indicate, traditional family development theory allows the health professional to view family development as a process, with specific phases attended by changes in role reciprocities and role conflicts. Role reciprocities are defined in the traditional manner of husband–father, wife–mother, daughter–sister, and son–brother. Role conflicts evolve from changes in role relationships that may be predicated on interface with the wider social system or may include family system changes in terms of communication, affection, and decision-making.

Duvall's (1977) classic family developmental stage theory includes the following stages: (1) getting married or the joining of families; (2) childbearing families; (3) families with preschool children; (4) families with school-aged children; (5) families with teenagers, (6) families launching young adults; (7) middle-aged or empty-nest families; and (8) aging families. The

problems attendant with this type of framework involve issues related to definition of family (which only applies to childbearing families), varying ages of members comprising the modern family, and explanatory power related to how the stages are accomplished.

For instance, family developmental stage theory as it has been proposed does not allow for the continued development of married partners without children, nor for other unmarried persons who may consider themselves families, such as gay or lesbian couples or blended or reconstituted families. The framework was originated when marriage was the norm for men and women; childbearing was universally valued and occurred not long after establishment of the marital dyad (Troll, 1985). Today families may not be established until both members are in their mid-30s, with childbearing occurring, if at all, in the late 30s or early 40s. In such cases, the launching family is past middle-age, and empty-nest families are already confronting the problems of aged families. Additionally, changes in the economy have necessitated the return to the parental home in early adulthood for many young adults unable to maintain independent living because of low earning ability or because of a change in financial status related to divorce (Clemens, Axelson, 1985).

Family constellations are more complex today. Many remarried men begin a second family when they are in their 50s and are already fathers of 20-year-old children from the first marriage. That "late fathers are great fathers" has been suggested by Nyedegger (cited in Troll, 1985) and serves to support our contention that the variability in timing of role transitions and family development makes the concept of formalized family developmental stages difficult to codify.

The issue related to the explanatory power of developmental stage theory is perhaps its greatest handicap. As Mederer and Hill (1983) have pointed out, most family development research has examined what occurs within stages rather than between stages or the process by which families move from one stage to the next. In addition, they note that an assumption is made that there are discrete differences in family roles and behavior from stage to stage, although other theorists believe that the stages instead move imperceptibly from one to another (Menaghan, 1982; Neugarten, Hagestad, 1976). Burr (1972) developed the concept of "ease of role transition," which attempts to explain the differences between families in their abilities to accomplish movement from one stage to the next. Another issue that has yet to be examined is that of role stability and role change from stage to stage. And last, family developmental theory assumes that roles change uniformly from stage to stage, although the structure of some roles, such as division of labor, may change when the wife and mother goes back to work, while other role structures (affection, decision-making, and communication) may remain the same. Changes in roles that are precipitated by changes in health status may have a greater impact than changes precipitated by the movement from one developmental stage to the next, indicating the importance of the many variables affecting family growth and development and the necessity of having a broader framework with which to assess families.

Consideration of a new schema from which to view families follows. This schema attempts to integrate both stage and transition approaches. Table 11–1 illustrates tasks of the family, characteristics and examples of the family at each stage, and transitions that are most likely to accompany each stage.

Emerging Families

Emerging families are those families constituted of two or more adults who are involved with tasks that concern the future of the particular family unit. During the emerging phase, the adults in the family unit are coalescing the relationship and usually are considering such decisions as marriage and childbearing. An example of an emerging traditional family would be the young couple in their early 20s who met in college, lived together for three years while establishing careers, and then made the decision to marry and have children. If the family unit is not traditional, then decisions related to such issues as permanency of the relationship, contractual obligations regarding living accommodations, and responsibility for financial management are primary. (The reader will note that issues for traditional and nontraditional families are frequently similar.) An example of a nontraditional couple in the emerging stage might be two women who decide to live together in a lesbian relationship, buy a house together, and consider the possibility of artificial insemination for one of the women.

Decisions related to childbearing and childrearing are perhaps the most crucial that are made during this period. The traditional marital couple has a number of options available. They may choose to bear their own children or, if unable, may choose to adopt. The decisions related to couple assumption of this identity are covered in Chapter 12. Additionally, the couple may choose not to assume the parental role at all, a decision that is being made more often (Fullerton, as cited in Rexroat, 1985).

Nontraditional couples, whether heterosexual or homosexual, also face issues related to childbearing. For example, an unmarried heterosexual couple may choose to have children outside of marriage. This couple may experience a stable, ongoing relationship or may separate and form other relationships in the future.

The homosexual couple, whether male or female, also must make decisions related to childbearing. In some instances, children are adopted and in others, options such as artificial insemination are exercised. For instance, the *San Francisco Chronicle* (1986) reported that 400 Bay Area lesbians had tried artificial insemination in recent years in order to achieve parenthood. One author who facilitates groups for lesbian women considering parenthood states that about 15% of the women decide to have children (Pies, 1985). The last and most common option facing ho-

Table 11-1 Developmental Family Framework and Common Family Transitions

Family Type	Tasks	Characteristics/Examples	Common Transitions
Emerging	Finding suitable partners	Formalization of marital bond	Change in personal relationships—addition of spouse or significant other. Loss of friends, changes in family relationships
	Constitution of meaningful adult relationships	Decision to live with person of opposite or same sex with nonformalized bond	Changes in roles and status—unmarried to married status, addition of parental role. Possible changes in job, career, related to change in personal relationships
	Decisions related to childbearing and infertility	Traditional or nontraditional family pattern, that is, opposite sex partners obtain in vitro fertilization or same sex partners adopt	Change in familiar environment—moving households
	Decision to remain childless	Opposite or same sex partners	
Solidifying or Reconstituting	Solidification of adult partners' bonds Childrearing and required interface with schools, health care institutions, and other societal institutions	Stable, nondivorcing families Childrearing tasks involve nurturance, education, socialization, and provision of climate suitable to development of responsible individuals. Characteristics of families with children are similar whether the family is traditional or not	Change in roles and status—loss or change in marital role through divorce and/or remarriage. Continued career changes Changes in personal relationships—potential loss of significant other, that is, mate, child. Loss of parents in family of origin Changes in physical and mental capacities—major health change
	Reconstitution of family bonds with integration of new family members and loss of old ones	Divorced families and blended families	Changes in possessions—loss or acquisition of loved possessions necessitated by change in income or catastrophic occurrences
Contracting	Launching and release of children to environments separated from family	Traditional nuclear family releases young adult children to armed services, college, marriage, or work	Change in personal relationships—loss of spouse, children, siblings
	Adjusting to loss of adult partner	Death, late-in-life divorce	Change in roles and status—retirement
	Adjusting to loss of work, parental roles	Enforced retirement with consequences of lowered standard of living	Changes in physical and mental capacities—exacerbation of chronic problems, onset of acute episodes
	Integration of leisure time and adjustment to lack of responsibility for children and/or occupation. Development of avocation Adaptation to caregiving	Younger, healthy retired couples. Older, healthy workers who choose to continue employment	Changes in familiar environment—moves required by decreased income, loss of spouse, or health problems

mosexual couples involves questions of custody pertaining to children of a previous heterosexual relationship. It is not clear that children raised by gay fathers or lesbian mothers tend to a specific sexual preference, and reports by these parents indicate that their relationships with their children have not been affected by the children's knowledge of their parents' sexual preference (Bell, Weinberg, 1978). Much of the research that examines the origins of homosexuality indicates that its genesis is most likely to lie in neuroendocrine conditioning (Gladue et al, 1984), indicating that the sexual preference of parents or intrafamilial family climate would have little effect on children's preferences. Because issues involved in parenting are similar across sexual preference lines—that is, effective and emotionally healthy parenting results in physically and psychologically healthy offspring—health professionals direct involvement with these families toward client-specified issues rather than issues related to sexual preference.

Important transitions confronting emerging families involve changes in environment, in roles and status, and in personal relationships. A change in familiar environment is the norm when a new family unit is constituted and may also change with the birth of children. The change in environment may be accomplished relatively simply, or it may include a cross-country move. The changes in role and status that accompany formation of a new family unit are usually salutary and desired, although the loss of old roles in the family unit of origin may be of concern to some clients (Boss, 1983). Movement into parental roles may or may not be desired, depending on the couple's age, economic circumstances, and whether the pregnancy was planned or unplanned. The changes brought about in personal relationships are perhaps the most difficult to integrate. When a new family unit is created, there are both gains and losses in terms of personal relationships. Friendships are sometimes lost or displaced, and relationships with in-laws or others important to the

partner must be attempted. Additionally, the changes wrought by the birth of children are manifold and require constant attempts to adapt.

The emerging phase in the life of the traditional family is equivalent to the stages Duvall (1977) and others have recognized as stage one, getting married, and stage two, families with infants or birth of the first child. Because norms related to childbearing are changing and varied, a family unit may enter this stage when the adults are in their early 20s and exit by their late 20s, or they may not enter until their mid 30s and exit in their early 40s. As noted, however, we have also included those relationships that meet the definition of family suggested earlier in the chapter but are not necessarily inclusive of marriage.

Important transitions that occur prior to and during the emerging phase have been mentioned. The transition that usually signals movement into the solidifying or reconstituting stage is, again, change in personal relationships. Rather than view the family as developing according to the growth of the oldest child, we are instead considering the transitions in personal relationships that require movement and growth. For example, the next stage for some families may be a solidifying of personal relationships with adult family members, making the choice to continue the family unit intact. At this same juncture, other families may separate and reconstitute new families.

Solidifying or Reconstituting Families

When families move into the solidifying or reconstituting phase, the transition may be subtle, or it may be accompanied by changes in personal relationships that have consequences for all family members for years to come. Indeed, this stage may occur more than once as the incidence of marriage-divorce-remarriage-second divorce becomes more common. The child and adult developmental stages continue unwinding as the family approaches and enters this stage.

When families respond to the transition from the first stage to this next stage by solidifying, primary tasks involve the concretion and stabilization of adult partners' bonds and socialization of children if they are involved in the family system. Socialization of children requires interface with schools, health care institutions, and community agencies and institutions. These families, moving along the paths of solidification, are the nondivorcing families and as such may include traditional or nontraditional family systems.

Frequently, the developmental stage of the adults involved in the family may affect the family's development. The work by Gould (1972), Levinson (1977), and Lowenthal et al (1975) is especially important to the understanding of personality development during middle age. It is possible that the two developmental levels may conflict with one another. For example, in the case of timing of illness episodes, we observe that the greater the needs and tasks of the family unit in regard to children, the greater the upheaval of the family in response to the illness. In addition, the greater the developmental tasks of either adult in the family unit, the greater the disruption of the family caused by timing of the illness event. Young families experiencing the disruption caused by cardiac surgery are a good example of this phenomenon. The confluence of adult developmental transitions, family transitions, and the event of a major illness can cause such disequilibrium that continuity of the family system as previously configured is jeopardized. The impact of coronary artery bypass graft surgery on young men carries completely different meanings and implications for future lifestyles than for older men and their families. The younger men view the surgery as a portent of their own mortality, and older men view it as a means of guaranteeing a longer life. Additionally, the role transitions required by adjustment to illness may be of such magnitude that the relationship of the adult partners may not survive the assault.

Family units that reconstitute themselves because of changes in personal relationships such as death or divorce continue to have the same responsibilities to children that the solidifying families have. However, they also may have to accommodate new family members, as is the case in blended families (Visher, Visher, 1983), or they may have to adjust to the absence of a parent or adult partner, as in situations of divorce or death. Besides changes in personal relationships, the nurse can expect these families to encounter changes in roles and status and perhaps changes in environment and psychologic functioning. In essence, the reconstituting family must complete the same tasks and contend with the same child and adult developmental stages as the solidifying family, but they also must cope with the loss of old members and perhaps the addition of new ones. As Wallerstein (1984) and the Center for the Study of Families in Transition have noted, children of divorce often carry the residue of the loss for years, demonstrating an inability to form lasting relationships as young adults and exhibiting a higher incidence of depression than children from intact families.

Less is known about the length and stability of gay and lesbian relationships than about heterosexual, traditional marriages. The mean length of time spent in a homosexual relationship is reported to be 8.9 years (McWhirter, Mattison, 1984). As with the traditional heterosexual relationship, a reconstituted nontraditional gay or lesbian family may also be involved with problems related to loss of old members and the addition of new ones.

The solidifying or reconstituting period of family life tends to be the longest in duration and is followed by the final category of family transitions, the contracting family. The solidifying or reconstituting stage usually lasts from 10 to 30 years, depending on the ages of the adult partners when the family unit formed. When compared to the traditional family developmental paradigm, this phase encompasses the stages that include families with preschool-aged children through middle-aged families.

Contracting Families

Contracting families encounter tasks related to the launching and release of children (Duvall, 1977), if children were part of the family unit, and also to the loss of adult partners through death or, as is becoming more common, through late-in-life divorces (Berardo, 1982). In addition to transitions in personal relationships, changes in roles and status and in physical and psychologic functioning must be successfully integrated during this stage.

Adjusting to the loss of parental roles and the "empty-nest syndrome" has been frequently mentioned as one of the more difficult transitions for adult family members. Although popular belief has supported the notion that depression accompanies the empty-nest syndrome, especially for women, available research indicates that the early childrearing years are instead the most stressful, and that the launching phase signals new freedom and a chance for growth for women (Abbott, Brody, 1985; Neugarten, 1979; Rollins, Feldman in Heckerman, 1980). Similar to beliefs held about the empty-nest syndrome are those related to retirement. Loss of work roles for younger men and women are indeed difficult to integrate, but persons over age 65 not only desire retirement more than was previously thought (Atchley, 1982) but also enjoy an enhanced standard of living since a sizable portion of this group possesses the greatest percentage of expendable income of any age group (Aldous, 1987).

Other tasks that families in this phase must accomplish include integration of leisure time and adjustment to the lack of responsibility for both children and careers. Those older people who are able to continue with avocations developed in younger years often find these avocations, or the development of new interests,

a helpful adjunct to adaptation to decreased responsibility (Atchley, 1982).

Health and illness demands attain greater importance during this stage, with middle-aged children and spouses frequently involved in caregiving activities. Caregivers are typically women, with middle-aged women delivering care to their own parents or parents-in-law (Brody, 1981; Fengler, Goodrich, 1979; Soldo, Myllyluoma, 1983) and with elderly women delivering care to their spouses (Cantor, 1983; Oliver, 1983; Poulshock, Deimling, 1984; Worcester, Quayhagen, 1983). The emotional and physical demands of caregiving are now being considered in terms of the social policy implications for women, the unpaid caregivers (Evers, 1985).

As the population ages and the proportion of people over age 65 increases, the strengths and deficits of these families must be considered to a greater extent than they are now in terms of health policy and planning. The fact that 95% of individuals over age 65 and 75% of individuals over age 85 are not institutionalized but instead are supported within the community and family (Miller, 1985; Shanas, 1979) suggests that nursing should exert additional efforts to better serve older families. For instance, advocacy of respite care to support family caregivers would be a possible route nurses could take to better serve older families. Additionally, nursing might consider the supports needed by older and less traditional families, such as gay couples and older couples living together outside of legal marital bonds. For example, the regressive nature of the Social Security system makes it difficult for many older couples who desire to marry to do so without fear of losing existing Social Security benefits. Again, nursing's advocacy of this population at the federal health care policy level could add stability to the lives of this group. Lastly, the same diversity of lifestyle and belief systems that is becoming more apparent in younger families today will be seen in the older families of the future.

Summary

That transitions and change are predictable within families has been well established. The patterning of these transitions and the development of families of varying structures is less well known. Parkes's psychosocial transitions are suggested as a beneficial aid for examining the transitions that propel families through their own personal histories. Transitions are recognized as occurring within developmental stages and also as being the impetus for movement to the next stage. The psychosocial transition deemed as most important in families is that of change in personal relationships.

This chapter has introduced a flexible framework for examining family development. The framework suggests that family development may be better understood from the perspective of the adults who influence the direction and stability of the family than simply from the perspective of the oldest child. Family development, as outlined in this chapter, is guided primarily by the adults in the family unit and secondarily by the interaction of the parents and children. This framework also allows for the inclusion of families without children, families in which there are not two parents, and nontraditional groups of adults who consider themselves families.

Families develop and change at their own rates, and what may be a major transition for one family may be barely noticed by another. The question of why is yet to be answered. It is important that nurses be aware of potential for transition problems, such as those found during the birth of a child or death of a parent, but at the same time also be aware that not all families need the same types of intervention or even desire intervention. Families have tremendous strengths, and we are only beginning to understand their abilities to cope with transitions creatively and to grow healthfully.

Issues for Further Investigation

1. Which of the following changes in personal relationships are most likely to require nursing intervention and which types of intervention—preventive, supportive, or therapeutic—are best suited: birth of an infant, suicide of an adolescent, sudden death of a middle-aged father?

2. How do sex-role development and cultural norms affect the changes in role and status necessitated by adaptation of patient and family members to chronic illness?

3. What impact do changes in physical and psychologic functioning of parents have on school-aged children and adolescents?

References

Abbott DD, Brody GH (1985): The relation of child age, gender, and number of children to the marital adjustment of wives. *J Marr Fam, 47*(1): 77–84.

Aldous J (1987): New views on the family life of the elderly and the near-elderly. *J Marr Fam, 49:* 227–234.

Atchley RC (1982): Retirement: Leaving the world of work. *Ann Am Acad Pol Soc Sci, 464:* 120–131.

Bell AP, Weinberg MS (1978): *Homosexualities: A Study of Diversity Among Men and Women.* New York: Simon & Schuster.

Berardo DH (1982): Divorce and remarriage at middle age and beyond. *Ann Am Acad Pol Soc Sci, 464:* 132–139.

Boss PG (1983): The marital relationship: Boundaries and Ambiguities. In: *Coping with Normative Transitions,* McCubbin HI, Figley CR (eds.). New York: Brunner/Mazel.

Brody EM (1981): 'Women in the middle' and family help to older people. *Gerontologist, 21*(5): 471–480.

Burr W (1972): Role transitions: A reformulation of theory. *J Marr Fam, 34:* 407–416.

Cantor MH (1983): Strain among caregivers: A study of experience in the United States. *Gerontologist, 23*(6): 597–604.

Carter E, McGoldrick M (1980): The family life cycle and family therapy. In: *The Family Life Cycle: A Framework for Family Therapy,* Carter E, McGoldrick M (eds.). New York: Gardner.

Clark NM, Rakowski W (1983): Family caregivers of older adults: Improving helping skills. *Gerontologist, 23*(6): 637–642.

Clemens AW, Axelson LJ (1985): The not-so-empty-nest: The return of the fledgling adult. *Fam Relations, 34:* 259–264.

Deutsch M (1968): Field theory in social psychology. In: *Handbook of Social Psychology,* Lindzey G, Aronson E (eds.). Menlo Park, CA: Addison-Wesley.

Duvall E (1977): *Family Development,* 5th ed. Philadelphia: Lippincott.

Duvall E, Hill R (1948): Dynamics of family interaction. From National Conference on Family Life (First White House Conference on Family Life). Washington, DC: GPO.

Evers H (1985): The frail elderly women: Emergent questions in aging and women's health. In: *Women, Health, and Healing,* Lewin E, Oleson V (eds.). New York: Tavistock.

Fengler AP, Goodrich N (1983): Wives of elderly disabled men: The hidden patients. *Gerontologist, 19*(2): 175–183.

Gladue BE, Green R, Hellman RE (1984): Neuroendocrine response to estrogen and sexual orientation. *Science, 225:* 1496–1499.

Gorman ML (1966): Towards a definition of intervention: In: *Interpersonal Relations,* Maloney EM (ed.). Dubuque: William C Brown, pp. 54–72.

Gould RL (1972): The phases of adult life: A study in developmental psychology. *Am J Psychiatry, 129*(5): 521–531.

Hatton CL, Valente SMcB (eds.) (1984): *Suicide: Assessment and Intervention.* East Norwalk, CT: Appleton-Lange.

Heckerman CL (1980): *The Evolving Female: Women in Psychosocial Context.* New York: Human Sciences.

Hill R (1949): *Families Under Stress.* New York: Harper & Row.

Hull D (1979): Migration, adaptation, and illness: A review. *Soc Sci Med, 13:* 25–36.

Kelly RF, Voydanoff P (1985): Work/family role strain among employed parents. *Fam Relations, 34*(3): 367–374.

Kolitz S, Pimm JB (1984): Crisis intervention and coronary bypass surgery. In: *Psychological Risks of Coronary Bypass Surgery,* Pimm JB, Feist JR (eds.). New York: Plenum.

Lear M (1981): *Heartsounds.* New York: Simon & Schuster.

Levinson DJ (1977): The mid-life transition: A period in adult psychosocial development. *Psychiatry, 40:* 99–112.

Lipson JG, Meleis AI (1983): Issues in health care of middle eastern patients. *West J Med, 139:* 854–861.

Lowenthal MF, Chiriboga D (1972): Transition to the empty nest: Crisis, challenge, or belief? *Arch Gen Psychiatry, 26.*

Lowenthal MF, Thurnher MT, Chiriboga D (1975): *Four Stages of Life.* San Francisco: Jossey-Bass.

McWhirter DP, Mattison FM (1984): *The Male Couple: How Relationships Develop.* Englewood Cliffs, NJ: Prentice-Hall.

Mederer H, Hill R (1983): Critical transitions over the family life span: Theory and research. In: *Social Stress and the Family,* McCubbin MB, Sussman MB, Patterson M (eds.). New York: Haworth.

Meister SB (1977): Charting a family's developmental status for intervention and for the record. *Am J Mat Child Nurs, 2:* 43–48.

Menaghan E (1982): Assessing the impact of family transitions on marital experience: Problems and prospects. In: *Family Stress, Coping, and Social Support,* McCubbin HI, Cable AE, Patterson J (eds.). Springfield, IL: Charles C Thomas.

Miller DB (1985): Women and long-term nursing care. *Women and Health, 10*(1): 29–38.

Montgomery RJV, Gonyea JG, Hooyman NR (1985): Caregiving and the experience of subjective and objective burden. *Fam Relations, 34:* 19–26.

Neugarten BL (1979): Time, age and the life cycle. *Am J Psychiatry, 136:* 887–894.

Neugarten BL, Hagestad G (1976): Aging and the life course. In: *Handbook of Aging and the Social Sciences,* Binstock R, Shanas E (eds.). New York: Van Nostrand Reinhold.

Oliver J (1983): The caring wife. In: *A Labour of Love,* Finch J, Groves D (eds.). London: Routledge & Kegan Paul.

Parkes CM (1971): Psycho-social transitions: A field for study. *Soc Sci Med,* 5: 1010–1015.

Pearlin LI (1983): Role strains and personal stress. In: *Psychosocial Stress: Trends in Theory and Research,* Kaplan H (ed.). New York: Academic Press.

Pies C (1985): *Considering Parenthood: A Workbook for Lesbians.* San Francisco: Spinsters.

Portner J (1983): Work and family: Achieving a balance. In: *Coping with Normative Transitions,* McCubbin HI, Figley CR (eds.). New York: Brunner/Mazel.

Poulshock S, Deimling G (1984). Families caring for elders in residence: Issues in the measurement of burden. *J Gerontol,* 39(2): 230–239.

Pratt CC et al (1985): Burden and coping strategies of caregivers to Alzheimer's patients. *Fam Relations,* 34: 27–33.

Rankin SH et al (1986): Improving recovery from cardiac surgery: A profile of the elderly patient's needs and caregiver response. Proceedings of the International Nursing Research Conference, Edmonton, Alberta, Canada.

Rexroat C (1985): Women's work expectations and labor market experiences in early and middle family life cycle stages. *J Marr Fam,* 47(1): 131–142.

Rowland KF (1977): Environmental events predicting death for the elderly. *Psychol Bull,* 84(2): 349–372.

San Francisco *Chronicle* (1986): UC seeks lesbians for AIDS study. January 18, p. A6.

Shanas E (1979): The family as social support systems in old age. *Gerontologist,* 19: 169–174.

Soldo BJ, Myllyluoma (1983): Caregivers who live with dependent elderly. *Gerontologist,* 23(6): 605–611.

Stevenson JS (1983): Adulthood: A promising focus for future research. In: *Annual Review of Nursing Research: Vol 1,* Werley H, Fitzpatrick J (eds.). New York: Springer-Verlag.

Treischmann RB (1978): *Spinal Cord Injuries: Psychological, Social, and Vocational Adjustment.* New York: Pergamon.

Troll LE (1985): *Early and Middle Adulthood.* Pacific Grove, CA: Brooks/Cole.

Visher E, Visher J (1983): Stepparenting: Blending families. In: *Coping with Normative Transitions,* McCubbin HI, Figley CR (eds.). New York: Brunner/Mazel.

Wallerstein JS (1984): Children of divorce: Preliminary report of a ten-year follow-up of young children. *Am J Orthopsychiatry,* 54(3): 444–458.

Wolanin MO (1978): Relocation of the elderly. *J Gerontol Nurs,* 4(2): 47–50.

Worcester MI, Quayhagen MP (1983): Correlates of caregiving satisfaction: Prerequisites to elder home care. *Res Nurs Health,* 6: 61–67.

12

CHILDBEARING AND ITS EFFECT ON MARITAL QUALITY

Brooke P. Randell, RN, DNSc

Most research in family nursing focuses on dyadic relationships. With the exception of the mother-child dyad, the marital pair is the most frequently studied dyad. This chapter reviews the marital dyad during the childbearing phase of the family life cycle, and offers a historic perspective on the transition from dyad to triad. It also provides a brief review of the research literature on marital quality and childbearing, simultaneously raising research questions with special significance to nurses as care providers for the marital dyad undergoing a transition.

Brooke Randell, director of Special Projects at the UCLA Neuropsychiatric Institute and Hospital, has many years of experience working with families with disturbed children as a psychiatric nurse specialist. She has also taught nursing theory and child mental health at the UCLA School of Nursing.

Introduction

The literature on relationships is replete with descriptors like cohesion, mutuality, and intimacy. In Western culture the marital dyad is the ideal model, the relationship that is said to exemplify the processes associated with the above descriptors. The dyad has been described as the locus of intimacy, with both partners being necessary for the unit's continued existence (Simmel, 1950), a circumstance that does not occur in groups of other sizes. Bowen (1959) suggests that this interdependence makes the dyad inherently unstable, often requiring the addition of other persons for its maintenance over time.

Despite the fact that nurses are charged with meeting the needs of individuals who are part of a marital dyad or who as a dyad provide care for a child, the marital relationship has historically been the province of the sociologist and the psychologist and has less frequently been linked to nursing. However, as caregivers to families, nurses must understand the relationship of the marital couple if they are to grasp the complex matrix of the family.

The marital dyad has special significance when examining the experience of childbearing. Childbearing irreversibly alters the marital dyad, increasing its complexity. Contemporary research has demonstrated that the quality of the marital relationship is often predictive of successful childbearing outcomes (Belsky, Spanier, Rovine, 1983; Grossman, Eichler, Winickoff, 1980; Porter, Demeuth, 1979; Richardson, 1981; Shereshefsky, Yarrow, 1973; Wenner et al, 1969; Westbrook, 1978).

Lewis and Spanier (1979), in a review of research on the quality and stability of marriage, suggest that in this time of record high divorce rates, it is essential to build at least a partial theory of marital stability that identifies many of the conditions under which a marriage may remain intact or be dissolved. The transition from dyad to triad is thought to be one of the major threats to marital stability, which allows the nurse caring for the childbearing family the unique opportunity to contribute to the theory of marital stability.

Barnard (1980) suggests that we can question whether nursing care is family-centered, for although such care is espoused, there is a lack of scientific literature in this area to document this supposition.

The Intimate Dyad: A Historical Perspective

The social meaning of interpersonal closeness suggests that intimate relationships are a product of the rapid urbanization and industrial development associated with the early decades of the 19th century (Gadlin, 1977; Goode, 1963). Gadlin bases his argument on the shifting nature of the intimate relationship from public to private and on a belief that many of the changes in social life reflect a need to preserve social cohesion and diminish the power of the exclusive relationship.

Gadlin traces intimate relationships from the colonial period of the mid-1600s to the contemporary period, which he identifies as beginning post-1940. The distinctive feature of intimate relationships during the colonial period was their public nature. Marriages were entered into because they were functional, and it was hoped emotional attachment and connection would occur at some future time. During the early decades of the 19th century, however, the nature of relationships changed from public to private.

Gadlin suggests that personal identity was a product of the 19th century, and with this focus on the personal it became necessary to also acknowledge the interpersonal. With industrialization, people became isolated and were no longer part of enduring communities or kinship networks. As a result, they sought interpersonal relationships to replace old social networks. Marriage provided a vehicle for reconnection, but unlike the colonial period, unions were based on personal feeling and attraction as opposed to social function. The marriage relationship became part of private life, removed from the public sector.

The intimacy of the interpersonal relationship and the move to the private sector are seen as threatening social cohesion. The addition of a child to the intimate dyad then may be viewed as a social mechanism that pulls the dyad back toward the larger aggregate and diminishes social anxiety. Gadlin suggests that the movement of the intimate relationship from the public to the private sphere has necessitated the formation of social institutions mediating against the power of this dyad. The ultimate control over the intimate dyad, however, is embodied in the institution of the family (Gadlin, 1977).

Slater (1963) states that the intimate, exclusive dyad is essentially playful and nonutilitarian. The organized societal intrusion of marriage, childbirth, and childrearing is required to convert the intimate dyad into a socially useful relationship. The question then arises: What is the relationship between marital quality and the conversion of the intimate dyad into the socially useful relationship embodied in the family?

The Marital Dyad: A Brief Overview

Current research on the marital dyad indicates that marital satisfaction, marital quality, and marital happiness are of great interest to researchers in the area of marital and family theory. Despite the interest and research, there remain many overlapping definitions and a multiplicity of variables as well as methods for operationalizing them. In addition, considerable uncertainty remains about the linearity versus curvilinearity of many of the concepts as well as about the general course of relationships across the life span.

Despite these methodologic and conceptual concerns, there are some consistent findings regarding marital satisfaction and marital quality. In addition, new questions are posed and others remain unanswered. Men and women appear to be different in their participation in and experience of marriage (Argyle, Furnham, 1983; Eastman, 1958; Kiernan, Tallman, 1972; Ryder, 1970). Other authors suggest there is no real difference in the male and female experience (Argyle, Furnham, 1983; Gilford, Bengston, 1979). It is indicated that women put more into marriage and are required to change more and be more flexible (Eastman, 1958; Hansen, 1981; Kiernan, Tallman, 1972; Rhyne, 1981; Ryder, 1970). The male's unique emotional contribution to marriage remains uncertain (Bowen, Orthner, 1983; Kiernan, Tallman, 1972; Ryder, 1970). The marital relationship is seen to be both highly satisfying and highly conflictual (Argyle, Furnham, 1983; Gilford, Bengston, 1979). Finally, it has been demonstrated that objective characteristics like age and socioeconomic status account for little variance in marital satisfaction, but subjective experiences like perceived friendship or affection are key factors in explaining satisfaction (Spanier, Lewis, 1980; Rhyne, 1981).

With this brief review of the literature on the marital dyad, it seems apparent that there are many issues and unresolved questions in the field of marital research. When one adds to these existing problems the complex physical and psychologic experience of first pregnancy, it seems safe to assume the difficulties will be compounded. Research that is directed toward the impact of childbearing on the family will be examined next, with a focus on marital quality, dependence, and intimacy.

The Marital Dyad in First Pregnancy

According to Caplan (1959), pregnancy is a biologically determined psychologic crisis. In addition, Caplan suggests that if there is a disordered husband–wife relationship, the result is likely to be a disordered mother–child relationship. Caplan allocates to the husband the task of "charging the wife's battery" through love in order to prevent difficulties, especially in later pregnancy. The following review will examine research that focuses on the relationship between first pregnancy and early postpartum and the marital relationship. The review will examine as a central focus the impact of childbearing on marital quality, an overriding theme in this body of research literature. In addition, the concepts of intimacy and nurturance will be reviewed, as these concepts are seen as recurrent threads in this literature and are relevant to the theoretical perspective suggesting that childbearing alters the exclusive nature of the intimate dyad, providing it with a societal link and function.

Marital Quality

In the early studies that described the transition to parenthood as an extensive crisis, Le Masters (1957) attributed these findings to the subjects' romanticized view and inadequate knowledge of parenthood. In a later study however, Hobbs and Cole (1976) found lesser but significant levels of crisis and also sought to identify variables that differentiated subjects or couples on the amount of difficulty experienced. It was found that prebirth and postbirth ratings of marriage were relevant for fathers and that none of the identified variables were relevant for mothers. It has also been noted that disruption of the marital relationship is perceived as creating severe problems in adjustment to pregnancy (Helper et al, 1968) and that a strong desire for pregnancy is associated with wives who are most satisfied with their husbands and their lives in general (Grimm, Venet, 1966).

Marital quality has been examined as an outcome variable, viewed as changing in either a positive or a negative direction following childbearing, or as a predictor variable, having a

positive or negative outcome on the experience of childbearing. By far the majority of research focuses on this latter formulation, but a brief review of data concerning the positive and negative effects of childbearing on marital quality are worthy of examination.

Marital Quality as an Outcome Variable

The reported positive impact of childbearing on marriage is tenuous and seems overbalanced by studies describing the negative outcomes. Only two of the studies reviewed here specifically identify the positive impact of childbearing. In a multidimensional study of 60 families, Shereshefsky and Yarrow (1973) concluded that pregnancy has a greater intrapsychic than social impact, but they also suggested that marital adaptation improves between the first and the third trimester of pregnancy, thus implying pregnancy serves a positive role in marital adaptation. In another multidimensional longitudinal study, Grossman, Eichler, and Winickoff (1980) found that couples reported enrichment and enhancement of their marital relationship when they became parents. Women in this sample demonstrated at one year that they had regained their previous level of satisfaction, and the marriage remained their central source of support, but it seemed that the marriage never would attain the focal position it had before birth.

The negative impact of childbearing is more frequently documented. Meyerowitz and Feldman (1966) studied 400 primiparous couples from several geographic areas of the United States using a short-term longitudinal approach. Their findings revealed that the marital relationship prior to pregnancy was recalled as having been more positive than the marital relationship during pregnancy. The decline in quality was more significant for the husband than for the wife. In a study of 47 first-time fathers, Wandersman (1980) also found that fathers reported a small but significant decrease in marital satisfaction. Miller and Sollie (1980) examined the experience of 109 couples using a short instrument with questionable construct validity to measure personal well-being, personal stress, and marital stress at three time intervals. They concluded that new parents typically experience modest declines in personal well-being and some increase in personal stress over the first year of parenthood. Generally mothers reported steadily increasing marital stress scores; fathers' marital stress scores remained essentially the same (Miller, Sollie, 1980). Harriman (1983), using a stratified random sample drawn from birth records, conducted a retrospective study of married couples who had recently given birth. Harriman concluded that, in general, wives experienced more personal change, whereas husbands experienced more marital change. Finally, Belsky, Spanier, and Rovine (1983), on examination of 72 predominately Caucasian, well-educated, middle-class families, of whom 41 were bearing first children, concluded that there is a small but generally unfavorable change in the marital relationship as evidenced by the linear decline in the mean Dyadic Adjustment Score.

What is perhaps most interesting about these findings, in addition to the obvious sparsity of positive effects, is the repeated difference noted for mothers and fathers. Lipps (1981) specifically examined attitudes toward childbearing held by men and women expecting their first child. She concluded men and women have different attitudes about pregnancy in general, and these differences, especially for women, remain consistent even within the couple relationship. For example, men who had been married longer tended to have a more positive expectation, whereas women who had been married longer tended to question whether becoming pregnant was desirable and were more able to envision a satisfying life without children. As Lipps (1981) and Richardson (1983) have identified, the childbearing process tends to have the greatest impact on the personal lives of women

and the marital lives of men. These findings suggest that questions regarding marital quality might provide valid information regarding the male partner but do not completely tap the woman's experience of childbearing. Despite this, the following review suggests that marital quality is a good predictor of positive childbearing outcomes.

Studies using marital quality as an outcome variable seem to suggest that the child's impact on the marital dyad is more frequently negative than positive. It is significant, however, that studies reporting positive outcomes are large, multidimensional, longitudinal studies as opposed to studies with limited measures at a single time period. This suggests that perhaps we need to consider the complexity of the transition to parenthood and the number of individuals involved when selecting a design. A simple design is not likely to capture the richness of the experience. The studies also consistently report a difference between the mothers' and fathers' perceptions of their experience. We know a great deal more about the woman's experience than we do about the man's; therefore studies that include fathers are essential. When marital quality is viewed as an outcome variable, it would seem important to undertake a study that would generate a typology of marital patterns early in pregnancy and at one year postbirth that uses both couple and individual data. Such a study could use existing typologies or could generate an original format. Such data would be valuable in that they would provide information on the marital dyad and would demonstrate the existence of a pattern across the transition, suggesting further research questions regarding the hazards inherent in this transition for the various types of dyads.

Marital Quality as a Predictor of Childbearing Outcomes

Wenner et al (1969), in an examination of women receiving psychotherapy during pregnancy, found that an uncomplicated pregnancy depended to a great extent on the success of the marital relationship. These authors found a parallel between the degree of marital satisfaction and neuroticism; as marital conflict increased, so did neurotic symptoms and difficulties in the pregnancy. Contrary to these findings, Shereshefsky and Yarrow (1973) found little correlation between husband variables and pregnancy adaptation, but these variables were highly correlated with maternal adaptation. Thus these authors concluded that the husband plays a crucial role in the mother–infant relationship but not in the pregnancy.

In a retrospective study of 200 Australian women who had borne a child two to seven months previously, Westbrook (1978) hypothesized that the quality of a woman's marital relationship would be significantly associated with her experience of childbearing. Westbrook concluded that there is a significant association between marital relationship and maternal reaction to childbearing. Women with positive marital relationships believed that their marital satisfaction had increased. Women with ambivalent marital relationships felt that children increased marital satisfaction. Finally, women with negative marital relationships were unlikely to feel that children enhanced the marital relationship.

Gladieux (1978) studied married couples undergoing first pregnancy. Subjects in this study were described as traditional or modern based on sex-role behavior scores. Gladieux's findings suggested that traditional women were likely (1) to have mates who had similar viewpoints regarding sex-role behavior; (2) to expect satisfaction from motherhood; and (3) to have husbands who tended to reinforce this view. Modern women were less likely to anticipate motherhood would be fulfilling, and their uncertainty was often amplified by the husband. These results tend to suggest that it is not so much the quality of the marriage but the attitudes toward childbearing mediated through

the relationship that affect the reproductive experience.

Porter and Demeuth (1979) examined the relationship between marital adjustment and pregnancy acceptance using Spanier's Dyadic Adjustment Scale and Grimm's Pregnancy Acceptance Questionnaire. These authors concluded that as marital adjustment increases, so does pregnancy acceptance. In addition, the authors concluded that spouses are less similar in their experience of the pregnancy than of the marriage. Wandersman (1980) and Wandersman, Wandersman, and Kahn (1980) examined the role of parenting groups on fathers' adjustment to their first baby. In this study, the quality of the marital relationship was correlated with the father's general well-being and parental sense of competence. Wandersman (1980) concluded that the quality of the marital relationship played a central role in fathers' adjustment to parenthood. Mothers, however, seemed more influenced by the temperament of the baby than by the marital relationship. These findings seem consistent with research on the marital dyad that suggests that the male and female experience and sources of satisfaction are different (Argyle, Furnham, 1983; Rhyne, 1981; Ryder, 1970).

Grossman et al (1980) conclude that from a woman's perspective, the marriage is like a barometer; when the marriage is going well, other things go well. Richardson (1981) viewed marriage in a different light, describing the marital relationship as problematic; one-third of her subjects described their relationships with spouses as unsatisfactory.

Given these diverse findings, it is clear that many questions remain to be answered. Comparisons need to be made of marital quality for couples who have varying degrees of success in enactment of the parental role. Additionally, we need to look at the interaction between the variables of culture, socioeconomic status, marital quality, and childbearing. In this technologic age, we need to determine if marital quality is a mediator of the stress associated with the diagnostic uncertainties of the contemporary pregnancy experience.

It appears that marital quality is a complex phenomenon that is indeed intertwined with the experience of childbearing. Particular characteristics of the marriage or individual qualities of the spousal pair might offer more insight regarding the impact of the marital relationship than the more global measure of marital quality. The concepts of intimacy and nurturance will be briefly reviewed in an effort to determine if research thus focused adds dimension to our understanding of the impact of the childbearing experience on the marital relationship.

Intimacy as a Concept in the Childbearing Literature

Although intimacy is not a concept that has informed the research on childbearing, an exploration of the data available lends support to Gadlin's (1977) formulation that childbearing weakens the exclusivity of the intimate dyad and suggests that more rigorous examination of intimacy as a variable might prove informative.

In Meyerowitz and Feldman's (1966) study of 400 primiparous couples, the most frequent complaint among spouses related to sexuality, with women expressing more dissatisfaction than men. The authors found these data confusing in view of the fact that the male usually reports less satisfaction with the frequency of sexual activity (Ammons, Stinnett, 1980; Rhyne, 1981). Female subjects reported less desire and consequently felt that they were being bad wives by not being more sexually active (Meyerowitz, Feldman, 1966). Consequently, the wives' dissatisfaction seems to be a measure of a different dimension than that usually implied by the

husband. Her concern could be construed to be her failure to respond to her husband's needs, whereas his concern is usually over not having his needs met, a self-versus-other orientation.

Grimm and Venet (1966) also examined sexuality and concluded that early in pregnancy, sexual adjustment was related to satisfaction with the husband but late in pregnancy, there seemed to be little correlation between sexuality and satisfaction with the spouse. Harriman (1983) identified that there is a mutual change in the area of sexual responsiveness; both the husbands and wives agreed that the wives' declining sexual responsivity was a negative change.

Using a broader definition of intimacy, the ideas of cohesion and mutuality have some explanatory power. Wandersman (1980) attributed any decrease in marital satisfaction to the fathers' feelings that their needs were being put aside because of the baby and that it was taking longer than they had anticipated to reestablish intimate contact with their wives. Using a canonical analysis procedure to determine a set of measures of support that best predicted the measures of adjustment, Wandersman et al (1980) found that a quality they label "marital cohesion" was a significant factor. These authors suggest that this subjective dimension of cohesion may play a more general role in accounting for overall postpartum adjustment. Similarly, Richardson (1981) concludes that there must be some degree of stability or cohesion in the marriage for the relationship to withstand the intensity of the reorganization process. Grossman et al (1980) suggest that some of the best-adjusted couples had a quality of giddiness—a shared anxiety and excitement that made the changed relationship a shared experience, not something inflicted on one by the other. A mutuality is described that seems to allow for nondestructive change. Intimacy, conceived as cohesion or mutuality, seems to be a significant quality of the marital relationship that warrants further study.

Nurturance as a Concept in the Childbearing Literature

Like intimacy, nurturance is a quality inherent in our understanding of the marital relationship. Recently this concept has been appearing in the childbearing literature and appears to offer an expanded view on the impact of marital quality. These findings suggest that the ability of both partners to nurture and be nurtured has significant effects on childbearing outcomes.

Wenner et al (1969) found most adaptive couples had collaborative relationships characterized by "adult–husband and adult–wife" configurations. These relationships were often associated with mature dependency, meaning that the subjects were well differentiated, or aware of their separateness from others; they did not expect their needs to be intuitively sensed nor their demands to be totally gratified.

Shereshefsky and Yarrow (1973) specifically examined a nurturance factor that was considered a personality measure for the woman. In general, they describe this factor as a measure of the woman's responsiveness and giving qualities. Although there are some general items within the factor, it appears to be derived almost exclusively from the marital relationship. This nurturance factor correlated significantly with pregnancy adaptation. This would seem to imply that the capacity to be nurturant within the marital relationship has a significant impact on childbearing outcomes.

Shereshefsky and Yarrow also found that 41% of the husbands were competitive with their wives in an attempt to see who could be the best parent. This behavior was most obvious in the husbands whose wives had the most difficulty with the mother role. These men were the least supportive during pregnancy and had the most anxiety, but were more competent and loving in the handling of the babies than their wives. Nurturance has also been identified as an attribute that must be possessed by the male partner. In a

psychoanalytically based interview study, Ballou (1978) concluded that in optimal circumstances, the husband functions to facilitate adaptation to the dependency and regression associated with pregnancy. It is suggested that problems arise when the husband is unable to assume the more nurturant role. Ballou concludes that when husbands can be empathetic yet remain separate, the wife further reconciles with her mother and experiences further resolution of Oedipal issues. Grossman et al (1980) offer a similar view but from a less theory-embedded perspective, suggesting that men who have a strong sense of their masculinity do not have difficulty providing nurturance and dealing with increased dependence of their wives. In addition, men who perceive themselves as having been positively mothered and who identify with their own mothers have more positive pregnancy experiences.

Richardson (1981) examined relationships during pregnancy. One-third of the women in the study described their marital relationships as unsatisfactory. In a follow-up study, Richardson (1983) examined changes in the husband–wife relationship in more depth and suggested that changes involved either task or affective performance. The women reported a slight change in the husband's willingness to do household chores, but marital reorganization focused primarily on the affective dimension. Most of the women wanted greater demonstrations of affection; they wanted acceptance of themselves and of the child they were expecting. If the husband demonstrated adequate affection, women evaluated the relationship as satisfactory, and with satisfactory evaluation of the relationship, the husband's involvement in the pregnancy experience increased.

Many questions remain to be answered. The construct of nurturance and its relationship to marital quality would seem of significance to nursing. We need to determine if there are areas of agreement between couples concerning what constitutes nurturing behavior. What spousal behaviors are perceived as nurturing by pregnant and newly parturitient women? What nurturing behaviors do husbands identify engaging in during pregnancy and early parturition? Cohesion (Olson et al, 1979) is a construct receiving considerable attention in the family literature; with concept clarification, it would appear to have explanatory power in relationship to the nature of intimacy and nurturance within the marital dyad.

Future Directions

As caregivers who have long professed a family-centered perspective, nurses would be wise to join the efforts of family researchers, bringing a nursing orientation to the variety of methodologic and conceptual issues. We must participate in the effort to bring meaning to these findings and plan future research that will elucidate the complex phenomena involved in the transition from the intimate dyad to the expanding family.

First we must address issues of instrumentation, timing, and data sources. When evaluating the previous studies, comparisons were often difficult because the topic was frequently examined from different time perspectives, ranging from early in the first trimester of pregnancy to late in the first postpartum year. Some studies were retrospective (Meyerowitz, Feldman, 1966; Westbrook, 1978), and others were prospective (Grossman et al, 1980; Porter, Demeuth, 1979; Shereshefsky, Yarrow, 1973). Data were often based on a measurement made at one time interval (Harriman, 1983; Porter, Demeuth, 1979), using a single instrument (Harriman, 1983; Miller, Sollie, 1980), and other data were generated from interviews and multiple instruments spread over several time intervals (Grossman, et al, 1980; Shereshefsky, Yarrow, 1973; Wenner, et al, 1969). Frequently, studies purported to assess the marital relationship but used only the wife as a data source. Although other studies did not use couple data, they did include both partners (Belsky et al, 1983; Lipps, 1981; Shereshefsky, Yarrow, 1973; Grossman et al, 1980). These studies occasionally lacked methodologic rigor, employing poorly standardized instruments or failing to report critical demographic variables (Lipps, 1981; Harriman, 1983; Porter, Demeuth, 1979; Westbrook, 1978). Finally, almost all the data relates to white, middle-class, educated couples in their mid- to late twenties, a notable exception being the work of Richardson (1981, 1983), who reports on a small sample of women, half of whom are Mexican-Americans.

Perhaps even more significantly, we must engage in conceptual clarification. Conceptually, the studies often appear to measure the same variable; however, there is wide divergence in the definitions of marital quality. Multiple instruments have been used, and to date there seems to be little agreement concerning what constitutes a good measure of marital quality. The literature on marriage and childbearing seems to lack the conceptual and theoretical sophistication of the general marital relationship literature. None of the childbearing literature has addressed the issues of linearity versus curvilinearity, nor has the multidimensional nature of marital quality been examined. Although the research on marital relationships seems to have benefited from the use of exchange theory, the research on childbearing seems to have bypassed this potentially useful conceptualization.

Concepts such as nurturance, which can be generated from existing data, would appear to focus the direction of research on specific qualities of the marital relationship that have special significance to the childbearing process. In addition, there has been considerable effort expended in attempts to generate marital typologies (Goodrich, Ryder, Raush, 1968; Ryder, 1970). Similar efforts or collaborative efforts are not evident in the childbearing literature, with the possible exception of Westbrook (1978), Gladieux (1978), and Richardson's (1981, 1983) beginning attempt. It would appear that the exploration of the association between the marital relationship and the childbearing experience would be enhanced by a stronger connection to the developing body of knowledge in the area of marital relationships in general.

Summary

As in the research on marital relationships in general, the research on marital relationships during childbearing offers conflicting and overlapping perspectives. It seems clear that there is a positive relationship between marital quality and childbearing (Shereshefsky, Yarrow, 1973; Westbrook, 1978; Gladieux, 1978; Grossman et al, 1980; Wandersman, 1980; Richardson, 1983; Belsky et al, 1983). Much of the data suggest that like marriage in general, the marital relationship in the transition to parenthood is experienced differently by females than by males (Belsky et al, 1983; Harriman, 1983; Lipps, 1981; Porter, Demeuth, 1979; Wandersman, 1980). Other authors conclude that the primary function of the marital relationship is the provision of nurturance and the satisfaction of emergent, mutual dependency needs (Ballou, 1978; Grossman et al, 1980; Wenner et al, 1969). Still others suggest that changes in sexual responsivity contribute to the change in marital quality during pregnancy (Grimm, Venet, 1966; Harriman, 1983; Meyerowitz, Feldman, 1966). These conflictual and interrelated findings can be attributed to the variety of methodologic and conceptual issues inherent in a research review of this nature.

The nurse engaged in the care and understanding of the childbearing family is in the unique position of being able to join the multidisciplinary efforts of family researchers, contributing an additional perspective on the significance of the marital dyad in the transition to parenthood and childbearing outcomes.

Issues for Further Investigation

1. What factors differentiate those couples whose marital quality is reduced following childbearing from those whose marital quality is improved or unchanged? Is there a relationship between parenting success and marital quality in early parenting?

2. How is marital quality following childbearing differentially affected across socioeconomic status, age or culture?

3. Does uncertainty associated with pregnancy (maternal–fetal health outcomes, sustaining pregnancy to term, gender of the fetus) contribute to changes in marital quality following childbearing?

4. Are couples experiencing a chronic illness at higher risk for reductions in marital satisfaction following childbearing than couples whose health is not impaired?

5. To what extent does prepregnancy marital quality predict post-childbearing marital quality?

6. How does marital quality change in subsequent childbearing episodes?

References

Ammons P, Stinnett N (1980): The vital marriage: A closer look. *Fam Relations*, 29:37–42.

Argyle M, Furnham A (1983): Sources of satisfaction and conflict in long-term relationships. *J Marr Fam*, 45(3), 481–493.

Barnard KE (1980): Knowledge for practice: Decisions for the future. *Nurs Res, 29:*208–212.

Ballou J (1978): *The Psychology of Pregnancy.* Lexington, MA: Lexington Books.

Belsky J, Spanier GB, Rovine M (1983): Stability and change in marriage across the transition to parenthood. *J Marr Fam, 45*(3):567–577.

Bowen M (1959): The family as the unit of study and treatment. *Am J Orthopsychiatry, 31*(1):40–60.

Bowen G, Orthner D (1983): Sex-role congruency and marital quality. *J Marr Fam, 45*(1):223–230.

Caplan G (1959): Concepts of mental health and consultation. U.S. HEW.

Eastman D (1958): Self acceptance and marital happiness. *J Consult Psychol, 22*(2):95–99.

Gadlin H (1977): Private lives and public order: A critical view of the history of intimate relations in the United States. In: *Close Relationships,* Levenger G, Raush HL (eds.). Amherst: University of Massachusetts Press, pp. 33–72.

Gilford R, Bengston V (1979): Measuring marital satisfaction in three generations: Positive and negative dimensions. *J Marr Fam, 41:* 387–398.

Gladieux JD (1978): Pregnancy—the transition to parenthood: Satisfaction with the pregnancy experience as a function of sex role conceptions, marital relationship and social network. In: *First Child and Family Formation,* Miller WB, Newman LF (eds.). Chapel Hill: Carolina Population Center, University of North Carolina.

Goode WJ (1963): Industrialization and family structure. In: *The Family,* Bell NW, Vogel EF (eds.). New York: Free Press, pp. 113–120.

Goodrich W, Ryder RG, Raush HL (1968): Patterns of newlywed marriage. *J Marr Fam, 30:*383–390.

Grimm ER, Venet WR (1966): The relationship of emotional adjustment and attitudes to the course and outcome of pregnancy. *Psychosom Med, 28:* 34–50.

Grossman K, Eichler LS, Winickoff SA (1980): *Pregnancy, Birth, and Parenthood.* San Francisco: Jossey-Bass.

Hansen C (1981): Living in with normal families. *Fam Process, 20:*53–75.

Harriman LG (1983): Personal and marital changes accompanying parenthood. *Fam Relations, 32:* 387–394.

Helper MM et al (1968): Life-events and acceptance of pregnancy. *J Psychosom Res, 12:* 183–188.

Hobbs DF, Cole SP (1976): Transitional parenthood: A decade of replication. *J Marr Fam, 38:* 723–731.

Kiernan D, Tallman I (1972): Spousal adaptability: An assessment of marital competence. *J Marr Fam, 37*(2): 263–275.

Lewis RA, Spanier GB (1979): Theorizing about the quality and stability of marriage. In: *Contemporary Theories About the Family, Vol 1,* Burr WR et al (eds.). New York: Free Press, pp. 268–294.

LeMasters EE (1957): Parenthood as crisis. *Marr Fam Liv, 19:* 352–355.

Lipps H (1981): Attitudes toward childbearing among women and men expecting their first child. *Int J Wom Stud, 6*(2): 119–129.

Meyerowitz JH, Feldman H (1966): Transition to parenthood. *Psychiatr Res Report, 20:* 78–84.

Miller BC, Sollie DL (1981): Normal stresses during the transition to parenthood. *Fam Relations, 29:* 459–465.

Olson DH, Sprenkle DH, Russell CS (1979): Circumplex model of marital and family systems. I. Cohesion and adaptability dimensions, family types and clinical applications. *Fam Process, 18*(1): 3–28.

Porter L, Demeuth BR (1979): The impact of marital adjustment on pregnancy acceptance. *Maternal–Child Nurs J, 8*(2): 3–28.

Rhyne D (1981): Bases of marital satisfaction among men and women. *J Marr Fam, 43:* 941–955.

Richardson P (1981): Women's perception of their important dyadic relationships during pregnancy. *Maternal–Child Nurs J, 10*(3): 159–174

Richardson P (1983): Women's perceptions of change in relationships shared with their husbands during pregnancy. *Maternal–Child Nurs J, 12*(1): 1–20.

Ryder RG (1970): A typology of early marriage. *Fam Process, 9*(4): 385–402.

Shereshefsky RN, Yarrow LJ (1973): *Psychological Aspects of a First Pregnancy and Early Postpartum.* New York: Raven.

Simmel G (1950): In: *The Sociology of Georg Simmel,* Wolff KH (ed.). New York: Free Press.

Slater P (1963): On social regression. *Am Sociol Rev, 28*(3): 339–364.

Spanier GB, Lewis RA (1980): Marital quality: A review of the seventies. *J Marr Fam, 42:* 825–839.

Wandersman LP (1980): The adjustment of fathers to their first baby: The roles of parenting groups and marital relationships. *Birth Fam J, 7*(3): 155–161.

Wandersman LP, Wandersman A, Kahn S (1980): Social support in the transition to parenthood. *J Comm Psychol, 8*(4): 314–342.

Wenner NK et al (1969): Emotional problems in pregnancy. *Psychiatry, 32*(4): 389–410.

Westbrook MT (1978): The reactions to childbearing and early maternal experience of women with differing marital relationships. *Br J Med Psychol, 51:* 191–199.

13

THE PERINATAL FAMILY

M. Colleen Stainton, RN, DNSc

The dynamics of the perinatal family are often fluid during the period of emotional acceptance of a new member into a family system that may include multiple generations. This chapter offers an understanding of the family during the prebirth and postbirth phases of family integration. An overview of knowledge about individual and dyadic relationships during the perinatal experience is provided, as well as a macroframework for family-focused practice.

Colleen Stainton is Associate Dean of Research and Scholarly Development at the University of Calgary School of Nursing in Alberta, Canada. She is also an associate professor in the Faculty of Nursing, and is known for her expertise in perinatal family dynamics.

Introduction

The experience of integrating a baby into an already existing set of attachment relationships in a family creates a need for change and adaptation. Study of this phenomenon focuses mainly on the individuals involved—primarily mothers —with the family as the context for the maternal experience (Ballou, 1978; Leifer, 1980; Mercer, 1985; Rubin, 1975, 1984).

Nursing the perinatal family as a unit requires merging of separate and expanding bodies of knowledge to develop a macroframework for family-centered practice. Pregnancy, birth, and the postpartum period have attracted investigators from many disciplines. Fathers and siblings have been of only recent interest. There is a dearth of information about the experience of grandparents, aunts, and other relatives. Nonintegrated literature is available for the interactive behavior of the unborn, newborn, and infant. There are numerous studies of the maternal–infant dyadic interaction. Because families consist of many sets of relationships and individual change, these studies provide the microtheory on which to develop perinatal family theory.

The Family as the Unit of Care

Conceptualization, assessment, and analysis of the family as a unit poses many problems (Gilliss, 1983). Wright and Leahey (1984) have presented a framework for the family as the unit of care. The childbearing family continues to be addressed through the expectant or new mother as the focus of care (Duvall, 1977; Rubin, 1984).

The perinatal family can be conceptualized as usually including three generations, extending past the nuclear household to extended family members. The internal and external structure of the family is an important consideration when assessing the childbearing family. Extended family members are important as role models and support systems.

The life cycle concept was introduced into the family literature by Duvall in 1957 and continues to be one of the core concepts in family theory (Duvall, 1977; Wright, Leahey, 1984). Duvall's framework suggests that the family proceeding through an emotional transition of accepting new members into the system must achieve three second-order changes for developmental progression: (1) adjusting the marital system to make space for child(ren); (2) taking on parenting roles; and (3) realigning relationships with extended family members to include parenting and grandparenting roles. This paradigm has not been used extensively by nursing in either clinical or scientific work with childbearing families. The woman remains the unit of care, with her mate and other family members included in aspects of care as the mother's support system and context.

The Pregnancy Experience

Family interaction with caregivers may begin with the care needs of one or more members who may be self-referred or referred by another family member or member of the health care team. One set of care needs that frequently brings families and caregivers into therapeutic interaction is the potential or actual event of pregnancy.

The Childbearing Decision

The motivation for pregnancy is complex and not well understood. Studies of premarital decision-making about childbearing strongly suggest that marriage and childbearing are two distinct decisions (Miller, 1974; Oakley, 1985). The decision to have or not have a child has become a possibility with the development of effective birth control measures. Childbearing can theoretically be planned to coincide and fit with other life events for the couple as a couple and as individuals. A relatively new phenomenon—a sequelae of the women's movement—has been the lengthening of the marital family stage of the family life cycle by postponing parenthood until marital, career, and financial stability are established for both potential parents. Some women find it easier to begin parenthood rather than a career at a later date (DeVore, 1983).

Cultural and family mores influence the parenthood decision. Extended family members often influence or try to influence decisions about pregnancy. Western women probably have more cultural choice about if and when to have children than other cultural groups. Cultures also identify the conditions under which pregnancy is considered appropriate and welcomed.

The Psychodynamics of Pregnancy

The family as a unit of people encompasses varied personalities, stages of development, and needs, all attempting a mutually satisfying set of relationships and functions (Hill, 1970). When family membership changes, these relationships and functions undergo change as well. These changes may create stress in the family system, and in some families a crisis state may result. The stress or crisis of pregnancy can be maturational in nature, and can be temporary if adequate support or intervention are available.

Pregnancy studied from the perspective of the pregnant woman has been variously described as a period of disequilibrium (Deutsch, 1945), a crisis (Bibring et al, 1961; Caplan, 1959; Pines, 1972), symbiosis (Benedek, 1949; Deutsch, 1945), or a turning point for the woman (Bibring, 1959; Entwisle, Doering, 1981). Each of these conceptualizations implies change and adaptation.

In her classic study of the meaning of motherhood for women, Deutsch (1945) set the stage for the study of the processes whereby a woman integrates an unborn and newborn infant into her life. Her descriptions were based in the psychoanalytic tradition in which the fetus was known to the pregnant woman as a part of her narcissistic self.

This work became the foundation of Rubin's seminal clinical nursing studies, extending over almost three decades. These studies described the maternal experience and elaborated a theory of maternal identity development that includes psychobiologic, maternal–infant, and some family variables and processes that integrate the maternal experience into the woman's life (Rubin, 1961, 1963, 1967, 1970, 1972, 1975, 1977, 1984). Rubin (1975) identified four interdependent developmental tasks of the pregnant woman: (1) ensuring safe passage for herself and her child; (2) gaining acceptance of significant others for the unborn child; (3) binding-in to the unborn child; and (4) giving of oneself. These tasks motivate changes in self-concept and relationships that propel the pregnant woman toward the maternal role and identity as a mother of the infant. Much of the subsequent study of the maternal experience is grounded in Rubin's work (Chao, 1979; Highley, 1967; Mercer, 1974, 1981, 1985, 1986; Richardson, 1981, 1983; Stainton, 1981). Research, education, and practice in the field of maternity care have been enriched by the theoretical base provided by Rubin's numerous field studies of the maternal experience.

Relationships during Pregnancy

Another group of studies of the pregnant woman describe her in dyadic relationships with others. The relationships the pregnant woman has with significant others and her mate appear to exert a strong influence on her responses to pregnancy and to motherhood (Arbeit, 1975; Ballou, 1978; Bibring et al, 1961; Entwisle, Doering, 1981; Richardson, 1981; Rubin, 1970, 1975). These studies describe a set of developmental tasks of pregnancy variously to include the ability of a pregnant woman (1) to be concerned for the embodied infant as well as for herself; (2) to reconcile tensions with her own mother; (3) to feel positive toward herself in developing the role of mother to this infant; and (4) to prepare physically and psychologically with her mate to incorporate another person into the attachment system while maintaining their marital relationship (Stainton, 1985a). The accomplishment of these tasks is dependent on the extent to which the social system is perceived as nurturing and supportive during pregnancy. Although a complete social system will include other persons such as friends and relatives, a reconciled mother–daughter relationship and a harmonious relationship with the mate form the basis for attachment to the infant. These dyadic relationships have been studied with the family context as the as background.

The mother–daughter theme pervades the pregnancy literature. It seems vital for the woman, particularly in the first pregnancy, to view her own mother positively as a role model in order to commit to the maternal role (Arbeit, 1975; Ballou, 1978; Lederman, 1984; Mercer, 1986; Rubin, 1984). The mother–daughter relationship is reshaped by the pregnant woman and her mother into a collegial-style relationship as they both prepare for the next generation.

The husband's role during pregnancy has had little attention until recently. Ballou (1978) found the husband's role in pregnancy to be one of nurturance and responsiveness to his mate's feelings of vulnerability in both her biological state and in her relationship with her mother. The husband's support during pregnancy is thought to be an indicator to his wife of his acceptance of the pregnancy and preparation for attachment to the child (Caplan, 1959; Grossman, 1980; Leifer, 1980; Shereshefsky, Yarrow, 1973). The husband's style in experiencing his mate's pregnancy ranges from being highly involved to being a detached observer (May, 1980). The readiness for parenthood also varies among men (May, 1982).

These relational dynamics during pregnancy have been studied mainly from the perspective of the primigravida; less is known about the multigravida. The multigravida experiences changes in her relationships with previous children as part of the preparation for and incorporation of another child into the family unit (Jenkins, 1976; Ulrich, 1982; Walz, Rich, 1983). The preparation of the first-born for the birth of a second child is an additional and major task of the secundigravida (Richardson, 1983). Secundigravidas express intense concern about having enough love for an additional family member (Richardson, 1983; Stainton, 1985a). Mothers expecting a third or fourth child do not express this concern as intensely (Stainton, 1985a).

The Unborn Family Member

Conception is the beginning, not only of the infant but also of the family with an additional member and with changed relationships (Grossman et al, 1980). A mother becomes increasingly focused on the unborn child during the course of pregnancy, forming opinions, attitudes, and a mental image of the child within her (Benedek, 1959; Deutsch, 1945; Klaus, Kennell, 1982; Leifer, 1980; Lumley, 1980a, 1980b, 1982; Rubin, 1970). She believes the child will come into being and begins to develop a relationship to the unseen infant.

Caplan (1959) was the first to differentiate the attitude of the mother toward the fetus as more of a determinant of the mother–child relationship than a woman's attitude toward her pregnancy. Bibring et al (1961) and later Rubin (1977) identified that a specific developmental task of the pregnant woman was to form a sense of the embodied infant as a separate person prior to birth. Leifer (1977, 1980) differentiated anxiety about the fetus from anxiety about self, concluding that the major psychologic task of pregnancy was forming an emotional attachment to the fetus and that the success with this task was predictive of early maternal behavior and attitudes.

Four phases in developing a sense of the unborn infant as human and separate can be extrapolated from the studies of pregnancy. These four phases occur in concert with the developmental tasks of pregnancy: (1) incorporation of the fetus into body- and self-image; (2) differentiation of the fetus from self; (3) attainment of a sense of the child; and (4) attachment.

The maternal–fetal relationship has only begun to be studied systematically (Cranley, 1981a, 1981b; Fuller, 1984; Lumley, 1980a, 1980b, 1982; Rees, 1980a, 1980b; Stainton, 1985a, 1985b). These studies show variability in trimesters and in maternal style. The mate's interest in the fetus has been associated with a positive maternal attitude toward the unborn child (Ballou, 1980; Leifer, 1980) and with fetal movements (Entwisle, Doering, 1981). Lack of husband support or interest has been shown to negatively affect maternal–fetal attachment (Lumley, 1980a).

These studies all virtually ignore the behavior of the unborn infant as a participant. The fetus is able to hear external sound by the fifth month of pregnancy (Liley, 1972) and is selective in its response to music (Clements, 1977) and human voices (Als, Lester, Brazelton, 1979; Brazelton, 1982). The unborn infant will startle and move away from cold and brightness and will move toward soft light and warmth (Als, Lester, Brazelton, 1979). Timor–Tritsch et al (1976) identified three behavioral states—active, quiet, and sleeping—using ultrasonic observation of the fetus. The responsiveness and interactive behavior with parents has been described (Stainton, 1985b).

The degree to which maternal–fetal attachment is a precursor to maternal–newborn attachment is unclear. Research requires refinement of the definitions, instruments, and analysis used through replication and retesting of instruments. The existing paradigm does integrate relationships with major figures in the pregnant woman's family with her ability to relate to the unborn infant as a developing member of the established attachment matrix.

Postpartum Changes and Processes

Maternal Role Attainment

Another large body of literature describes the processes whereby a woman becomes the mother of the infant and the variables affecting the quality of the relationship. Maternal and infant variables that affect the mothering role have been identified, such as maternal age, self-concept, perceptions of the birth experience, infant illness, and maternal–infant separation (Rubin, 1967; Mercer, 1981, 1985, 1986; Mercer, Stainton, 1984).

Less clear is the importance of various family variables, with the exception of the husband's role. The literature generally refers to social support or the support system. Social support, particularly that of the mate, continues to be considered a major contributor to functional mothering (Ballou, 1978; Leifer, 1980; Shereshefsky, Liebenberg, Lockman, 1973). Less is known about the effect of sibling behavior, grandparent response, and what is perceived as supportive behavior of others. The woman and other family members establishing a relationship with an infant are influenced and supported by cultural norms and mores, financial stability, and status within the community.

The Mother–Infant Dyad

The maternal–infant relationship has been studied for more than three decades. Two major approaches have emerged. One describes interactive behaviors as traits, behaviors, and cognitive operations considered representative of a special relationship between a mother and her infant (Affonso, 1976; Bowlby, 1958; Chao, 1979, Condon, Sander, 1976; Klaus, Kennell, 1976).

The other approach concerns transactional processes in maternal and infant adaptation to each other, which are described in qualitative terms such as *cue sensitivity, mutuality, reciprocity,* and *synchrony* (Brazelton, Koslowski, Main, 1974; Caudill, Weinstein, 1969; Field, 1978; Packer, 1983; Stainton, 1985a). Both schools of thought virtually ignore the context of the family in which the interaction takes place and fail to account for the variability in maternal and infant styles of interaction.

Father–Infant Interaction

The father–infant dyad became more accessible to research during the upsurge of interest in a phenomenon described as *bonding* (Klaus, Kennell, 1970) and the established importance of the husband's supportive role to the pregnancy outcome and maternal–infant attachment (Ballou, 1978; Leifer, 1980; Rubin, 1977). These findings generated major changes in birth practices and maternity care to facilitate mother–infant contact and husband involvement. Greenberg and Morris (1974) reported the fathers' response to the newborn at birth to be one of engrossment, with preoccupation and intense interest in their newborn. Studies of father–infant interaction do not show consistent patterns in the relationship postbirth (Ricks, 1985). Ricks suggests this may be due to the application of methods generally used for dyadic research to the father's interaction, which more often occurs in triadic situations.

Sibling Response

The birth of a sibling creates changes in the mother–child relationship with other children. In a series of studies of mother–child dyads in families introducing a second child, Dunn et al found that maternal attention and play are decreased and more confrontation occurs (Kendrick, Dunn, 1982; Dunn, Kendrick, MacNamee, 1980). The first-born child's behavior also changes, with increased tearfulness, clinging, and sleep disruptions (Dunn et al, 1980). In transactional studies of the family as a whole, the father's participation in care of the older children was crucial in modifying the stress on both mother and child after birth of a second child (Belsky, 1981; Kreppner, Paulsen, Schuetze, 1982).

The Newborn's Contribution

The human newborn is highly oriented to human interaction, most specifically toward the mother. Cry prints of the infant correspond to the maternal voice print (Truby, Lind, 1965), and the just-born infant will turn toward its mother's voice (Brazelton, 1982). The newborn has a number of engaging features that attract the mother, such as softness of the skin, an expressive human face, familial characteristics, and dependency (Rubin, 1961, 1963; Brazelton, 1982). The infant also has various soliciting behaviors that bring the mother into proximity. These include crying, reaching and touching with the hands, imitating facial expressions, and being consoled when near the mother.

The available research on the impact of the single variable or combination of variables provides insight into the complexity of the experience for the individuals and specific dyads within a family unit. The dynamics of the perinatal family as a whole are an interwoven set of patterns that are more than a composite of the individual and dyadic experiences occurring within it.

Perinatal Family Dynamics

To understand the perinatal family as a whole, it is important to conceptualize the individual tasks and psychodynamics as occurring within the structure and function of the family unit that adapts to accommodate these specific processes. The family dynamics neither dispute nor replace previous work on the individual or dyadic experiences. These experiences create and are created by a context that fosters family functioning and the mutually satisfying meeting of needs while achieving developmental tasks.

This section will describe the family dynamics uncovered in a study of 16 American families during the pre- and postbirth period (Stainton, 1985a). Interview and photodocumentation are augmented with examples from a current collaborative perinatal practice.

The Prebirth Period

During the prebirth period, three major themes emerge as guiding the practices of the childbearing family: (1) the pregnant woman as centerpiece; (2) the infant as focal point; and (3) narrowing of the social world. These themes intensify as birth approaches.

The Pregnant Woman as Centerpiece of the Family A specific feature of the perinatal family is the mother–infant unit. Once pregnancy is confirmed and announced, the family begins to orient toward the integration of a new family member into the family system and household. As the infant is embodied in one family member, the others assume roles and tasks that complement and provide support for the biopsychosocial processes that the mother of the infant undertakes. Visible maternal body changes create a reality about the infant, who gradually becomes the focal point of the family by the time of birth. Concomitantly, the pregnant woman becomes the centerpiece of the family unit.

In a culture highly oriented toward individualism, control, success, and self-reliance in its practices, contemporary pregnancy implicitly becomes a project oriented toward producing a perfectly formed, healthy newborn with maximum potential for achievement (Stainton, 1985a; Winslow, 1985). The operational tenet is that rational manipulation and control of the circumstances in which pregnancy occurs and of the internal and external environment in which

infant development takes place can override luck or fate. Within this cultural milieu, the woman's body is regarded as the incubator for the developing infant. Women modify or change dimensions in their lifestyles in order to protect the vulnerable infant from influences considered dangerous, such as cigarette smoke and alcohol. Eating, rest, and exercise patterns may be changed. As one mother summarized:

> I am very conscientious. I mean, no coffee, tea, or liquor and I maintain a healthy diet. I am not compromising in any way. I am unbending about prenatal exercise class and swimming. I take a nap each day no matter what else is going on. I feel this is number 1 priority.

Women varied in the extent to which they modified their lifestyles, from total abstention, as in the example above, to "occasional sips or one cup of tea." Increasingly, women change their habits when planning to conceive.

This giving over of one's body is required only of the mother, who harbors and later breastfeeds the infant. Interestingly, the male body's contribution to the pregnancy is minimized, with little concern for the possible effects of alcohol on sperm. Other family members do not have to modify or change daily body habits to the same extent, even though smoking may be restricted or sexual relations adapted. It is the woman's body that has to maintain the healthy environment and be presented for regular scientific assessments of the "incubator" and infant development. It is her body that must prepare for labor and infant feeding.

The woman's degree of acceptance and enthusiasm for the pregnancy affects the family. A woman in the first trimester of an unplanned third pregnancy was upset at the thought of "another boy. I can't accept that." She regarded the infant as an unwanted intruder. Considerable distance in the marital relationship resulted with frequent blaming and fighting. She was disinterested in her two sons. Difficulties in her relationship with her own mother were rekindled. Her husband was already doing more child care than before, preferring to be with his sons than with his wife. Family therapy, supportive care, and second trimester evidence of the infant's presence with movement and audible heartbeat promoted a progression toward maternal acceptance of the infant and less troubled family relationships. Other women stated feeling empowered by the presence of the developing baby in their bodies (Stainton, 1985a). One said, "There is this new feeling of empowerment or potency. Now if I can't lift or move something, I get someone to do it for me."

Once pregnant, the mother assumes almost total responsibility for the unborn child. The continuous harboring and sensing of the unborn infant as an individual also leads to protectiveness and possessiveness in maternal practices. As the end of pregnancy approaches, family relationships begin to shift as plans are made to facilitate the postbirth mother–infant relationship.

Structural changes in the family occur to provide support for and meeting of members' needs. In first pregnancies, the expectant father may help more with household chores, providing more rest and introspective time for his mate. In families expecting a second or subsequent child, the family may take the form of two subgroups, with the father and older child(ren) aligning in more interaction, providing interpersonal space for the mother–infant unit. This realigning can be controlled by the older child(ren) who have to be cooperative in order for it to work. The older child may become more attached to the introspective mother, creating tensions in meeting the child's needs and in conserving maternal energy. Fathers describe enjoyment in their increased access to the older children and willingness to help run the household either by paying for help or by providing help themselves (Stainton, 1985a).

The Infant as Focal Point of the Family   The first communication from the embodied infant is compelling in nature. The ambivalence that is common in early pregnancy (Rubin, 1970) is re-

duced and leads to confirmation of another's presence. Although the expectant father cannot yet experience the sensation, the report of the felt movement provides confirmation for him as well. The felt infant's presence transcends a rational, intellectualized approach and begins to draw the parents into a reshaping of their social world to accommodate new relationships and responsibilities.

By the eighth month of pregnancy, both parents can experience their unborn infant's movements and patterns of response. Time is spent in trying to get the unborn infant to respond to touch and voices. The infant's behavior is interpreted as happy or distressed, sleeping or awake, and responsive or unresponsive. By late pregnancy, expectant parents are congruent in describing the infant's sleep–wake cycle, temperament, preferences, gender, and size. Some parents interact with their unborn infant during the last trimester of pregnancy and perceive the infant to respond to tactile, verbal, and other environmental stimuli, such as warmth and light, in an individualized, personalized manner. Parents with other children were able to compare this embodied infant with previous ones.

Only mothers reported sensing the infant's emotional state as shared with their own, with statements such as "When I get angry, it does. It gets all tense in there and my lower back will hurt." Another described the infant's strong kicking as indicative of distress when she and her husband raised their voices in argument, causing them to stop. Another mother worried that her unborn infant would feel her distress from severe pancreatic pain and "feel badly."

In later pregnancy, other family members may make tactile and verbal contact with the infant through the abdominal wall. Mothers described trying to get the fetus to respond "for" the father. Fathers generally are more playful in their interaction and mothers more instructive (Stainton, 1985b). Second-time mothers especially encouraged the first child to interact with the unborn more than mothers with more than one other child. The amount of access other family members had to the unborn infant was controlled by the mother. As one father said, "I know it is there, but it is part of her right now."

Mothers sensed a difference in the unborn infant's response to family members. One said, "I want my husband to feel it moving, but if he puts his hand on my side, it stops. I wonder if it senses a difference." Another, whose husband was away for two to three days at a time, described the infant as hesitant to respond when the husband returned and tried to make contact, "as if he was a stranger again." Second-time mothers reported fetal responsiveness to be higher toward the sibling than to either parent (Stainton, 1985a). These parental descriptions of the unborn infant's behavior are consistent with experimental evidence of fetal sensory capacity and behavior.

During pregnancy, the amount of information acquired about the individual responsiveness and behavioral patterns of the unborn varies. Neldam (1982) found that an anterior placenta reduced the number of felt movements mothers reported when compared to ultrasound visualization of movement. Pregnant women with career or family responsibilities, or both, reported not paying attention to fetal movement when busy. Women report an inner communication with the infant when alone—an experience unavailable to the others. Women vary in the amount and type of interaction with their unborn. Some women are often verbally interactive and others are seldom verbally interactive, with a self-reported pattern of consistency between pregnancies. Thus, overt interaction seems to be more a style than a feeling about or toward the infant (Stainton, 1985b). Sensations from the intrabody relationship between mother and child accumulate to provide a sense of and information about the unborn infant that is part of a continuum of experience with the infant, leading to cue sensitivity and attachment.

Body-related relationships with others in the attachment matrix change as the awareness of the unborn increases. Fathers may avoid sexual intercourse because, "it might hurt the baby," or "the baby really has first claim to her body now." A multipara described decreased body contact with her children:

> I am not as cuddly toward the other kids. I don't know if it is a maternal process because you have to kick the birds out of the nest a little bit when you bring a new one in.

In recognition of the infant's autonomy as a person, preparation for the infant's birth includes reorganization of space in the home. Apart from the gathering of necessary supplies and clothing, families may plan a separate room for the newborn, requiring reallocation of rooms or selection of a larger home. Some place a crib in an older child's room approximately a month before the infant's birth as part of preparing the other child.

Narrowing of the Social World Toward the end of pregnancy, the family energy is directed toward the approaching birth. The social world is narrowed by the focus on the infant and the needs of the pregnant woman. Attending prenatal classes, purchasing, and making arrangements for career, child day care and household management become the main goals and conversation themes. Family energy is directed toward being prepared and able to successfully proceed through birth and the postbirth period.

Birth is a highly focused event. The bodily processes of the mother and the coaching and supportive function of the father draw them together in an intense dyadic experience and transition. Other children and grandparents may be involved in maintaining family functions. As the father realigns himself as a protector of the mother–infant unit by creating space for the infant both emotionally and physically, the marital dyad is paradoxically and simultaneously closer and more distant. The maternal focus is on the infant within her, and the paternal focus is on the responsibilities and assistance with childcare and household management. Both members of the marital dyad are focused on the impending labor from different perspectives. The loosening of the dyad provides space for the infant to enter into a relationship with each parent at a time when both feel vulnerable and dependent on each other for coping with labor and integration of the infant. This may create a sense of disconnectedness and fear of disruption of the marital relationship, requiring reassurance and support from caregivers and family members. By the time of birth, the family is a tightly knit, cohesive group of persons focused on the infant, with energy directed toward supporting the mother–infant unit (Figure 13-1).

The Postbirth Period

During the postbirth period, the themes are similar: (1) the infant as centerpiece; (2) the mother as essential caregiver; and (3) widening of the social order.

The Infant as Centerpiece   Fascination and preoccupation with the newly born infant dominate maternal practices during the first weeks

postbirth. The infant is visible and can affirm that the pregnancy has gone well. Recognition of familial characteristics facilitates acceptance and responsiveness to the infant. New cues about the infant's behavior are available and occupy the mother in interpreting and responding to them. Similarities to previous children dominate the initial impressions of multigravidas, who then begin to differentiate (Stainton, 1985a, p. 167).

Maternal attention to other family duties is accomplished within a focus of maintaining close body contact between mother and infant, caregiving, and studying the infant's behavioral cues. The infant's dependency, softness, and smallness elicit strong tugs on the maternal emotions. The infant's preference for the mother engages her and keeps her close. The attention of others is directed toward the other children, often with instructions about how to effectively meet their needs or interpret their behavior. Fathers continue to help with the household management and care of other children, and grandparents may be actively involved in helping. The mother carries out household management with constant awareness of the infant. Family members negotiate and manipulate in order to have time alone with the infant.

By eight weeks, maternal sensitivity to the individual patterns in the needs and style of the infant is evident in maternal practices. The infant's increased physical and social competence is appreciated, and maternal sensitivity to the infant's needs has become habit. The infant's vocalization in interaction becomes the most significant infant behavior and is interpreted as reciprocal:

> If I talk to him and concentrate on him and really talk to him, he will make little sounds back to me. It is really cute.

The mothers in the study group described their infants at this stage as "fun." New evidence of self-reliance with self-quieting and more predictable patterns of sleeping and waking liberated the mother from the intense focus.

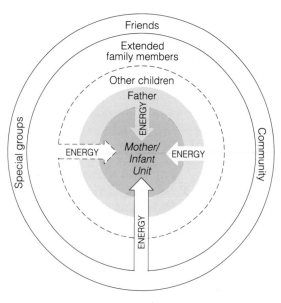

Figure 13–1 The mother/infant unit as centerpiece.

The Mother as Essential Caregiver An attitude of generosity and tolerance pervades the first four weeks of interrupted sleep and changing interfamily relationships. The style of handling the mother's preoccupation and involvement with the infant within the established matrix of relationships varies. Some fathers extend their working hours. Their wives may feel relieved by the moratorium this provides on the marital relationship; others feel deserted and frightened. Some used humor to tide them over:

> Time alone is minimal between us, and that has created an underlying tension. You laugh about it because there is really nothing you can do about it.

Another commented: "Mostly, we have been missing each other, and that's nice to know. I think you miss each other a lot after having a baby." These tensions function to bring the marital dyad into awareness. Previous stressors may become paramount by four weeks, when all are sleep-deprived and feeling somewhat alone. Four weeks is a vulnerable time for the marital dyad, requiring considerable tolerance for tension, disorganized family life, and sleep deprivation.

Sibling response to the new infant is both interesting and troublesome for the postbirth family. Young siblings solicit the mother's attention, and the father attempts to monitor, protecting the mother–infant unit and assisting in meeting the other child's needs for attention. Parallel parenting begun in late pregnancy continues as time and emotional support is reallocated. Sibling rivalry is most intensive with one other child. The mother's prebirth concern of having enough love for both children is manifested in negotiating cooperation with the older child and trying to equalize time and attention. Equipment for carrying the infant that keeps the mother's hands free is used to keep the infant close while attending to other children, shopping, and performing other activities. The mother feels sympathy and guilt in creating stress for the older child, who is upset, while at the same time feeling pressured and diverted from the infant with whom she is so involved. Her love for the older child prevails, although time and energy are limited. Within a month postbirth, children in the study group were more settled and by eight weeks had a visible physical and social growth spurt. They were more verbal and more independent in behavior.

Within this tension, the infant provides rewards and support for the stress experienced by the family. Growth and strengthening of the body are visible. The infant responds to other human beings in recognizable human ways such as smiling and reaching that are compelling to all family members. By four weeks, the infant is showing recognition and preference for the mother that generates energy in her for a continuing commitment.

Widening of the Social World Throughout the first four weeks postbirth, the family is involved with grandparents and friends who, while coming to see the infant, provide validation for the successful project and contact with the outside world. Mothers find this shift in attention from themselves as pregnant to the infant both confirming and disarming. "I felt so significant when I was pregnant. Now, the baby seems to be most significant!"

Eight weeks seems to be time when the infant's physical strength and interactive capability motivate the mother to release the infant and let it become accessible to others. She begins to widen the infant's context, involving others in the infant's care. Siblings, if any, have become more interactive than reactive with the new infant and may have achieved a growth spurt in social and physical abilities. The marital relationship becomes a higher priority, and the family "rounds off again." In the words of one mother:

> It's hard work to get to know a baby. I put him in his own room last night. It was time my husband and I had some time alone. I know

the baby is OK, and we have to get it back together.

New family dynamics are evident at eight weeks. The mother, now attached to the infant in a secure, reciprocal relationship, is ready to share and wants others to participate in the care and fun. She feels the infant is ready for other involvements, and she wishes to do other things. She may be returning to work. However, her possessiveness and intensiveness of the first weeks make her the expert with the infant. She may be impatient with the other family members who know the infant less well. One mother described her husband as "always thinking the baby's hungry. I wonder where he has been the last eight weeks that the kid has been here!" A husband described having had little time with the infant "until now. I have to learn to break the code." Husbands felt they had the first real access to the infant at eight weeks. Mothers in the study group were generally unaware of how possessive they had been, expressing concern that their husbands may not be interested in the infant. When asked, they agreed it would be hard for the husband to know the baby well. One mother stated, "I think it is very natural to keep your new kid away from everybody until it has a chance to be big enough so that you are not afraid it is going to break."

The Changing Shape of the Perinatal Family

The perinatal family undergoes a reshaping of space, time, and interpersonal relationships that provides the possibility for individual and dyadic tasks to be accomplished. This reshaping takes an "hourglass" form (Figure 13-2). The social and individual world of the family becomes increasingly focused on the mother–infant unit before birth and gradually widens again during the first eight weeks postbirth. The processes involved generate exaggerated personal needs of the family members and the dyads and triads within it.

Tensions created by the intensive mother–infant unit are offset by reducing the context of the family, by parallel parenting, and by the complementary nature of the mate's protectiveness of that unit and increased responsiveness to the household and other children. The mother maintains control over household management and childcare but is primarily focused on the infant. By eight weeks, the mother has acquired a sense of the infant as able to respond in interpretable, human ways, and she is ready to relinquish the infant to become a family member and rejoin the family group that now incorporates the infant.

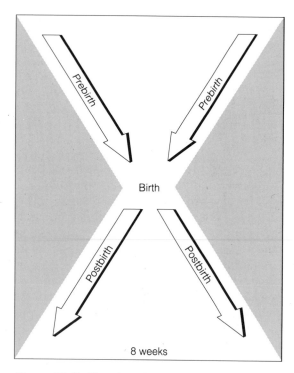

Figure 13–2 The changing shape of the perinatal family.

The Nature of Perinatal Nursing

The frameworks presented provide guidelines for understanding the perinatal family in relatively normative circumstances. The range of circumstances presented by families needing care during the perinatal period is wide and varied. Single women, teenagers, older first-time mothers, mothers combining pregnancy with chronic disease, and repeated pregnancy loss or diagnosed lethal fetal conditions are only some of the variations found in a day in clinic. The progressive nature of developmental tasks and goals of the family and each of its members is essential knowledge in providing appropriate nursing care in situations in which circumstances are less than ideal.

Case Studies

Lynne was brought to hospital by ambulance one afternoon from a rural community. She had begun to bleed heavily while making tea for a friend. A complete placenta previa was diagnosed at 22 weeks. She was to remain in the hospital for the remainder of the pregnancy. She had four further episodes of bleeding and each time was rushed to the labor area and put into intensive observation, and preparations were made for cesarean birth.

Lynne was angry and withdrawn. Her husband was taking exams, her 18-month-old would have her second birthday while Lynne was in the hospital, and her parents cancelled a planned trip to care for her daughter. In the second week, she began to verbalize her feelings, stating, "If we are going to lose this one, I just want to get it over with. People at home need me. My little girl is getting spoiled, and my husband very tired. This kid better make up its mind!"

In such instances, the family members are often separated in order to provide childcare. Husbands may be transporting young children to and from other caregivers during working hours and caring for them at night in order to keep some continuity in their lives. Daily visiting in the hospital under strange conditions creates strain in the relationship. Childrearing couples are not used to having long periods of time together without diversion. Overnight stays of the husband may be of assistance. They may be impossible if care of other children is required.

In the situation described above, the nurse assisted Lynne with progression in maternal–fetal attachment by helping her focus on the placenta as the offender. Reassurance of infant stability was quietly provided during daily fetal stress tests and heart rate monitoring. The nurse helped Lynne focus on another project by asking her if she had something she always had wanted to get done but had not had the time. By the third week in hospital, Lynne was able to mobilize energy to work on and finish an afghan she had started two years earlier. A telephone in her room and occasional overnight stays of her husband seemed to assist her to cope. She had a healthy infant at 38 weeks.

Working with families of a preterm infant also requires adaptation of the framework. This infant exaggerates the mother's concern for its survival and is a less rewarding participant in interaction. Identification is difficult for the mother because the infant does not have the same development of features to attract the mother and often is unavailable for her to hold and carry. Family dynamics progressing toward "rounding out" and viewing the infant as being fun are delayed.

A mother described her time with her hospitalized infant through three months as, "I am doing all this bonding and nothing is happening. She just lies there. She looks at me and all that, but it's not like a baby should be. I am doing it all!" Lack of reciprocity and organization of these infants prolongs the maternal intensity of focus and may decrease the feelings of integration of the infant into the family for an extended period. Reminders of the infant's real age helped to keep the abilities in perspective. Assistance in feeding and reducing the maternal tendency to overstimulate the infant was somewhat helpful. Two weeks after the infant's expected date of delivery, the mother called and said, "I have a human being here. She is a real baby now!"

These two examples of practice dimensions in perinatal nursing point out the need for using the framework with a repertoire of approaches to the perinatal family. Thomlison's (1984) review of the effectiveness of various approaches to practice with families is helpful for all disciplines in pointing out the strengths and deficits in current practice. Calkin's (1982) delineation of the characteristics of advanced practice provides guidelines for graduate education and practice within areas of specialization.

The most common issue in nursing care of these families is the lack of continuity of caregivers. Prenatal care, birth, and postnatal care may all be given by different groups of persons. This has precipitated a movement toward home births, midwifery practice, and flexible hospital environments. Supporting the family dynamics required to successfully integrate the infant as a family member needs more attention to continuity in caregivers and caregiving. This area of practice needs to include a home-based model, where the family dynamics can be appropriately assessed and interventions planned.

Future Directions

Nursing the entire family is the hallmark of perinatal practice, even though the whole family may not be present. As pointed out throughout the chapter, further inquiry with the entire family from a transactional perspective is needed to provide the appropriate theoretical basis for practice. Small, isolated projects do not generate a significant, integrated body of knowledge. Programs of research directed at defining the appropriate questions and designing appropriate methods for perinatal family research are needed. The designing and testing of interventions directed at supporting or treating family dynamics is an important next step. Basic questions should include the following:

1. How do we conceptualize the family as a unit composed of all members that the family experience as members, whether in or out of the household?

2. Is the family a legitimate area of advanced nursing practice?

3. Under what conditions do the variables of culture and social context need to be treated as foreground or background when studying the family?

Summary

Dynamics within the perinatal unit create and are created by the needs of each member while focused on successful development of the infant and attachment processes. Study of the transactional processes occurring in the family during the perinatal period provides meaningful understanding of the normal tensions and critical points that foster change and growth in the family and its members. Assessment from this transactional persepctive brings indicators of stress into prognostic focus for the practitioner who can determine to what extent they are adaptive. Interventions designed for the family as a group would seem most appropriate.

Issues for Further Investigation

1. What adjustments are made in the marital system to make space for a child? How do these adjustments vary between Anglo-American, Chicano and Black Americans?

2. To what degree does the father's attitude toward the unborn infant influence maternal response to the infant at birth?

3. What is the influence of addictive substances, (i.e. drugs, alcohol or nicotine) on the quality and quantity of sperm?

4. Does the participation of both parents in the patterns of movement and responses of the unborn infant facilitate the incorporation of the newborn as a member of the family post delivery?

References

Affonso D (1976): The newborn's potential for interaction. *J Obstet Gynecol Neonat Nurs*, 5: 9–14.

Als H, Lester BM, Brazelton TB (1979): Dynamics of the behavioral organization of the premature infant: A theoretical perspective. In: *Infants Born at Risk.* T.M. Field, A.M. Sostek, S. Goldberg, & H. H. Shuma (Eds.), New York: Spectrum, pp. 173–192.

Arbeit SA (1975): A study of women during their first pregnancy. Unpublished doctoral dissertation, Yale University, New Haven, CT.

Ballou JW (1978): *The Psychology of Pregnancy.* Lexington, MA: D.C. Heath.

Belsky J (1981): Early human experience: A family perspective. *Dev Psychol*, 17(1):3–23.

Benedek T (1949): The psychosomatic implications of the primary unit: Mother–child. *Am J Orthopsychiatry*, 19:642–653.

Bibring GL (1959): Some considerations of the psychological processes in pregnancy. *Psychoanal Study Child*, 14:113–121.

Bibring GL et al (1961): A study of the psychological processes in pregnancy and the earliest mother–child relationship. *Psychoanal Study Child*, 16:9–44.

Bowlby J (1958): The nature of a child's tie to his mother. *Int J Psychoanal*, 39:350–373.

Brazelton TB (1982): Joint regulation of neonate-parent behavior. In: *Social Interchange in Infancy: Affect, Cognition, and Communication*, Tronick EZ (ed.). Baltimore: University Park Press.

Brazelton TB, Koslowski B, Main M (1974): The origins of reciprocity. In: *The Effect of the Infant on its Caregiver*, Lewis M, Rosenblum L (eds.). New York: Wiley.

Calkin JD (1982): A model for advanced nursing practice. *J Nurs Admin*, 1:24–30.

Caplan GS (1959): Concepts of mental health and consultation: Their application in public health social work. Washington, DC: U.S. HEW.

Caudill W, Weinstein H (1969): Maternal care and infant behavior in Japan and America. *Psychiatry*, 32:12–43.

Chao YM (1979): Cognitive operations during maternal role enactment. *Maternal-Child Nurs J*, 8:211–274.

Clements M (1977): Observations on certain aspects of neonatal behavior in response to auditory stimuli. Paper presented at the Fifth International Congress of Psychosomatic Obstetrics and Gynecology, Rome.

Condon WS, Sander LW (1974): Neonate movement is synchronized with adult speech: Interactional participation and language acquisition. *Science*, 183:99–101.

Cranley MS (1981a): Development of a tool for the measurement of maternal attachment during pregnancy. *Nurs Res*, 30:281–284.

Cranley MS (1981b): Roots of attachment: The relationship of parents with their unborn. In: *Perinatal Parental Behavior: Nursing Research and Implications for Newborn Health*, Raff BS, Carroll P (eds.). Birth Defects: Original Article Series: Vol 17. New York: Liss.

Deutsch H (1945): *Psychology of Women: Motherhood* (Vol 2). New York: Grune & Stratton.

DeVore NE (1983, August): Parenthood postponed. *Am J Nur*, 1160–1163.

Dunn J, Kendrick C, MacNamee (1980): The reaction of first-born children to the birth of a sibling: Mothers' reports. *J Child Psychol Psychiatry*, 22:1–18.

Duvall E (1977): *Marriage and Family Development*, 5th ed. Philadelphia: Lippincott.

Entwisle DR, Doering SG (1981): *The First Birth: A Family Turning Point*. Baltimore: Johns Hopkins University Press.

Field T (1978): The three Rs of infant-adult interactions: Rhythms, repertoires, and responsivity. *J Pediatr Psychol*, 3:131–136.

Fuller JR (1984): The development of maternal attachment from fetal affiliation to infant interaction. Unpublished master's thesis, Dalhousie University, Halifax, NS.

Gilliss CL (1983): The family as a unit of analysis: Strategies for the nurse researcher. *ANS*, 5(3):50–59.

Greenberg M, Morris N (1974): Engrossment: The newborn's impact upon the father. *Am J Orthopsychiatry, 44*(4):520–531.

Grossman FK, Eichler LS, Winickoff SA (1980): *Pregnancy, Birth and Parenthood.* San Francisco: Jossey-Bass.

Highley BL (1967): Maternal role identity. In: *Maternal–Child Health Nursing,* Highley BL et al (eds.). Boulder, CO: Western Interstate Commission for Higher Education, pp. 31–43.

Hill R (1970): *Family Development in Three Generations.* Cambridge, MA: Schenkman.

Jenkins PW (1976): Conflicts of a secundigravida. *Maternal–Child Nurs J, 5*:117–126.

Kendrick C, Dunn J (1982): Protest or pleasure: The response of first-born children to interactions between their mothers and infant siblings. *J Child Psychol Psychiatry, 23*(2):117–129.

Klaus MH, Kennell JH (1970): Mothers separated from their newborn infants. *Pediatr Clin North Am,* 4:1015–1017.

Klaus MH, Kennell JH (1976): *Maternal–Infant Bonding.* St. Louis: Mosby.

Klaus MH, Kennell JH (1982): *Parent–Infant Bonding.* St. Louis: Mosby.

Kreppner K, Paulsen S, Shuetze Y (1982): Infant and family development from triads to tetrads. *Hum Dev, 25*:373–391.

Lamb ME (1975): Fathers: Forgotten contributors to child development. *Hum Dev, 18*:245–266.

Lederman RP (1984): *Psychosocial Adaptation in Pregnancy: Assessment of Seven Dimensions of Maternal Development.* Englewood Cliffs, NJ: Prentice-Hall.

Leifer M (1977): Psychological changes accompanying pregnancy and motherhood. *Genet Psychol Monographs, 95*:55–56.

Leifer M (1980): *Psychological Effects of Motherhood: A Study of First Pregnancy.* New York: Praeger.

Liley AW (1972): The foetus as a personality. *Aust NZ J Psychiatry, 6*:99–105.

Lumley J (1980a): The development of maternal-foetal bonding in first pregnancy. In: *Emotion and Reproduction,* Zichella L (ed.). New York: Academic Press.

Lumley J (1980b): The image of the fetus in the first trimester. *Birth Family J, 7*:5–14.

Lumley J (1982): Attitudes to the fetus among primigravidae. *Aust Pediatr J, 18*:106–109.

May KA (1980): A typology of detachment/involvement styles adopted during pregnancy by first-time expectant fathers. *West J Nurs Res, 2*:445–461.

May KA (1982): Factors contributing to first-time fathers' readiness for fatherhood: An exploratory study. *Fam Relations, 31*:353–361.

Mercer RT (1974): Mothers' responses to their infants with defects. *Nurs Res, 23*(2):133–137.

Mercer RT (1981): A theoretical framework for studying factors that impact on the maternal role. *Nurs Res, 30*(2):73–77.

Mercer RT (1985): The process of maternal role attainment over the first year. *Nurs Res, 34*:198–204.

Mercer RT (1986): *First-Time Motherhood.* New York: Springer-Verlag.

Mercer RT, Stainton MC (1984): Perceptions of the birth experience; A cross-cultural comparison. *Health Care for Women Int, 5*:29–47.

Miller WB (1974): Relationships between the intendedness of conception and the wantedness of pregnancy. *J Nerv Ment Dis, 159*:396–406.

Neldam S (1982): Fetal movements: A comparison between maternal assessment and registration by means of dynamic ultrasound. *Dan Med Bull, 29*:197–199.

Oakley D (1985): Premarital childbearing decision making. *Fam Relations, 34*(4):561–563.

Packer MJ (1983): Communication in early infancy: Three common assumptions examined and found inadequate. *Hum Dev, 26*:233–248.

Pines D (1972): Pregnancy and motherhood: Interaction between fantasy and reality. *Br J Med Psychol,* 45:333–343.

Rees BL (1980a): Maternal identification and infant care: A theoretical perspective. *West J Nurs Res,* 2:666–706.

Rees BL (1980b): Maternal identification with the mothering role. *Res Nurs Health, 3*:49–56.

Richardson P (1981): Women's perceptions of their important dyadic relationships during pregnancy. *Maternal-Child Nurs J, 10*:159–174.

Richardson P (1983): Women's perceptions of change in relationships shared with children during pregnancy. *Maternal-Child Nurs J, 12*:75–89.

Ricks SS (1985): Father–infant interactions: A review of empirical research. *Fam Relations, 34*(4):505–511.

Rubin R (1961): Basic maternal behavior. *Nurs Outlook*, 9:683–686.

Rubin R (1963): Maternal touch. *Nurs Outlook*, 11:828–831.

Rubin R (1967): Attainment of the maternal role: Part 1. Processes. *Nurs Res*, 240:237–245.

Rubin R (1970): Cognitive style in pregnancy. *Am J Nurs*, 70:502–508.

Rubin R (1972): Fantasy and object constancy in maternal relationships. *Maternal-Child Nurs J*, 1:101–111.

Rubin R (1975): Maternal tasks in pregnancy. *Maternal-Child Nurs J*, 4:143–153.

Rubin R (1977): Binding-in in the postpartum period. *Maternal-Child Nurs J*, 6:67–75.

Rubin R (1984): *Maternal Identity and the Maternal Experience*. New York: Springer-Verlag.

Shereshefsky PM, Yarrow LJ (1973): *Psychological Aspects of a First Pregnancy and Early Postpartum Adaptation*. New York: Raven.

Shereshefsky PM, Lubenberg, Lockman (1973): Maternal adaptation. In: Psychological aspects of a first pregnancy and early postnatal adaptation, Shereshefsky PM, Yarrow LJ (eds.). New York: Raven, pp. 165–180.

Stainton MC (1981): *Parent-Infant Interaction: Putting Theory Into Nursing Practice*. Calgary: The University of Calgary.

Stainton MC (1985a): *Origins of Attachment: Culture and Cue Sensitivity*. Unpublished doctoral dissertation, University of California at San Francisco.

Stainton MC (1985b): The fetus: A growing member of the family. *Fam Relations*, 34:321–326.

Thomlison RJ (1984): Something works: Evidence from practice effectiveness studies. *Soc Work*, 29:51–56.

Timor-Tritsch IE et al (1978): Studies of antepartum behavioral state in the human fetus at term. *Am J Obstet Gynecol*, 132:524–528.

Truby H, Lind J (1965): Cry sounds of the newborn infant. In: Newborn infant cry. Lind J (ed.). *Acta Paediatr Scand*, 163 (Suppl.).

Ulrich SC (1982): Psychosocial work of a secundigravida in relation to acceptance of her baby. *Maternal-Child Nurs J*, 2(1).

Walz BL, Rich OJ (1983): Maternal tasks of taking-on a second child in the postpartum period. *Maternal-Child Nurs J*, 12(3).

Wright LM, Leahey M (1984): *Nurses and Families: A Guide to Family Assessment and Intervention*. Philadelphia: Davis.

Winslow W (1985): Pregnancy as a project: 12 women's experience of a first pregnancy after age 35. Unpublished master's thesis, University of British Columbia, Vancouver.

14

THE PROCESS OF GRIEF IN THE BEREAVED FAMILY

Sandra McClowry, RN, MS

Catherine L. Gilliss, RNC, DNSc

Ida M. Martinson, RN, PhD, FAAN

The grief experienced by bereaved families is more than a reaction to the loss of a family member. It is a process that involves familial and extrafamilial role alignment and reorganization. This chapter presents the unique role of nursing during the grief process and explores, through a review of existing literature, controversial issues of current bereavement theory and research. The process of bereavement is illustrated through a case study of a family experiencing the death of a child from cancer.

Sandra McClowry, a former member of the faculty in pediatric nursing, is a doctoral candidate at the Department of Family Health Care Nursing at the University of California at San Francisco. Her current research focus is on the effect of temperament and the environment on the behavior of hospitalized school-aged children.

If he was only here . . . to see what he would be like. How tall he would be; what he'd be doing for a living; what girls he would have dated and who he would have married; whether he'd have kids already.*

Introduction

The potential for significant relationships that provide meaning and structure to daily living exists within the family unit. The loss of a cherished family member causes pain, for as Marris (1982) explains, each relationship is unique and cannot be exchanged for another. When someone in the family dies, the family changes, not only because the person is gone but also because the loss of that particular relationship forces each individual to rethink the purpose of life as well as to contemplate each other's vulnerability.

> I think Charlie's death had a lot to do with the changes in our lives. It really makes you start questioning things. I think the first two years, you can't really judge what your life is going to be like because you really are still just trying to cope. It's not until after the first year, year and a half or so that you start saying, "OK, now what am I going to do with my life? Am I going to go on or am I just going to sit here?"

Grief is more than a reaction to the loss of a person. Parkes (1972, p. 21) describes it as a "process, not a state."

Family Tasks in the Process of Grief

Spinetta and Deasy–Spinetta (1981) emphasize the potential of the family for mitigating the pain individual members experience while grieving. They propose that, when functioning effectively, the family aids in individual coping. However, when the family cannot reduce the stress, not only are additional obstacles created for the members but the family's very existence is jeopardized.

According to Goldberg (1973), there are several tasks that should be fulfilled by the family during the bereavement process. These include: (1) permission to grieve; (2) realignment of intrafamilial roles; (3) intrapsychic role reorganization; (4) extrafamilial role realignment; (5) increased solidarity; and (6) object replacement. A discussion of these tasks follows.

Permission to Grieve

Families that demonstrate effective communication encourage open expression of emotions, and can thereby better handle the stress of bereavement (Kaplan, Grobstein, Smith, 1976; Goldberg, 1973). Those who express sadness, as well as anger, guilt, and relief, are more successful in adjusting to the loss (Vollman et al, 1971). The surviving children gain comfort through the shared responsibility of mourning and should be included in family discussions (Kubler-Ross, 1969). In contrast, families who are unable to communicate or express emotions experience isolation and diffusion, especially if preexisting conflicts remain (Vollman et al, 1971).

Realignment of Intrafamilial Roles

The death of a member leaves a gap in family functioning. Rather than assigning one particular individual to replace the person who has died, responsibilities and needs should be redistributed among the members. For example, a replacement pregnancy may be used to deny the child's death and interrupt the grieving process (Lewis, 1976; Poznanski, 1972). Or, one of the surviving children may be designated or may assume the roles previously occupied by the deceased sibling (Krell, Rabkin, 1979). However,

---

*In a study by Martinson (1987), families were interviewed eight years after they each had experienced the death of a child from cancer. Their comments are included throughout the chapter to illustrate some of the major points in bereavement theory. The study was funded by the California Division, American Cancer Society, Grant No. 2-210-PR-14

neither of these responses allows the process of grief to continue. Rather, a substitute person only provides distraction and often causes the replacement child psychologic harm (Krell, Rabkin, 1979; Poznanski, 1972). On the other hand, having another child can be a useful strategy if the child is viewed not merely as a replacement for the deceased child but is desired for more appropriate reasons (Videka-Sherman, 1982).

Intrapsychic Role Reorganization

In addition to reassigning familial roles is the related task of role changes for the individual members. Perceptions of self require adjustment in relation to the current family unit. For example, on the death of her husband, the wife no longer is a spouse; or parents who have lost their only child find themselves no longer in the active role of parents. Even when the family has surviving children, the loss of a child requires an intrapsychic role reorganization.

> There's always one missing. For a long time after Greg died, I used to stop at the store near here and get four candy bars for the kids. And Doris, the lady at the store would say, "Betty, you only need three now."

Extrafamilial Role Realignment

Family members must also examine their extrafamilial roles. Prior roles, such as involvement as a parent helper in the Cub Scouts, must be evaluated and either discontinued or approached with a different focus. Relationships with friends and relatives may also change as the family renegotiates how it will expend its energy and time. Changes in roles and commitments, such as taking a new job or beginning school, may also prompt a reevaluation.

Persons outside the immediate family, whether professionals, friends, or extended family, may assist or hinder the bereavement tasks (Bozeman, Orbach, Sutherland, 1955; Martinson, Moldow, Henry, 1980). For example, widows who were pressured by friends to deal with the present and future experienced less adjustment than those who were allowed to express their feelings and review the past (Maddison, Walker, 1967). Families who did not receive support during their grief process felt stigmatized, isolated, or angry, which only exacerbated their distress (Benfield, Leib, Volman, 1978; Parkes, 1972).

> Q: How do you wish your friends had treated you?
>
> A: I wish they would have let me talk about it. I wish they would have said they were sorry. They just acted like nothing happened.

Increased Solidarity

Families may become emotionally closer during bereavement. Growth of individual members or the family unit may occur. Parents whose child has died may develop a better relationship, especially if they previously had a foundation of good communication (Helmrath, Steinitz, 1978; Strauss, 1975).

Even when the stress of a child's death precipitates marital problems, some couples emerge with a renewed sense of commitment and maturity. Such growth is exemplified by this response from a couple who stayed together despite serious marital problems after the death of their child:

> Q: Have there been any changes in the quality of your relationship?
>
> A: It's a more mature way of feeling. I don't know how to explain it. It was like we were in love before, but that was cute love. Now it's deep.

Object Replacement

If the family has taken the time and energy necessary to process their grief, the energy and insight necessary to restate the meaning of life finally occurs (Marris, 1982). Goldberg (1973) describes this as object replacement, which he says enables the family to have a new child or to invest additional energy in its surviving children. However, whether most parents ever replace the deceased child is debatable.

Controversial Issues in the Field of Bereavement

Replacement versus Integration

Although bereavement theorists have been helpful in describing the process of grief, clinicians frequently recognize the limitations of applying the current literature to bereaved families. Goldberg's (1973) family task of object replacement is a description that does not appear to apply to the majority of grieving families. *Integration*, rather than object replacement, seems a more appropriate term since the dead person is not necessarily replaced by someone or something; rather, the loss is integrated into the changed person that the bereaved individual has become. Furthermore, whereas object replacement implies that pain at some point ceases, never to return, integration does not. Indeed, as the Committee for the Study of Health Consequences of the Stress of Bereavement states (Osterweis, Solomon, Green, 1984), for some individuals the pain of loss may continue for a lifetime, even after successful adaptation. As one of the mothers expressed during an interview, she still experienced pain when thinking of her son, but the passage of time made it a more "comfortable pain," which she actually did not want to end because with the pain came many memories.

> I don't ever want to forget. I want to remember every bit of it. I don't think I'll ever forget. It's as vivid in my mind as if it were yesterday. I can close my eyes and see the unit. I can see the nurses. I can see the doctors. I can see Anne. No, I won't ever forget any of it.

Of paramount importance in understanding the concept of integration is recogniz-ing another controversial issue regarding the process of grief that has been erroneously afforded credibility. Unfortunately, many persons dealing with the bereaved, including clinicians, researchers, and theorists, believe that bereavement is a programmed set of stages with recovery as the final stage.

Stages Approach

Relying on the work on Lindemann (1944), who was the first to describe grief in stages, Engle (1961) proposes that "uncomplicated grief" follows a predictable course with generalizable phases. Others, such as Kubler-Ross (1969), who proposed the stages that dying individuals experience, and Parkes (1972) present hierarchical steps that, if ascended, lead to resolution. Although it facilitated the beginning of a systematic investigation into bereavement, the use of the phasal conceptualization has had several unfortunate consequences.

The danger in describing bereavement in pristine, preconceived stages rather than acknowledging individual patterns of coping and integration is the assumption that the bereavement process is universal and predictable for everyone in all situations. On the contrary, Bugen (1977) asserts that the centrality of the relationship and the preventability of the death are important determinants in the intensity of grief. For families who have lost a child, the loss may be profound. In a comparison of those experiencing the death of a spouse, child, or parent, Sanders (1979, 1980) found higher grief scores among parents who lost a child than those among the other groups. As Schiff (1977) notes: "When your parent dies, you have lost your past. When your child dies, you have lost your future."

Another danger in viewing grief as a series of stages rather than as a process is the assumption of hierarchy. Stages are not discrete entities completed in a progressive pattern but rather involve considerable overlap and frequently a return to earlier phases (Bugen, 1977). To be distinguished from chronic grief, which the Commission (Osterweis, Solomon, Green, 1984) defines as persistent grieving that does not diminish in time and is a deterrent to finding new meaning or purpose in life, is the profound sadness families periodically experience. Poznanski (1972) refers to an "anniversary reaction," an intense level of grieving on special days like holidays or the deceased child's birthday.

> Q: When would you say was the most intense time of grieving?
>
> A: Mine as on Christmas and Mother's Day.
>
> Q: The Mother's Day immediately following?
>
> A: Every Mother's Day after . . . and Christmas. There's still one missing. I think it will always be that way. There's always one missing.

It is not unusual for the family to grieve for different reasons over time. As the years pass and as siblings grow older, mourning occurs for whom and what the child might have become.

> Last year, Laura's best friend got married. We went, and it was the most beautiful wedding. I never cried at a wedding before, but I just thought: "God, that could be my sister." It was really hard.

Nor does the process of grief limit the bereaved to one particular emotion at a time. Indeed, there may be a variety of feelings occurring simultaneously (Osterweis, Solomon, Green, 1984). Or, depending on individual personality characteristics, some people may experience certain emotions consistently and not experience others (Bugen, 1977).

> I was very angry . . . very angry . . . and bitter at everything, just everything. I didn't think it was fair. I still don't think it's fair. You know, I don't think that will ever change for me. Not children. Anybody but children. I don't think it's fair. They don't deserve it. They don't.

Because individual patterns differ, family members are unlikely to follow uniformly the same bereavement schedule. Therefore, applying stages to families becomes at best a questionable exercise. Although DeFrain, Taylor, and Ernst (1982) found no differences in length of grieving between fathers and mothers, other studies indicate that fathers experience grief symptoms less acutely and for a shorter duration (Cornwell, Nurcombe, Stevens, 1977; Helmrath, Steinitz, 1978; Rando, 1983). Whether fathers grieve as intensely as mothers is difficult to determine because societal expectations still discourage a male's expression of feelings (Martinson, Moldow, Henry, 1980). Fulfilling the appointed male role responsibilities is explained by one of the fathers:

> I think a guy is a lot luckier in that respect because of work. It's more than just work with the guy; you've got to be the rock or whatever . . . for security. You kind of bury yourself. You've got to keep going.

Another danger in viewing bereavement as an ascending progression of stages is the expectation that grief should be completed at some specific point in time (Kubler-Ross, 1983). Passage of time after death, however, does not appear to change the emotional state of parents (Kennell, Slyter, Klaus, 1970) or siblings (Davies, 1983). Studies also disagree whether length of illness before death changes the subsequent length of the grief process. "Anticipatory grief" is viewed as useful in reducing the pain of bereavement (Friedman et al, 1963; Rando, 1983). However, Miles (1985) did not find this relationship to be so.

Probably the most conclusive argument against using a phasal model is that empirical evidence does not support this premise (Cowan, Murphy, 1985; Bugen, 1977). What is needed rather than specific and altogether too rigid categories or stages is a clarification of the various ways individuals and families handle grief. Once the functional or dysfunctional patterns are known, interventions to mitigate adverse consequences can be planned and examined.

Consequences of Grief

Beginning with Engel's provocative 1961 article, "Is grief a disease?," the relationship between bereavement and the development or exacerbation of physical illness or emotional problems has been discussed in health and medical research (Osterweis, Solomon, Green, 1984). Understandably, the multiple losses and changes that occur when someone in the family dies subjects the bereaved to an intense level of stress. From a physiologic perspective, illness can be expected because during grief, immune responses are depressed (Parkes, Benjamin, Fitzgerald, 1969; Frederick, 1983). Regarding the psychologic impact, Marris (1982) maintains that processing grief requires, for all persons, "retrieving, consolidating, and transforming the meaning of their relationships to the person they lost, not by abandoning it, but, by becoming obsessed with it" (p. 195). Any effort, then, to distract, delay, or prevent discussion of memories is counterproductive to negotiating through the grief process. Because many people find it difficult to listen to those who have experienced the death of someone they loved, the bereaved frequently lack the opportunity to express their pain.

Lindemann (1944) reports many reactions, psychologic and physical, which he cites as common in uncomplicated grief:

- Somatic distress
- Preoccupation with the image of the distress
- Guilt
- Irritability, anger, and hostile reactions
- Loss of usual patterns of conduct
- Tendency toward sighing
- Lack of strength, exhaustion
- Digestive upset
- Altered sensorium
- Loss of warmth in relationships with others

- Quick speech, restlessness, inability to sit still, but without organization of behavior

Additionally, Bowlby (1960, 1961) emphasizes crying and yearning as a frequent response during the grief process, particularly during acute grief.

In agreement with Klein (1948), Bowlby (1960, 1961) recognizes depression as a normal part of mourning. In fact, the absence of depression in those who experience a significant loss may be an abnormal response (Lindemann, 1944; Osterweis, Solomon, Green, 1984; Parkes, 1972). On the other hand, what appears as inertia and purposelessness, an inability to self-organize and participate fully in life, is, in fact, an adaptive response to the psychic demands of bereavement (Bowlby, 1960). The reflective nature of depression permits the mourner to be preoccupied with memories of the past. Rather than plan for the future without the loved one, the depressed survivor's inability to think shelters the individual temporarily from that responsibility. Bowlby (1961) maintains that mental disorganization through depression is crucial in order that reorganization can occur.

Depression coupled with an unaccountable oscillation of emotions (Bowlby, 1960) may be frightening to grieving persons. Mothers whose newborn died were surprised by the intensity of their feelings and worried whether their feelings were abnormal (Helmrath, Steinitz, 1978). In a support group for bereaved parents, Macon (1979) noted bizarre responses, regressive behavior, and suicidal thoughts among the participants. These studies suggest that the bereavement process takes a longer time and may be more difficult than is commonly thought by many professionals and by the bereaved themselves. Clayton (1974) found that 17% of bereaved widows demonstrated depressive symptoms a year after their husbands died. Rando (1983) reported a decrease in grief symptoms the second year but an increase during the third year.

The possibility of other negative consequences also exists. Bereaved families demonstrate more emotional distress and problems as compared to those who have not experienced a loss (Miles, 1985; Parkes, Benjamin, Fitzgerald, 1969; Polak et al, 1975). Other researchers have found a high percentage of marital discord, divorce, or other family-related difficulties, particularly if problems existed prior to the child's illness or when other extenuating circumstances occurred concomitantly (Jurk, Ekert, Jones, 1981; Kaplan et al, 1976; Lansky et al, 1978; Miles, 1985; Strauss, 1975; Cornwell, Nurcombe, Stevens, 1977; Vollman et al, 1971). Especially if used previously, an increase in alcohol, drug, and tobacco use frequently occurs (Clayton, 1974; Helmrath, Steinitz, 1978; Parkes, 1964; Parkes, Brown, 1972). In some instances, behavioral problems and related school difficulties were increased among bereaved siblings (Davies, 1983; Tietz, McSherry, Britt, 1977). Also, a long-term consequence appears to be that children whose sibling died during childhood have a tendency toward depression in adulthood (Blinder, 1972; Hilgard, 1969).

The consequences of bereavement need not be negative. Figley (1984, p. 18) lists the characteristics of families functionally coping with stress that may lead to positive outcomes. These characteristics can be applied to the bereaved family:

• Ability to identify the stressor
• Ability to view the situation as a family problem rather than merely a problem of one or two of its members
• Ability to adopt a solution-oriented approach to the problem rather than simply blaming
• Ability to show tolerance for other family members
• Clear expression of commitment to and affection for other family members
• Open and clear communication among members

• Evidence of high family cohesion
• Evidence of considerable role flexibility
• Appropriate use of resources inside and outside the family
• Lack of overt or covert physical violence
• Lack of substance abuse

The Committee also points out that although no agreement exists on either normal outcomes or ways to assess normal outcomes, some favorable outcomes include a "reduction of depression-like symptoms, return to usual level of social functioning, reduction in frequency of distressing memories, the capacity to form new relationships and to undertake new social roles, and other functional outcomes such as return to work" (or school) (Osterweis, Solomon, Green, 1984, p. 18). However, when discussing positive outcomes, individual differences and goals must be considered. What may be a satisfactory outcome for one individual may not be an adequate solution for another.

Nevertheless, the potential for growth exists. Bowlby (1961) describes a personal reorganization that may eventually occur "by maintaining values and pursuing goals developed in association with the deceased." Moreover, this occurs partly as a method of maintaining the connection with the deceased person and partly from the personal reorganization the bereaved person has undergone as a result of the loss (Bowlby, 1960).

Other signs of continued growth may become visible. Relationships, new and renewed, may be pursued and nurtured. Familial tasks, formerly the responsibility of the now deceased, may be tackled with greater ease. New roles and commitments can commence yet with a qualitative difference and perhaps a greater depth of empathy and appreciation for life.

> I think they [the siblings] learned a lot more about life, living, and dying than I think a lot of children do. I don't know if that's good or bad, but I think it made them stronger and more mature.

Clinical and Research Implications

Despite the fact that bereavement literature is expanding, methodologically sound research remains sparse. Yet such research is critical in order to understand the process of grief, functional patterns of coping, and interventions to assist in achieving integration. Until such knowledge is obtained, clinicians should be concerned that some interventions may produce a negative impact (Osterweis, Solomon, Green, 1984).

Bereavement research is complex and will require years of further investigation. Meanwhile, clinicians will continue to rely on what is currently known and what appears compassionate and appropriate. However, the importance of sound research on which to base interventions cannot be overemphasized. Moreover, the involvement of clinicians in research is critical if bereavement theory is to have clinical relevance.

The Nurse's Role

The Committee recognized the role of nurses in the care of the dying and the bereaved. "The concepts of loss, grief, crisis, dying, death, and bereavement are basic to the nursing curricula. So, too, are the acquisition of communication and interpersonal skills required to apply that knowledge" (Osterweis, Solomon, Green, 1984, p. 232). In a variety of settings, nurses care for the dying and their families. As hospices and home care for the dying continue to develop in communities, nurses will be needed for the planning, administration, and direct care of the families who have dying members. Programs such as the "Home care for dying children" developed (Martinson, Moldow, Henry, 1980) in St. Paul, serve as models for the development of other programs.

The death of a child is a tremendously painful experience for families. In addition, the daily stress of having a sick family member compounds the burden the family experiences. Hospital technology and pace, as well as disruptions in family functioning, can cause the family to feel powerless and helpless in comforting and caring for its dying child. Martinson, Moldow, and Henry (1980) have demonstrated that with nursing support many families can be assisted in caring for their dying child at home. Parents and the other children have the opportunity to be responsible for the child's care, to provide a more familiar environment than the hospital, and to continue functioning as a family unit. The experience may also help the siblings understand and accept the death of their brother or sister (Lauer et al, 1985; Martinson, Kersey, Nesbitt, 1987).

Summary

This chapter reviewed the current knowledge of family bereavement with an emphasis on clinical significance. Rather than accepting the phasal model of bereavement, grief was described as a process that can result in either positive or negative outcomes. The difficulty of losing a family member was viewed with the acknowledgment that for many individuals, even after successful adaptation, pain continues and is integrated into the person the bereaved person has become. Although successful adaptation is desired and possible, bereavement is difficult, and mourners are susceptible to a variety of physical or emotional sequelae. The role of support appears to mitigate the pain of loss but needs systematic verification. Ironically, although death is a universal phenomenon, relatively little about the reaction to it has been empirically tested. Of the research related to bereavement, methodological and theoretical flaws reduce its credibility. The need for sound research on which to base interventions is critical.

When death becomes imminent and talk of cure is replaced by a primary concern for comfort, family needs for support and assistance require the specialized skills of professional nurses. Family needs for those skills continue during the process of grief. Nurses as care providers have the necessary skills to support and assist families through the process of bereavement.

Q: How often do you think about your brother?

A: I think about him . . . I don't think a day goes by that I don't think about him.

Issues for Further Investigation

1. What are the patterns of grieving families following the death of one of their members?

2. Do families whose members use divergent patterns of grieving experience more discord and other negative consequences?

3. Do family members experience a resolution in their grief within two years of a child's death from cancer?

4. What are the immediate physical responses of surviving children following the death of a significant other?

5. What types of support are viewed by families as most helpful?

References

Benfield G, Leib S, Volman J (1978): Grief response of parents to neonatal death and parent participation in deciding care. *Pediatrics, 62:* 171–177.

Blinder B (1972): Sibling death in childhood. *Child Psychiatry Hum Dev, 2:* 169–75.

Bowlby J (1960): Grief and mourning in infancy and early childhood. *Psychoanal Study Child, 15:* 9–52.

Bowlby J (1961): Processes of mourning. *Int J Psychoanal, 42:* 317–340.

Bozeman MF, Orbach CE, Sutherland AM (1955): Psychological impact of cancer and its treatment. *Cancer, 8*(1): 1–19.

Bugen LA (1977): Human grief: A model for prediction and intervention. *Am J Orthopsychiatry, 47*(2): 196–206.

Clayton PJ (1974): Mortality and morbidity in the first year of widowhood. *Arch Gen Psychiatry, 125:* 747–750.

Cornwell J, Nurcombe B, Stevens L (1977): Family response to loss of a child by sudden infant death syndrome. *Med J Aust, 1*(18): 656–658.

Cowan ME, Murphy SA (1985): Identification of postdisaster bereavement risk predictors. *Nurs Res, 34:* 71–75.

Davies EM (1983): Behavioral responses of children to the death of a sibling. Unpublished doctoral dissertation, University of Washington.

DeFrain J, Taylor J, Ernst L (1982): *Coping with Sudden Infant Death.* Lexington, MA: Lexington Books.

Engel GL (1961): Is grief a disease? *Psychosom Med, 23:* 18–22.

Figley CR (1984): Catastrophes: An overview of family reaction. In: *Stress and the Family,* Figley CR, McCubbin HI (eds.). New York: Brunner/Mazel.

Frederick JF (1983): The biochemistry of bereavement: Possible basis for chemotherapy. *Omega, 13:* 295–303.

Friedman SB et al (1963): Behavioral observation on parents anticipating the death of a child. *Pediatrics, 20:* 610–625.

Goldberg SB (1973): Family tasks and reactions in the crisis of death. *Social Work, 54:* 398–405.

Helmrath TA, Steinitz EM (1978): Death of an infant: Parental grieving and the failure of social support. *J Fam Pract, 6*(4): 785–790.

Hilgard JR (1969): Depressive and psychotic states as anniversaries to sibling death in childhood. *Int Psychiatry Clinics, 6:* 197–207.

Jurk IH, Ekert H, Jones HJ (1981): Family responses and mechanisms of adjustment following death of children with cancer. *Aust Paediatr J, 17:* 85–88.

Kaplan D, Grobstein R, Smith A (1976): Predicting the impact of severe illness in families. *Health Soc Work, 1*: 71–82.

Kennell J, Slyter H, Klaus M (1970): The mourning response of parents to the death of a newborn infant. *N Engl J Med, 283*: 344–349.

Klein M (1948): *Contributions to Psycho-analysis, 1921–45*. London: Hogarth.

Krell R, Rabkin L (1979): The effects of sibling death on the surviving child: A family perspective. *Fam Process, 18*: 471–477.

Kubler-Ross E (1969): *On Death and Dying*. New York: Macmillan.

Kubler-Ross E (1983): *On Children and Death*. New York: Macmillan.

Lansky SB et al (1978): Childhood cancer: Parental discord and divorce. *Pediatrics, 62*: 184–188.

Lauer ME et al (1985): Children's perceptions of their sibling's death at home or hospital: The precursors of differential adjustment. *Cancer Nurs, 2*: 21–25.

Lewis E (1976): The management of stillbirth—Coping with an unreality. *Lancet, 2*: 619–620.

Lindemann E (1944): Symptomotology and management of acute grief. *Am J Psychiatry, 101*: 141–149.

Macon L (1979): Help for bereaved parents. *Social Casebook: The Journal of Contemporary Social Work, 11*: 558–565.

Maddison D, Walker WL (1967): Factors affecting the outcome of conjugal bereavement. *Br J Psychiatry, 113*: 1057–1067.

Marris P (1982): Attachment and society. In: *The Place of Attachment in Human Behavior*, Parkes CM, Stevenson-Hinde J (eds). New York: Basic Books.

Martinson I (1987): A longitudinal study of family bereavement after childhood cancer. Final report. Grant no: 2-210-PR-14, American Cancer Society, California Division.

Martinson I, Kersey J, Nesbitt M (1987): Children's adjustment to the death of a sibling from cancer. In: *The Pediatric Nurse and the Life-Threatened Child* series, Bushman P, Schowalter J, Kutscher A (eds.), *6*(1): 15–21.

Martinson I, Moldow D, Henry W (1980): *Home care for the child with cancer: Final report* (Grant no. CA19490), U.S. Department of Health and Human Services. Washington, DC: National Cancer Institute.

Miles MS (1985): Emotional symptoms and physical health in bereaved parents. *Nurs Res, 34*: 76–81.

Osterweis M, Solomon F, Green M (eds.) (1984): *Bereavement: Reactions, Consequences, and Care*. Washington, DC: National Academy Press.

Parkes CM (1964): Recent bereavement as a cause of mental illness. *Br J Psychiatry, 110*: 198–204.

Parkes CM (1972): *Bereavement*. New York: Penguin.

Parkes CM, Benjamin B, Fitzgerald RG (1969): Broken Heart: A statistical study of increased mortality among widowers. *Br Med J, 1*: 740–743.

Parkes CM, Brown RJ (1972): Health after bereavement. *Psychosom Med, 34*: 449–461.

Polak P et al (1975): Prevention in mental health: A controlled study. *Am J Psychiatry, 132*: 146–148.

Poznanski E (1972): The "replacement child": A saga of unresolved parental grief. *J Pediatr, 81*: 1190–1193.

Rando T (1983): An investigation of grief and adaptation in parents whose children have died from cancer. *J Pediatr Psychol, 8*: 3–20.

Sanders C (1979–1980): A comparison of adult bereavement in the death of a spouse, child and parent. *Omega, 10*: 303–322.

Schiff HS (1977): *The Bereaved Parent*. New York: Penguin.

Spinetta JJ, Deasy-Spinetta P (eds.) (1981): *Living with Childhood Cancer*. St. Louis: Mosby.

Strauss A (1975): *Chronic Illness and the Quality of Life*. St. Louis: Mosby.

Tietz W, McSherry L, Britt B (1977): Family sequelae after a child's death due to cancer. *Am J Psychother, 31*: 417–425.

Videka-Sherman L (1982): Coping with the death of a child: A study over time. *Am J Orthopsychiatry, 52*: 688–698.

Vollman RR et al (1971): The reaction of family systems to sudden and unexpected death. *Omega, 2*: 101–106.

15

CHILD DAY CARE FOR HEALTHY YOUNGER FAMILIES

Roberta S. O'Grady, RN, DrPH

Meryl Glass, MA

It is anticipated that by 1990, 75% of mothers will be working outside the home, and young families throughout the world are already faced with the dilemma of child day care outside the home. Nurses may often assume the role of counselor to families during the child day care decision-making process. This chapter will present critical issues in child day care in the areas of policy, legislation, licensing, health, and family support. The chapter is followed by a photographic gallery that depicts a photodocumentary study of child care designed to reveal the philosophy of care at a child day care center.

Roberta O'Grady is Associate Field Program Supervisor in the Department of Social and Administrative Health Sciences at the University of California at Berkeley School of Public Health. Also an Adjunct Lecturer in the Program in Maternal and Child Health, she has particular expertise in the areas of maternal–child public health services and the needs of disabled youth making the transition to adult life.

Meryl Glass is the Director of the Marilyn Reed Lucia Child Care Study Center at the University of California at San Francisco, as well as Assistant Clinical Professor in the Department of Family Health Care Nursing at UCSF. Her areas of interest include play as a way of learning, and the role of the director at a child day care study site.

Introduction

Child day care by an adult other than parents for some part of each day has become a necessary service for many families. These are families in which both parents are employed, families headed by single parents, and families with special needs, such as families with adolescents, families with parents at risk of neglecting or abusing their children, families with emergency needs for child day care who lack traditional family supports, and families with a physically or emotionally disabled child.

This chapter has two major purposes. The first is to prepare nurses and other health professionals for their role in supporting and guiding a family who must make decisions about child day care in the context of their goals for themselves and their children. The second is to provide information on other roles for the health professional in child day care. The health professional may serve as advocate for adequate child day care; as advisor to state and local health, welfare, and educational organizations responsible for health standards in child day care; and as consultant to providers on the health program for staff and children in child day-care settings.

The Need for Child Day Care

The need for child day care is evident in employment trends for women. Data from the current population survey (U.S. Department of Labor, 1985) show that 53.5% of women with children under five years of age are in the labor force, and 50.5% of these women have children less than three years of age. By 1990, it is expected that three out of four mothers will be working, and 66.7% of all two-parent families will have both parents employed (U.S. Department of Commerce, 1984). The fastest rise in women in the labor force has been among mothers of children under three years of age. This trend has major implications for child day care licensing, which traditionally made no provision to meet the health and safety needs of children under two years of age, particularly in group settings.

Mothers of school-aged children are also participating in the labor force at an increasing rate, indicating a pressing need to provide for children between 5 and 14 years of age after school and during vacation. It is estimated that from 2 to 6 million school-aged children are left unsupervised for part of each day (Baden et al, 1982; California Senate Office of Research, 1983).

The option of not working in order to stay at home with young children does not exist for most single-parent families as well as for many two-parent families (Morgan, 1983). In addition to economic need, women want to complete their education and contribute to their own growth and that of their family through paid employment. Families are also interested in finding sources of nurturance and education for their children as a supplement to exclusive parental care, particularly in the absence of extended family members . It is these economic demands, parental expectations for self-fulfillment, and beliefs about optimum care for children that lead to the need for child day care.

Historical and Political Context of Child Day Care

Child day care, which involves persons other than parents or settings outside the home, has been provided in various ways and for special populations for over 150 years in the United States. The concept of child day care came from the industrialized countries of Europe, where it was fostered under certain conditions by communities. In general, these were the need for women in the work force; an interest in providing children with what was believed to be optimal cognitive and social learning for the improvement of society; and a perception that certain families were failing to acculturate their children to the accepted norms of society and were in need of assistance in childrearing (Steinfels, 1973; Baxandall, 1975; Marver, Larson, 1978).

These same conditions have led to the development of child day-care programs in the United States. For example, during the period of massive immigration in the late 19th century, child day care was used as a way to socialize both parents and children to the health and educational practices of the dominant culture. During World War II when women were needed in the work force, the federal government subsidized child day care for children aged three years and older for the duration of the war (Nelson, 1982).

The entry of women into the work force, especially married women with children, is making the relationship between work and family life an important policy issue faced by all countries (Newland, 1979). The child day-care policies of selected governments are briefly discussed as a basis for comparison with the United States policy response to the economic and childrearing functioning of the family.

Sidel (1972), the Socialist Child Care Cooperative (1976), and Otaala (1981) present views of family and child day-care policies in China, Cuba, Tanzania, and Seychelles. In these socialist societies, the government supports universal child day-care, beginning in infancy, to foster child health and development, to prepare children for citizenship in a socialist state, and to free both parents for productive work.

Israel has also experimented with a communal approach in childrearing, based on the view that the closely knit nuclear family may be an obstacle to the achievement of an ideal larger community. This philosophy supported the establishment of the Kibbutzim, but at no time has communal childrearing affected more than about 3% of families. Israel has a variety of policy approaches to support the need for full employment of women and to replace population lost to war through family allowances, housing assistance for families, and subsidized child day care (Kamerman, Kahn, 1978).

The status of child day care in the Federal Republic of Germany, the German Democratic Republic, France, Hungary, and Sweden has been surveyed because their female labor force participation rate is similar to that of the United States (Kamerman, 1980; Kamerman, Kahn, 1981). At the time of the survey in 1976, the government policies to support families in their childrearing functions differed markedly from United States policy. For example, all five countries provided paid maternity or parental leave for employed women or parents. All countries except Sweden provided cash or in-kind maternity benefits. In Hungary, this benefit was contingent on the receipt of prenatal care. Other benefits in these countries were the protection of the jobs of the parents while on maternity leave, special housing allowances or priorities for families with children, benefits for single-parent families, and entitlement to child health services.

In contrast, the United States has no statutory maternity-related benefits, no universal cash allowances for childrearing, and no universal maternal and child health service benefits. The basic income support program in the United States, Aid to Families with Dependent Children (AFDC), assures no uniform minimum cash benefit; is restricted, for the most part, to single-family, female-headed households; and is largely unavailable to employed women. The United States does provide tax benefits for families with children. These are (1) a tax exemption for children; (2) an earned income tax credit for one- and two-parent families with at least one wage earner and a child under 19, a full-time student, or a disabled child; and (3) a tax credit to cover some part of child day care expenses of working parents. Those who benefit from these programs must have sufficient income to pay taxes. For families who are eligible for AFDC, there is a work expense allowance for child day care costs. They may deduct these costs from their income when it is assessed for entitlement to benefits. Also, there are extensive non-statutory benefits covering maternity-related medical care, hospitalization, and paid leave. These vary, dependent on insurance and employer practices, and apply generally to employed women or to families with one employed wage earner (Kamerman, Kahn, 1981). In essence, childbearing and child day care have not been considered as appropriate for federal intervention unless such benefits were linked to welfare reform; that is, such benefits enable mothers who would otherwise be on welfare to enter the labor force (Grubb, Lazerson, 1982).

Just as there are differences in family benefits between the United States and other countries, there are differences in the policies for child day care. Finding care for children, particularly for children two and three years of age, and school entry is less of a problem in socialist and other European countries because of voluntary free or low-cost, government-subsidized, public preschool programs. It is beyond the scope of this discussion to evaluate the quality of child day care in other countries. This is a comparison only on availability of child day care and on an attitude prevalent in European countries that out-of-home care for young children is optimum for their development, regardless of whether parents are working (Kamerman, Kahn, 1981).

Regulation of Child Day Care in the United States

The regulation of child day care rests with the states, as efforts to have federal child day-care standards have failed (Nelson, 1982). When discussing the licensing of child day-care facilities with parents, it is important to keep in mind that states and local jurisdictions will vary in licensing requirements and that the majority of child day care in the United States is provided in unlicensed settings. Murray (1984) presents estimates of the number of unlicensed child day-care facilities, the impediments to licensure, and the factors such as provider ignorance, restrictive zoning laws, and licensing standards that are difficult to meet and act to keep child day care in the underground economy. To the extent that child day care arrangements are made outside a regulatory system, the public and private health sectors are limited in their influence on the health and safety of children in these settings. Their greatest impact on the protection of mental and physical health of children in child day care will be through education of parents to be informed consumers of child day-care services and advocates for improved public policy for child day care.

The authority to license child day-care centers and family day-care homes is granted by state legislatures to a unit of state government, usually the department of social services, education, or health. The components of a licensing system include standards for the physical environment; staff qualifications; staff–child ratios; inspection of facilities on initial application, on renewal, and on the basis of complaints; and a process for reviewing the denial of a license (Murray, 1984). It is recognized that application of such standards in family day-care homes would inhibit the growth of this type of child day care. Standards that take into account the special characteristics of family child day care may be found in California regulations (State of California Health and Welfare Agency, 1982). As an example of the differences in licensing regulations, there are no educational qualifications for the family day-care provider. He or she need only be 18 years of age or older and have no criminal record.

The licensing agency may provide educational materials and conferences for parents, the directors of centers, and family day-care providers to maintain compliance with the licensing regulations and to assure that parents are informed about the minimum health and safety regulations of child day care.

In addition to licensing, the child day-care information and referral services are provided by the state. These agencies have been supported by various federal initiations since the 1960s and by states. They bring the licensed day-care provider and the interested family together. They may enhance the activities of the licensing agency by bringing unlicensed providers into the system and by maintaining a consultation service to licensed providers, which may not be possible for the licensing agency (Levine, 1982). Their staffs may include social workers, nurses, and early childhood educators, and their activities may range from providing childrearing education classes for parents to helping child day-care staff to achieve better working conditions and employee benefits.

Other important national sources* that can inform and support health professionals who wish to play an active role in child day care are:

1. The American Academy of Pediatrics, a primary resource on standards for the protection of children's health in child day care (American Academy of Pediatrics, 1987; The American Academy of Pediatrics, Northern California Chapter 1, 1984)

2. The Children's Defense Fund, a private charity organization that sponsors a nationwide network of advocates who monitor Congress and support bills pertaining to child day-care services and other issues of importance to children and their families

3. The National Association for the Education of Young Children, a nonprofit association representing people in a diverse range of services to young children, with over 200 affiliates; their publication is *Young Children*

4. The National Black Child Development Institute, Inc., a nonprofit, national, charitable, and educational organization that focuses on childcare, child welfare, and education

---

*See the Appendix at the end of this chapter for addresses of these associations.

Models of Child Day Care

Goals that child day care programs attempt to meet can determine the types of philosophical models they represent. The following is an attempt to categorize models of child day care. These are not mutually exclusive, as programs can perceive their purpose as multifaceted. Usually, however, one pattern will emerge and predominate.

The Deprivation–Education Model

This model attempts to provide the child with a head start on formal schooling through successful experiences with learning skills that will carry over into the lower and intermediate grades. Child day care is viewed as preparation for school. Reading and mathematical readiness, attention to teacher direction, cooperation and verbal sharing in small and larger groups, and a sense of group identity are emphasized.

Examples of the deprivation–education model of child day care are Head Start (Hubbell, 1983; Brown, 1985) and other programs described by Ramey, Dorval, and Baker–Ward (1981) and Schweinhart and Weikart (1980). These reports are of interest because of the extensive review of research on the impact of child day care on cognitive ability, mother–child relationships, and social behavior. The report by Schweinhart and Weikart (1980) includes a long-term follow-up of children enrolled in their preschool program, showing decreased incidence of delinquent acts and teenage pregnancy and improved likelihood of employment.

The Empowerment Model

This model can be viewed as an extension of the deprivation–education model, in that the child is perceived to be at risk for school failure, but this is not necessarily due to the child or to the home environment. The problem is believed to be inherent in the school, which does not acknowledge and validate culturally varied backgrounds or promote self-esteem, cultural pride, and the accomplishments of the child's ethnic group. The parents, the neighborhood, or the community respond to this perception by seeking to empower the child, without conforming or attempting to acculturate the child to the dominant system for as long as possible (Moore, 1982). Child day care sponsored by the Black Muslims and the Black Panthers in the 1960s and 1970s and the more recent growth of child day care under the direction of Christian Fundamentalist churches are examples of this model.

The Surrogate Parenting Model

These programs are attempts to nurture children who are considered to be at risk because of faulty or immature parenting skills. Examples are programs for teenage mothers attempting to finish high school or programs that target families identified to be victims of child abuse or neglect (Friedman, Sale, Weinstein, 1984). This model can include care for the parent as well as for the child, and the more effective programs do this through parent education, counseling, peer support, and vocational guidance (Provence, Naylor, Patterson, 1977, pp. 42–60). Respite care for disabled children can also be included in this category (Association for the Care of Children's Health, 1984).

The Acceleration Model

In this model, the child is viewed as developmentally competent, and the major purpose of the child day care program is to accelerate the learning process. Activities usually associated with kindergarten may begin at age four, such as prereading or premathematics games. Fein and Clarke-Stewart (1973, pp. 207–212) give examples of curricula that may be used in child day-care programs that focus on academic concepts and school-appropriate behaviors.

The Custodial Model

The primary purpose of child day care is viewed as physical care and the provision of emotional comfort. Safety and health standards are upheld. The parent is seen as the primary and appropriate educator and molder of values, and the child day care setting is a place where the child is kept comfortable and safe until reunion with the parent. Custodial care can be pleasing to the child for a period of time, but it is usually not very stimulating beyond the social contact with other children. When incidental learning occurs, there is no structure to use and build on. Custodial child day-care models and their attendant problems are discussed by Suransky (1982).

The Cognitive-Play Model

Play is viewed as the child's mode of learning, and attempts are made to optimize, enrich, and extend the level of play. Staff are trained to use moments of incidental learning that arise through the play and are there to assist a child who gets "stuck" or confused, guiding him or her to a more appropriate activity. The cognitive-play model's theoretical basis is described by Almy (1968), and curricular examples are given. Many state college and university programs follow this model to some degree.

Infant Programs

Child day-care settings that serve infants will be guided by any of the philosophical models described above. However, infants in child day care are most likely to be in care of relatives, unlicensed homes, or licensed family day care because few centers have the facilities and staff to provide a physically safe and emotionally appropriate environment for children under two years of age.

Those who have proposed group care for infants (Provence, Naylor, Patterson, 1977; Provence, 1982; Gerber, 1984) describe developmentally supportive environments. Providers are particularly attentive to needs of parents to become familiar with their infant and to enjoy caregiving activities. The impact on the infant's physical and emotional well-being of infant–provider interactions in play, bodily movement, and communication in group settings is also discussed. These programs focus on infants' interests in looking, moving and grasping, mastering developmental tasks such as sitting or standing, becoming aware of themselves and others, and on the benefits of having a speaking social partner, an adult who is comfortable talking to infants and who can also serve as a resource for rest, replenishment, and security.

Helping Families Select a Child Day Care Program

Supporting the Choice for Child Day Care

Families facing the need of selecting appropriate child day care can experience anxious and negative feelings. An assumption, based on the authors' experiences with parents, is that most parents attempt to do what is in the child's best interest within the framework of their own understanding. If parents have read widely in the field of child day care, they will encounter professional opinion on the threats to the young child's development when separated from the mother or parents for the majority of the day (Fraiberg, 1977; Blum, 1983). The attention in the media to reported cases of abuse in child day-care centers and day-care homes also adds to the fear and guilt. Mothers, in particular, can experience considerable guilt if they believe, or are made to believe by spouse and friends, that they are choosing love of work over love of their child. These feelings, combined with fear of the unknown, can lead parents to delay planning for child day care.

Health professionals can be most helpful when they assist the family in the process of selecting child day care as early as possible—before the birth of the child or before the mother is compelled to return to work for financial or other reasons. The health professionals' knowledge of existing child day-care resources, information and referral agencies, and overall quality and availability of child day care in a community will be of great help.

It is not desirable for the health professional to make the family's decision for them; foregoing of the parental obligation and responsibility could be damaging and could erode the family's future decision-making confidence, particularly in future choice of schools. Therefore, without recommending specific programs or types of care, the health professional can listen and help families explore their options as they perceive them. This may include discussion of whether the mother wishes to and can lengthen her stay at home, whether she can participate in job sharing* or return to work part-time for a while, or whether the father may wish to stay at home with the child for a period of time.

The health professional also needs to listen closely for fears the parent may have. The parent may be angry that she or he seems to be giving up primary control of the child or fearful that the provider will impart cultural or moral values that the parent finds repugnant or strange. The potential provider may appear to be so competent as to not need the parent as a partner in the child day-care arrangement. The parent needs to find a child day-care provider or program that includes him or her as a partner in care and integrates parental values and needs into the total program.

In the case of a minority family or family in which English is a second language, it is essential that the child day-care situation not threaten or alienate the family as an integral unit. Similar

---

*Two people voluntarily share the responsibilities of the full-time position with prorated salary and benefits (Burud, Aschbacher, McCroskey, 1984).

cultural background and language is very often what minority families seek for their young children.

Anxiety about what a program will be like can be answered simply by encouraging the parents to visit prospective providers and programs. Just as they would comparison shop when preparing to buy a car or house, parents should visit as many programs as possible while deciding which one to choose. Familiarity with the variety of care will demystify the process of selection and provide a base for a knowledgeable choice.

To avoid being overwhelmed by the bombardment of impressions when visiting child day-care centers or homes, parents need to be prepared with certain simple and basic questions.* Parents need to take into account proximity to work or home, cost, and meal service and to ask questions that enable them to deepen their understanding of quality components that they have a right to expect. In other words, one goal is for the parent to become an informed consumer.

The parent should be able to ask such questions as: How are staff who work with children trained (in a center setting)? Does the provider have a family day-care license? Is there attractive, safe, and well-planned indoor and outdoor play space? Do the children currently using the child day-care program look relaxed, happy, and industrious? Do the children seem crowded or hovering about? Are the toys and materials appropriate for the age served? If meals and snacks are served, what is the food like and how is it prepared? What will the provider do in case of an accident or illness? Is there a physician or emergency service on call to the center or family day-care home?

Potential providers or program directors can unintentionally cause a parent to feel ill at ease. Is the parent comfortable enough to sort out his or her own feelings and not begin to wonder if the family and child are "good enough" or cooperative enough for the program? Maintaining self-confidence is as crucial to the child day-care selection process as when job-hunting or seeking a place to live; it is actually more crucial because the most essential relationship of parent to child and feeling good about that relationship is at stake. A crucial contribution that the health professional can make is to emphasize that no decision is made once and for all. Child day-care choices will change based on changing conditions at home or at the child day-care setting; indeed, the child may outgrow a particular setting or exhibit needs not met by existing care. Other reasons for changing child day-care settings are that parents may need more flexibility in scheduling hours for child day care; more time for warmer or longer greetings and good-byes; or more detailed information about the child's day away from the parent. Providers sometimes forget how helpless the parent feels away from the child without knowledge of the important events in the child's daily life. Even older, articulate children cannot give an adequate description of information a parent wants to know, such as what was for lunch and how much they ate.

At the time a change in child day care is being considered, parents are concerned about the child's need for stability and security and the bond that may have developed with the child day-care provider. The parents and the provider can work together to make the move to a different setting gradual and give the child the sense that he or she is "graduating" or going to a place that offers more opportunities for development.

In summary, the health professional does not make the actual child day-care decision for the family but provides problem-solving strategies. He or she suggests to the family as many site visits to child day-care providers and programs as possible. This creates a realistic expectation of what is actually available and provides practical knowledge of what programs look like.

---

*As an example, the Northern Alameda County Resource and Referral Agency (BANANAS) has free publications such as *Choosing Family Day Care, Choosing a Child Care Center* and *Leaving Child Care: Developing a Plan for Everyone.*

The health professional can suggest that the parents bring certain basic questions to ask of providers and programs. These questions establish some criteria whereby informed comparisons and matching of family to program or provider can be made. The health professional also emphasizes that child day-care decisions may be changed.

Supporting Concerns, Needs, and Values of Minority Families

Minority families have concerns with their choice of child day care particular to their cultural identity and values (Moore, 1982). When minority families encounter potential providers and teachers who reflect the majority or white culture, they have questions such as, Will the teachers adequately represent what I am? Will they interfere or attempt to negate the culture I am trying to give my child? Will the teacher misrepresent or belittle my background? Will my child feel different from or inferior to a child from the majority culture? If English is not the first language at home, the parent might ask, Will my child lose his or her lingual heritage? These questions are sometimes not expressed openly for fear of reprisal or embarrassment.

Some parents may see advantage in integrating their child into the white culture, but issues of identity and values remain. Majority providers do not understand this "us/them" dynamic unless they too have had some similar life experiences or unless they have been sensitized by others they have cared for and known.

The health professional can help the minority family in sorting out these sensitive issues, validate their importance, and offer assistance in formulating minimal acceptable standards. The community may offer multicultural programs and teachers who reflect the family's language and cultural background. Questions can be formulated for the family to present when investigating programs. The family can note by observation how other minority children behave and are treated in the program. The family can be as-

sured that if the program does not live up to expectations, the child can be moved from that setting.

Types of Child Day Care

If an immediate family member is not available to care for a young child, the family must decide on the remaining child day-care options. Family-based care is care from a provider, usually in her own home, with several other children. In the case of the licensed child day-care home, the adult–child ratio is specified. Center-based care is at a business site rather than a home and is usually licensed by the state. It serves a predetermined number of children and has a mandated adult–child ratio and square footage of space per child.

Whether a family will choose family-based or center-based day care will depend on many factors, such as availability, cost, and closeness to the child's home or parent's place of work. Other considerations in parents' choices are whether or not the facility is licensed and the parents philosophy or beliefs about childrearing.

The age of the child is a primary consideration. Family-based care, because of its intimacy and small number of children, is believed to be especially well suited to infants and toddlers. One reason is that infants are particularly vulnerable to infections that may be spread in settings where there are large numbers of children and few staff (Kendall, 1983). The small number of children in family-based care may also permit expressions of physical caring between the adult and child, which foster mutual enjoyment and social learning. Examples of these interactions are described by Provence, Naylor, and Patterson (1977, pp. 90–144) and Gerber (1984). *Resources for Infant Educarers* (see the Appendix at the end of this chapter) is an excellent resource for the preparation and ongoing education of adults who wish to provide infant care and for health professionals who may be consulting with infant care providers in the areas of physical and mental health of infants in groups.

Clarke-Stewart (1982) presents advantages of family child day care and center child day care. The advantages of center care are the educational opportunities, the variety and accessibility of activities, and the social development that may accrue from interaction in a group of children and adults. Centers may be more easily monitored by parents, and they are more likely to have staff trained in early childhood development.

Choice of Staff and Staff–Child Ratios

In the process of assisting families with their child-care decisions, the health professional will need to be informed about the educational and other requirements of a director, teacher, aide, or family child day-care provider.

The process of regulating child day care, as previously described, includes specification of the educational background of the staff and the ratio of numbers of staff to numbers of children. It has also been explained that in the United States, regulation of child day care rests with the states, and this leads to regional differences in types of staff and staff–child ratios. However there are recommended standards for federally supported child day-care facilities, and these standards influence state licensing decisions. Federally recommended staff–child ratios for centers are as follows (Clarke-Stewart, 1982; p. 127):

AGE	MAXIMUM GROUP SIZE	STAFF–CHILD RATIO
0–2	6	1:3
2–3	12	1:4
3–6	16	1:8

Staff–child ratios for homes are:

AGE	MAXIMUM GROUP SIZE	STAFF–CHILD RATIO
0–2	10	1:5
2–6	12	1:6

It should be kept in mind that these are minimum standards. Provence, Naylor, and Patterson (1977, pp. 196–198) believe that optimum care for infants and children under three years of age occurs with a staff–child ratio of one adult to two children.

Standards of education and experience are minimal for directors, teachers, and aides in the child day-care field and vary by state. In general, some college or equivalent education in early childhood education and administration is required for directors, but there are states that specify completion of high school only or no educational requirement (Provence, Naylor, Patterson, 1977, pp. 187–196). Teachers may also have some postsecondary educational requirements in early childhood education, and teacher aides may complete high school only or be currently enrolled in an occupational program in a high school. Many states have options for completion of educational requirements after a person accepts the child day-care position.

There are no standards of education or experience for the person who operates a family child day-care home. However, with current public concern for recent exposures of child abuse in centers, there is now particular attention to police clearance for all child day-care workers so that known child abusers will be barred from the child day-care field.

Hiring child day-care workers will remain problematic as long as the field remains underpaid and overtaxing work conditions continue. Three recent surveys of convenience samples of child day-care workers, most of whom were members of the National Association for the Education of Young Children, reveal that they are in the lowest 10% of adult wage earners (Whitebook et al, 1982; Pettygrove, Whitebook, Weir, 1984; National Association for the Education of Young Children, 1984). In addition to low salaries, only one-third of respondents received health insurance, and less than 10% received maternity benefits as part of employment. High turnover of staff, due in part to low wages, remains one of the chief impediments to maintenance of quality programming, especially for infants and preschool children, who need lasting significant adult relationships in the absence of a parent in the home. These problems will not be resolved until there is equitable pay for labor in the field.

The Child Day Care Environment

An initial intake interview between parents and the director is essential to introduce parents to the policies and procedures of the program, to sign necessary papers, and to discuss parental expectations and participation at the center. In the initial interview, the director attempts to establish the first bonds of trust between parents and the center. Through initial conversation about topics such as policies, procedures, routines, and parent participation, the director will attempt to bring out as many questions and concerns as the parent may have about the child day-care experience. Given the attention to child abuse in the media, California has developed a guide to be used by child day-care directors to help in informing parents on the prevention of child sexual abuse (State of California, 1984). Other topics for discussion are the center's methods of discipline, toileting, and diapering, dressing and undressing, naptime procedures, and daily routines.

Daily routines that are comfortable, realistic to accomplish, and age appropriate should be made available to parents at all centers. Routine schedules are, in fact, an informal contract of understanding and a component in the establishment of trust between the family and the programs. Developmentally focused programs will also be able to furnish parents with a plan of the daily routine that incorporates what is considered to be "curriculum"; that is, the plan includes age-appropriate and sequenced activities that foster and assure cognitive and social learning. Provence, Naylor, and Patterson (1977) de-

scribe routines and their rationales at length, with examples. If, after discussion, a parent is truly reluctant to use the child day-care service, the director should suggest other options.

Discussion of and preparation for the transition into center life is particularly critical for parents of infants and toddlers under three years of age, for parents and children who have not yet been separated for any considerable period of time, and for parents whose children have had unpleasant or unstable and changing child day care in the past.

Health Program for Infants and Children in Child Day Care

The health program of a child day-care center or family day-care home should foster the physical and mental development of the children by promoting the health of the staff; providing health education, preventive health, and illness care; and helping the children and families to have access to community health services that are compatible with cultural and personal preferences. Physicians, nurses, and other health professionals who provide direct services to children in child day care or who serve in an advisory capacity to the staff or families should understand the potential of child day care for promoting child health. They must be familiar with child day-care licensing laws, standards for programs, the usual heath problems encountered in the children, and the potential dangers to children, staff and parents if services are poor in quality.

The Health Needs of Child Day-Care Workers

Health professionals may find that a good way to provide for the health of children in child day care is to become aware of the health needs of the staff (Whitebook, Ginsburg, 1983). Child day-care employees are exposed to the respiratory and gastrointestinal infections found in child day-care settings. They are at risk for head lice and skin infections, and they may work daily with a variety of toxic substances, such as the silica in dry clay, solvent-based glues, and toxic substances in cleaning agents. The design of the workplace, although appropriate for small children, can result in back problems for adults who may be lifting children and objects improperly. Noise can reach stressful levels, particularly in spaces that were not originally designed for children. Child day-care workers may also be subject to a variety of emotional stressors such as low pay; no sick days with pay; no health benefits; insufficient education in child development to understand the behavior of the children; inadequate staffing, leading to physical and mental hazards for the children; inability to understand the needs of parents; and a lack of opportunity to have influence on their own working conditions. Staff may have difficulty considering their own health needs without the consultation of a health professional. The National Association for the Education of Young Children and other private foundations have been a source for funding educational materials, counseling, and advocacy programs for child day-care workers. Licensing laws may also assure that the provider is free of contagious disease and does not have a criminal record (State of California, Health and Welfare Agency, 1982, 1984).

The Health Needs of Infants and Children

The components of a health program for children are based on their health needs and the special features of the center or family day-care environment. In essence, these are injury control, the prevention and management of infectious diseases, and the evaluation of unique needs of individual children. Assuring a regular source of health care for children, a procedure for emergency care, and a plan for the care of mildly sick children are also part of the health program.

Injury Control

Sources of health hazards in day care are the potability, pressure, and temperature of water; the location and height of handwashing facilities and the safety of the sewage system; food service facilities and the risk of food-borne diseases; the location of caustic cleaning substances; the heating system; and the paint used in fixtures, equipment, and walls. Other considerations are the safety of indoor and outdoor play areas, accessibility of exits, and access for emergency vehicles. The local and state health departments and local fire department can inspect facilities to assure conformance to building regulations and the licensing authority (American Academy of Pediatrics, 1987; Educational Facilities Laboratory, 1972). An Early Childhood Environment Rating Scale (Harms, Clifford, 1980) is also available and is particularly useful in increasing the sensitivity of the staff to the importance of providing a safe environment for the children. Staff require training for emergencies, including resuscitation, control of bleeding, and first aid for minor accidents and injuries. Written guidelines for emergency procedures, which are reviewed by the health consultant, are recommended (American Academy of Pediatrics, 1987). However, the extent of compliance with these procedures is limited (Chang, Zukerman, Wallace, 1978; Chang, 1979; Aronson, Aiken, 1980).

Licensed centers are required to develop and update their plans for safety and emergencies. Parents need to ask for this information if it is not given during the intake interview. They need to ask what happens in case of fire or other disaster; how parents will be contacted; where medical care will be given; whether the staff is trained in first aid; whether there are frequent fire drills; and whether there is an evacuation plan. Health professionals can be of assistance to centers in reviewing their procedures and making recommendations for improvement.

The environment and all materials within reach of children should be scrutinized for general cleanliness and safety. Attentive supervision of children should preclude unnecessary accidents. Rest times for children and staff should be built into the daily routine, so that fatigue does not compound the accident rate.

Prevention and Management of Infectious Diseases

There is controversy regarding whether children in child day care, particularly those under three years of age, have an increased incidence of infections in comparison with home-reared children (Loda, Glezen, Clyde, 1972; Strangert, 1976; Doyle, 1976; Kendall, 1983). However, there is evidence that certain types of infections are frequently found in child day-care facilities. These are various respiratory viruses, *Hemophilus* influenza type B, *Giardia,* shigella, hepatitis A, bacterial infections, fungal skin infections, and infestations of head lice, scabies, and pinworms. Factors that contribute to the spread of these infections are prolonged, close personal contact; poor hygiene and sanitation, particularly in diapering infants and toddlers; and insufficient education of child day-care workers.

Information on the problem of communicable diseases in general and findings from epidemiological studies of specific infections indicate ways in which health professionals can assist child day-care staff in minimizing risk for infectious diseases (The Child Day Care Infectious Disease Study Group, 1984; Silva, 1980; Sealey, Schuman, 1983; Pickering et al, 1981; Granoff, Daum, 1980; Jacobson, Holloway, 1977; Haskins, Kotch, 1986). The publication *Morbidity and Mortality Weekly Report* (*MMWR*), from the Centers for Disease Control in Atlanta, is an important source of current information on infectious diseases in child day care. The epi-

demiology of the specific infection is explained, and measures for control of spread are recommended. This publication is helpful when trying to decide whether or not to exclude a child with a particular infection.*

Recommendations for prevention and control of infections in child day-care centers are published by the American Academy of Pediatrics (1987), by the Committee on Infectious Diseases, Northern California Chapter 1 of the American Academy of Pediatrics (1984), and in publications for parents and child day-care workers distributed by local health departments and advocacy groups for safe childcare.**

Another facet of the health care component in child day care is the provision for the care of the children who arrive with symptoms of illness or who become ill during the day. Traditionally, licensing regulations have prohibited child day-care programs from accepting children who are ill, in order to protect the other children and staff from the possibility of infection (Logue, 1978). Nevertheless, a child who is excluded from child day care presents a problem to working parents. Parents may have to lose a day's pay or be in jeopardy of losing a job if they stay at home to care for the child. Although state child day-care regulations may not clearly define a child day-care center's responsibility for the child with a minor illness (California Administrative Code, 1980), some programs have demonstrated that with proper precautions, contagion is minimized (Keister, 1975). With medical consultation, good communication between staff and parents, and parent–staff education, a program of care for sick children can be successfully implemented (Loda, Glezen, Clyde, 1972; Logue, 1978; Peters, 1976).

---

*Recent publications have discussed the following infections: measles (*MMWR* [1980] 29:426–427); shigellosis (*MMWR* [1986] 35:753–755); cryptosporidosis (*MMWR* [1984] 33:599–601); cytomegalovirus (*MMWR* [1985] 34:49–51).

**See *What You Should Know About Contagious Diseases in the Day Care Setting: A Handbook for Child Day Care Center Directors, Caregivers, and Parents.* Center for Disease Control, Atlanta, 1984.

Mohlabane (1984) has reviewed options for the provision of care for sick children, citing their advantages and disadvantages, and presented examples of care programs for sick children. In-home care, with the parent receiving a paid leave from work to care for a sick child, is an option in several countries (Kamerman, Kahn, 1981). In the United States, employers are being encouraged to work with employees' care programs for sick children to support working parents (U.S. Department of Labor, 1982; Burud, Aschbacher, McCroskey, 1984, pp. 203–212). A related option is in-home care in which a child day-care worker from the care program comes into the home to care for the child, freeing the parent to continue working throughout the course of the child's illness (Peters, 1976; Roby, 1973; Children's Defense Fund, 1982, pp. 95–99).

Primary Health Care

There is no question that emergency services, protection of the child from acute illness, and provisions for care of the sick child are of utmost importance in the child day-care health care program. Nevertheless, the health care programs that may affect lifelong health status are the preventive health services, including health education, health screening program, and primary care and the related nutritional, dental, and mental health services. Staff health needs must also be met through education, screening, and physical examinations at the time of employment and at periodic reevaluations of health status.

The primary health program requirements may be met by child day-care centers in a variety of ways (American Academy of Pediatrics, 1987). The first obligation of the staff is to promote the parent's effort to secure primary care from a regular provider in the community. If health supervision is not available in the community, the child day-care center may consider providing primary care as part of its program (Peters, 1976; Gururaj et al, 1974; Mohlabane, 1984).

The child day-care health component, which has as its focus prevention and education, takes many different forms dependent on the size of the center and the resources of the community. With the advent of the Head Start program, guidelines for the content and implementation of health promotion programs in child day-care centers and family day-care homes were made available by the federal government (North, 1971; Richmond, Janis, 1982). Current recommendations are published by the American Academy of Pediatrics (1987).

The health services director may be a physician or nurse with education and experience in the health supervision of young children. This individual may be paid or may volunteer, and a variety of arrangements are made for the director to consult with the staff or see selected children on a part-time basis. (Appalachian Regional Commission, 1970). With consultation from a health services director, the health program is written for clear understanding by the parents and staff. It should include the policies on health appraisal for admission to the program, the persons responsible for ongoing medical care, the management of acute illness or accidents, and the provision for the child who is ill. Other features of the written health plan may be to specify the health education objectives, roles of other professionals such as nutritionist or dentist, and plans for ensuring follow-up of any children referred for specialty health care (North, 1971; American Academy of Pediatrics, 1987).

Frequently, child day-care health programs assure that the children receive the minimum screening tests as recommended by the Early, Periodic Screening, Diagnosis and Treatment Program (EPSDT), the comprehensive plan for screening and treatment services for children under Title XIX of the Security Act (Medicaid) (U.S. Department of Health, Education and Welfare, 1972; U.S. Department of Health and Human Services, 1984). The department that administers the EPSDT program within each state can provide information on the EPSDT screening program, eligibility of children, costs, and consultation on implementing the program or making the ongoing screening accessible to the child day-care population.

Families and Children with Special Needs

In this discussion, children with special needs are those with physical, mental, or emotional disabilities, and abused and neglected children.

The integration of disabled children into nondisabled child day-care settings has been fostered for many years. The beliefs that guide this effort are that disabled children should be given a chance to play and learn with able-bodied children and that both groups benefit most from being together during the years when children can more easily learn to understand and accept the range of human differences (U.S. Department of Health and Human Services, 1981; Guralnick, 1976; Cooke et al, 1981; Apollini, Cooke, 1975; Heekin, 1984). Federal policy supports these beliefs in the Education for All Handicapped Children Act of 1975, mandating integrated education for the disabled (Select Panel for the Promotion of Child Health, 1981; American Academy of Pediatrics, 1973, 1987; Sommers, 1982). Leadership in the movement to integrate the disabled into preschool settings has come from Project Head Start, which, in 1972, mandated enrolling disabled children who were otherwise eligible for Head Start (U.S. Department of Health and Human Services, 1981). This is the largest child day-care program to integrate the disabled. The private child day-care sector has not been successful in serving disabled children, despite the excellent example of Head Start in demonstrating the feasibility of integration (Chang, Teramoto, 1984; Abelson, 1976; Berk, Berk, 1982). It is apparent that, unlike Head Start, private child day-care centers do not have the financial resources to enable them to hire and

train staff and provide appropriate physical facilities for integration of the disabled. However the Children's Defense Fund (1982, pp. 25–32, 90–94) presents a child day-care model that has been successful in integrating the disabled. This is a centralized service, coalition, or consortium of all child day-care programs in a community, which permits the centralization of technical assistance, training, purchasing of supplies and equipment and the provision of health consultation or special education at costs shared by all programs.

The analysis of the position of disabled children in our society by Gliedman and Roth (1980) is instructive in understanding why child day care has been slow to respond to legislative mandates and professional encouragement to admit the disabled into integrated child day-care settings. There must be a political perspective, that is, advocacy for child day care for all children, and an ethnographic perspective, that is, understanding disabled children in terms of their own norms and social situations.

Another group of children with special needs are the abused and neglected. Their parents need child day care, as do any parents who must maintain jobs and provide for children either all day or after school. However these parents require a child day-care setting that is sensitive to the parents' needs for help as well as to the children's needs for protection.

The type of child day care that may benefit an abusive family must be given as careful consideration as any other mode of treatment. A long-held belief is that child day care provides relief for parents who are frustrated or experiencing family crises that precipitate abusive acts (Alexander, 1972). However, the type of child day care (center or in-home care) that will be most protective of the child and at the same time work toward meeting the abusing parents' needs will differ based on such factors as type of abuse, age of the child, presence of other supportive persons in the family, and whether or not legal action is being taken for temporary or permanent termination of parental rights to raise the child (Crittenden, 1983). The State of California Commission on Crime Control and Violence Prevention (1983) and Oates (1982) present models of child abuse programs that include primary prevention services, respite care, emergency shelters, treatment programs, and programs that combine these approaches.

All community efforts to improve availability of child day care will benefit families who have the potential for or who have been identified as child abusers. Center-based child day care and family day care are resources for the detection of child abuse and primary prevention of abusive childrearing practices through strengthening staff–parent relationships and identifying sources for referral and treatment (Barber–Madden, 1983). If a child is identified as abused while enrolled in a center, the center may be an important source of respite. This placement should not be ended while the child abuse investigation proceeds until careful consideration is given to the meaning of the center or family day-care home to the child and the abusing parent.

The Future of Child Day Care

At a time when the demographic and social changes in the American family point to an increased need for a variety of child day-care arrangements, there is no national policy to support child day care, and there are no federal financial provisions, other than Aid to Families with Dependent Children for families in poverty, to enable parents, particularly the mother, to stay at home to care for an infant. In the absence of direction on the national level on how to support the childrearing function of families, the future of child day care will be in the hands of local and state child day-care constituencies made up of parents, early childhood educators, health professionals, teachers and school administra-

tors, and employers. Entrepreneurs who view child day care as a profit-making enterprise have also entered the field.*

These groups have a profoundly difficult task balancing their beliefs about the importance of the family in day-to-day childrearing, the compelling need for mothers to work in a society without a child allowance or programs of income support, and the need for mothers and fathers separated from their own parents or relatives who traditionally helped and taught the new family about parenting, to find other resources for learning. They will also be faced with monitoring the child day-care-for-profit industry, which is likely to reduce costs through increasing the ratio of children to staff.

The Children's Defense Fund (1982) has published a number of case studies of successful child day care under varying types of sponsorship and models of care that illustrate the strengths to be found in community-based, parent-controlled programs. Baden et al (1982) present case studies of successful programs that meet the specific needs of school-aged children for care after school and during school vacations.

It is instructive to study the operating methods of these programs in the areas of conducting needs assessments, building community coalitions, seeking public and private funding, and training staff. The sponsors of these programs range from private and public corporations to voluntary associations. They serve children from infancy through elementary school age. These groups have in common an ability to break down what may seem like an overwhelming task, when viewed as a national problem, into manageable activities appropriate to their own corporate interests or local needs.

Another development that promises sup-

---

*See Magnet M: What massed produced child care is producing. *Fortune* (Nov) 1983; 108(10–13): 157–174, for a discussion of the marketing and cost-saving techniques of childcare chains.

port to employed parents is employee-sponsored child day care. This includes on-site, company child day care; reimbursement of child day-care costs to employers; information and referral services; provision of family day-care homes, after-school care, and care for the sick child; corporate contributions to community child day-care agencies; and various flexible time- and job-sharing provisions that reduce the need for out-of-home care. The status of employee-sponsored child day care, the financial benefits to companies, and the tax advantages to both employees and industries are described by Burud, Aschenbacher, and McCroskey (1984). These authors include a survey of existing programs and a guide to industry in selecting the appropriate child day-care options in relation to needs of employees and children, community resources, and cost–benefit analyses.

A major consideration for the future of child day care is the preparation and reimbursement of child day-care staff. At present, in some states, child day-care staff are receiving only a minimum wage and no health or other job-related benefits. It is frequently impossible for a child day-care provider to offer a competitive salary for a director or teacher who has completed an undergraduate or graduate program in early childhood education or a related field. Adequate financial compensation may not be available for health and mental health, health education, or nutrition consultation. Whitebook et al (1982) report that the work environment and salary structure in child day care lead to frequent staff turnover, thus depriving children of consistency in the program. It is not uncommon for child day-care workers to spend unpaid time with parents or in such activities as fund-raising, curriculum-planning or continuing education. Upgrading salaries is crucial for the survival of good child day care, but at the same time, it is necessary to develop the public's perception of the importance of child day care to family life and child development.

The Child Care Employee Project is an example of a local effort to improve conditions for child day-care workers through public education and legislative advocacy (see Appendix). This organization has publications available on such topics as policies for substitute child day-care workers, breaks while working, health coverage, worker compensation, and employee rights under the Fair Labor Standards Act (Child Care Employee Project, 1983).

Summary

It is anticipated that by 1990, 75% of mothers will be working outside the home. The fastest growing segment of working mothers will be those with children under two years of age. Child day-care services are not keeping up with the number of children in need of services. Of the presently estimated 13 million children under age 13, the care of 7 million cannot be accounted for by the available places in child day-care centers and relative or nonrelative homes (U.S. Department of Labor, 1982).

These demographic facts compel health professionals to become informed about child day care in order to guide and support families and to make available to child day-care consumers and providers their particular knowledge and skills in physical and mental health and safety, disease prevention, and health promotion. Together with parents, the health professional can monitor state and federal initiatives for child day care and support public funding for economically disadvantaged families and children with special needs.

Issues for Further Investigation

1. Are there significant differences in behaviors (other than parent–child relations and stranger anxiety) between children who have spent two to three years in a child day care center and children who spent their first five

years in the home when they enter the public school system? For example, are there differences in self-esteem, independence, socialization, aggressiveness, and self direction?

2. It is generally accepted that the children of a nation represent its future. To what degree do child day care centers contribute to the formation of national character?

3. Assuming that child day care centers do contribute to the transmission of cultural values, what are the differences in the values transmitted in centers that serve populations of different socioeconomic groups, such as housing project centers in the ghetto and upper-class child day care centers?

4. To what degree is health education incorporated into the curriculum of child day care centers? What is the frequency distribution of health behaviors that are taught and practiced in such centers?

5. How does cultural background influence parental attitudes toward the acceptability of out of home placement for child day care? What other factors influence parental attitudes toward and adjustment to out of home child care?

6. What are some of the patterns of behavior of children when they return to their homes during the first two weeks following placement in a child care center?

7. How does family style influence selection of and use of a child day care facility?

References

Abelson AG (1976): Measuring preschools' readiness to mainstream handicapped children. *Child Welfare, 55:* 216–220.

Alexander H (1972): The social worker and the family. In: *Helping The Battered Child and His Family*, Kempe CH, Helfer RE (eds.). Philadelphia: J.B. Lippincott.

Almy M (ed.) (1968): *Early Childhood Play: Selected Readings Related to Cognition and Motivation.* New York: Simon and Schuster.

American Academy of Pediatrics, Committee on Children with Handicaps (1973): Day care for handicapped children. *Pediatrics, 51:* 948.

American Academy of Pediatrics, Committee on Early Childhood, Adoption and Dependent Care (1987): Health in day care: A manual for health professionals. Elk Grove Village, IL: American Academy of Pediatrics.

American Academy of Pediatrics, Northern California Chapter 1. (1984): *Infections in Day Care Centers: Recommendations for Prevention and Control for Physicians.* San Rafael, CA: American Academy of Pediatrics, Northern California Chapter 1.

Apollini T, Cooke TP (1975): Peer behavior conceptualized as a variable influencing infant and toddler development. *Am J Orthopsychiatry, 45:* 4–17.

Appalachian Regional Commission (1970): *Programs for Infants and Young Children.* (3 vols.) Washington, DC: U.S. GPO.

Aronson S, Aiken LS (1980): Compliance of child care programs with health and safety standards: Impact of program evaluation and advocate training. *Pediatrics, 65:* 318–325.

Association for the Care of Children's Health (1984): Home care for children with serious handicapping conditions: A report of a Conference. Washington, DC: Association for the Care of Children's Health, pp. 50–53.

Baden RK et al (1982): *School Aged Child Care. An Action Manual.* Boston: Auburn House.

Barber-Madden R (1983): Training day care program personnel in handling child abuse cases: Intervention and prevention outcomes. *Child Abuse Negl,* 7:25–32.

Baxandall RF (1975): Who shall care for our children? The history and development of day care in the United States. In: *Women: A Feminist Perspective,* Freeman J (ed.). Mountain View, CA: Mayfield

Berk HJ, Berk ML (1982): A survey of day care centers and their services for handicapped children. *Child Care Quarterly, 11:* 211–214.

Blum M (1983): *The Day Care Dilemma.* Lexington, MA: D.C. Heath.

Brown B (1985): Head Start: How research has changed public policy. *Young children, 40:* 9–13.

Burud SL, Aschbacher PR, McCroskey J (1984): *Employer Supported Child Care: Investing in Human Resources.* Boston: Auburn House.

California Administrative Code (1980): Title 22 of the social security act, Sections 31275, 31277.

California State Senate Office of Research (1983): *Who's Watching Our Children? The Latchkey Child Phenomenon.* Sacramento, CA: Senate Office of Research.

Chang A (1979): Health services in licensed family day care homes. *Am J Public Health, 69:* 603–604.

Chang A, Teramoto R (June, 1984): Services for children with special needs in private day care centers. Los Angeles, California: Division of Population and Family Health, School of Public Health, University of California, Mimeographed.

Chang A, Zukerman S, Wallace H (1978): Health service needs of children in day care centers. *Am J Public Health, 68:* 373–377.

Child Care Employee Project (1983): Health and safety resources for child care workers. Berkeley, California 94705: Child Care Employee Project, P.O. BOX 5603.

Children's Defense Fund (1982): *The Child Care Handbook.* Washington, DC: Children's Defense Fund.

Clarke-Stewart A (1982): *Daycare.* Cambridge: Harvard University Press.

Commission on Crime Control and Violence Prevention (1983): Taking root: An overview of violence prevention programs in California. Sacramento, CA: J.D. Franz Research.

Cooke TP et al (1981): Handicapped preschool children in the mainstream: background, outcomes and clinical suggestions. *Topics in Early Childhood Special Education, 1:* 73–83.

Crittenden PM (1983): The effect of mandatory protective day care on mutual attachment in maltreating mother-infant dyads. *Child Abuse Negl, 7:* 297–300.

Doyle A (1976): Incidence of illness in early group and family day care. *Pediatrics, 58:* 607–613.

Educational Facilities Laboratory (1972): Found spaces and equipment for children's centers. New York: Educational Facilities Laboratory.

Fein GG, Clarke-Stewart A (1973): *Day Care in Context.* New York: Wiley.

Fraiberg S (1977): *Every Child's Birthright: In Defense of Mothering.* New York: Basic Books.

Freidman DB, Sale J, Weinstein V (1984): Child care and the family. Chicago, Illinois 60604: National Committee for Prevention of Child Abuse, 332 South Michigan Avenue, Suite 1250.

Gerber M (February, 1984): Caring for infants with respect. In *Zero to Three: Bulletin of the National Center for Clinical Infant Programs* IV, (3): 1–3.

Gliedman J, Roth W (1980): *The Unexpected Minority: Handicapped Children in America.* New York: Harcourt Brace Jovanovich.

Granoff DM, Daum RS (1980): Spread of hemophilus influenzae type B: Recent epidemiological and therapeutic considerations. *J Pediatr, 97:* 854–860.

Grubb WN, Lazerson M (1982): *Broken Promises: How Americans Fail Their Children.* New York: Basic Books.

Guralnick MJ (1976): The value of integrating handicapped and nonhandicapped preschool children. *Am J Orthopsychiatry, 46:* 236–245.

Gururaj VJ et al (1974): Health care for day care children. *NY State J Med, 74:* 340–343.

Harms T, Clifford RM (1980): Early childhood environment rating scale. New York: Teachers's College, Columbia University.

Haskins R et al (1981): Minor illness and the social behavior of infants and caregivers. *J Appl Dev Psychol, 2:* 117–128.

Haskins R, Kotch J (1986): Day care and illness: evidence, costs and public policy. *Pediatrics, 77* (6) part 2, Supplement: 951–982.

Heekin S (1984): New friends. *Children Today,* Sept/Oct:8–13.

Hubbell R (1983): A review of head start research since 1970. Washington DC: Administration for Children, Youth and Families, Office of Human Development Services, Department of Health and Human Services.

Jacobson JA, Holloway JT (1977): Meningococcal disease in day care centers. *Pediatrics, 59:* 230–299.

Kamerman, SB (1980): *Parenting in an Unresponsive Society.* New York: The Free Press.

Kamerman SB, Kahn AJ (1978): *Family Policy: Government and Families in Fourteen Countries.* New York: Columbia University Press.

Kamerman SB, Kahn AJ (1981): *Child Care, Family Benefits and Working Parents: A Study in Comparative Policy.* New York: Columbia University Press.

Keister ME (1975): The good life for infants and toddlers. Washington, DC: National Association for the Education of Young Children.

Kendall ED (July, 1983): Child care and disease: What is the link? *Young Children,* 39: 68–77.

Levine JA (1982): The prospects and dilemmas of child care information and referral. In: *Day Care: Scientific and Social Policy Issues,* Zigler EF, Gordon EW (eds.). Boston : Auburn House.

Loda FA, Glezen WP, Clyde WA Jr. (1972): Respiratory disease in group day care. *Pediatrics, 49:* 428–437.

Logue PL (1978): Should the physically ill child attend day care? *Child Care Quarterly,* 7: 236–241.

Marver JD, Larson MA (1978): Public policy toward child care in America: A historical perspective. In: *Child Care and Public Policy,* Robins PK, Weiner S (eds.). Lexington, MA: Lexington Books.

Mohlabane N (1984): Infants in day care centers in sickness and in health. Oakland, California; 94609: BANANAS: Child Care Information and Referral and Parent Support, 6501 Telegraph Ave.

Moore E (1982): Day care: A Black perspective. In: *Day Care: Scientific and Social Policy Issues,* Zigler EF, Gordon EW (eds.). Boston: Auburn House.

Morgan G (1983): Child day care policy in chaos. In: *Children, Families and Government.* Zigler EF, Kagan S, Klugman E (eds.). Cambridge: Cambridge University Press.

Murray KA (September, 1984): Child care standards and monitoring. In: *Day Care, Report of the Sixteenth Ross Roundtable.* Columbus, Ohio: Ross Laboratories.

National Association for the Education of Young Children (1984): Results of the NAEYC survey of child care salaries and working conditions. *Young Children,* 40: 9–14.

Nelson JR (1982): The politics of federal day care regulation. In: *Day Care: Scientific and Social Policy Issues,* Zigler EF, Gordon EW (eds.). Boston: Auburn House.

Newland K (1979): *The Sisterhood of Man.* New York: W.W. Norton.

North FA (1971): Day care-health services: A guide for project directors and health personnel, U.S. Department of Health and Human Services, Pub. No. (OHDS) 78: 31060. Washington, DC: GPO.

Oates K (ed.) (1982): *Child Abuse: A Community Concern.* London: Butterworths.

Otaala B (1981): Day care in eastern Africa: A survey of Botswana, Kenya, Seychelles and the United Republic of Tanzania. Addis Abada: United Nations Economic Commission for Africa.

Peters AD (1976): A plan for the health care of children. In: *Child Care: A Comprehensive Guide* Vol. II, Chapter 7, Auerbach S (ed.). New York: Human Sciences Press.

Pettygrove W, Whitebook M, Weir M (1984): Beyond babysitting: Changing the treatment and image of child care givers. *Young Children,* 39: 14–21.

Pickering LK et al (1981): Diarrhea caused by shigella, rotavirus and giardia in day care centers: Prospective study. *J Pediatr,* 90: 51–56.

Provence S, Naylor A, Patterson J (1977): *The Challenge of Day Care.* New Haven: Yale University Press.

Provence S (1982): Infant day care: Relationships between theory and practice. In: *Day Care: Scientific and Social Policy Issues,* Zigler EF, Gordon EW (eds.) Boston: Auburn House.

Ramey CT, Dorval B, Baker-Ward L (1981): Group day care and socially disadvantaged families: Effects on the child and the family. In: *Advances in Early Education and Day Care,* Kilmer S (ed.). New York: JAI Press.

Richmond JB, Janis JM (1982): Health care services for children in day care programs. In: *Day Care: Scientific and Social Policy Issues,* Zigler EF, Gordon EW (eds.) Boston: Auburn House.

Robinson NM et al (1979): *A World of Children: Day Care and Preschool Institutions.* Monterey, CA: Brooks/Cole.

Roby P (1973): *Child Care: Who Cares? Foreign and Domestic Infant and Early Childhood Development Policies.* New York: Basic Books.

Schweinhart LJ, Weikart DD (1980): Young children grow up: The effects of the Perry Preschool Program on youths through age 15. High/Scope Educational Research Foundation, Monograph No. 7, Ypsilanti, Michigan: The High/Scope Press.

Sealey DP, Schumann SL (1983): Endemic giardiasis and day care. *Pediatrics, 72:* 154–158.

Select Panel for the Promotion of Child Health (1981): Better health for our children: A national strategy Vol. II, Analysis and Recommendations for Selected Federal Programs. The U.S. Department of Health and Human Services. Washington, DC: GPO.

Sidel R (1972): *Women and Child Care in China.* Baltimore, MD: Viking-Penguin.

Silva RJ (1980): Hepatitis and the need for adequate standards in federally supported day care. *Child Welfare, 60:* 387–400.

Socialist Child Care Cooperative (1976): *Changing Child Care: Cuba, China and The Challenging of Our Own Values.* London: Writers and Readers Publishing Cooperative.

Sommers PA (1982): Day care, public education and exceptional children. *Early Child Dev Care, 10:* 29–40.

State of California, Health and Welfare Agency, Department of Social Services (1982): Manual of policies and procedures: Family day care homes for children. Title 22, Division 6, Chapter 8.5. Sacramento, CA: Department of Social Services.

State of California, Health and Welfare Agency (1984): Facing the facts: A parent's guide to the understanding of child sexual abuse. Sacramento, CA: Department of Social Services.

State of California, Health and Welfare Agency, Department of Social Services (1984): Manual of Policies and Procedures: Child Care Centers. Title 22, Division 6, Chapter 2. Sacramento, CA: Department of Social Services.

Steinfels MO (1973): *Who's Minding the Children: The History and Politics of Day Care in America.* New York: Simon and Schuster.

Strangert K (1976): Respiratory illness in preschool children with different forms of day care. *Pediatrics, 57* (2): 191–196.

Suransky VP (1982): *The Erosion of Childhood.* Chicago: University of Chicago Press.

The Child Day Care Infectious Disease Study Group (1984): Public health considerations of infectious diseases in child day care centers. *J Pediatr, 105:* 683–701.

U.S. Department of Commerce, Bureau of the Census (1984): Money income of households, families and persons in the United States: 1983. *Current Population Reports,* Consumer Income, Ser P-60, No. 149, Washington, DC: GPO.

U.S. Department of Health, Education, and Welfare (1972): Medicaid: Early and periodic screening, diagnosis and treatment for individuals under 21, PRG-21 SRS, Medical Services Administration.

U.S. Department of Health and Human Services (1981): The status of handicapped children in Head Start programs. Washington, DC: Office of Human Development Services, Administration for Children, Youth and Families, Head Start Bureau, p. 21. U.S. Department of Labor. Bureau of Labor Statistics (1985) Unpublished Data Current Population Survey.

U.S. Department of Labor, Women's Bureau (August, 1982): Employers and child care: Establishing services through the workplace. Pamphlet 23, LAB-441, Washington, DC: GPO.

U.S. Department of Health and Human Services. (October, 1984): Early and periodic screening, diagnosis and treatment program. *Federal Register, 49* (212): 43654–43667.

Whitebook M, Ginsberg G (1983): Warning: Child care work may be hazardous to your health. *Day Care and Early Education, 11:* 22–26.

Whitebook M et al (1982): Caring for the caregivers: Staff burnout in child care settings. In: *Current Topics in Early Childhood Education,* Vol. IV, Katz L (ed.). Norwood, NJ: Ablex.

APPENDIX: CHILD DAY CARE RESOURCES

Organizations

American Academy of Pediatrics A primary resource on standards for the protection of children's health in child day care. Publications Department, P.O. Box 927, Elk Grove Village, IL 60009-0927, (800) 433-9016.

BANANAS Child Care Information and Referral Maintains files on licensed centers and homes, publishes a newsletter, a questionnaire for parents' evaluation of child day care, and free information handouts and publications in the areas of care for sick children in centers, employer-supported child day care, and identifying and caring for children with special needs. 6501 Telegraph Avenue, Oakland, CA 94609, (415) 658-7353.

Child Care Employee Project A nonprofit support, resource, and educational organization that provides consultations, workshops, and materials focused on improving the status of people working in the child day care field and on child day care working conditions. P.O. Box 5603, Berkeley, CA 94705, (415) 653-9889.

Child Care Law Center A nonprofit legal resource for local, state, and national child day care communities. Publishes a variety of useful handouts. 22 2nd Street, 5th Floor, San Francisco, CA 94105, (415) 495-5498.

Children's Defense Fund A public charity organization that sponsors a nationwide network of advocates who monitor Congress and sponsor bills around the issues of child day care, nutrition, child abuse, education, welfare, and other issues of importance to children and their families. 122 C Street NW, Suite 400, Washington, DC 20001, (202) 628-8787.

National Association for the Education of Young Children A nonprofit association representing people in a diverse range of services to young children throughout the United States. 1834 Connecticut Avenue NW, Washington, DC 20009, (800) 424-2460.

National Black Child Development Institute A nonprofit, national, charitable, educational organization dedicated to improving the quality of life for Black children. 1463 Rhode Island Avenue NW, Washington, DC 20005, (202) 387-1281.

Resources for Infant Educarers A nonprofit organization that publishes *Resources for Infant Educarers (RIE Manual); Educaring,* a quarterly publication mailed to members of the association, and provides parent-infant guidance classes, training courses in skills in working with parents and infants, and workshops and films. 1500 Murray Circle, Los Angeles, CA 90026, (213) 663-5330.

Publications

Beginning Books A book series written for teachers of young children. P.O. Box 2890, Redmond, WA 98073, (206) 883-9394.

Child Care Information Exchange A publication for child day care center directors. P.O. Box 2890, Redmond, WA 98073, (206) 883-9394.

Day Care and Early Education A publication on issues in working with young children. 72 Fifth Avenue, New York, NY 10011, (212) 243-6000.

School Age Notes A publication for child day care staff who work with school-age children. P.O. Box 120674, Nashville, TN 37212, (615) 292-4957.

Texas Child Care Quarterly A publication that covers many topics in child day care from infants to adolescents. Some of the articles are written in Spanish. Corporate Child Development Fund for Texas, 4029 Capital of Texas Highway South, Suite 102, Austin, TX 78704, (512) 440-8555.

Young Children A publication of the National Association for the Education of Young Children. NAEYC, 1834 Connecticut Avenue NW, Washington, DC 20009, (800) 424-2460.

Zero to Three A publication from the National Clinical Center for Clinical Infant Programs, 733 15th Street NW, Suite 912, Washington, DC 20005, (202) 347-0308.

CHILD DAY CARE

By Betty L. Highley

The photographs in this gallery are from a documentary study of child care that has been in progress since 1982. The central question was: Is the philosophy of care visible?

This study was the first in the evolution of Visual Media Research. The design, simulated qualitative field work, carried with it the expectation that design, methodology, and analysis issues would be illuminated. The search for the visibility of philosophy of care was as much a way to learn more about the use of photography for study purposes as it was to learn about child care.

Over 1500 photographs were taken over an eight month period. Content analysis of the proofs led to the identification of the visible concepts.

Several procedures were used to address the need for verification and to create a model for future research. Selected images were presented to a panel of experts in child day care and early childhood education. Their readings of the photographs indicated that philosophy of care was, indeed, visually perceptible.

The collection of photographs has served as a baseline data bank fulfilling a number of purposes, including comparative studies. The work has been extended to encompass several countries, including Israel, Egypt, China, and Denmark. Centers caring for children of families of similar socioeconomic status have been sampled. Cultural values and strategies in early child day care designed to transmit these values became visually apparent. This work is still in progress.

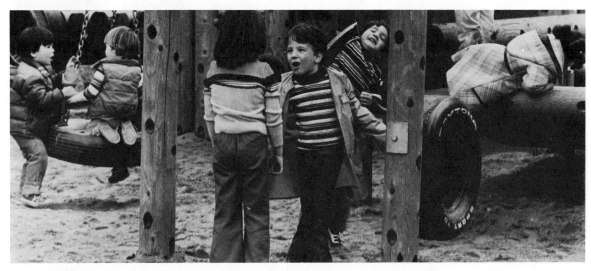

Funding for the study on the Marilyn Reed Lucia Child Care Center came from the Van Loben Sels Foundation in San Francisco.

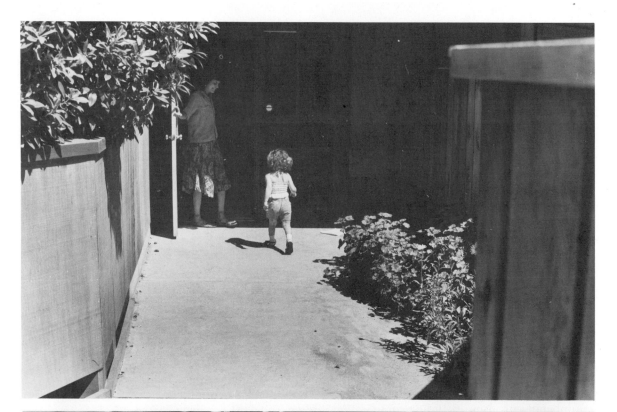

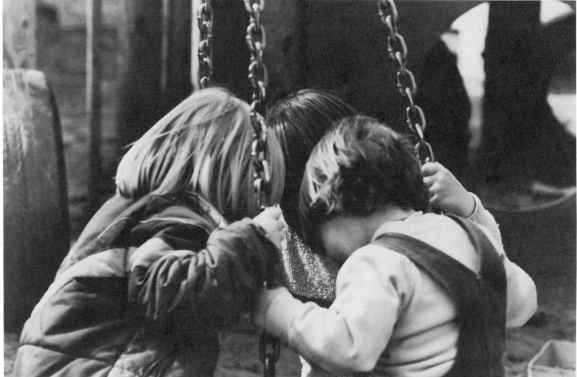

Intimacy

1–2

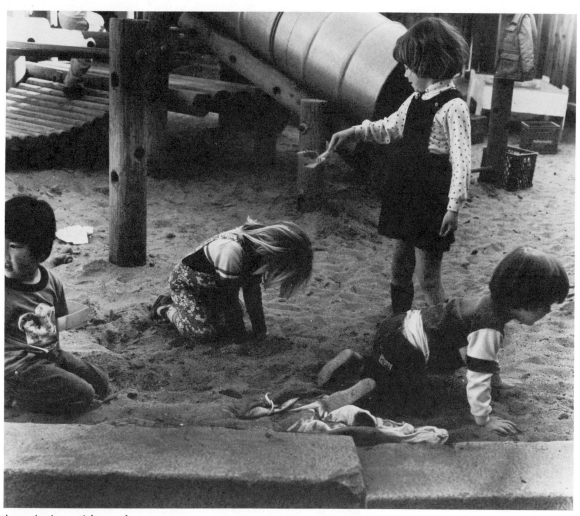

Annointing with sand

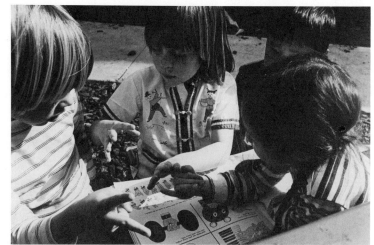

Learning signing through self-directed play

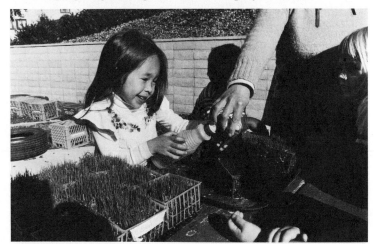

Growing grass for Easter baskets

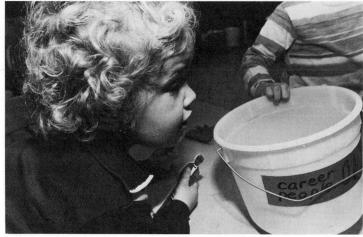

Structured play

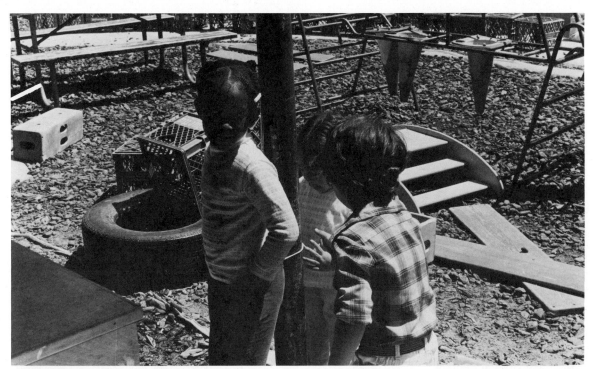

The hostage

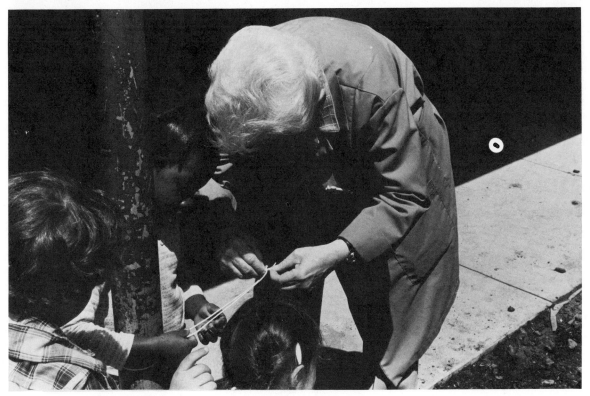

Intervention when needed

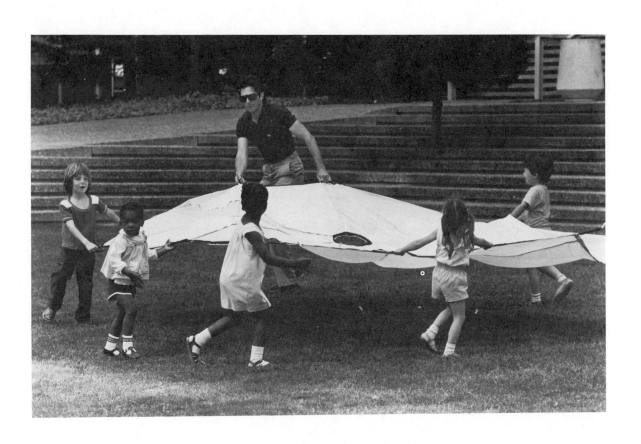

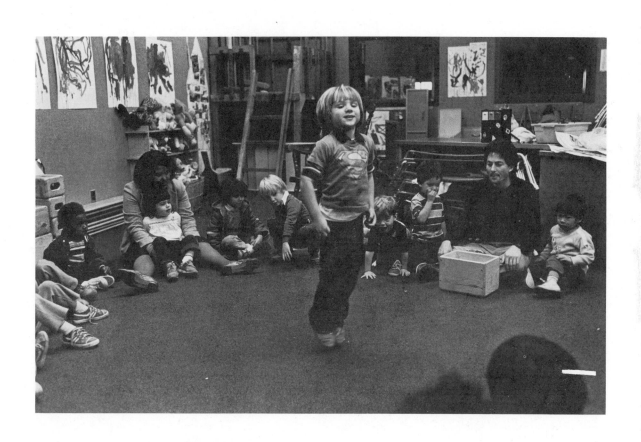

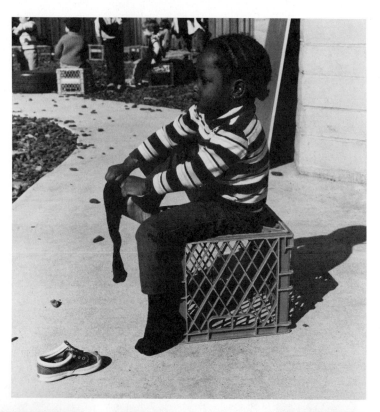

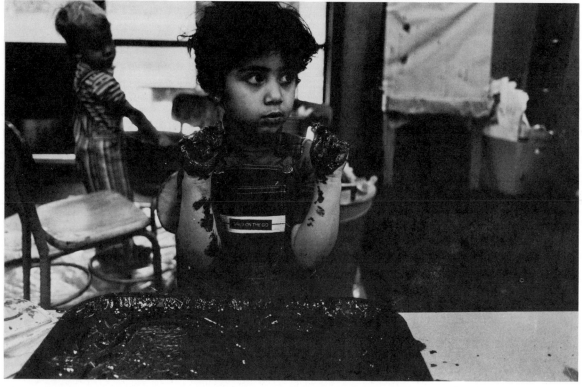

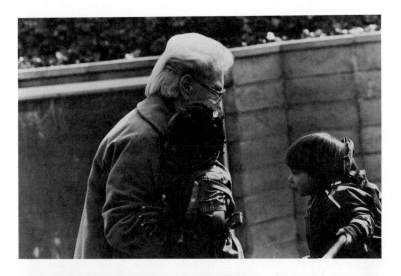

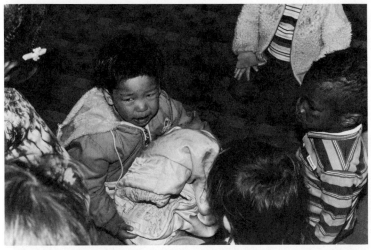

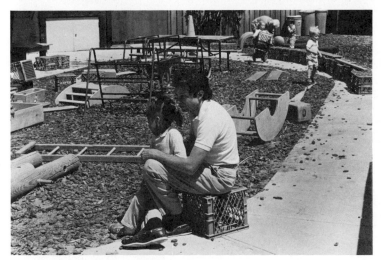

Nurturance and empathy

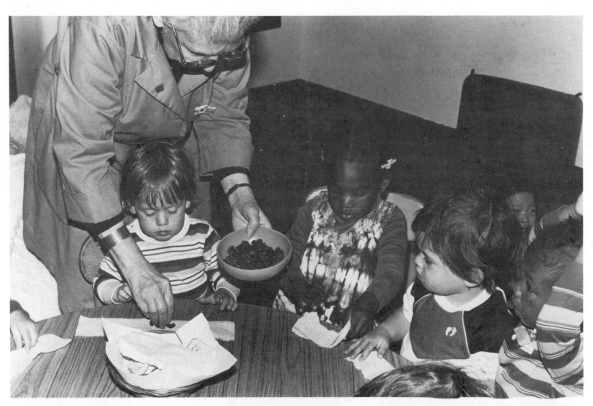

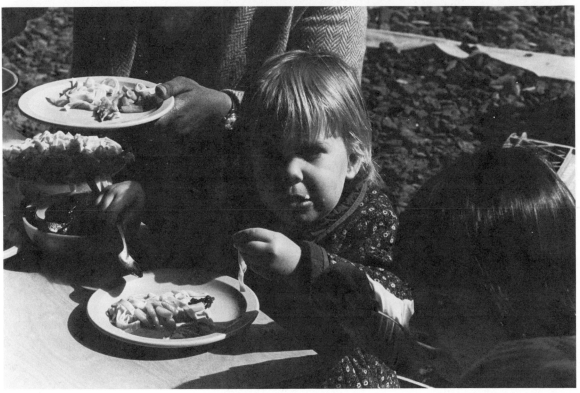

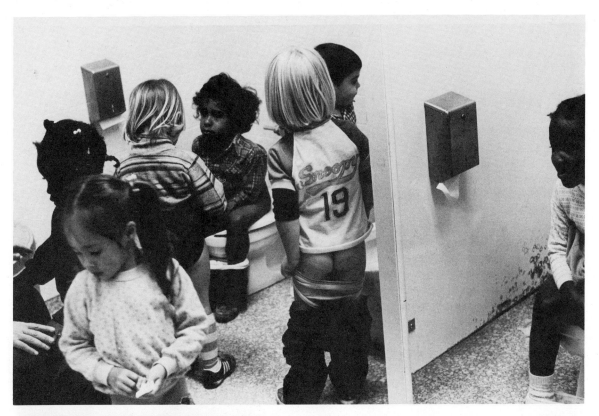

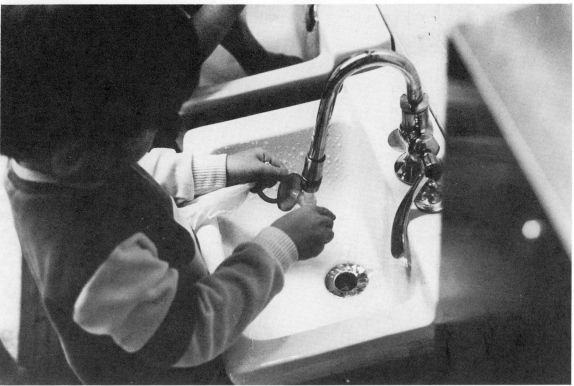

Preparing for naptime

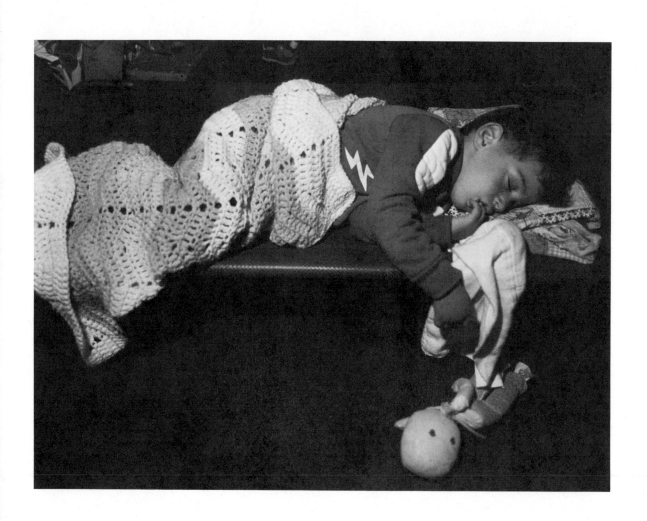

16

THE FAMILY WITH A HOSPITALIZED CHILD

Carol Hardgrove, MA

Brenda M. Roberts, RN, MS

Knowledge about the need for family support during a hospital stay and about the dangers of separation has influenced institutions and parents to increase the level of parents' involvement in the hospitalization of their children. This chapter discusses the history of family involvement with the hospitalized child, including a presentation of the early studies showing the negative effects of separation, the transition to a more enlightened period, and the current trends.

Carol Hardgrove is Clinical Professor Emeritus at the University of California at San Francisco School of Nursing. Known for her work with other health care professionals to emphasize family support of children during hospitalization, she was a pioneer in the development of programs for parent involvement in the care of their hospitalized children. She is the co-author of Parents and Children in the Hospital: The Family's Role in Pediatrics.

Introduction

A walk through a pediatric unit today gives a different view from that of 20 years ago. Where there is an infant or preschooler, there is usually a rocking chair with someone special to hold the child or keep him or her company. The relationship between family and staff has changed from adversarial to collegial. It is more informal, and parents are more likely to be consulted than interrogated. The young child alone in the hospital is cause for concern, and efforts are made to help the parent who is unwilling or unable to be with a youngster. It is recognized that not only is the child's health in jeopardy but the family unit is jeopardized as well. Bonding is a two-way street, requiring communication and interplay among all members, especially in time of crisis. When a child is hospitalized, the entire family is affected and needs to be involved. Knowledge about the need for family support and stimulation during a hospital stay and about the dangers of separation has moved institutions and parents to change. This revolution brings new attitudes, architecture, role descriptions, and definitions to the concept of health care. The word *patient* includes the family. *Family* includes significant others, related by blood or not. The nurse's role includes teaching and supporting the family, and the site of care delivery extends to home, school, and community. It is gratifying to note that there are successful programs that incorporate these new dimensions. These programs evolved from a coalition between families and professionals, and were forged in response to professional education about the family and to consumer groups joining together, often in indignation at being excluded from their own children's care, first to demand and later to assist in creating humanistic settings and policies within the health care system.

History

In 1971 Hardgrove received a World Health Organization Travel Study grant to examine family inclusive policies and facilities in England, Sweden, and Denmark. In the office of the Chief Nursing Officer in the Ministry of Health in London was an engraving of the children's ward of Great Ormand Street, the world's first pediatric hospital. Children dressed in fashions of the day were playing: A little girl in the foreground was astride a rocking horse, and a boy in the background played with a train. Beside each child was a hoop-skirted mother, and nurses busied themselves in the background. "This was the scene when Great Ormand opened its doors," the Nursing Officer told me. "But within 10 years, all that spirit was gone. Children were restricted to their beds and all the mums were banished."

"What happened?" this author asked.

"I'm afraid it was our Ms. Nightingale," was the answer. Families were excluded to prevent the spread of contagion and to maintain discipline and quiet.

"A mother should never be allowed to remain on the ward and thus demoralize the discipline of the hospital and the other children," warned a 1907 text. How many thousands of children's lives were saved by the new knowledge of contagion and antisepsis? Certainly no one wanted to return to the former pest houses. However, new dangers to children caused by separation became apparent as children were hospitalized.

Levy (1945) noted three stages of adjustment to the hospital situation where children were hospitalized without a parent: protest, despair, and denial. During the period of protest, which lasted a few hours to several days, children cried loudly, shook their cribs, threw themselves about, and rejected the nurses. Despair was characterized by longing for the mother, combined with a hopeless feeling that the child would never see her again. During this period, the child withdrew from the ward personnel. During the period of denial, the child superficially showed more interest in the surroundings and even appeared happy. This was taken as an encouraging sign by the staff: in former days it was called settling in, yet actually it indicated that the child was resigned to the situation, suppressing feelings of grief and fear. In the 1940s, it was a common practice in pediatric hospitals to forbid the parents to visit for a month in order to encourage a process of "settling in."

Bowlby et al (1951) wrote:

> Essential for the infant is a warm, intimate, and continuous relationship with mother in which both find satisfaction and enjoyment. Prolonged deprivation of young children of maternal care may have grave and far-reaching effects on his character and so on the whole of his future life. A bad home is better than a good institution.

Douglas et al found in 1975 that repeated hospitalizations correlated to family discord and posthospital pathology of disturbed and delinquent behavior and difficulty in learning. Prugh et al found in 1953 that despite the kindest nursing care, children younger than four years of age, without a parent to accompany them, misinterpreted their surroundings, assumed that the hospital events were punishment, and reacted with regression, hostility, withdrawal, or apathy (Prugh, Jordan, 1975). On return home, the child may have expressed his or her disturbance with temper tantrums, clinging, and regression. Although numerous studies documented the importance of the maternal–child bond for infants and young children, few studies focused on the importance of the bond to the mother and family and to the long-term disruption that could occur to a family deprived of contact. Many parents inferred from the enforced separation that they were inadequate to care for their own child. In many families, bonds were not only broken, they were never formed (Lozoff et al, 1977).

The work of Robertson and Robertson in London dramatically brought attention to the plight of parents and young children separated during hospitalization (Robertson, 1970). Robertson went onto the wards with a movie camera and filmed scenes that demonstrated children's protest, grief, and withdrawal and posthospital behavior. In 1956, the Department of Health in Britain studied arrangements for children in hospitals in response to the need for a change in policy. The recommendations of this committee were published in 1959 in a report entitled, "The Welfare of Children in Hospital," known as the Plat report. In 1961 Robertson's film "A Two-Year-Old Goes to the Hospital" was shown on television, and a series of newspaper articles were written in which Robertson urged parents to unite to push for changes in hospital policies. Under his guidance, a group of mothers organized, calling themselves "Mother Care for Children in Hospitals." They surveyed hospitals, both those that admitted parents with their child and those that did not, and worked to persuade hospitals that childcare with the parent was worthwhile and workable. Meanwhile, they informed parents through public meetings, posters, and advertising of the parents' important role in the care of their sick children. Mother Care's contact with the Ministry of Health and with individual professionals led to a name change for the organization. In 1965 it became the National Association for the Welfare of Children in Hospitals (NAWCH), a name reflecting its change in membership, which now included professional staff workers. NAWCH continues to offer public information, educational conferences, and supervision of hospitals to ensure that the policies of preparation and support are enforced. NAWCH has maintained close links with the Association for the Care of Children's Health in the United States since that group's formation in 1965.

In 1965 Meadow interviewed mothers regarding their feelings about staying in the hospital with their sick children. Boredom, she found, was prevalent, and boredom made many normal emotions and worries loom larger than they ordinarily would. But she found that mothers in the hospital worry less about the sick child than if they had stayed home. Their major complaint was lack of information; this exacerbated their worry and resentment. Parental fears were sometimes difficult for staff to identify with, but the staff did discover that answering questions and finding time to listen to concerns reduced the anxiety. Parents' principal complaints were that they were not told the results of tests. They worried until their requests for information were heard and answered. Many mothers felt too ill at ease to demand more information. Some felt themselves to be on trial, guilty, and responsible. Inadequately oriented to care and procedures, they often hesitated even to touch their own child. But despite these difficulties, mothers who stayed usually gained confidence and reported a better posthospital adjustment on their return home (Meadow, 1969).

Fagin, a nurse educator and a mother, stayed with her own child in the hospital and following that experience wrote the article, "Why not involve parents when children are hospitalized?," advocating the usefulness of parents in their child's care both during the hospital stay and following it (Fagin, 1962). Plank (1962) discussed the importance to the children at home (especially if a twin) of keeping in close touch with the child in the hospital. Most research, however, focused on the hospitalized child. Not until recently has much attention been paid to the adverse effects on the burgeoning family of separating members from each other at such a stressful and sensitive time as hospitalization of a family member.

Transition

As the plight of the hospitalized child became dramatized and publicized, a mounting body of literature urged hospitals to become healthy environments for children. The Association for the Care of Children in Hospitals (ACCH) was founded in the early 1960s by educationalists who were developing a few play programs. The focus was on more interesting environments, preparation, play, education, and activity programs (ACCH, 1985). Nurses donned colored smocks and in some hospitals, they wore street clothes. Volunteers came through the ward with toy carts. Playrooms opened, although they were not always supervised or equipped. Parents were still discouraged, however, and little in the way of preparation or education about their children's state was routinely offered.

When the idea of allowing parents to visit was broached in one hospital, a supervisor said, "We're too crowded now. What would it be like with all those parents?" It was shown that despite the hordes of doctors, students, technicians, nurses, volunteers, foster grandparents, social workers, dietitians, and visiting entertainers, children unaccompanied by parents averaged 20 minutes of procedure-free attention in a 24-hour period. Individual attention for purposes of companionship was, therefore, minimal.

Studies showed that the best way to reduce stress and prepare an infant or young child for the hospital experience was to prepare the parent (Skipper, Leonard, 1968). Parents given information about what their child would experience and what was expected of the parents were found to be more cooperative; their children were better adjusted; and their posthospital recovery was smoother, with fewer questions back to the hospital than those not so prepared. Wolfer and Visintainer (1975) indicated that short orientations to parents at particular stress points rather than a longer orientation in the beginning reduced anxiety and increased cooperative behavior both of parents and of children.

Franklin (1976) aptly describes how, in making procedures the priority for care, hospitals become antifamily in orientation. Although not intended, routines create indifference, and "human needs are grafted onto the procedures rather than vice versa." He asks that we meet the challenge of adapting routines to meet patient needs. For example, Mrs. J, rooming in with her 2-year-old daughter, had finally gotten her child to sleep after a restless, fretful night. At 5:30 AM the child was awakened by the nurse to be weighed, a task the mother could have performed at a more appropriate time, if allowed.

McCarthy, an English pediatrician who was convinced by Robertson's work, began admitting family members with young patients and wrote an article describing his program (McCarthy, Londsay, Morris, 1962). For nurses unaccustomed to children's normal reactions of protest and grief, it appeared that parents upset their children and were consequently bad for them. Limited to proscribed and sparse visiting hours, children either sobbed and screamed when parents left or pretended to ignore them, thus giving nurses who were not schooled in normal child behavior the impression that the children could be better cared for in a calmer, more professional style. As one nurse in McCarthy's hospital said:

> There's only one way I would have changed my attitude toward the parents. That was with the direct order from the Chief that parents be brought in. It was only after I saw the difference in the children in the ward, saw children acting alive, saw how much more quickly they recovered, that I became a convert. In all the hospitals that have opened up their doors to parents, the nurses feel this way. We had thought we were giving excellent care, and we were, excellent *nursing* care. We didn't realize because we hadn't seen the difference that mother care made. Having seen it, we would never go back. We were worried that there wouldn't be enough room. Now we know the room is in your head.

Change of Focus

The Association for Care of Children in Hospitals, an organization founded and dedicated to humanizing health care for children, at first fo-

cused primarily on the child. In the early conference program indexes, the word *family* was not mentioned once. The transitional period saw a change of focus to the family. The 20th program index, in 1986, listed *family* 89 times as the subject of workshops, speeches, and roundtables.

Research indicating that the young child suffered as much from sensory deprivation and inactivity as from the separation from the family led to the hiring of more play staff or other parent substitutes. In the early phase of the transition movement, consideration focused on the child's need for play, education, and preparation. Play staff, social workers, nurses, and volunteers directed their activities in these areas. There were preparation puppet shows conducted by volunteers, tours of the hospital with play hospital sessions for preschool and kindergarten children, and all manner of well-meaning visitors, often in costume. When possible, companionship was provided by volunteers, students, foster grandparents, or paid sitters. Parents were not yet considered able or willing to spend much time with their children. Consequently, the corridors in many institutions were teeming with people even as parents were restricted to specific short hours. It was generally assumed family members would not be suitable for the tasks necessary for psychologic support.

Consumer Groups as a Change Force

Some of the pressure for change has come from consumer groups—usually mothers—who are often disgruntled about the rebuff they encountered in the hospital. La Leche League, an organization for breastfeeding mothers, formed out of their membership an organization called Children In Hospitals (CIH) to bring hospital policies in the Boston region into line with good child development practice. Originally their concern was for breastfeeding mothers who had to hospitalize their children and who were then told they were not allowed to be present, so the child had to be weaned abruptly. CIH now works to convince hospital professionals that parents should be informed before admission or on admission of the psychologic hazards that face the unsupported, inactive young child in the hospital.

CIH surveyed institutions in the region regarding family-inclusive policies. Their surveys helped communicate ideas and information among the hospitals and resulted in numerous changes. Hospitals—discovering that other hospitals in their same area had very different policies and were admitting parents, conducting sibling programs, and so forth—quickly modified their own policies. Meanwhile, CIH's newsletter kept parents informed about various policies and about the parents' experience and advice. Like a number of consumer advocate networks that started out in an adversarial stance, CIH is now viewed by the local hospitals as a valuable ally. Representatives of CIH serve on the hospitals' parent advisory boards and consult regarding hospital design as well as other topics.

Parent Programs as a Change Force

In 1967 only 28 of the 5000 general hospitals in the United States had any facilities for parents to spend the night with their child. Of the 132 children's hospitals, only 20 permitted living-in and, of these, 15 admitted only mothers from upper socioeconomic groups (Haller, Talbert, Dombro, 1967). A follow-up study conducted in 1978 (Hardgrove, Kermoian, 1984) identified a gap between research-based rationale encouraging parents to stay with their hospitalized child and the style of implementing "living-in" programs. Results of the survey indicated that institutional support of parental presence was, for the most part, limited to providing beds. There were almost no facilities for well children to play while parents visited, and cooking for the hospitalized child or eating with the child was forbidden. Few hospitals provided services for psychologic and family support or helped with parent-to-parent peer support groups. This sur-

vey was conducted with only a sample of those hospitals who responded to a questionnaire by expressing positive regard for their philosophy of and accommodations for family-centered care. Answers to questionnaires revealed that parents were barred from supporting their child during the most stressful as well as the most homelike routines, such as administering treatments or eating together; siblings were excluded from the pediatric unit, and few hospitals made any proviso for their care in other areas of the hospital. Large signs were prominently posted saying, "No one under the age of 14 allowed." This was despite the 1971 recommendation of the American Academy of Pediatrics (AAP) (1971) that the hospital should provide facilities and attitudes to promote the well-being both of the parents and of the child. The Academy's report recognized the need for continuing contact of the pediatric patient with his or her parents and recommended generous visiting privileges. The need for contact with siblings and other children was also recognized and supported.

The AAP (1971) stated, "For a child to leave the hospital emotionally impaired is a serious failure of professional responsibility." The AAP proposed that in order to avoid emotional damage, hospitals should offer liberal visiting hours and overnight parent facilities and should change rules to allow children to visit. The American Civil Liberties Union (Annas, 1975) contends that barring parents from accompanying the child is an infringement of the informed consent. How can parents assess the child's condition if they are not with the child to observe?

During the transitional period, several versions of parent programs emerged. A Kentucky pediatrician had observed pediatric care in Japan during the war and had been impressed with the calm he observed when mothers sat by the bedside of each child. He wondered how effective it would be to have parents stay with their child and at the same time involve themselves in their own child's care. The Japanese mothers just sat; the nurses performed the care activities. When this doctor returned to Kentucky, he opened a care-by-parent unit with the idea that certain patients could be better and more economically cared for by parents and that parents could master some concepts of health and care that would be needed on the child's discharge. The unit was located on the pediatric floor between the outpatient clinic and the pediatric unit. It was manned by childcare aides, with the clinic physician and nurse making daily rounds. A telephone connected the unit to 24-hour emergency service. Parents had an apartment with a bedroom with enough sleeping space for family members, including the husband and a sibling, and a bathroom. The care-by-parent unit had a living/play room and a kitchen where parents cooked for themselves and their child. They were also responsible for administering their child's medications and escorted their child to other parts of the hospital for needed tests. The families in residence were mostly from Appalachia, people who lived far from health care facilities and would never have permitted treatment that required separation (Hardgrove, Dawson, 1972).

On the top floor of the old Boston floating hospital was a tuberculosis unit that was no longer needed; it became the Family Participation Unit (Hardgrove, Dawson, 1972). This was a modified care-by-parent program in that a nurse was present at all times during the day with a hot line to the rest of the hospital for night emergencies. There was also a part-time social worker affiliated with the unit and available for parents. Not all of the child's care was expected to be given by the parents in the Family Participation Unit, and parents were supervised and taught by the nurse before they did take over. This unit too had a room for the family, and there was no hospital furniture in the room. There was a laundry room, a common room that served both as a center for health services and as a place for parents to congregate, a kitchen, and a common bath.

Still another type of care was care-through-parent or care-with-parent, where parents were welcomed as supporters or companions of their child, and the nursing care was the responsibility of the nursing staff, who evaluated the parents' desire and ability to give care and then provided individualized supervision to enable them to do so. Programs like these were more informal, more common, and no special services, other than perhaps a mat, rollaway, or cot to sleep on, were offered. A few hospitals that wanted to encourage parents to come offered beds for them and created a special staff position for a care provider for parents. The nurse responsible for parents was called the Parent Living-In Coordinator.

Children's Hospital in Boston used the services of the adjacent motel, The Children's Inn, as a place where parents could stay. There was a nursing station on each floor and a connection to the hospital. Many of these programs were short lived, partly because of economics, partly because there was not yet a whole-hearted dedication, and partly because parents themselves had not yet become convinced or able to rearrange their lives and come and stay with their child, especially because there were few services available for the care of healthy siblings. A few hospitals offered professional assistance to families, hiring a special advocate for them. A gap still remained in terms of educating families preadmission that their child really needed them and that there was space for them. Allowing parents to stay with the sick child came quite a while before encouraging, inviting, and assisting them to stay.

Changing Perceptions of Families and Hospitals

Ideally the pediatric unit should offer a community of caring for the child patient. The staff should be encouraged to view parents as part of the family, as well as a valuable resource. This community of caring could begin with presence of the family on the unit. Parent education raises awareness of the parents' role but nothing is as motivating as direct observation of other parents participating in their child's care. For staff, the forced proximity to parents helps the parents to be known as individuals. Gradually, routines develop to maximize the usefulness of the family, whether as helpers or just as a supportive presence.

Before the care-through-parent program began at one hospital, parents waited outside the unit until 2 o'clock, when visiting hours officially began. While they waited, they talked to each other. Some of the staff members held these conversations in contempt, referring to them as "misinformation swaps." Today these exchanges are valued and used. Out of the grapevine networks of support and learning are fashioned. Staff encourages these parent-to-parent confidences and information swaps by having regularly scheduled coffee meetings, by helping parents network with other parents and by giving individual interviews. Orienting family members at the beginning of their stay is a great help in preventing the misinformation swaps (Hardgrove, Healy, 1984).

Parents, under the stresses of emergency, exhaustion, and worry, can be overwhelmed. Left to cope on their own, a family can shatter under the impact, each member expecting more from an equally overwhelmed partner, if there is one, than that person can give. At such times staff can serve as an extended family, supporting and enhancing the clinical role, helping without pushing until the family recovers and can resume some measure of support for their child with the knowledge that help is available. Parents can remain involved and take credit for and satisfaction in parenting while part of their load is shouldered by other caring people.

During this transitional phase, not every department in the hospital changed its perception of the family all at once. For example, during one stage of the transition in a large teaching hospital, the nurses and parents good-naturedly collaborated in a small masquerade. Parents were forbidden to accompany their child to several departments in the hospital, x-ray for example. Children, the rule stated, were to be accompanied only by a nurse, a volunteer, or a foster grandparent. The nurses therefore kept a volunteer smock in the nurses' station for any parent who wished to go with the child to x-ray. The following example from the same hospital shows one way of empowering parents through consciously bridging the gap between the health care system and the family system. During preadmission orientation for a cardiac catheterization for a 2-year-old girl, the pediatric cardiologist prepared the mother and child to expect many examinations and questions. He explained that the redundancy was because the hospital was a teaching hospital and asked her cooperation in assisting his residents and students to learn. However, he also gave her permission to protect her daughter, if need be, by asking that such examinations be paced according to the child's tolerance. If the mother sensed the child had had enough, she could ask the resident to come back later.

Family Adjustment

What happens to the family of the hospitalized child? What happens to the siblings when a brother or sister is critically ill in the hospital and taking the parents' time and attention? Payne reports on families with a child in treatment for cancer (Payne, 1981). She asked parents about the adjustment of siblings. Parents reported problems such as depressive withdrawal, school difficulties, and reluctance to see a doctor. Many families did not know how the children were coping. Parents were having such problems themselves that they did not notice their childrens' problems. Payne's study also showed that the longer the child was in treatment, the greater the chance of marital problems.

The influence of fathers, an area neglected by research, was found to be equally important. At an Atlanta hospital that pioneered rooming-in, fathers stayed overnight with their children as frequently as mothers (Shore, 1970). Fathers were not invited or expected as routinely as other family members, but when they were invited, they usually came.

Studies illustrate the need for communication with the family. Korsch (1978) notes that compliance with treatment following discharge is correlated positively with open family communication and support. Noncompliance correlates with poor patterns of family communication. The communication style of the health care staff strongly influences these patterns within the family.

Current Trends

Family Support

The United States lags behind many countries in providing for family support. There are few organizations that have paternity leave policies, and there has been little research in this area. There is no national policy (as there is in England) requiring a certain number of parent beds for every child bed on the unit, and there is no general policy granting sick leave to workers when a child is ill or hospitalized. The gap between the nation's economic and social policies and family health care needs is great. Several excellent care-through-parent programs have been discontinued.

Hospital Design

New hospitals frequently do not have facilities for parents. Increased building costs make space for parents a premium most hospitals cannot afford. On the other hand, a growing trend in hospital design gives the child and family a sense of mastery. St. Louis Children's Hospital, for example, has an entrance with an outdoor walk bordered by shrubs leading to an ordinary door that opens onto an intimate space decorated in soft colors. A low, curved counter allows child and receptionist to see each other. Only one or two strangers are there to serve as

receptionist and to direct patient and family to the appropriate service. This design gives the child a favorable initial impression of the hospital. The pediatric units have a parent chair-bed for every patient bed in a pleasant room with window seats. There are several circular, glass-enclosed playrooms. The large parent lounge has a number of couches and chairs, and there is a shower and toilet basin for parents.

Separate Housing for Parents There is a growing number of "living-in" houses affiliated with and contiguous to hospitals. There are now, for example, over 100 Ronald McDonald Houses in the United States. These houses allow entire families to be together in a home-like environment in close proximity to the sick member. In San Francisco, a group of professionals and parents of children with cancer formed a board to purchase a large building, which is now known as the Koret Family House, adjacent to the Moffitt–Long Hospitals. Koret Family House is not part of the hospital, but the links are very strong. The house has a library with books and videotapes to help families understand cancer. It has playrooms and rooms for families to be together. There is a kitchen and an eating area on each of the three floors. A core of volunteers is available to families.

The need for Koret Family House is so great and the appeal of it is so strong that the house thrives, and in 1986, at the invitation of the hospital administration and pediatricians at UCSF, the Koret Family House board was approached to explore creation of a Family House Annex on the pediatric floor itself. The design that evolved allows the conversion of two spaces that are used by day for other purposes plus one room that is designed solely for the use of parents to sleep and shower. This participation by Family House helps the University in its plans to design space that is receptive to families at a time when financial realities severely limit building funds. Family House designated space directly on the pediatric unit with salary assistance for a person to serve as parent coordinator or concierge–host to facilitate maximum support for the family and to troubleshoot for the program. Families will still be welcome across the street at Family House. Those who prefer to stay in the unit may use Family House to do their laundry, use the library, or drop in to relax and chat, but they will also have accommodation at the hospital

The Child Life Movement

In 1965 a small group of teachers, now known as child-life workers, organized the Association for the Care of Children in Hospitals now known as the Association for the Care of Children's Health (ACCH). They joined together to form a support network for professionals in all disciplines concerned about children's emotional health and well-being during hospital care. This group has had tremendous impact on humanizing health care. Chief among the contributions of the ACCH has been their assistance in facilitating communication among those people who wish to make changes in their institutions and those who have developed interesting and effective ways to make such changes. This networking has effectively changed pediatric units so that today pediatric care is assumed to include the family. Various publications can be obtained through the Association.*

The ACCH's checklist for health care facilities summarizes and supports some of the services described in this chapter. They recommend policies that support family togetherness, including the following:

1. Twenty-four-hour visiting rights for parents (some hospitals object to the term *visiting*, in that the parent is not visiting his/her own child)
2. "Rooming-in" accommodations for parents
3. Parent participation in patient care
4. Parents' presence during anesthesia induction and recovery room

*Association for the Care of Children's Health, 3615 Wisconsin Avenue NW, Washington, DC 20016.

5. Sibling visitation whenever possible
6. Preparations for specific procedures, admission to hospital, and return home
7. A child-life program staffed with professionals and an appropriately equipped playroom
8. Out-patient one-day surgery whenever possible
9. Intermediate or step-down units as alternatives to the intensive care unit
10. Supportive design of facilities to enhance comfort
11. Facilities geared to the needs of different age groups and families
12. Ronald McDonald-type housing
13. Ambulatory care as an alternative to hospitalization

The Association's recommendations for health care professionals and educators include development of curricula to specifically address child development, family dynamics, and effective communication skills. Also recommended are greater effort toward cooperation with community agencies to help families cope with extended hospital stays or chronic illness; long-term support for families; respite care; and continuation of schooling. When appropriate, hospice care concepts should be included. The ACCH recommends that parents participate more generally in the child's hospital care and work with parent support groups.

Basic Principles for Family-Centered Care

Farkas (1983) polled 25 experts regarding their recommendations for family-centered care. Following are some of the basic principles for family-centered care. Once again, the predominant need is for information communication. In order to manage their own stress and to comfort their child, parents must have information and help in the hospital.

1. Parents need medical knowledge regarding the child's illness and the treatments. This reduces anxiety and helps parents explain to their child what is happening.

2. Parents must prepare their child for hospitalization and procedures, so they must be prepared themselves.

3. Parents need knowledge about child development and common emotional reactions to illness so they can provide appropriate and practical emotional support.

4. Parents must have access to their children. This includes rooming-in when necessary.

5. Parents must be helped to see how they can bridge hospital, home, and school life for their child. Parents and patients must be given as much control as is medically possible. In the emergency room, for example, staff can ask children whether they want their parents to come with them or not.

6. Hospitals must recognize their role in treating the whole child; there must be someone in administration who understands the importance of this approach and incorporates it into the institution.

7. Hospitals must directly and indirectly address the stress parents experience.

8. There must be provisions for parents to help each other, as with self-help groups.

9. Family involvement does not just mean mothers and fathers. The child's relationship with siblings and extended family members must be considered.

10. There must be attention to cultural differences and individual situations of families.

11. There must be a systematic way for parents to have input into policy and practice decisions through advisory committees and evaluation.

The hiring of patient advocates is recommended by the group of experts in the Farkas report. These can be patient representatives or ombudsmen whose job is to help patients and their families negotiate with the hospital system and personnel and coordinate the child's care. Also recommended is continuous in-service training to help staff know what information to provide families, how to communicate effectively with families, and how to involve families in their child's care.

Some of the barriers to institution of family-inclusive policies are a result of staff misconceptions. One study showed that the staff of one hospital believed the reasons for the lack of parental visits were jobs, family responsibilities, or simply lack of interest; when in fact some parents did not visit frequently because they perceived their child as temperamental or difficult, or they felt they were not needed. (Farkas, 1983). Families must be told how important and necessary their presence is to their child's adjustment to the hospital environment.

Still another barrier to optimal care is that only about 10% of children are served in pediatric hospitals; the rest are in pediatric wards of general hospitals. Recently there has been a trend to close pediatric units and admit children to the adult wards, where their unique needs and those of their families are not met.

Summary

There has been a revolution in children's health care during the past twenty years. The pediatric patient is no longer seen as a single entity to be admitted, treated, and returned home. Instead, the child is acknowledged as part of a living family, who needs to continue to function as part of that family.

Parents feel more welcome on pediatric units today; they can form an alliance with the staff for the benefit of the child. There is, however, an added challenge because more parents are in the work force than ever before, and there is not a formal system in this country for homemaker services for the care of the family at home. As a nation, we have not established the assistance other governments offer, such as sick leave when a child is ill, paternity leave, home care for an ill child who must stay home while parents work outside the home.

Families must become active participants in the hospital system; the institutions and their staff are empowered to help families to achieve this goal. The changed view of parent-as-intruder to parent-as-resource has extended the influence of both professionals and parents in creating a circuit of caring.

Issues for Further Investigation

1. What medical and nursing knowledge needs to be given to parents before treatments?

2. How can parents be helped in their preparation of their child and themselves for hospitalization?

3. What are the emotional reactions to various illnesses and treatment regimens?

4. Under what circumstances should parents not be present with their child?

5. What stress management activities should be given to parents?

6. What cultural differences influence the child's hospitalization experience?

References

American Academy of Pediatrics (1971): Care of children in hospitals, pp. 4, 11, 14.

Anderson B (1985a): Parents of handicapped children as collaborators in health care. *Coalition Quarterly, 4*(5): 2–3.

Anderson B (1985b): Impact of a parent advisory committee on hospital design and policy. Federation for Children with Special Needs, 312 Stuart Street, Boston, MA 02116.

Annas GJ (1975): *The Rights of Hospital Patients: The Basic American Civil Liberties Guide to Hospital Patients' Rights.* New York: Avon, pp. 136–144.

Association for the Care of Children in Hospitals (1985): A quiet revolution: The first 20 years. Videotape.

Azarnoff P, Hardgrove C (1981): The family in pediatrics. In: *The Family in Child Health Care,* Azarnoff P, Hardgrove C (eds.). New York: Wiley.

Barnett C et al (1970): Neonatal separation: The maternal side of deprivation. *Pediatrics,* 45: 197–205.

Belson P (1981): Parents advocacy for parents. In: *The Family in Child Health Care,* Azarnoff P, Hardgrove C (eds.). New York: Wiley, pp. 217–231.

Bowlby J, Robertson J, Rosebluth D (1952): A two-year-old goes to the hospital. *Psychoanal Study Child,* 7: 82–94.

Brain DJ, McClay I (1968): Controlled study of mothers and children in hospital. *Br Med J,* 1: 278–280.

Brazelton TB (1976): *Doctor and Child.* London: Allen & Unwin.

Dew T (1977): Parents in the pediatric recovery room. *Assoc Oper Room Nurs J,* 26: 2.

Douglas JWB (1975): Early hospital admissions and later disturbances of behavior and learning. *Dev Med Child Neurol,* 17: 476.

Fagin C (1962): Why not involve parents when children are hospitalized? *Am J Nurs,* 6: 78–79.

Farkas S (1983): The family's role in care and treatment. Family Impact Seminar, National Center for Family Studies, Catholic University of America, Washington, D.C.

Franklin J (1976): Institutional barriers to the family. In: *The Family: Can It Be Saved?,* Vaughn VC, Brazelton TB (eds.). Chicago: Year Book Medical Publishers.

Freiberg K (1977): How parents react when their children are hospitalized. *Am J Nurs, 11*(8): 1270.

Garrand S et al (1978): A parent-to-parent program. *Fam Commun Health, 11:* 103–113.

Green M (1979): Parent care in the ICN. *Am J Dis Child, 133:* 1119–1120.

Green M (1986): Riley hospital. *The Indianapolis News,* September 16, p. 4.

Greenberg M, Morris N (1974): Engrossment: The newborn's impact upon the father. *Am J Orthopsychiatry,* 44: 520.

Haller J, Tralbert J, Dombro R (1967): *The Hospitalized Child and His Family.* Baltimore: Johns Hopkins University Press.

Hardgrove C (1972): Care through parent: Creating space in pediatrics. University of California at San Francisco Media Center. Film.

Hardgrove C, Dawson R (1972): *Parents and Children in the Hospital.* Boston: Little, Brown.

Hardgrove C, Healy D (1984): The care through parent program at Moffitt Hospital, University of California. *Nurs Clin North Am,* 19(1): 145–160.

Hardgrove C, Kermoian R (1984): Parent-inclusive pediatric units: A survey of policies and practices. *Am J Public Health,* 68(9): 847.

Heagarty M (1975): The pediatric clinics: A challenge. *J Assoc Care Child Health,* 3(3): 3–4.

Jones D (1978): Home early after delivery. *Am J Nurs, 8:* 1378–1380.

Kennell J, Trause M, Klaus M (1975): Evidence for a sensitive period in the human mother. Parent–infant interaction, Ciba Foundation Symposium 33, Amsterdam. Essenier, 87–101.

Korsch B (1976): Chronic illness in childhood and family functions. In: *The Family: Can It Be Saved?,* Vaughn VC, Brazelton TB (eds.). Chicago: Year Book Medical Publishers.

Korsch B et al (1978): Non-compliance in children with renal transplants. *Pediatrics,* 61(8): 872–876.

Levy D (1945): Psychic trauma of operations in children. *Am J Dis Child,* 69(7): 7–25.

Lozoff B et al (1977): The mother-newborn relationship: Limits of adaptability. *J Pediatr,* 91(1): 1–12.

Mahaffey P (1964): Nurse-patient relations in living-in situations. *Nurs Forum,* 111(2): 53–64.

Marino B (1980): When nurses compete with parents. *J Assoc Care Child Health,* 8(4): 94–98.

Mason EA (1965): The hospitalized child: His emotional needs. *N Engl J Med, 272:* 406–414.

Mason E (1978): Hospital and family cooperating to reduce psychological trauma. *Community Ment Health J,* 14(2): 153.

McCarthy D, Londsay M, Morris I (1962): Children in the hospital with their mothers. *Lancet, 16:* 306–308.

Meadow SR (1969): The captive mother. *Arch Diseases Child,* 6: 362–367.

Oremland J, Oremland E (1973): *The Effects of Hospitalizations on Children.* Springfield, IL: Charles C Thomas.

Payne J (1981): Family adaptation after death of a child. In: *The Family in Child Health Care,* Azarnoff P., Hardgrove C (eds.). New York: Wiley.

Plank EN (1962): *Working With Children in Hospitals.* Cleveland: Western Reserve Press.

Prugh D, Jordon K (1975): Physical illness or injury: The hospital as a source of emotional disturbance in child and family. In: *Advocacy for Child Mental Health,* Berlin IN (ed.). New York: Brunner/Mazel.

Robertson J (1970): *Young Children in the Hospital.* London: Barnes & Noble.

Schaeffer HR, Callender WM (1959): Psychologic effects of hospitalization in infancy. *Pediatrics,* 24: 528–539.

Shore M (1970): Red is the color of hurting. U.S. HEW, publication no. 583.

Simons W (1985): Loss of parental support: A form of emotional child abuse. In: *Psychological Abuse of Children in Health Care: The Issues,* Azarnoff P, Lindquist P (eds.). Santa Monica: Pediatric Projects.

Skipper JK, Leonard RC (1968): Children, stress, and hospitalization: A field experiment. *J Health Soc Behav,* 9(4): 68.

Solnit A (1960): Hospitalization: An aid to physical and psychological health in childhood. *Am J Dis Child,* 99: 155–163.

Spence JC (1946): *The Purpose of a Family: A Guide to the Care of Children.* London: Epworth.

Spitz R (1945): Hospitalism: An inquiry into the genesis of psychiatric conditions in early childhood. *Psychoanal Stud Child,* 1: 53–74.

Sundstrom-Feigenberg K (1983): Parenthood education: A reform to support the family. Current Sweden, Svenska Institute, Box 7434, S=10391 Stockholm.

Thompson R (1986): Where we stand: 20 years of research on pediatric hospitalization and health care. Children's Health Care, *J Assoc Care Child Health*, Spring, 200–210.

Vernon DTA, Foley JM, Schulman JL (1967): Effects of mother-child separation and birth order on young children's responses to two potentially stressful experiences. *J Pers Soc Psychol*, 5: 162–174.

Vernon DTA et al (1965): *The Psychological Responses of Children to Hospitalization and Illness: A Review of the Literature*. Springfield, IL: Charles C Thomas.

Wolfer JA, Visintainer M (1975): Pediatric surgical patients and parent: Stress responses and adjustment. *Nurs Res*, 24(4): 244–255.

17

TRANSITION TO ILLNESS

The Family in the Hospital

Maribelle B. Leavitt, RN, MS

The family's visibility in the hospital has increased in recent years. From changes that permitted the rooming-in of parents with young hospitalized children in the late 1960s, we now appear to be in an era of family-centered care. Concern for families has become visible in published works; however, the recognition of and response to the problems and concerns of families during hospitalization requires continued attention. This chapter reviews and integrates the findings of recently published health care literature pertaining to the experience of families in the hospital setting

Maribelle Leavitt is a doctoral candidate in the Department of Family Health Care Nursing at the University of California at San Francisco. She has a long-standing career interest in family stress and coping processes with the hospital and major illness. She is the author of Families at Risk: Primary Prevention in Nursing Practice.

Introduction

The family's experience in the hospital has only recently become an issue of concern for health care providers. The increasing attention to the family in the last decade and the relative dearth of family-focused care studies or papers before 1975 has been noted in the more recent literature (Daley, 1984; Feetham, 1983; Leavitt, 1982).

Professional attention to families in the hospital had its first major impetus with the case of the hospitalized child. Family-centered care of the hospitalized child became a major trend by the early 1960s (Hardgrove, Healy, 1984; Shapiro, 1983). The field of family therapy, which emerged in the 1960s, also helped to focus professional attention toward families as units of care for delivery of health care services. Evidence to support the contention that the family should be considered a basic unit of health and medical care in the health care arenas was gathered and critiqued (Litman, 1974). Features of families conducive to health, such as compliance (Schmidt, 1979) and activism or effectiveness (Pratt, 1976), were studied. The role of the family in illness and illness care, the intimate and complex interaction between the ill family member and the rest of the family, and the health care system's ability to effectively respond to families' needs are topics of major critiques and literature reviews (Schwenk, Hughes, 1983; Shapiro, 1983; Young, 1983).

Technologic advances in medical treatment have substantially altered the life–death trajectory for seriously ill patients and their families, ushering in a new host of treatment considerations. These include an increase in serial, episodic admissions in the course of a chronic illness (Ferraro, Longo, 1985; Scott, Goode, Arlin, 1983); the exhaustion of family resources (Mailick, 1983; Scott et al, 1983); increased contact with providers; and more specialized care and discrete units of specialists for patients and their families to deal with (Dracup, Breu, 1978). Quality of life, a multifaceted construct, has assumed increasing importance in deliberations of treatment (Spinetta, 1984), bringing with it the need for a more behavioral approach and consideration of the whole life constellation around the illness.

Although there are many parallels, the family's perspective and problems coping with serious illness may be quite distinct from the patient's. In addition, the family needs to be viewed as more than a refuge or "first line of defense" for the patient; rather, they need to be viewed as the unit facing illness (Giaquinta, 1977). The complexities of this view for study and practice are only now emerging.

The recognition that the family's perspective of hospitalization and its stresses, rather than professional assumptions about what is stressful or helpful, characterizes the hospital course for the family as a relatively recent phenomenon. Even minor inpatient procedures can be extremely distressing for parents of hospitalized children (Shapiro, 1983).

The intention of the family as a unit of care is not yet realized in practice (Schwenk, Hughes, 1983), although excellent examples of family-focused care do exist. Along with recognition of the need for a broader scope of care delivery and for the family's view of care, the perspectives, concerns, and needs of the providers must be examined. Lack of time and other institutional factors, such as a lack of recognition for efforts to attend to families' needs or the lack of a systematic approach to the family as a unit of care, are major deterrents to implementation (Geary, 1979). Lack of skills and knowledge of how to deal with families also contributes to this dilemma (Leavitt, 1982, 1984; Temple, 1983; Yoder, Jones, 1982). Families pose unique challenges as targets of care in several dimensions and may require a completely different professional armamentarium of provider skills, personnel, and methods (Schwenk, Hughes, 1983; Shapiro, 1983) than the traditional object of health care: the individual, identified patient. Families do not naturally seek attention for themselves, do not always want it, and do not always need it.

Along with technologic advances, the rapidly escalating costs of hospital care and concern for cost containment have also provided impetus for investigation into the family's experience of illness and treatment and its role in illness care. Hospital stays are shorter and more critical. The human experience of and accommodation to such an intense, fast-paced, important event has obvious implications for the ultimate recovery or well-being of the family, the intimate human group surrounding and surrounded by the serious illness of one of its members.

Family involvement in hospital care may have economic as well as therapeutic outcomes, and may increase the chances of continued recovery after discharge. The downsizing of health programs can be accomplished by innovations in health care, specifically ones that make better use of existing resources, such as families and relevant social networks in the patient's natural environment (Toth, 1984; O'Connor, 1984).

The task of this paper is to review and integrate the findings of recently published health care literature pertaining to the experience of families in the acute-care (hospital) setting. The purposes of the review include the following:

1. To ascertain the major foci of inquiry regarding families in hospitals; that is, is the inquiry primarily disease oriented, as in helping a family deal with cancer or a family with a member recovering from heart surgery, or is it primarily setting bound, such as critical care, or care-stage bound (for example, the time of admission or discharge)?

2. To examine the focus of theoretical and clinical papers about family-focused care and questions they raise for inquiry.

3. To summarize and integrate the substantive findings of research pertaining to family experience and care in hospitals toward a tentative statement of major correlates of the family's experience or adaptation to hospitalization and, perhaps, the family's recovery from serious illness.

Method

Health care literature relevant to families in hospitals was reviewed for 1983 through 1986. Sources of the literature reviewed were the *Index Medicus* and the *Cumulative Index of Nursing and Allied Health*. Other, earlier references were retrieved for their relevance to the development of a particular issue or topic in the current review, and will be cited as they are included in discussion. The effort was to broadly examine the topic of families in hospitals.

The first objective was to ascertain the major substantive foci of the published papers. The largest group of papers (17 out of 55) were general in focus; that is, they explored general questions or problems of family care and family needs in the hospital setting, such as a description of models of family-centered care in a major medical center (Pearlmutter et al, 1984). Some of these papers discussed family response in theoretical terms, such as a paper on the complexity of families' psychologic and cognitive adaptation (Melito, 1985) or they investigated the practice and research realities of the current status of the family as a unit of care (Schwenk, Hughes, 1983).

The family and critical care, and the family and cancer formed the next largest groups (12 and 9 articles, respectively). Pediatric family-focused care articles, not including childhood cancer (8 articles) and the family perspective of heart disease (recovery from myocardial infarction, bypass surgery), were the next in frequency (6 articles). Four articles addressed a variety of family care problems, such as managing the family's anger when death occurs, the family's needs and experience in psychiatric care (Rose, 1983), or the care of ill family members by adult children as a type of normative family stress (Brody, 1985).

The second objective was to examine the source of data about the family. The largest number (26 out of 55) were clinical papers. Clinical papers are those that discuss uncontrolled clinical observation and practice experience in the framework of family care (family needs and strategies to meet these). The next largest group (21 out of 55) of papers were research reports, and of those, the majority (18) were nursing studies. Two studies were multidisciplinary; one of these included a nurse investigator; and one was primarily a social work study. One study was a combined effort of a sociologist and a psychologist. A variety of methods were used, including surveys, longitudinal designs, correlational studies, grounded theory, qualitative/factor analysis, and controlled experiments.

Theory papers explored research and practice applications of theoretical frameworks, or reviewed the literature on a topic to determine the current level of knowledge and speculate about questions that remain to be explored. These accounted for approximately one-fifth (8 out of 55) of the papers reviewed.

In this review, some commentary on method will accompany the analysis of findings. Reasons for this will become more apparent, but evaluation of a finding's validity and reliability for its contribution to a knowledge system for intervention efforts or of other research must be considered.

Family Needs

A series of studies has addressed the topic of needs of family members of critically ill patients (Daley, 1984; Mathis, 1984; Norris, Grove, 1986; Stillwell, 1984). These studies are replications and expansions of Molter's (1979) study of needs of relatives of critically patients. Molter's descriptive, exploratory study sought to identify what personal needs these relatives of critically ill patients perceive, the importance of these various needs, and whether and by whom these needs were being met. A structured interview was used to collect data. This interview, however, is described as a list of 45 "need" statements, assembled on the basis of a review of lit-

erature and a survey of 23 graduate nurses. The need statements were read to the family members, who were asked to rank each statement's importance to them on a scale from 1 to 4. They were then asked if the need was met and by whom. Although some findings were highly interesting and valid (that is, the rankings themselves; the fact that relatives frequently stated that they did not expect health care personnel to be concerned about them; that most of the needs were being met by nurses, although informational needs concerning treatment and prognosis were chiefly met by physicians; and that families in this study seemed to have many resources available to them), one questions the validity of the families' identification of their needs when they were actually being asked to rank need statements presented to them. The fact that they were given an opportunity to add to the list after the ranking procedure and no new needs were mentioned is not sufficient to establish validity, although this was claimed as such. This data is in contrast to Hampe's (1975) study of the needs of grieving spouses, in which content and concurrent validity were specifically addressed. The literature was used to develop areas of concern for the otherwise open-ended interviews. That the investigator noted spouses' eagerness to talk is another indication that they were allowed to do so. Dracup and Breu's (1978) controlled field experiment to apply Hampe's findings to the care of spouses of acutely ill terminal patients with cardiovascular disease found significant differences in baseline and postintervention responses of the spouses who were recipients of a standardized care plan that incorporated Hampe's findings.

Welch (1981) assessed family needs and perceptions of care using an open-ended questionnaire format as well as a Likert scale rating of investigator-constructed statements. The stated effort was to obtain "a broader picture of preexisting psychosocial stressors" for families of cancer patients, but findings were limited to fear of leaving the patient at home, fear of other family members being lost to cancer, lack of friends, reactive illness in the family, and the need for work changes. These findings' validity can be questioned on similar grounds to Molter's (1979) because the report states that families "checked" these items. The study is rather inconsistent in its stated objectives, design, and findings, although the importance of the nurse's attitude and behavioral cues for the family's coping was supported in the families' statements.

Of the studies that have used Molter's (1979) work, Stillwell (1984) found no significant association between the ranked importance of the visiting needs, taken as a subsample of the whole of Molter's needs list, and socioeconomic status, social support (operationalized as having someone accompany the family member when they visit the patient), religious preference, and church attendance. Significant correlations existed between the severity of the illness and the need to visit frequently; close to significant correlations existed in favor of older relatives indicating less need to freely visit. The need for privacy and to have someone accompany them at the bedside were not ranked as important.

Another study compared the needs of families with a brain-injured member to Molter's population and to a new population similar to Molter's (Mathis, 1984). Although there existed the possibility of type I, or alpha, error due to large frequency counts, significant differences were found for all three populations. Spearman rank correlations, however, suggested that the groups were similar. Four items were ranked as not important in all groups: to have visiting hours changed, to talk about negative feelings, to be encouraged to cry, and to have another person at the bedside. Seven items were ranked as very important by all groups: to have questions answered honestly, to feel that staff care about their relative, to feel there was hope, to have the facts about progress, to receive reassurance that the best care possible was being given, to know they would be called at home about any changes in the condition, and to receive information about their relative at least once a day. Low ranks

are in the emotional intervention arena, and these coincide with Molter's (1979) findings. The statistically significant difference in the rankings of the brain injured versus the nonbrain injured suggests that different populations have different needs, and the author attributes this difference to an increased sense of separation for families of the brain injured. The needs that were similarly ranked across the three groups constitute the more important findings, since the differences may be accounted for by type I error.

Another study of 40 family members of ICU patients during the first 72 hours after admission also used ranking of needs statements, based on Molter's (1979) and Hampe's (1975) findings, as well as on the investigator's experience (Daley, 1984). The ranking of needs was analyzed by category; needs pertaining to the relief of anxiety were ranked highest, and the next highest need was the need for information. Categories had considerable conceptual overlap, but the specific items within the categories were presented as data. Items dealing with the need to be with or to stay nearby hospitalized relatives were also rated highly.

Personal needs as a category—which included privacy and physical comforts such as coffee or food—received the lowest ratings. The top ten most highly ranked needs were perceived as being met by physicians. These were all in the categories of relief of anxiety, need for information, and need for ventilation and support. In Molter's (1979) study, nurses met most of the families' needs; in this study, physicians met most of the families' needs. The fact that this study sampled the first 72 hours may account for this. (Molter's sample was taken from relatives of patients who had been in the intensive care unit more than three days and in the general care unit for less than 48 hours.)

Needs identified by families were compared with nurses' perception of family needs in a study by Norris and Grove (1986). The study used Molter's items but refined them in a pilot study through the use of median score cut points to delete and revise items. The perceptions of needs by intensive care nurses differed significantly from needs expressed by the family members. The differences were accounted for by nurses' lower rankings of family needs, particularly informational needs about care. The authors speculate that nurses have different assumptions about family needs and that nurses do not perceive their own importance to families. Key needs of families identified in this study, as in the other studies, were for honesty, caring, information, and hope. Talking about feelings (an item changed from "talking about negative feelings"), talking about the possibility of the patient's death, and changing visiting hours had the lowest family ratings. This study was undertaken to examine the validity of professionally constructed assessment or needs assessment. Its conclusion supports the view that professionals can and do have different assumptions of family needs, and that additional grounding of professional assessment criteria in the words and deeds of the families themselves is necessary.

It appears that Molter's (1979) needs statements have provided a convenient basis for comparison of the needs of family members of the critically ill at different time points and in different populations. In spite of the questionable validity of these items, the consistency across studies and populations provides evidence to support the importance of certain features of the family care experience. These are the family's need for information, for confidence, for assurance that their relative is receiving the best care possible (a caring attitude), and for hope. In spite of the importance of the need to relieve anxiety—a category represented by the need for information and a caring attitude—families consistently gave low ratings to the need to talk about feelings or the possibility of the patient's death. These findings suggest that a "frontal assault," that is, an explicit invitation to talk about feelings in a nonspecific or nondirected sense, would not be helpful. It may even be detrimental to family's coping for a variety of reasons, one of which may be that certain essential family defenses are threatened by such an open invitation. Other reasons will be explored later in the chapter, along with findings concerning the family's need to normalize their situation and experience and to accentuate their successful strategies.

Family's anxieties are tightly bound to the realistic threats of their frightening, painful, and uncertain situation. Families' needs for their own personal comfort, such as privacy, coffee and food, changed visiting hours, or to be accompanied to the bedside, were not perceived as important. Low family ratings for these "family-only" needs may be a reflection of the primacy of the patient's condition to the family's well-being and of the need to abnegate family needs out of care and concern for the patient. It is as if families might be afraid to take away precious resources from their ill relative.

Family Strengths

A call for a tentative, cautious approach to family intervention, one that looks first to the family's strengths and needs for particular defenses, has emerged recently and complicates the call for more assessment instrumentation (Feetham, 1984; Lasky et al, 1985) and for rigid conceptualizations and systematization of family intervention efforts.

The family's vital concern with normalcy and dignity and the need to feel successful in its coping and management of severely disruptive and painful events, and the professional's need to acknowledge this in assessment and intervention efforts have been addressed in several studies and clinical papers. Thorne's (1985) remarks serve as an introduction:

> Much of our understanding of the family cancer experience is predicated upon professionally derivedconstructs such as crisis intervention or adaptation theory. The everyday life of the cancer patient from the perspective of those involved is a relatively untapped information source (p. 285).

Thorne's qualitative, phenomenological study of families whose middle-aged relative was undergoing treatment for cancer uncovered three explanatory layers of the families' experience. The first was the family's depiction of themselves as coping well in spite of major upheavals and overwhelming emotional repercussions: "these families adamantly described themselves as coping well. Clearly the belief that they did not need outside help was a source of dignity to the families" (p. 287). These families valued normalcy and perceived themselves as having retained it, although most were leading lives that health care professionals might well describe as severely disrupted by the illness. Normality, however, was measured by criteria unique to the family's values, or style, and seemed to reflect an almost desperate attempt in some cases to continue to perceive normalcy in their lives.

Anderson's (1981) ethnographic study of the family's construction of illness focused on the issue of the family's need to normalize coping with chronic illness in their children, pointing out the rather glaring inconsistencies between the family's "nonnormal" adjustments to the illness and its demands in their daily life and their continued insistence that their life was quite normal. Anderson's interpretation of her findings focused on the family's desire to minimize the deviant disease label in spite of realistic accommodation to the special care needs of its child. "Coping well" was defined by the families as managing their lives, including their children's illness demands, with equanimity.

Building on Anderson's (1981) study, Ferraro and Longo (1985) argue that the employment of crisis intervention strategies may be counterproductive for families of hospitalized chronically ill children. These authors apply Miller's (1983) Family Power Resources Model to assess family strengths and resources and coping strategies. Maintaining a positive self-concept through normalization processes is seen as a major and necessary adaptive strength for families in this model, and the findings of four other studies are cited to support this conclusion. These authors emphasize that normalization should not be seen as or confused with denial, although studies (Breznitz, 1983) have brought to light the adaptive qualities and effects of certain types and levels of denial at points in time throughout the coping process (Cohen, Lazarus, 1979), suggesting that normalization and denial have conceptual overlap.

Barbarin and Chesler (1984), in their stratified sample of 55 families, describe the family's "often valiant efforts to cope in ways that retain vestiges of normalcy in family life" as a major theme in family strategies for coping with childhood cancer. They conclude that effective coping should not be viewed as stress reduction but rather as the means by which people go on with their lives in the presence of highly distressing conditions. They also note that family self-evaluations are made on the basis of social comparison with those who are less well off.

The Role of Stigma

Barbarin (1986) explored the central role of stigma in families coping with illness, which may be a major explanatory construct accounting for the need for normalization. Families are highly embedded in the culture of the larger society, taking cues for their sense of competence and identity in its values and norms, which, in our culture, are highly idealized (Fleck 1975; Hill, 1965; Huston, Robins, 1982; Offer, Shabshin, 1974; Walters, 1982).

Stigma as a social process may also operate in the interactions of the family and the staff in the hospital setting. Estroff (1981), Erickson (1973), and Barbarin (1986) have described the "Catch 22" of being on the receiving end of patient care and the social cues attached to that status. Health professionals hold a special position as stigmatizers and destigmatizers of disease (Volinn, 1983). In his paper on psychosocial transitions, Parkes (1971) proposes the intriguing idea that hospitals can be viewed as communities whose purpose is to facilitate the process of psychosocial transition. One of these transitions would include the management of identity and status changes for families and patients adjusting to major change in their assumptive worlds. The family–health professional interface constitutes as yet uncharted scientific waters but may well yield some crucial knowledge for health care providers who focus on families as units of care.

In Thorne's (1985) study, family capacity to identify and articulate successful coping strategies was remarkable. These coping strategies, in turn, showed remarkable variation: open and closed communication patterns, shifts in responsibility for emotional support from the patient to the family and back again, and a need to maintain faith in the medical care, sometimes to the point of rationalizing and developing elaborate explanations for negative experiences. Rasie (1981) also observed a fear of criticizing and a compulsion to defend the quality of care. The family philosophy, different from family to family and articulated as family mottoes or slogans, dictated characteristic coping style and was used by the families to explain their positive attitude. The fit between the family philosophy and the specific strategic choices was seen as allowing them to maintain a sense of normalcy and dignity.

Leavitt (1982, pp. 28–29) described the need to maintain dignity and a positive self-concept in theoretical terms as the coping strength of family pride. Supporting the formulation of the centrality of self-esteem and pride in family coping are reports of families' satisfaction in their extension of help to others in the context and in the midst of their own situation (Thorne, 1985; Barbarin, Chesler, 1983; Rose, Finestone, Bass, 1985). Gift giving and negotiating a personal relationship with health care providers (Robinson, Thorne, 1984; Drew, Stoeclke, Billings, 1983) are other family efforts to tip the balance in favor of maintaining status and reciprocity and, thus, maintaining the family's pride

and dignity, as well as simply gaining better treatment and more attention.

Family Intervention

Levels of Intervention

A longitudinal family intervention study (Kupst et al, 1982) tested the differential effects of three levels of intervention for 64 non referred, or apparently well-functioning, families of pediatric leukemia patients. The study was well controlled by randomized design, multiple data sources, and carefully operationalized and standardized experimental protocols. Of particular interest are the findings that, beyond the initial phase intervention at diagnosis and the first few weeks afterward, there were no significant differences in the two intervention comparison groups: the total intervention, or most active, group and the moderate group. These two differed in degree of outreach and frequency of contact. At one year there was no significant difference in the intervention groups or the control (no intervention) groups, and 72% of all subject families were coping well, based on composite ratings by physicians, nurses, and psychosocial staff. Mothers' self-ratings were that they were doing better than at the time of diagnosis, and mothers' coping evaluation contributed most of the variance at the first two measurement points. At two years the results were the same.

Intervention techniques found to be helpful in the initial weeks were using an indirect approach, emphasizing topics related to the management of the illness, acknowledging the difficulties of the situation, and acting as liaison between the family and the physician. Like in the family needs studies, in which families gave lowest ratings to direct emotional care, most families in this study avoided direct discussion of emotional issues. The investigators note that "most families were friendly but distant and did not respond openly to the (active) intervention" (p. 37). In the second phase, one to three months postdiagnosis, interventions included anticipating possible emotional sequelae, supporting the need for information, strengthening the family's own resources, returning to school, and other activities. More frequent and shorter visits worked best. Family sensitivity to the "fine line between empathy and pity" (p. 39) was noted, as well as the patients' and families' need to feel that they were handling the crisis well. Perceptions of pity undermined their sense of mastery. A tentative, nondirective approach, sensitive to the family's receptiveness, was employed.

This rich and excellent study helps to delineate some of the parameters and considerations of family-level intervention. It seems that families can use some intervention, at least in the first stages of diagnosis and early treatment; that this intervention should focus on the treatment and information needs, rather than the family's emotional needs per se; and that most families will eventually do well, with or without intervention. Ninety-one percent of the families were coping well at three months, and 72% were coping well at one year. No group had more poorly coping families than the other.

We have yet to discover how to be of real benefit to those who "fall out" and why they do not do well. This study identified the ill child's age, other family supports, and lack of additional stresses as major moderators of the illness course for the family. The investigators did not speculate on why the intervention groups did not seem to manage better than the nonintervention groups by the end of the first year. The variation in illness course, life events, and family dynamics may overcome the variation due to intervention by that time.

Fallacies of Family-Centered Services

In a far-ranging, theoretically based clinical paper, Lewis (1983) discussed five fallacies of family-level services for families with cancer patients. These fallacies are not specific to cancer, however. Lewis's points echo and serve to integrate and summarize findings of other family studies reviewed here.

One fallacy is the fallacy of causal simplicity. Lewis states:

> It is inappropriate to adopt simplistic interventionist models in research with families experiencing cancer; at a minimum many of these models involve two-way feedback loops in which factors cause or effect each other (p. 195).

Functioning or dysfunction is caused by a composite of variables and is not a linear, cause-effect outcome. This issue is also explored by Young (1983), who argued against simplistic formulations of assumed family disruption. Families are not passive, and the family–illness intermesh has much mutuality. Leading family theorists (McCubbin, 1979; McCubbin, Patterson, 1981) have acknowledged this and have revised the classic ABCX model of family stress and coping to account for and to integrate the family's active role.

The family's definition of its situation seems to be the major key to understanding how it responds to illness (Schwenk, Hughes, 1983). Knafl's (1985) study of parents' management of their child's hospitalization supports and refines this conclusion. The centrality of the family's definition in coping with illness is also supported by Robinson and Thorne's (1984) work in the area of family "interference" as a phenomenon representing the family's efforts to negotiate a working alliance with professional health care providers and to have its criteria for viewing illnesses acknowledged as different but nevertheless valid.

The family's definition of its situation has both stable and reactive features. These need to be examined separately and together. More stable features might refer to the clarity of community norms for family behavior under stress and the family's fit with these (McCubbin, 1979). Reactive features might refer to the integration and effect of a positive or negative experience or event in the longer trajectory. Thorne (1985) concluded that a major dimension of the family's experience of cancer is the fit of its strategies with their collective family consciousness. That effort to distinguish generally effective from ineffective coping responses represents an overly simplistic approach to a complex experiential phenomenon.

Another, related fallacy discussed by Lewis (1983) is the fallacy of warranted intervention. This may have particular relevance for cancer, where a cure is not always possible and change-oriented strategies of intervention are not appropriate, but it must certainly have relevance for families coping with illness in many contexts. Affirmation and acknowledgement can help without hurting, as the findings about normalization and the family's self-concept have illuminated.

The other three fallacies discussed by Lewis (1983) are the fallacy of provider-timed services, the fallacy of informality, and the fallacy of diffused effect. Families have their own schedules for coping and for receiving or accepting "outside" help, as Lewis points out and others have noted. It is, however, possible to make some generalizations, to establish some guidelines for the illness trajectory or for the kinds of families who need certain levels of services, based on careful studies, such as those of Kupst et al (1983) and Knafl (1985).

The fallacy of informality refers to the provider's unstructured efforts to respond to the family's needs, depending on the family's spontaneous request for assistance. It is argued that systematic efforts "capture" families who do not ask for assistance, and socialize families to the concept of family-level services. Systematic intervention does not have to be rigid or overdone. With enough empirical knowledge of family coping, interventions can be appropriately timed and "packaged."

The fallacy of diffused effect is directed truly toward family rather than toward individual-level care. Thorne (1984) interviewed whole families, not family members. Her data

were different, with family mottoes, strategies, and family strengths coming into focus. Diffusion of positive intervention outcome for an individual throughout the family system cannot always be assumed but warrants further investigation. (When and under what conditions might there be a diffused effect? Is a diffused effect different from a direct effect?)

Group Support Strategies

Other intervention studies have contributed answers as well as questions about the family's needs and experiences in the hospital and in coping with serious illness. Pearlmutter et al, (1984) found group support strategies for families to be effective and economical for learning to deal with hospitalization and illness. Dracup et al (1984) report the effectiveness of group support for families managing cardiac rehabilitation. Benefits of group participation for families included obtaining and imparting information and hope, redefining wellness through the confirmation of a reference group, and having the opportunity to experience the healing forces of altruism. Rose et al (1985), in their study of a support group's effect for families of psychiatric patients, also report that helping others helped families. Sharing an experience and comparing and contrasting reduced isolation and allowed group participation in solving issues of management, including the family's relationship with the health care system (increased assertiveness was one solution), the family's relationship with the patient, and ways to take care of themselves. Disparate stages in the illness process and experiences seemed to balance one another rather than to alienate or isolate members.

Brown et al (1984), however, separated patients from their families in group intervention following open heart surgery after they determined that the relatives' issues became secondary to those of the patients', that families were reluctant to focus on themselves in the presence of the patients, and that concerns were not necessarily mutual. These were one-session groups that were held during the recovery period, in anticipation of discharge. The groups helped patients to absorb their experience and express their fears about separation from the hospital. Patients admitted that they hide feelings from their families. Relatives discussed the patients' emotional ability and narcissism and the conflicts that evolved from the family's monitoring of the patient. Both patients and families needed orientation to the use and conduct of group meetings. An earlier study reported problems arising from differing needs for support for families in different phases of coping, necessitating the formation of subgroups (McHugh et al, 1979). The question of homogeneity in group support intervention remains to be answered. The only study that did not support group work with families was Welch's (1981), in which 51% of the subject families gave "least helpful" ratings to the establishment of support groups. This was explained as a possible artifact of having to rate a limited number of items of equal importance.

Daily telephone contact and volunteers are used to help families of patients in intensive care as a part of the Family Crisis Intervention program described by Hodovanic et al (1984). The program includes an assessment of family informational needs, (for example, explanation of visiting hours, notification of patient's condition). Providing information and establishing a trusting relationship between the family and the professional staff are the goals of the program, which is being evaluated.

Watson and Hickey (1984) described a decrease in anger and tension as results of a program of perioperative support for families waiting for relatives undergoing cancer surgery. This program is also being evaluated.

The Coping Trajectory

Studies of the coping trajectory provide insights into families' experiences over time and guidance for intervention efforts during hospitalization and after discharge. Dhooper (1983) has reported a study of 40 families coping with the crisis of a heart attack from the time of hospitalization through three months after discharge. A new instrument, the Family Adjustment to Crisis Scale, whose reliability had been established in preparatory trials, was used in the study. Anxiety, but not insecurity, characterized the early period for families. Spouses reported many symptoms, such as sleeplessness, headache, lack of concentration, forgetfulness, and shortness of breath. Children aged 6–12 were most adversely affected. Social life was affected for most of the families, other than those who described themselves as homebound and not socializing before the illness. One month after discharge, most families reported moderate as opposed to high degrees of anxiety and persistent social life disruption. All children seemed to be coping quite successfully by this time. The incidence of reactive illness in family members, considered to be a result of the strain, increased. Life was described as back to normal by three months.

This study reports financial strain becoming a major issue for families by the third month. Strain in household management was greatest in the first month, due to visiting the hospital, and then care needs and accommodation to the illness and recovery created additional stress. Role reversal and new care routines such as diet and exercise disorganized the household. This was largely under control by the third month. Coping strategies used by spouses were passive acceptance, talking to others, seeking information and reassurance, and praying. The overall picture of the family's functioning was evaluated by the families as worse at three months than at two. The families by this time are coping with the rest of their lives, not just recovering from the heart attack. This study looks at certain dimensions along a trajectory, but does not provide sufficient explanation or interpretation from the family's viewpoint.

The variation of family needs at different stages of illness with cancer was explored in a cross-sectional study by Wright and Dyck (1984). Using a semistructured interview and a Likert scale questionnaire, four major concerns were identified. These were, in order of frequency, problems associated with symptoms of the disease, fear of the future, waiting, and obtaining information. A higher mean score was found for the four major identified needs for families at hospitalization for recurrence. Welch (1982) studied anticipatory grief reactions of families in all stages of cancer, noting that family grieving takes place on a continuum from the time of diagnosis. Conceptual relationships in this study, that is, the association of unresolved grief with discharge panic and other study conclusions, however, were not sufficiently developed to consider these as valid findings.

Patient versus Family Coping Trajectories

Differences in patient versus family experience and coping trajectories are seen in several studies. Gilliss (1983), in a longitudinal, descriptive study, compared subjective stress of spouses and patients and found the spousal stress level to be significantly higher at the time of hospitalization for open heart surgery. An earlier study found spouses' anxiety scores to be higher than surgical patients' mean scores, including those undergoing heart surgery (Silva, 1979). Patients and families focused on different problems and were more able to explore these when they attended separate groups (as in the Brown et al [1984] study of group intervention for open heart surgery patients and their families, discussed earlier in this chapter).

Differences in the recovery trajectory for 40 spouses and patients after cancer surgery were examined by Oberst and James (1985). This study used a combination of measures, qualitative and quantitative. Interviews were deemed the richest source of the study data.

The patient's health remained the primary concern for both patients and spouses throughout the first 30 days. After that time, spouses began to focus on their own health and the impact of the illness on their own lives. While patients are coping with pain and discomfort of surgery, the spouses are coping with disruption in their lives, travel to and from the hospital, interruptions of work and other schedules, and changes in social activities. For more than one-third of the spouses, these disruptions continued into the third month and were accompanied by anger and resentment. Spouses were involved in physical care activities in the first few weeks at home, but this dropped off sharply thereafter.

Symptom distress continued after discharge for most of the patients; it was unexpected and, thus, more disturbing. Spouses had their own symptom distresses. During hospitalization, spouses suffered fatigue and inability to eat. Later, in the first and second months after discharge, spouses had increased incidence of physical illness, including diffuse aches and pains, indigestion and food intolerances, exacerbation of previous medical conditions, and upper respiratory conditions. Dhooper (1983) documents similar spouse symptomatology during hospitalization and increased incidence of reactive illness in the family during the first month. Patients were unaware of the spouses' distress and spouses expressed exasperation at the patients' egocentricity.

Spouse anxiety during the predischarge period was significantly higher than that of the patients. Spouses were grappling with the suddenness of the events, along with lowered emotional reserves brought on by exhaustion. Spouses described a need to maintain a cheerful, optimistic demeanor during the hospitalization but recognized that they were not coping well and felt disturbed by this. Spouses were seen as initially having to cope with a sudden release of emotions that overwhelms coping resources, followed by exhaustion.

At each postdischarge interview, spouses continued to have a higher incidence of emotional problems than the patients. At 10 days, spouses felt fairly positive and more in control and derived considerable satisfaction at being able to manage, but thereafter, they experienced a steady decline in their emotional state. This finding coincides with that of Dhooper (1983). Depression took the place of anxiety, and anger at the patient's egocentricity was accompanied by guilt. Guilt also accompanied spouses' efforts to take care of themselves. Patients and spouses were extremely well informed during the hospitalization but were upset by the unexpected distresses experienced after discharge. Unexpected distress was also found by Gilliss (1983). Spouses in this study experienced anger and frustration about the lack of support from professionals and the perceived lack of support from all sources. The authors suggest that the period immediately following the return home is the time of greatest vulnerability for spouses and therefore is the time for supportive interventions.

Issues raised by families of psychiatric patients in their group sessions included the need for learning practical coping skills and strategies for caring for their relative, negotiating with the health care system, and caring for themselves. Family fatigue and self-neglect was addressed, along with the need for obtaining supportive services (Rose, Finestone, Bass, 1985).

Mailick (1984), in an article describing the reactive depression of hospitalized patients resulting from dependency conflicts and separation and from the intrusions of and adaptation to strangers and removal from normal identity and status supports, also addresses the role and needs of the family. Parallels in the patient and family experience are acknowledged, but the complexities of the family's reaction are explained as being derived from preexisting emotional disturbances and the role of illness or the ill person in the family dynamics.

Mailick (1984) notes that repeated episodes of illness and hospital admissions can exhaust the family's physical, economic, and emotional resources. Family members need to deal with their own anxiety, resentment, shame, anger, guilt, and depression. Mailick advocates encouraging the expression of these feelings to assist

with the reestablishment of familial coping patterns. This advice is contradicted by other studies cited and reviewed here and may represent untested professional assumptions or the unique expertise of this clinician-investigator to work directly with families' emotions.

Family members' exhaustion, conflict, and need for their own support is documented in a fine, detailed case analysis by Scott, Goode, and Arlin (1983). The patient's need to maintain control was at times in opposition to the family's need and desire to monitor and participate in care of the patient. The wife in this case had the need to create emotional distance between herself and her husband at different intervals in order to continue to cope with his illness and to prepare for his loss. These investigators agree that previously existing unresolved family issues surface and add to the present burdens. Preexisting and usually unstated family "contracts" about decision-making, behavior, and interactions with others are a major determining factor in how things get done or in how conflicts are associated with these processes.

The Effect of Multiple Remissions on the Coping Trajectory

With multiple remissions, the death trajectory is altered, and with its interruption, uncertainty and ambiguity are increased. Welch (1982) examined anticipatory grieving and factors associated with unresolved grief in family members. The factors included specialized treatment settings or treatments (such as bone marrow transplantation), and death occurring at a younger age.

Related, but not limited, to the situation of multiple remissions, Boss and Greenberg (1984) have explored family boundary ambiguity as a new and important variable in family stress. Briefly, they propose that uncertainty or ambiguity about the loss of family members rather than the event itself is most predictive of family stress. The system is held in limbo and cannot reorganize. Uncertainty can extend beyond the simple presence or absence of members to include uncertainty or ambiguity about role performance. The degree of loss is determined by the family's perception or construction of that reality, and this in turn will determine the degree of ambiguity. Cultural belief systems also determine the family tolerance for boundary ambiguity, such as the family membership status of divorced spouses or the personhood of stillborn children. Length and interpretations of the hospitalization event's significance influence the family boundary ambiguity and are predictive of family stress and restructuring. The hospital can be considered a place, or way station, where issues of boundary ambiguity can be addressed.

Clinical Intervention Guidelines

Papers describing guidelines and principles for family-focused care, outside of the context of reporting research findings' implications for practice, included the Lewis (1984) paper on fallacies of family-level intervention for cancer patients' families, discussed earlier; a paper on dealing with family anger when a patient dies (Poster, Betz, 1984); and a paper on application of general features of stress and coping theory to interventions for families of critically ill patients (King, Gregor, 1985). Lust (1984) outlined assessment and intervention techniques for families with patients in the intensive care unit. Family meetings, flexible visiting arrangements, and environmental considerations, such as available, working telephones and sleeping accommodations, were discussed. It is interesting to note that this was the only paper that examined and recommended environmental accommodation for families. This was a major feature of the pediatric movement to incorporate the family into hospital care.

Other papers describing guidelines focused on the special vulnerability of single parents during hospitalization (Burns, 1984); on the use of crisis intervention as the basis for intervention with families as trauma victims (Braulin et al, 1982); on care of the family in the unknown period between admission and diagnosis–prognosis conference (Curtis, 1983); and on stress reduction after coronary bypass surgery (Gilliss, 1984). Institutional family-focused care programs are described by Hodovanic et al (1984), discussed earlier in this chapter, and by Pearlmutter et al (1984). The role of the psychiatric liaison nurse with families (Minarik, 1984), parent involvement in pediatric care (Hardgrove, Healy, 1984), parent support in neonatal care (Thornton et al, 1984), and an ambulatory infusion pump program's effects on family life (Butler, 1984) are other topics of clinical papers.

The specific content of these papers deserves more discussion than this chapter allows. Most are well written and well documented and contribute to our knowledge and understanding of family-focused care. They serve to bridge the research–intervention gap and in some cases themselves serve to generate clinical research questions. For example, Butler's (1984) short paper about families' responses to the use of ambulatory infusion pumps for chemotherapy prompts an examination of ways to measure the effect on family functioning and quality of life, or to collect descriptive data pertaining to the educational needs of families for living with the infusion pump.

In some instances, interventions were increasingly refined as they were examined in different papers. Review, the systematic reexamination of upsetting events as a family-focused intervention, is described by Rasie (1981), Leavitt (1982), King and Gregor (1985), and Clements (1986). All but Clements cite the others' work. Clements calls the intervention *reminiscence* and uses a different body of knowledge to develop the paper, but the therapeutic goals are the same. The continued interest in this intervention strategy lends support to its clinical validity and calls for research to add to our understanding of its effects.

Implementation of Family-Focused Care

A major review of the literature and theory examined the gap between family care as rhetoric and as reality (Schwenk, Hughes, 1983). In this review, medical care of the individual in the context of the family was differentiated from the family as a fundmental unit of diagnosis and treatment. The authors explained the relative lack of research and development of knowledge about the family unit as a function of the relative dearth of valid and accurate definitions of family health, ill health, or "family diagnosis," compared to the large amount of study of the individual's effect on the family or the family's effect on the individual. These reviewers conclude that the state of the art is still somewhat primitive for the prevention and treatment of family disease, particularly the questions of which families and when and how they deteriorate or thrive as units, although these questions are now being approached by the stress and coping theorists.

The Schwenk and Hughes (1983) review also addressed the ethical and practical issues in health care delivery to families as opposed to individuals. Tradition and individual rights to privacy and primacy in care are potential areas of resistance to implementation of family-focused care. More outreach and different providers (teams rather than individuals) will be necessary. The specific instances, or indications, for family-centered care have yet to be sorted out. When and by what mechanisms family care is superior to individual care is an important question asked in this chapter.

Shapiro (1983) concludes her review of family coping with a physically ill or handicapped child with the call for increased awareness of the evidence that supports the critical role of the family for health outcomes, for attitudinal changes, and for skill and tool development for family-coping assessment and intervention. She notes that medical education at present neglects development of a knowledge base for family care and that the family is an underused resource that could be mobilized for medical care.

Barriers to Implementation of Family-Focused Care

The major barriers to the implementation of family-focused care in nursing are lack of educational preparation, not in family theory but in skill development (Temple, 1983), and role perception (Yoder, Jones, 1982). Nurses acknowledge the family as an important aspect of care but do not acknowledge their exclusive domain (Lust, 1984). Nurses complain that they do not have sufficient time or system support (institutional) to attend to family needs (Lust, 1983; Yoder, Jones, 1982). Nurses' educational level was positively correlated with comfort and preparedness to deal with families (Porter, 1980; Yoder, Jones, 1982). An earlier study of deterrents to crisis intervention in the hospital revealed that more than the institutional factors (time, reward), it was the nurses' lack of expertise that accounted for their lack of implementation of psychosocial care for patients and families (Zind, 1974).

Family assessment tools are being developed (Feetham, 1984; Lasky et al, 1985; Hymovich, 1981), but family intervention skills and strategies also need to be developed and tested. A major rationale for a textbook on the subject of family-focused preventive intervention was the development of family-level skills and intervention strategies. The book (Leavitt, 1982) was largely a clinically and theoretically oriented description of strategies employed in the clinical supervision of family-care courses in a baccalaureate school of nursing. More studies and reports of educational strategies for family-focused care, such as Jerrett and Ross's (1982) and Chafetz and Gaillard's (1978), are needed, as is systematic follow-up of graduates of these programs, if the implementation gap is to be filled. In turn, these courses must incorporate and contribute to the growing body of knowledge of the field. More program and intervention evaluation in controlled trials of interventions, supported by careful research—such as Dracup and Breu's (1978) study of a family intervention protocol or Meleis and Swendsen's (1978) role supplementation strategy for new parents—would advance the field's clinical knowledge and provide needed intervention guidance. The testing of interventions more often results in more questions than answers, but knowledge is advanced with questions as well as answers.

Family Care as a Tripartate Construct

The complexity of the patient–family–health care systems' interaction in the context of critical care is described by Ragiel (1984). The conflicting agendas, needs, expectations, and mutual influence of each system are explored. Ragiel describes the triangulation process of power shifts as the patient and family alternate membership in the power dyad, since a three-way power split is almost impossible to maintain. Information-hoarding is a way to maintain power, and changes brought about by recovery and care phases initiate renegotiation of relationships. Information control was also explored in Wright and Dyck's (1984) study of expressed family needs. The conceptual overlap of this and other recent papers—such as Robinson and Thornes' (1984) explanation of family "interference" as a family strength and an expression of the family's expectations and evolving relationships with the providers, the phase-specific changes in family needs and concerns, and the distress of the family's unmet expectations described by Oberst and James (1985), Kupst et al (1983), and Gilliss (1983)—support the need to examine family care as a three-system construct.

The tripartate construct is also supported by evidence that the family's construction and experience of hospitalization and the illness of its family member is perceived differently by the family and the providers (Lust, 1984; Norris, Grove, 1986; Robinson, Thorne, 1984; Thorne, 1985). Earlier theoretical work by Kleinman et al (1978) and Kleinman (1978) on the distinction of illness and disease or the biomedical versus the cultural construction of clinical reality has given impetus to these explorations and to a recent exploration of a theoretical model of health based on emic and etic distinctions (Tripp–Reimer, 1984).

Methodologic Implications

The implications for method in investigations of explanations and constructions of family illness and the determination of family need are evident. The family's view must be obtained in open-ended strategies for data collection, and the family's construction of its experience must be tapped. The family's view as a whole may be differently constructed than that of the individual member's view.

Spinetta (1984) discussed methodologic validity issues in relation to culture, that is, cultural differences in expression of private feelings and concerns, social class distinctions of interviewer and family, openness, role of religion, and explanation of illness in family-illness research. Litman and Ventners (1979) point out that health diaries are subject to bias of norms of relevance, social desirability, privacy, and decency. This bias might be more profitably considered as data, since the family's construction of reality for itself is subject to these norms. Family well-being is tied to the family's own sense of itself. Independent access to many clinically essential kinds of family phenomena might not be possible or desirable.

One might ask what constitute objective family data and what the clinical applications of such data are. Concurrent observational data that check for discrepancies in families' self-reports can reveal the specific effects of the norms of social desirability, the family's resources, the family's need for power over the family's behavior, and the family's construction and description of these to others. Studies of family anxiety (or stress) levels as outcome criteria, as Barbarin and Chesler (1983) have discovered, do not sufficiently discriminate between families that are coping well and those who are coping poorly. State anxiety evaluations may discriminate at a certain point in time, but the mechanism of effects of interventions are not clear and are "washed out" over time. Kathol (1984) attempted to examine the mechanisms of family members' anxiety reduction by contrasting a videotape intervention with a staff–family interaction and a videotape intervention alone. Both time and videotape produced main effects, but it is not known which was more influential. Staff interaction increased perceived support from the nurse, as did the combination, but anxiety levels were not the discriminating factor. Silva's (1979) study also showed no significant treatment effect of orienting information on anxiety scores per se. Family attitudes were positively affected as measured by the Spouses' Perception Scale. Attitudes are complex social and psychologic constructs. A multivariate, social–interpersonal definition of coping appears to be necessary for assessing families.

The Effects of Culture on Family-Centered Care

Cultural consideration of the family's experience of hospitalization is examined on another level of abstraction by Eldar and Eldar (1984). Their thesis is that the family's responsibility for the care of its sick members is a deeply rooted and cross-cultural phenomenon and is not taken into account sufficiently by most hospitals. The research implications of this thesis are myriad and include investigation of the effects of the family's role performance disrup-

tion and continuity and investigation of task-specific competencies for family involvement and participation in the hospital. Role integration as a model for predicting the family's adaptation to medical crisis with researchable propositions is presented by Fife (1985). This model could be strengthened by a broader view of role that accounts for the norms of the culture surrounding the family.

Families' participation in care is addressed by Hardgrove and Healy (1984). The role of specific cultural dictates, as well as variables in individual families' capability and motivation in regard to family participation, deserve more attention.

Research Conclusions

The needs of families with hospitalized relatives have been studied from the perspective of need statements developed by health professionals and from the statements and accounts of the families themselves. The family accounts reveal the influence of cultural norms and expectations on family perceptions of coping and the centrality of the family construction of their experience on their coping patterns and strategies.

Although different methods yield different kinds of data, the presence of overlapping findings with different methods strengthens the case for their validity. For example, the studies in which the families ranked needs statements consistently resulted in lowest ranks for talking about feelings. The longitudinal intervention study for families coping with childhood leukemia (Kupst et al, 1982) also found families cool to a direct discussion of emotional issues. Thorne's (1985) phenomenologic study reiterates this finding and explains and expands its meaning in relation to the family's need to maintain a sense of normality and competence.

It is interesting that simple controlled experiments to test discriminating effects of interventions, such as Kathol's (1984), do not really explain how, why, or why not an effect occurred. Perhaps this is because the study was not sufficiently located in a body of knowledge (the literature review), and therefore, the hypotheses were not sufficient to explain the findings. Elegance is not the same as simplicity. An elegant study is spare, but it is utterly and clearly sufficient; the study's results fit or do not fit a position carefully prepared for them. A more complex hypothesis testing study by Eberly et al (1985) concurrently sought broader explanation with other measures but was still left with some conjecture at the end concerning the interpretation of the findings. Simple criteria, such as anxiety reduction as outcome measures at one point in time, do not really tell us how the family is doing. The family's interactions with care providers and among themselves, and the effects of their social comparisons have more of a story to tell.

Over and over, the family's need to preserve and identify the normality of its experiences and management of highly (objectively speaking) disruptive and distressing experiences with illness was manifested. The maintenance of a sense of competency, mastery, and family self-esteem as central is seen in the constant social comparison noted in several studies (Barbarin, Chesler, 1983; Anderson, 1981) and in the families' need to give as well as to receive help (Rose et al, 1985; Thorne, 1985).

Longitudinal studies (Dhooper, 1983; Kupst et al, 1982; Oberst, James, 1985; Gilliss, 1983) had overlapping findings about the recovery trajectory, although measurement and data collection differed. Common findings include: the leveling off of the disruption and stress after the first few weeks of cancer surgery and heart attack or bypass surgery; the increase in spousal and family reactive illness; the differences in spousal and patient stresses and experience; the exhaustion and stress for family members while a relative is hospitalized for life-threatening surgeries; the rapid discharge and "let down" afterward for spouses; and the difficulty coping with the patient's narcissism or self-centered-ness (also noted by Brown et al's [1984] group intervention study). Other correlates of the family's experience in the hospital and in coping with serious illness include previous experiences; expectations; evolving relationship with providers; stage and length of illness; need for power; professional's comfort and skill in working with families; and institutional accommodation to family-focused care.

Rigid intervention protocols based exclusively on professional assumptions of family care and family needs will more than likely not hit the mark, since what helps one family can alienate another. It is not yet clear what approaches work best, or why they do or do not have an effect. This may be because the effects have not been appropriately measured. Data gathered from whole families appear to be different from data obtained from individual family members. Individuals complain more or more readily describe difficulties; families emphasize strengths and successes.

At this point, there seem to be more questions than answers, but how the parts fit with the whole is beginning to achieve some definition. One example of this definition, perhaps, is the connection of the family's information needs with the larger construct of the family's need to maintain its competency and exercise its particular strengths in a new and challenging situation rather than the construct of anxiety reduction.

Family coping over time is enormously complex and constantly reactive and evolving as families integrate their own successes and failures and redefine their experiences. Multiple events are encountered and managed by families as part of their normal, everyday lives. These enter into the hospital coping equation and may indicate which aspects of the hospital experience are seen as disruptive or unmanageable by the family.

Families seem to focus intensely on the patient and do not see a family focus as a part of the provider's role, except as pertains to their information needs regarding the patient and the patient's care. Why is this? Surely it is not simply that family-focused care is not institutionalized or that the family is not socialized to the idea. Even simple environmental comforts were not ranked in the higher levels of needs. Only one informal study of all the studies and papers reviewed examined environmental accommodations for families and found them relieved and grateful when these were provided. But they do not ask for these accommodations. Why is this?

Some of the answers to these questions may reside in the provider's role perceptions and skills in relation to family-focused care. The interactions of the family with health care personnel are colored by the cues they receive. Family behaviors that do not fit, or that seem to challenge or fight the cues received, are seen as interfering rather than as expressing family competency and need to maintain power. The family–health professional interface constitutes as yet largely uncharted waters but may well yield crucial knowledge for health care providers who deliver family-level services.

The question of which families and when and why they can benefit from family-level care remains to be examined. Or is a family focus simply part of humane care, integral to the nursing perspective of holism and humanism and therefore a necessary aspect of health care for all families?

Summary

This literature review has demonstrated some increases in sophistication in family study and care, although care seems to be lagging behind, using untested strategies that are based largely on professional assumptions. Crisis intervention is still a major theoretical basis for care. Self-care, role and systems theory, power models, exchange, and symbolic interaction frameworks may prove to be more fruitful in guiding family-level care research.

A last point for careful evaluation and use of research findings is both a warning and an invitation. There is a wealth of data, both as major and as peripheral findings, in the studies reviewed in this chapter. The data are not being used. For example, uncertainty and ambiguity as central aspects of family stress in hospitals is documented in several studies not directly addressing that dimension. Combining these findings with Mishel's (1984) causal modeling of uncertainty in illness and studies of stress and coping may yield some rewarding hypotheses for family research. Answers to many questions and data to support many hypotheses already exist.

Issues for Further Investigation

1. What is the natural course of family experience in adapting to demands during and following hospitalization? How do these responses vary from family to family and from disease to disease?

2. How and when can the nurse be most effective in intervening with hospitalized patients and their families to promote positive family functioning?

3. Who is at highest risk for family dysfunction after a distressing or demanding hospitalization? How can those at risk be identified during hospitalization?

4. How do families vary in pattern of responses to hospitalization, depending on the age and family role of the hospitalized member?

References

Anderson J (1981): The social construction of illness experience: Families with a chronically ill child. *J Adv Nurs* 6: 427–434.

Barbarin OA (1986): Family experience of stigma. In: *The Dilemma of Difference: A Multidisciplinary View of Stigma*, Ainlay S, Becker G, Coleman L (eds.). New York: Plenum.

Barbarin OA, Chesler MA (1984): Coping as interpersonal strategy: Families with childhood cancer. *Fam Syst Med*, 2: 279–289.

Boss P, Greenberg J (1984): Family boundary ambiguity: A new variable in family stress theory. *Fam Process*, 23: 535–546.

Braulin JL, Rook J, Sills GM (1982): Families in crisis: The impact of trauma. *Crit Care Quarterly*, 1: 38–46.

Breznitz S (1983): The seven kinds of denial. In: *The Denial of Stress*. Brenitz S (ed.). New York: International Universities Press.

Brody J (1985): Parent care as normative family stress. *Gerontologist*, 25: 19–28.

Brown DG, Glazer H, Higgins M (1984): Group intervention: A psychological and educational approach to open heart surgery patients and their families. *Soc Work Health Care*, 9(2): 47–59.

Burns CE (1984): The hospitalization experience and single parent families. *Nurs Clin North Am*, 19: 285–293.

Butler M (1984): Families' responses to chemotherapy by an ambulatory infusion pump. *Nurs Clin North Am*, 19(1): 139–144.

Chafetz L, Gaillard J (1978): The impact of a therapeutic nurse-family relationship on post graduate public health nursing students. *Int J Nurs Stud*, 15: 37–49.

Clements DB (1986): Reminiscence: A tool for aiding families under stress. *Am J Mat Child Nurs*, 11: 114–117.

Cohen F, Lazarus R (1979): Coping with the stresses of illness. In: *Health Psychology—A Handbook: Theories, Applications and Challenges of a Psychological Approach to the Health Care System*, Stone GC et al (eds.). San Francisco: Jossey-Bass.

Curtis NM (1983): Caring for families during the "unknown" period. *Dimensions Crit Care Nurs*, 2: 248–254.

Daley L (1984): The perceived immediate needs of families with relatives in the intensive care setting. *Heart and Lung*, 13: 231–237.

Dhooper SS (1983): Family coping with the crisis of heart attack. *Soc Work Health Care*, 9(1): 15–31.

Dracup K, Breu C (1978): Using nursing research findings to meet the needs of grieving spouses. *Nurs Res*, 21: 212–216.

Dracup K et al (1984): Family-focused cardiac rehabilitation: A role supplementation program for cardiac patients and spouses. *Nurs Clin North Am*, 19(1): 113–124.

Drew J, Stoeclke JD, Billings, JA (1983): Tips, status and sacrifice: Gift giving in the doctor-patient relationship. *Soc Sci Med*, 17: 399–404.

Eberly TW et al (1985, June). Parental stress after the unexpected admission of a child to the intensive care unit. *Crit Care Quarterly*, 57–65.

Eldar R, Eldar E (1984): A place for the family in hospital life. *Int Nurs Rev*, 31: 40–42.

Erickson K (1973): Patient role and social uncertainty. In: *Deviance: The Interactionist Perspective*, 2nd ed. Rubington E, Weinberg M (eds.). New York: Macmillan.

Estroff S (1981): *Making It Crazy*. Berkeley: University of California Press.

Feetham S (1984): Family research: Issues and directions for nursing. In: *Annu Rev Nurs Res*, Vol 2. H. Werley & J. Fitzpatrick (eds.). New York: Springer-Verlag.

Ferraro A, Longo DC (1985): Nursing care of the family with a chronically ill, hospitalized child: An alternative approach. *Image*, 17: 77–81.

Fife BL (1985): A model for predicting the adaptation of families to medical crisis: An analysis of role integration. *Image*, 17: 108–112.

Fleck S (1975): The family and psychiatry. In: *Comprehensive Textbook of Psychiatry*, Vol 1, 2nd ed, Freedman A, Caplan H, Sadock B (eds.). Baltimore: Williams & Wilkins.

Geary M (1979): Supporting family coping. *Superv Nurse*, 10: 52–59.

Giaquinta B (1977): Helping families face the crisis of cancer. *Am J Nurs*, 77: 1585–1588.

Gilliss C (1983): A comparison of patient and spouse stress associated with coronary artery bypass surgery. *Communicating Nursing Research*, Batey MV (ed.), 16: 33. Boulder, CO: Western Interstate Commission for Higher Education.

Gilliss C (1984): Reducing stress during and after coronary bypass surgery. *Nurs Clin North Am*, 19(1): 103–112.

Hampe SO (1975): Needs of grieving spouse in a hospital setting. *Nurs Res, 24*: 133–120.

Hardgrove C, Healy D (1984): The care-through parent program at Moffitt Hospital, University of California, San Francisco. *Nurs Clin North Am, 19*(1): 145–160.

Hill R (1965): Generic features of families under stress. In: *Crisis Intervention: Selected Readings,* Parad H (ed.). New York: Family Service Association of America.

Hodovanic BH et al (1984): Family crisis intervention program in the medical intensive care unit. *Heart and Lung, 13*: 243–249.

Huston T, Robins E (1982): Conceptual and methodological issues in studying close relationships. *J Marr Fam, 44*: 901–926.

Hymovich DP (1981): Assessing the impact of chronic childhood illness on the family and parent coping. *Image, 13*: 71–74.

Jerrett MD, Ross MM (1982): Learning to nurse: The family as a unit of care. *J Adv Nurs, 7*: 461–468.

Kathol DK (1984): Anxiety in surgical patients' families. *AORN Journal, 4*: 131–137.

King SL, Gregor FM (1985): Stress and coping in families of the critically ill. *Crit Care Nurse, 5*: 48–51.

Kleinman A, Eisenberg L, Good BG (1978): Culture, illness and care: Cultural lessons from anthropologic and cross-cultural research. *Ann Int Med, 88*: 251–258.

Kleinman A (1978): Concepts and a model for the comparison of medical systems as cultural systems. *Soc Sci Med, 12*: 85–93.

Knafl K (1985) How families manage a pediatric hospitalization. *West J Nurs Res, 7*: 151–176.

Kupst MJ et al (1983): Strategies of intervention with families of pediatric leukemia patients: A longitudinal perspective. *Soc Work Health Care, 8*(2): 31–47.

Lasky P et al (1985): Developing an instrument for the assessment of family dynamics. *West J Nurs Res, 7*: 40–57.

Leavitt M (1982): *Families at Risk: Primary Prevention in Nursing Practice.* Boston: Little, Brown.

Leavitt M (1984): Nursing and family-focused care. *Nurs Clin North Am, 19*(1): 83–88.

Lewis FM (1983): Family level services for the cancer patient: Critical distinctions, fallacies and assessment. *Cancer Nurs, 6*: 193–200.

Litman T (1974): The family as a basic unit in health and medical care: A social behavioral overview. *Soc Sci Med, 8*: 495–519.

Litman T, Ventners M (1979): Research on health care and the family: A methodological overview. *Soc Sci Med, 13A*: 379–385.

Lust BL (1984): The patient in the ICU: A family experience. *Crit Care Quarterly, 7*: 49–57.

Mailick M (1984): The short-term treatment of depression of physically ill hospitalized patients. *Soc Work Health Care, 9*(3): 51–61.

Mathis M (1984): Personal needs of family members of critically ill patients with and without brain injury. *J Neurosurg Nurs, 16*: 37–44.

McCubbin HI, Patterson JM (1981): Family stress theory: The ABCX and Double ABCX models. In: *Systematic Assessment of Family Stress, Resources and Coping.* McCubbin HI, Patterson JM (eds.). St. Paul: Family Stress and Coping Project, University of Minnesota.

McCubbin HI (1979): Integrating coping behavior in family stress theory. *J Marr Fam, 41*: 237–244.

McHugh M, Dimitroff K, Davis N (1979): Family support group on a burn unit. *Am J Nurs, 79*: 2148–2150.

Meleis A, Swendsen L (1978): Role supplementation: An empirical test of a nursing intervention. *Nurs Res, 27*: 11–18.

Melito R (1985): Adaptation in family systems: A developmental perspective. *Fam Process, 24*: 89–100.

Miller JF (1983): Patient power resources. In: *Coping with Chronic Illness: Overcoming Helplessness,* Miller JF (ed.). Philadelphia: Davis.

Minarik P (1984) The psychiatric liaison nurse's role with families in acute care. *Nurs Clin North Am, 19*(1): 161–172.

Mishel M (1984): Perceived uncertainty and stress in illness. *Res Nurs Health, 7*: 163–171.

Molter N (1979): Needs of relatives of critically ill patients: A descriptive study. *Heart and Lung, 8*: 332–339.

Norris LO, Grove SK (1986) Investigation of selected psychosocial needs of family members of critically ill adult patients. *Heart and Lung, 15*: 194–199.

Oberst MT, James RH (1985): Going home: Patient and spouse adjustment following cancer surgery. *Top Clin Nurs, 7*: 46–57.

O'Connor P (1984): Health care financing policy: Impact on nursing. *Nurs Admin Quarterly, 8*(4): 10–20.

Offer D, Shabshin M (1974): *Normality* (rev ed). New York: Basic Books.

Parkes M (1971): Psychosocial transitions: A field for study. *Soc Sci Med, 5*: 101–114.

Pearlmutter D et al (1984): Models of family-centered care in one acute care institution. *Nurs Clin North Am, 19*(1): 173–188.

Porter L (1980): Health care workers' role conceptions and orientation to family centered care. *Nurs Res, 28*: 330–337.

Poster EC, Betz C (1984): When the patient dies: Dealing with the family's anger. *Dimen Crit Care Nurs, 3*: 373–377.

Pratt L (1976): *Family Structure and Effective Health Behavior*. Boston: Houghton-Mifflin.

Ragiel CA (1984): The impact of critical injury on patient, family and clinical systems. *Crit Care Quarterly, 7*: 73–78.

Rasie S (1981): Meeting families' needs helps you meet ICU patients' needs. *Nursing, 80*: 32–35.

Robinson C, Thorne S (1984): Strengthening family "interference." *J Adv Nurs, 9*: 597–602.

Rose L (1983): Understanding mental illness: The experience of families of psychiatric patients. *J Adv Nurs, 8*: 507–511.

Rose L, Finestone K, Bass J (1985): Group support for the families of psychiatric patients. *J Psychosoc Nurs, 23*(12):25–29.

Schmidt D (1979): The family as a unit of medical care. *J Fam Pract, 7*: 303–308.

Schwenk T, Hughes C (1983): The family as patient in family medicine: Rhetoric or reality? *Soc Sci Med, 17*: 1–16.

Scott DW, Goode WL, Arlin Z (1983): The psychodynamics of multiple remissions in a patient with acute nonlymphoblastic leukemia. *Cancer Nurs, 6*: 201–206.

Shapiro J (1983): Family reactions and coping strategies in response to the physically ill or handicapped child: A review. *Soc Sci Med, 17*: 913–931.

Silva MC (1979): Effects of orientation information on spouses' anxiety and attitudes toward hospitalization and surgery. *Res Nurs Health, 2*: 127–136.

Spinetta JJ (1984): Measurement of family function, communication, and cultural effects. *Cancer, 53*: 2330–2338.

Stillwell S (1984): Importance of visiting needs as perceived by the family members of patients in the intensive care unit. *Heart and Lung, 13*: 238–242.

Temple P (1983): Using research in practice: The practice of family assessment by nurses who work with children: Implications for nursing. *West J Nurs Res, 5*: 194–196.

Thorne S (1985): The famiy cancer experience. *Cancer Nurs, 8*: 285–291.

Thornton J, Berry J, Dal Santo J (1984): Neonatal intensive care: The nurse's role in supporting the family. *Nurs Clin North Am, 19*(1): 125–138.

Toth R (1984): DRGs: Imperative strategies for nursing service administration. *Nurs Health Care, 5*: 197–203.

Tripp-Reimer T (1984): Reconceptualizing the construct of health: Integrating emic and etic perspectives. *Res Nurs Health, 7*: 101–109.

Volinn I (1983): Health professionals as stigmatizers and destigmatizers of diseases: Alcoholism and leprosy as examples. *Soc Sci Med, 17*: 385–393.

Walters LH (1982): Are families different from other groups? *J Marr Fam, 44*: 841–850.

Watson S, Hickey P (1984): Help for the family in waiting. *Am J Nurs, 84*: 604–608.

Welch D (1981): Planning nursing interventions for family members of adult cancer patients. *Cancer Nurs, 4*: 365–370.

Welch D (1982): Anticipatory grief reactions in family members of adult patients. *Iss Ment Health Nurs, 4*: 149–158.

Wright K, Dyck S (1984): Expressed concerns of adult cancer patients' family members. *Cancer Nurs, 7*: 371–374.

Yoder L, Jones SL (1982): The family of the emergency room patient as seen through the eyes of the nurse. *Int J Nurs Stud, 19*: 29–36.

Young R (1983): The family-illness intermesh: theoretical aspects and their application. *Soc Sci Med, 17*: 395–398.

Zind R (1974): Deterrents to crisis intervention in the hospital unit. *Nurs Clin North Am, 9*: 27–26.

PROMOTING FAMILY HEALTH DURING CHRONIC ILLNESS

18

THE FAMILY AND CHRONIC ILLNESS

Catherine L. Gilliss, RNC, DNSc

Debra B. Rose, RN, MS, PNP

Jeanne C. Hallburg, RN, PhD

Ida M. Martinson, RN, PhD, FAAN

Statistics suggest that the number of families with chronically ill members has increased in recent years. The family nurse plays a crucial role in the care of such families and often the need for family-focused interventions is critical. This chapter identifies ways in which chronic illness affects family life and describes how families problem-solve when a family member has a chronic illness. It also identifies nursing strategies to assist families experiencing chronic illness. The chapter is followed by a photographic gallery chronicling the home care of a man with amyotrophic lateral sclerosis.

Jeanne Hallburg is Director of the Diabetes Teaching Center at the University of California at San Francisco. Also a professor in the Department of Family Health Care Nursing, she has particular expertise in patient/family teaching, and in nursing care of the chronically ill.

Debra Rose prepared as a pediatric nurse practitioner and is a former clinical faculty member in the Department of Family Health Care Nursing at the University of California at San Francisco. She is currently a clinical research associate in the bioscience industry.

Introduction

Advances in public health, nutrition, and control of infectious disease have joined with dramatic increases in medical sophistication to produce a life span of ever-increasing length. A male born in 1984 is expected to live to the age of 71 years; a female will survive to age 78 (U.S. Census Bureau, 1984). In addition to the increased length of the life span, more vulnerable infants and vulnerable others are surviving. These survivors are likely to experience some yet unknown consequences of the treatment they have received. For instance, leukemic survivors of radiation and chemotherapy may experience learning disabilities or retardation of the growth of myaline as a result of their treatment (Moore, 1985). The eventual consequence of our public health progress and our medical masteries is that more and more people will live longer, and many of these will suffer from at least one chronic illness.

Statistics suggest that chronic illness is on the rise among children and elders. The number of families who have a child with chronic illness demands comprehensive nursing interventions. "Current estimates suggest that between 5 and 18 percent of all children suffer from some chronic illness or disability, and when new morbidities* are included, the prevalence estimates approach 30 percent or more" (IHPS, 1985). A yearly household survey, the National Health Interview Study, was begun in 1957 and has tapped 110,000 individuals, including 30,000 children under 17 years of age. According to this survey, the numbers of children with activity limitations related to health has doubled from 18 to 38 per 1000 within the past 30 years. More limitations of activity are seen among males than among females, and more limitations of activity are seen in the newborn to 5-year-old than in children from 6 to 16 years of age. In absolute

numbers, there are approximately 2 million children with chronic health problems (Budetti, Newacheck, 1985). Another source has described the disability rate in 1979 as twice the rate in 1962, affecting at least one million children (Harkey, 1983).

Severely disabled persons—those unable to carry on the major activities appropriate to their age group (attending school, working, housekeeping)—are estimated to comprise 3.7% of the population of 7.9 million Americans with a chronic illness. A significant rapid rise of severe disability has been reported in the yearly Health Interview Surveys. From 1966 to 1979, the prevalence of severe disability has increased by more than 70%, from 213 to 365 Americans per 10,000 (DeJong, Lifchez, 1983). Colvez and Blanchet (1981) have attributed rapidly rising causes of severe disability to hypertension (without heart involvement) and diabetes. These two causes of severe disability increased by 172% and 221% respectively from 1966 to 1976. In addition, about 1.5 million Americans have Alzheimer's disease, and 60% of the nursing home population is stricken with this "silent epidemic" (Burnside, 1982, 1983).

The significance of this increase to those who care for families is obvious. For with few exceptions, chronically ill persons are cared for by their family members. Organizing to provide care to a chronically ill person makes special demands on families. Therefore, these families are at risk for ill health. Fortunately, not all families who face the challenges of caring for a chronically ill member experience permanent disruption; however, we do know that these families differ from those in transition and that they have some common features.

Chronic Illness versus Transition

The family facing chronic illness differs from the family in transition. Chronic illness is a nonnormative event at any stage in the life cycle. There-

---

*The term *new morbidities* refers to problems associated with behavior, education, and families in general.

fore, the onset of a chronic disease represents a crisis. The crisis is often associated with the actual diagnosis of the problem, though it may follow by several weeks. The particular timing may vary with the characteristics of the disease, with those diseases with a rapid onset and immediate restrictions of behavior (for example, myocardial infarction) differing from those with an insidious and ambiguous onset (for example, hypertension). The crisis experienced by the family will result from the deficit that they experience in trying to meet new demands with old behavior patterns or without adequate information.

Change will be demanded of these families for an undetermined period of time. In that sense the family facing chronic illness also differs from the family in transition. These families will always be on their guard for expected and unexpected changes in the ill member. They will struggle to balance their need to be normal with their special needs. Families who are dealing with chronic illness require ongoing support from friends, health care providers, and communities.

Assumptions About the Family and Chronic Illness

Our overall assumption that we can be helpful to the family facing chronic illness is lodged in the following series of subassumptions, developed by Leahey and Wright (1985):

1. There are predictable points of family stress where there is a chronic illness.

2. Families vary in their level of tolerance for the patient's physical condition.

3. Families under stress tend to hold onto previously proven patterns of behavior, whether or not they are effective.

4. Families usually go through a grief–loss process following the diagnosis of a disabling condition.

5. Families play a significant role in the encouragement or discouragement of the family member with the chronic illness to participate in particular therapies.

6. Families react to particular illness behavior.

7. Many families have difficulty adjusting to a chronic physical illness because they either have incorrect or inadequate disease-related information.

8. Where there is a chronic illness, families must adjust to changes in expectations for each other.

9. A family's perception of the illness event has the most influence on their ability to cope.

These assumptions suggest that there is a common pattern to the experience of chronic illness in the family but that the pattern will vary somewhat between families. For instance, Assumption 1 suggests that there are predictable points of family stress in chronic illness. For each of the illnesses described in other chapters, these predictable points need to be identified. Further, they need to be particularized to the families who receive nursing care.

These assumptions, developed by clinician–scholars, direct the researcher to other fertile areas for exploration. Why do families vary in their tolerance for a patient's condition? Why can one family care for a schizophrenic member at home, but another cannot? In what ways does the family promote or discourage participation in treatment? And how is this ultimately useful for the family? What disease-related information is critical for the family to have to cope with the illness? Must everyone have this information, or are there particular members who must know? How does a family develop a perception of the illness event? Can nursing care influence that perception?

Inherent in Leahey and Wright's (1985) listed assumptions are a number of concepts and constructs that bear further examination. First, there is a notion of the family moving through space and time, having a life course of its own.

Assumption 1 suggests that this overtime trajectory will have some predictable points of family stress. Assumptions 2 and 6 suggest that there is significance to the characteristics of the illness, or the related illness behaviors. Family reactions, responses and coping, are all identified as functions of stress, illness features or perceptions of the illness. The identification of these concepts and constructs provides some direction in model-building about family behavior in response to chronic illness, and it may suggest why particular theories of family behavior have been popular with nurse scientists studying the family and chronic illness.

Family Frameworks Used in the Study of Chronic Illness

Though not intended to supplant Mercer's discussion of frameworks in Chapter 2, it is worth noting that several approaches to the study of families with chronic illness have been commonly employed by nurse scientists, notably family stress theory and the family paradigm.

Family Stress Theory

Family stress theory has developed from the general area of interaction, discussed by Mercer in Chapter 2. The interaction framework assumes the following to be true:

1. Humans live in a complex symbolic environment as well as a physical environment.
2. The interpretation of these symbol systems is taught by the family and other institutions.

This includes learning characteristic patterns of response to the physical, social, and emotional environments.

3. Social behavior is influenced by ideas in the mind.
4. Thinking is the process by which symbolic solutions are examined, assessed for their value to the individual, and chosen for action.
5. Humans are actors as well as reactors.
6. The family is an interacting and transacting organization.
7. The family has emergent properties; that is, it is greater than the sum of its parts.
8. Health behavior is a subset of human behavior that is best understood by studying the "mentalistic definitions people make of their unique situations" (Burr et al, 1979, p. 49).
9. Family health affects individual health, and individual health affects family health.

Using these assumptions, the relationship in Figure 18–1 may be proposed for the family. This equation was originally proposed by Hill (1949) and elaborated on by Burr (1973). Hill's work focused on the interaction of three variables: (A) a crisis-provoking event; (B) the family's resources; and (C) the meaning attached to the event to predict (X) the crisis-proneness of a family (Hill, 1949, 1958). The family was described by Hill as an interacting and transacting organization with internal roles, positions, and norms. These, in addition to the life experience of the family, comprise its repertoire of resources for dealing with life events, some of which are potential crises. According to Hill, a stressful

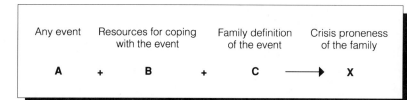

Figure 18–1 The ABC model of family stress (Hill, 1949).

event can be defined by the family alone. When the equation is reversed, we see that crisis-prone families (A) experience more frequent and severe stressful events; (B) have developed fewer resources for dealing with such events; or (C) define more of these events as crises than noncrisis-prone families.

A reworking of this formulation by Burr (1973) resulted in the identification of six variables that explain a family's behavior in response to stressors. Directly affecting the linear course between event and outcome are two variables: the amount of change and family vulnerability to stress. Affecting vulnerability are the definition of the seriousness of the event and family adaptability.

Mediating between family vulnerability to stress and family regenerative power (which characterize the family's ability to withstand the impact of a stressor and to recover if disrupted) are personal influence, positional influence, family integration, and family adaptability. Burr (1973) identified these as the core concepts in the study of family stress.

Fundamental to this framework is the development of stress as a concept distinct from stressor. Stressor is used to describe a particular external event or demand, and stress refers to the internal, subjective definition given to that event or experienced in response to a stressor. Therefore, a theoretical distinction is made between the event and the response to the event.

The A factor, the crisis-precipitating event, or stressor, is a "situation for which the family has had little preparation" (Hill, 1958) and must be viewed as problematic. Such events vary considerably from family to family, based on the individual family response to the event. Therefore, although theoretically distinct, the stress–stressor concepts are empirically interdependent.

The B factor, the family's crisis-meeting resources, is largely underdeveloped by Hill. He states that these resources lie within the family and must be distinguished from the attributes of the event itself. Burr's development of six new concepts actually serves to better describe the

family's abilities and structure that impinge on the outcome variable of X, the level of reorganization. These concepts are proposed as direct and indirect influences on the dependent variable, amount of crisis in the family social system. They include family vulnerability to stress; amount of positional influence of the family; amount of personal influence by the family; family definition of the seriousness of the changes; family externalization of blame for the changes; and regenerative power of families (Burr, 1973). Despite the fact that these concepts have been identified, little clarification has taken place. Hansen and Johnson (1979) have suggested that several of these concepts are distracting.

McCubbin (1979) has proposed that the B factor includes the family use of community resources, as well as its intrafamilial coping behaviors. He suggested that the family has been viewed only as a reactor to stressful events; yet the family has been shown to function proactively and to engage in transactions with the community as well. Specifically, McCubbin identified a need for familial development of integration and adaptability as internal resources and of a range of behaviors that strengthen the internal organization and functioning of the family, procure community and social supports, and reduce or eliminate sources of stress. McCubbin defined coping as a strategy for managing stress.

The stress variable is also referred to as "C factor" or "the definition the family makes of the event." In his early work, Hill distinguished between three types of definitions: (1) those formulated by an impartial observer; (2) those formulated by the community; and (3) those subjective definitions made by the family itself (Hill, 1949). Hill is careful to note that the latter description is appropriate to the C factor. Thus, the definition made by the family is viewed as a subjective, personal determination of one's own particular situation.

The X factor, or crisis-proneness of the family, is the dependent variable of the original

Hill equation. Again, the lack of clarity associated with the concept is evident by the many labels that have been used for this factor: type of adjustment (Cavan, Ranck, 1938); level of adjustment (Hill, 1949); recovery from crisis (Dyer, 1963); magnitude of crisis (Hill, 1958); and level of reorganization (Hill, Hansen, 1962). Burr (1973) has described the X factor as a continuous variable representing the amount of disorganization, disruptiveness, inefficiency, or crisis experienced by the family social system following a stressful event.

McCubbin and Patterson (1983) have proposed an elaboration, which they call the Double ABCX model. The Double ABCX model adds four additional factors to Hill's basic design that are believed to influence the course of a family's adaptation over time: (aA) the accumulation of additional stressors; (bB) family efforts to activate or acquire new coping resources; and (cC) modifications by the family of their perception of the total crisis situation. The entire set of variables is believed to be related and to contribute to a postcrisis level of family adaptation (xX), either bonadaptation or maladaptation (Figure 18-2). This level of adaptation is achieved through balancing of the reciprocal relationships that exist between individuals and the family system and between the family system and the community.

In a thoughtful critique of family stress theory, Walker (1985) acknowledges the heuristic value of the approach but addresses several crucial flaws. Notably, she challenges the existence of an event-specific stressor, recognizing the emergent properties of most stressful events. Additionally, Walker points out the operational interchangeability of individual resources with family resources, despite their conceptual distinction. She asks whether families ever share a perception of an event. Finally, Walker notes the omission of sociohistorical context from the family stress paradigm, claiming that it is impossible to understand the family outside of this context.

The Family Paradigm

The study of problem-solving in both clinical and nonclinical families has led Reiss and Oliveri (1980) to the development of a classifica-

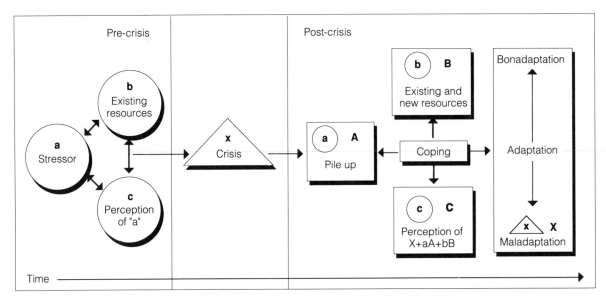

Figure 18–2 The double ABCX model (McCubbin, Patterson; 1983).

tion system that discriminates among families by problem-solving style. Based on the assumption that the family's intrinsic styles and capacities are manifest in the routines of typical, quiescent periods and that these behaviors may be viewed on the level of the family group, Reiss and Oliveri have proposed that the family paradigm is responsible for explaining the family's response to stressful events.

Consistent with the interaction approach, the family problem- solving framework assumes that each individual develops a personal system of social constructs and convictions about how these interrelate. These constructs and ideas guide behavior in novel, as well as familiar, situations. The shared system of family understanding results from reconciliation of the basic premises held by the involved individuals. Such reconciliation and integration must progress over time for a family to continue to develop. Conflict is viewed as a method undertaken by the family group to reconcile differences (Reiss, 1981).

Shared constructs may change throughout a family's history as a result of developmental and situational changes the family faces. Recovery from a crisis can result in reconstruction of premises and a change in the typical model of construing events. The sum of the family's constructs and premises is described as the family paradigm.

Reiss and Oliveri contend that knowledge of the family paradigm enables prediction of family response to moderately stressful events. The dimensions of this family paradigm are: configuration; coordination; and closure. *Configuration* refers to the degree to which a family can organize or discover patterns in a stimulus. *Coordination* is the aspect that describes the family membership's abilities to organize themselves to work together. Finally, *closure* specifies the amount of time spent by families in collecting all the available information pertaining to the awaited decision.

Three conceptual vantage points are identified for viewing the family response to a stress-ful event: (1) the definition and search for information; (2) the initial response and trial solutions; and (3) the final decision and the family's commitment to that position. These activities may occur in any order or simultaneously. The style within each phase is explained as a result of the dimensional qualities of the family paradigm (see Table 18–1).

Family stress theory and the family paradigm represent two explanations of family behavior that may be helpful when trying to understand the family and chronic illness. Both approaches attempt to address the family's process of responding to the demands for adjustment or change within it. Neither approach, however, speaks specifically to the relationship of the nurse or other health care providers with the family.

A Closer Look at Family Coping: What Does It Mean?

Coping functions are efforts to disregard distress or solve problems. Coping is not merely an adjustment to circumstances but often involves changing circumstances. Five individually oriented coping modes are described by Cohen and Lazarus (1979): (1) seeking information; (2) taking direct action; (3) inhibiting action; (4) using intrapsychic–cognitive processes; and (5) turning to others for help and support. Coping is best understood as involving multiple actions and thoughts that may change with time (Lazarus, Folkman, 1984). In the case of chronic illness, family members may need to employ different coping modes at different times. Family needs will evolve and change.

Similar coping modes have been described by Barbarin, Hughes, and Chesler (1985), who studied parents of children diagnosed with cancer. These modes included (1) information-seeking; (2) problem-solving; (3) help-seeking; (4) maintenance of emotional balance; (5) reliance on religion; (6) optimism; (7) denial; and

Table 18-1 Hypothesized Influence of Family Paradigm Dimensions on the Three Aspects of the Family's Response to Stressful Events

Paradigm Dimensions		Definition of the Event and Search for Additional Information	Phases of Family Coping	
			Initial Responses and Trial Solutions	Final Decision or Closing Position and Family's Commitment to This
Configuration: Mastery	High:	1. *Owning up.* Family takes responsibility for event and/or coping	2. *Exploration.* Family's initial responses are designed to seek information and outside resources or are in response to information and outside support	3. *Response to outcome.* The family is proud of accomplishment or feels it has learned something of value in failure
	Low:	Family feels victimized and blames outside forces	Initial reactions are unrelated to information or explanation	The family feels fortunate if successful or victimized if not
Coordination: Solidarity	High:	4. *Family identity.* Readily perceived as family issue; information exchanged quickly	5. *Organization or response.* Organized, integrated response by all family members; roles clear	6. *Consensus on decision.* Decision was reached with clear consensus and family remains committed to it
	Low:	Slowly or not perceived as family issue; information exchanged slowly; events are seen as happening to individual members	Individuals act on own; overt or covert conflict possible	The consensus was forced on the family by a single individual; the status of agreement unclear, or no consensus is reached
Closure: Openness	High: (Delayed)	7. *Reference to the past.* Focuses on current experiences; past family history unimportant	8. *Novelty of responses.* First responses include trying something new; individual experiences, intuitions, and guesses are encouraged	9. *Self-evaluation.* As a result of coping, family alters conception of itself in some way
	Low:	Past determines current perception and action; little interest in raw experience; more interest in convention or tradition	First responses mostly typical or familiar	As a result of coping, family confirms conception of itself

From Reiss D, Oliveri ME (1980): Family paradigm and family coping: A proposal for linking the family's intrinsic adaptive capacities to its responses to stress. *Fam Relations, 29:441.* Reprinted with permission of the authors and the National Council on Family Relations, 1910 West County Road B, Suite 147, St. Paul, MN, 55113.

(8) acceptance. Barbarin et al (1985) noted that parents who adopted more passive coping strategies tended to be those who were less well educated, but they enjoyed better relationships with medical staff than parents who were not passive.

The family faces additional demands in the presence of chronic illness. There are increased contacts with health professionals and the demands imposed by the disease itself. Pless et al, 1972, and Pless and Satterwhite, 1973, observed that certain characteristics of the disease seem to influence the family's ability to respond. These characteristics included age at onset, manner of progression, severity, prognosis, duration, and associated disability.

Family coping is distinct from the coping of individual family members, though it is often dependent on the coping of individuals. Family coping represents a group property that emerges from the interaction of the family members with their situation and their history. Family coping might be compromised when individual family members cope differently; however, this should not be assumed to be the case. The net effect of activity on the welfare of the family group must be evaluated. How can the nurse working with families experiencing a chronic illness promote coping of the family group?

The Role of the Nurse in Family Coping

Families experiencing a chronic illness have special needs. Nursing care can promote family coping through several strategies.

Families Need Coordination

Recent modifications in the health care delivery system have changed the nurse's role in caring for the chronically ill. More care is accomplished outside the hospital setting, both in clinics and at home. Nurses must help coordinate care for family members.

Coordination of care providers is one critical nursing responsibility in family care. The nurse's professional background in the requirements of care is of immense assistance for the family who may not be able to anticipate the care requirements or know where to find the resources to meet these needs.

Case Study Mabel is a 90-year-old woman who does not want to be admitted to a nursing home. The physicians have been urging nursing home placement because they believe she is unsafe at home. Mabel is a diabetic and dependent on daily insulin injections. An ulcer on her leg needs regular treatment. Her diabetes also needs close monitoring. Mabel's sister lives with her. She too is physically very weak, but with the help of various providers, the two sisters are able to manage at home. Mabel's daughter does the washing, cleaning, and shopping for her mother and aunt. Without the care providers, the daughter would not be able to let her mother be at home. The care needed includes the professional nurse from 15 minutes to 1 hour, 7 days a week; a home health aide 2 hours per visit for 3 to 4 times a week; and volunteers twice a month. The assignment of care to these providers is carefully coordinated by professional nurses, who identify and coordinate other resources from the community when needed.

Families Need Information

Families need a considerable amount of information to meet the demands of chronic illness. This information, properly offered, will serve as a source of support to the family.

Nurses provide information, based on physiologic and psychologic knowledge and on both health and care-related issues, such as maintaining skin integrity, preventing trauma, reducing possible sources of infection, promoting nutrition, promoting comfort, and recognizing and limiting side effects of medications. Providing feedback, altering interventions, and offering general encouragement to continue necessary protective measures over long periods of time are nursing activities.

Families need information about the illness and about how to care for the patient; they need to know how the care of the patient minimizes the patient's risk of complications. For instance, diet for a diabetic is important. The family who has a thorough understanding of the disease and the diet can be of great assistance to the diabetic.

Nurses also provide information about feelings. Some changes related to chronic illness are permanent, as in the case of amputation. Nurses expect grieving to occur in association with such losses and can aid the family in recognizing and normalizing this feeling. In addition, they must provide time, over a period of time and in accordance with patients' expressed concerns, for patients to discuss treatment-induced changes.

Families need information about resources. For instance, for the families of children having multiple congenital anomalies, physicians may provide information about the specific anomalies, but nurses might initiate referrals for genetic counseling or crippled children's services. Nurses also provide information regarding day-care centers for chronically ill children and adults. By collaborating and coordinating care plans with other health care providers, such as a physical therapist, social worker, or psychiatrist, and by having a functional knowledge of community resources, nurses advocate effectively for the needs of the individual and the family.

Families need information about their own responses. Informal teaching sources are increasingly available in the form of support groups. Identification and involvement of families who have a member with similar illnesses creates a unique sharing of experiences and feelings. Family members learn that their feelings are not unique. Providing nursing care by referring families or by facilitating group meetings is beneficial. Groups may involve only one nurse and a family discussing its ill member on a home visit or larger groups established by a foundation such as the Candlelighters or Alzheimer's Disease and Related Disorders Association.

Families Need to Communicate among Themselves and with Others

Communication is a complex process in families. Nurses help the chronically ill member and families to focus discussions of the diagnosis and impact of the illness on the family. Limited time may be available due to physical limitations of patient energy. Opening channels for discussions on a variety of topics may provide immense relief. Communication is a key concept in unlocking the doors to the stressors associated with chronic illness. Social isolation may adversely affect the individual and the family. It may be difficult for family members to discuss the impact of a chronic illness in terms of disability or even death. Exploring the patient's and family's understanding of the illnesses and necessary treatments is a vital area for nursing intervention, particularly with numerous specialists providing health care. Helping the family to determine the nature and content of discussions with children and other family members regarding chronic illness is an important nursing goal.

Families Need Advocates

Families need to be assisted by nurses to exercise their freedom of self-determination. Advocacy involves assessing the family's knowledge and understanding of the situation, clarifying and answering questions, and helping families to explore the concerns they were reluctant to discuss with the physician. The authors believe the professional nurse has a specific role in and responsibility for advocacy. Clearly the nurse needs to be more responsible for the health care delivery system. In an earlier study by Martinson (Martinson, Palta, Rude, 1977), a survey of registered nurses regarding home care for the dying, one surprising result concerned the nurses' self-understanding of their role. It was discovered that the nurses believed that their least important responsibility was the decision concerning whether home or hospital was the most appropriate site for the dying process and death event to take place. Nurses can be advocates for families when they desire to request a second opinion on treatment options. Clinical experiences reveal that the families, more so than the patients, are helped by the opinion of a knowledgeable second expert. In a recent case, the agreement among several experts about the best physician and treatment center for their only daughter, who was ill with a brain tumor, greatly relieved both parents.

Families Need Respite

Families may need to be reminded of the importance for respite. This is especially the case with chronic illness because the long-term demands of patient care can be exhausting. If the time is relatively short, as in the event of a dying child, the nurses need to be alert to the possibility that if respite care involves either the movement of the child to another setting or the bringing in of outside care providers, the family may not wish it. When respite care is not desired, support to the family must be more intense, and ready help for emergencies must be available. The sleep of family members each night is essential. There is no chance to make up for the loss of sleep the next day. Thus, symptom control is essential for the patient, in part to enable family members to get adequate rest. The simple knowledge that a visit is available at any time is one important form of respite for families. There are clearly situations where more respite care is needed. Although respite care can be provided in the home, there are a growing number of respite centers that will accept a seriously ill individual for one to two weeks at a time. This relief from the daily, unrelenting demands of a seriously ill family member can serve to sustain family members over a long period of time. Respite care can be given to family members in the home for short periods of time. For example,

relief for two hours a day, three times a week, can allow the family members to do other chores outside of the house or to get some relief from the intense care demands of the ill family member.

Summary

The role of family nurses in care of the family with a chronically ill member is of major importance now and in future decades. Essential services of support—through information, resources, and monitoring—enable many families to survive these demanding experiences that put them at risk.

In the next few decades, nursing research will need to focus on measuring the changes in families as a result of nursing interventions aimed at reducing or preventing complications. By generating new hypotheses and theories concerning risk factors, nurses can expand the scientific basis for family health care. A considerable number of unanswered questions face us. When can families most benefit from our help? What information is most critical? Prospective studies are needed to assess family coping strategies to describe characteristics associated with adequate adjustment to chronic illness. Persuasive empirical evidence is still lacking regarding family-focused interventions, in terms of prevention and treatment (Doherty, 1985). The family, however, influences both the patient's behavior and the provider-patient relationship. Therefore, the need for family-focused interventions is crucial. As "no one discipline owns family interventions, this area might serve as an example for professional collaboration between nurses and physicians" (Doherty, 1985). New theories are advancing the science and discipline of family health care, influenced by a multitude of patient and family needs. The challenge for future decades of nurses is to continue to develop innovative ways to understand families and to develop sensitive, personalized health care for them.

Issues for Further Investigation

1. At what point in the chronic illness trajectory can families most benefit from nursing interventions?

2. What is the nature of and timing of information needed by families living with chronic illness?

3. What are the individual and family characteristics associated with adequate adjustment to chronic illness?

4. How does the family influence both the patient's behavior and the provider/patient relationship?

5. What family coping styles and family-implemented interventions are the most helpful?

6. How do well-functioning families manage the demands of illness and meet their developmental needs?

References

Barbarin OA, Hughes D, Chesler MA (1985): Stress, coping, and marital functioning among parents of children with cancer. *J Marr Fam, 47:* 473–480.

Budetti PP, Newacheck PW (1985, July): Chronic disease and disability in children: Are the risks increasing? University of California, San Francisco, *IHPS Report, 5*(2).

Burnside IM (1982–1983): Editorial: If I don't worry, who will? *J Gerontol Nurs, 8–9:* 2.

Burr W (1973): *Theory Construction and the Sociology of the Family.* New York: Wiley.

Burr W et al (1979): Symbolic interaction and the family. *Contemporary Theories About the Family:* Vol. 2, Burr W et al (eds.). New York: Free Press, pp 582–603.

Cavan R, Ranck K (1938): *The Family and the Depression.* Chicago: University of Chicago Press.

Cohen F, Lazarus R (1979): Coping with the stresses of illness. In: *Health Psychology:* A Handbook.

Stone GC, Cohen F, Adler NE (eds.). San Francisco: Jossey-Bass.

Colvez A, Blanchet M (1981): Disability trends in the United States population 1966–76: Analysis of reported causes. *Am J Public Health, 75*(5): 464–471.

DeJong G, Lifchez R (1983, June): Physical disability and public policy. *Scientific American, 248*(6): 40–49.

Doherty WJ (1985): Family interventions in health care. *Fam Relations, 34:* 129–137.

Dyer E (1963): Parenthood as crisis: A re-study. *Marr Fam Living, 25:* 196–201.

Hansen D, Johnson V (1979): Rethinking family stress theory. In: *Contemporary Theories About the Family:* Vol. 1, Burr W et al (eds.). New York: Free Press.

Harkey J (1983): The epidemiology of selected chronic childhood health conditions. *Children's Health Care, 12:* 62–71.

Hill R (1949): *Families Under Stress.* New York: Harper & Row.

Hill R (1958): Social stress on the family. *Soc Casework, 39:* 139–150.

Hill R, Hansen D (1962): The family in disaster. In: *Man and Society in Disaster,* Baker G, Chapman D (eds.). New York: Basic Books.

Institute for Health Policy Studies (1985, July): Childhood chronic illness. University of California, San Francisco, *IHPS Report, 5.*

Lazarus RS, Folkman S (1984): *Stress, Appraisal and Coping.* New York: Springer-Verlag.

Leahey M, Wright L (1985): Intervening with families with chronic illness. *Fam Syst Med, 3*(1): 60-69. Copyright © Brunner/Mazel, Inc.

Martinson I, Palta M, Rude N (1977, April): Death and dying: Selected attitudes and experiences to Minnesota's registered nurses. *Commun Nurs Res, 9:* 197–206, Boulder Colorado Western Interstate Commission for Higher Education.

McCubbin H (1979): Integrating coping behavior in family stress theory. *J Marr Fam, 41*(2): 237–244.

McCubbin H, Patterson J (1983): The family stress process: The double ABCX Model of adjustment and adaptation. In: *Social Stress and the Family,* McCubbin H, Sussman M, Patterson J (eds.). New York: Hawthorne.

Moore K (1985): Late effects of childhood cancer on cognitive and psychosocial development. Unpublished doctoral dissertation, University of California, San Francisco School of Nursing.

Pless IB, Roghman K, Haggerty RJ (1972): Chronic illness, family functioning, and psychological adjustment: A model for the allocation of preventive mental health services. *Int J Epidemiol, 1:* 271–277.

Pless IB, Satterwhite B (1973): A measure of family functioning and its application. *Soc Sci Med, 7:* 613–621.

Reiss D, Oliveri ME (1980): Family paradigm and family coping: A proposal for linking the family's in-trinsic adaptive capacities to its responses to stress *Fam Rel, 29:* 431–444.

Reiss D (1981): *The Family's Construction of Reality.* Cambridge, MA: Harvard University Press.

Walker A (1985): Reconceptualizing family stress. *J Marr Fam,* 47(4): 827–837.

U.S. Census Bureau (1984), Washington, DC: U.S. GPO.

THE STORY OF BILL HANEY
Home Care of the Chronically Ill

by Tom Ferentz

What are the dimensions of home care? What improvisation and support does it take to normalize as much as possible the daily life of a severely handicapped and totally dependent person?

Bill Haney had amyotrophic lateral sclerosis (ALS). He would have spent his last few years shuttling between intensive care and a nursing home had not Gina (an old friend and former lover), who knew Bill would not survive for long under those circumstances, left her job and her own home and devoted herself entirely to Bill's care.

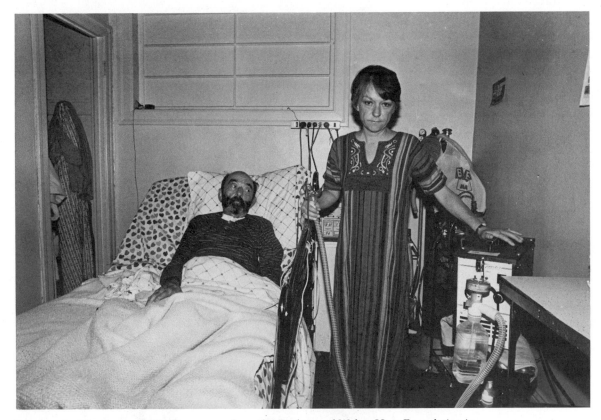

Funding for The Story of Bill Haney came from the Evelyn and Walter Haas Foundation in San Francisco.

Gina spent three months training at the Medical Center in the Pulmonary Unit. She learned how to operate respirator equipment, and she claimed she could even change Bill's trachea tube if she had the proper credentials.

Gina was Bill's primary caretaker. She was supported by a home health aide who came once a week to relieve her. Gina could then go out, do errands, have coffee, or just relax. Although she could have taken the whole day off, she usually didn't. She returned within an hour or didn't go out at all.

Walter, Bill's longtime friend, dropped by every day. He built a number of things for the house, including a call light system installed over Bill's bed.

This support system enabled Bill, who hated to be confined, to live at home and relate to his community in a reasonably normal way. This included engaging in simple activities, like going to the grocery store, the neighborhood bar, or just spending time in the back yard.

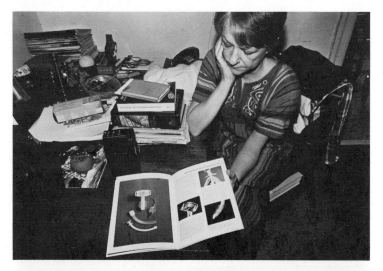

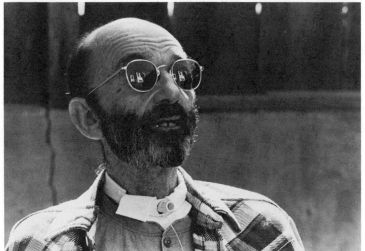

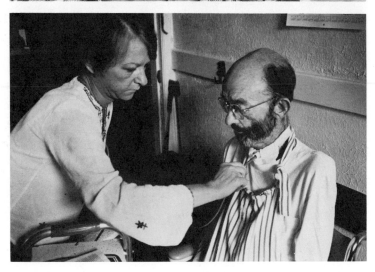

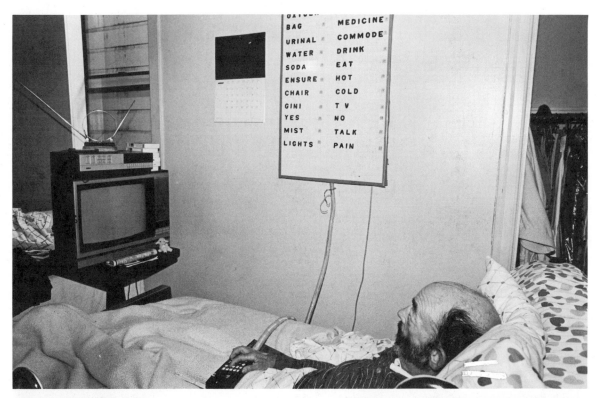

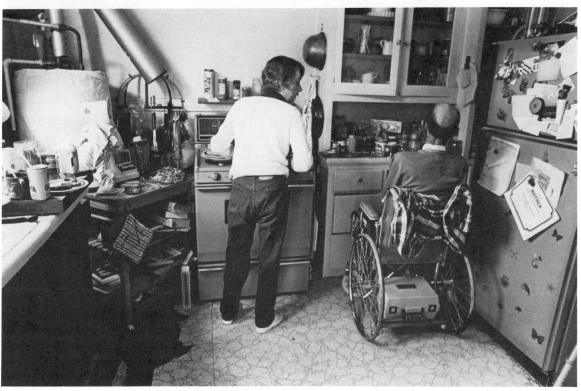

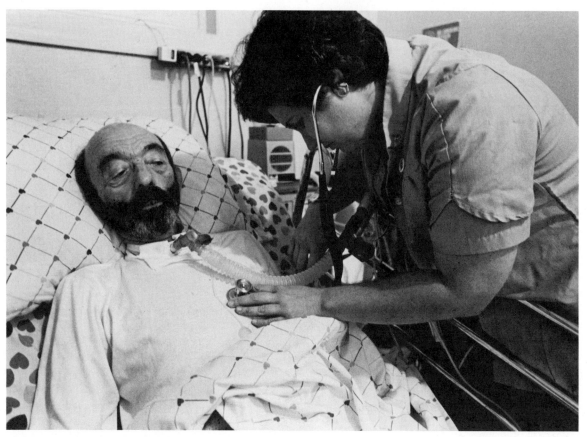

The VNA assigned a nurse to help set up Bill's home care situation. She visited once a week to assess Bill's condition and changed his trachea tube, with Gina's assistance, once a month.

The wheelchair ramp Walter built made it possible for Gina to wheel Bill down the long, narrow passageway from Bill's apartment to the street.

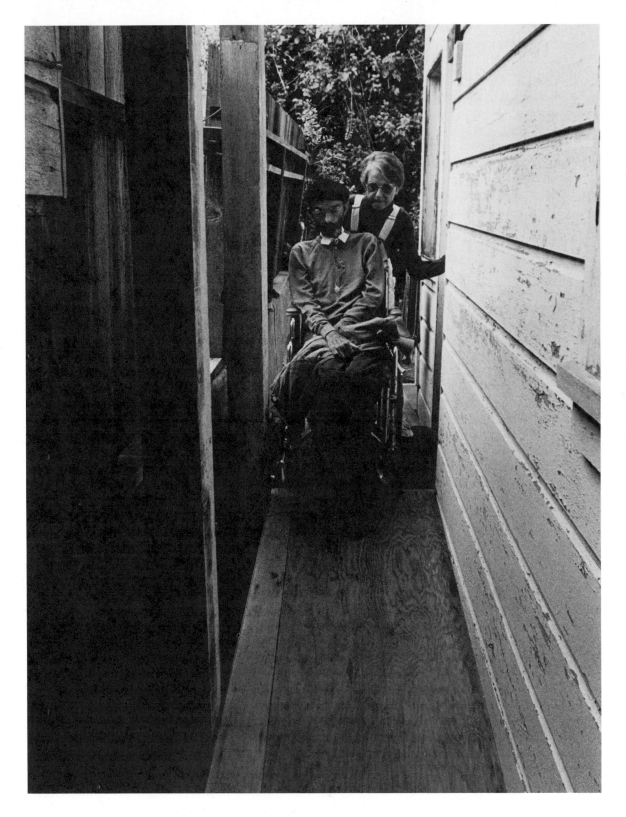

Bill and Gina often travelled in Walter's specially modified van, either to confer with Bill's doctors or simply to shop or visit the park, the aquarium, or the beach.

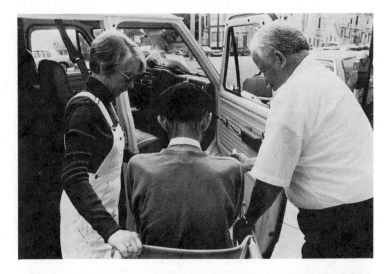

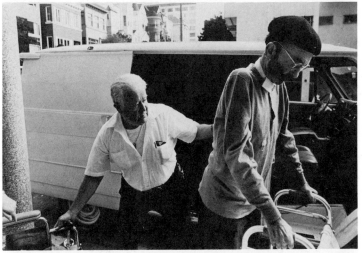

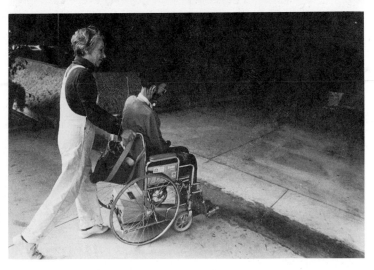

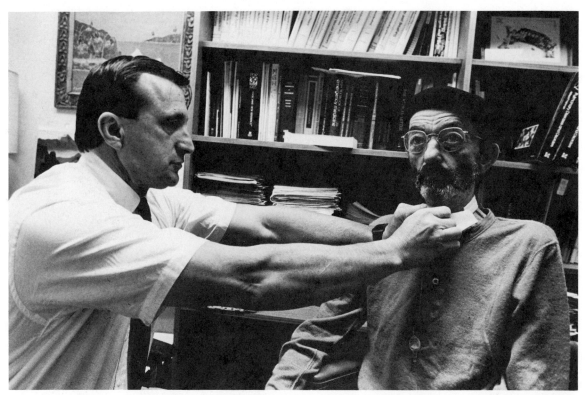

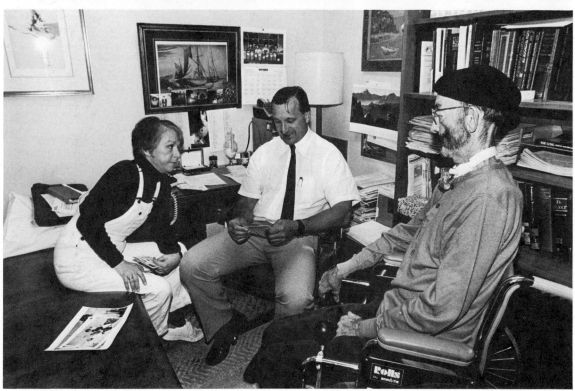

Health care professionals outside the home were important members of the team. Bill visited his pulmonary physician (previous page), the respiratory therapist, and the neurologist about once a month. Gina was always present as Bill's advocate.

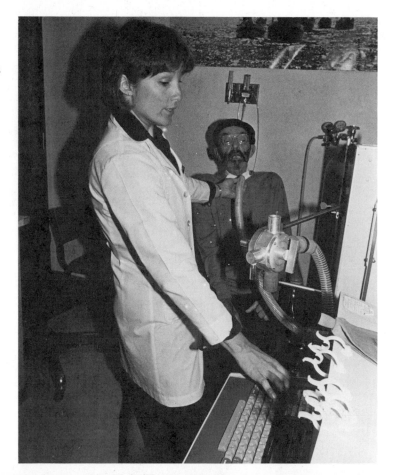

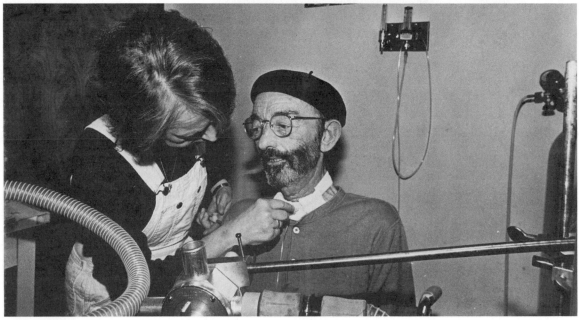

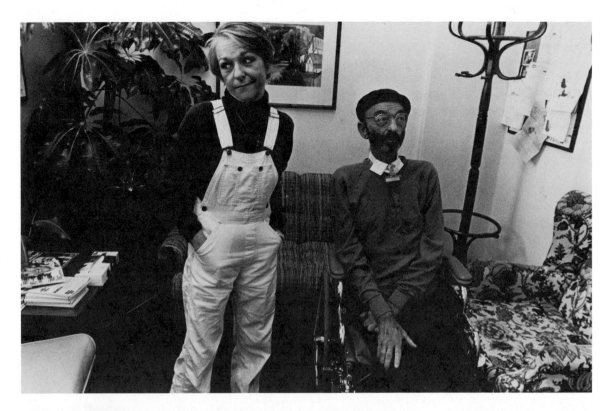

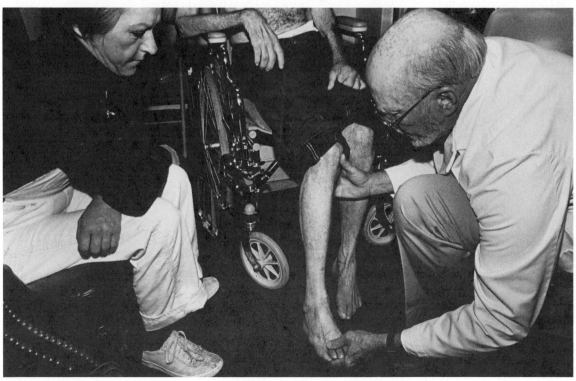

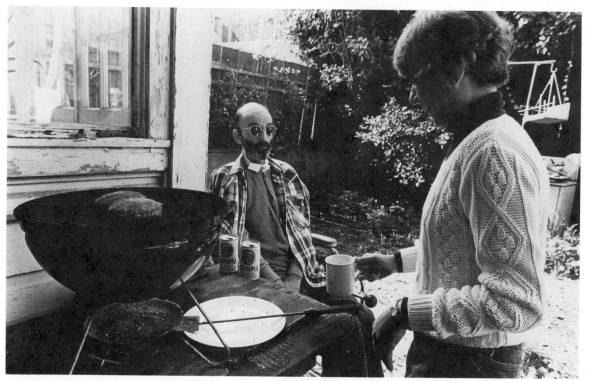

Despite the pressures of their daily life, Bill and Gina were able to relax and engage in "normal" everyday activities. Bill's doctors acknowledged that Bill's prognosis improved because he was able to remain in his own environment.

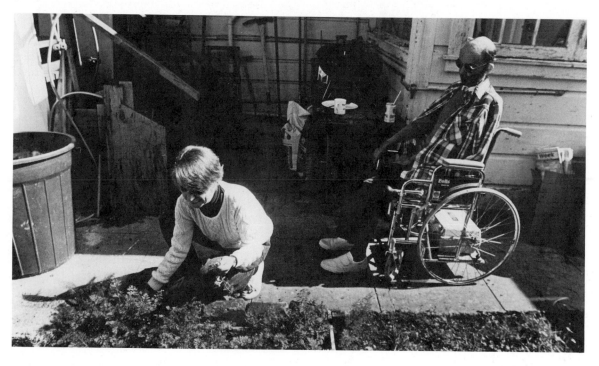

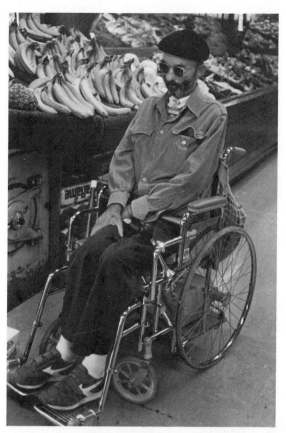

The method of having participants in a research study take photographs themselves ensures a record of their experience as seen through their eyes. It also yields photographs of events that the researchers could not attend. Finally, it involves the subject in the production of the project, which can be very therapeutic.

The group of photographs on pages 2-11 and 2-12 were taken by Gina, who used an automatic camera the researchers left with her. They also provided the film and processing. Gina's camera reveals poignant aspects of the story of Bill Haney that are unique to Gina and that add significant perspective to the overall impression of Bill's last two years of life.

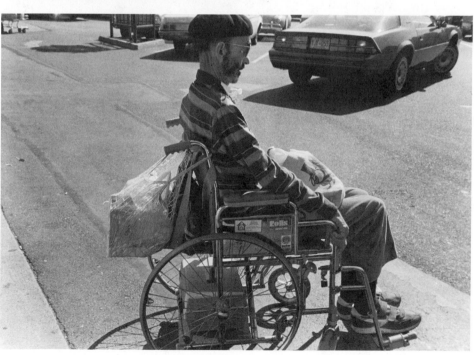

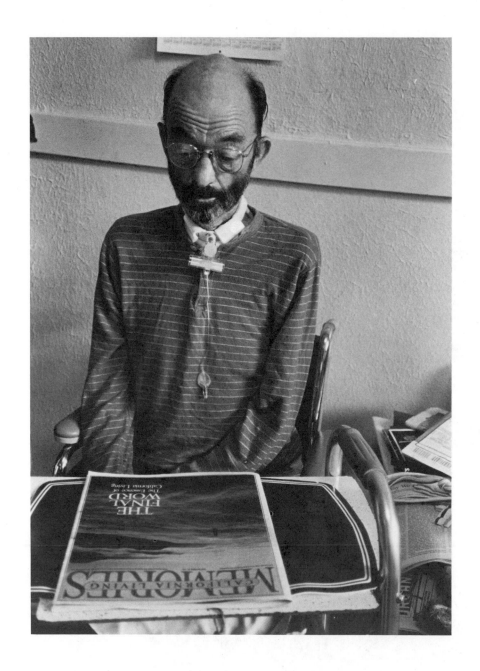

19

THE FAMILY WITH A CHRONICALLY ILL CHILD

An Interactional Perspective

Bonnie Holaday, RN, DNS

An interactional approach is often used to monitor the development of a chronically ill child. The interactional perspective focuses on the continuously ongoing, bidirectional interaction between the individual, the family, and the environment. This chapter provides an in-depth study of the family with a chronically ill child, and highlights developmental issues as well as the impact of the environment on the family and child.

Bonnie Holaday is an Associate Professor in the Department of Family Health Care Nursing at the University of California at San Francisco. She has extensive teaching experience in pediatric nursing at both the undergraduate and graduate levels. Her major research focus is childhood chronic illness.

Introduction

The purpose of this chapter is to consider the family with a chronically ill child from an interactional perspective. Basic to an interactional view is a focus on the continuously ongoing, reciprocal interaction between the individual, the family, and the environment (Magnusson, Endler, 1977). In the interaction process, person and environment are regarded as indispensably linked to one another. The individual, family, and environment, form in Bell's (1979) words, "a moving bidirectional system." Individual functioning in the process is not determined by inseparable person and situation interactions. The interactional view leads to the conclusion that models for individual or family functioning should focus simultaneously on person factors, environment factors, and the interaction between them. To illustrate the utility of this perspective, the impact of the chronically ill child on family functioning and the impact of the environment created by the family on the chronically ill child's functioning will be discussed. Attention will also be directed to specific developmental issues that can be examined from an interactional perspective.

The Newborn Experience

Parental Responses to the Birth of a Chronically Ill Infant

The birth of a chronically ill infant is often a stressful event, as evidenced by the studies describing the parents as shocked, angry, sad, anxious, and powerless (Darling, 1979; Drotar et al, 1975; Horan, 1982; Mercer, 1974). Specifically, Solnit and Stark (1961) characterized the reaction of parents to the birth of a defective child as consisting of several key elements. The first is that the infants do not match the expectations of the parents, so the parents must mourn the loss

of the perfect infant before relating to the real infant. The parents will experience guilt and anger, some of which is directed toward health care professionals. Drotar et al (1975) enlarged the ideas of Solnit and Stark and identified a sequence of five stages through which parents of children with congenital malformations may pass: (1) shock; (2) denial; (3) sadness, anger, and anxiety; (4) adaptation; and (5) reorganization. Other compensatory responses that the parents may experience are reported by Coda and Lubin (1973). They state that parents may experience responses of denial or of overacceptance; these reactions may prevent the parents from recognizing their own capabilities or the child's potential abilities, which can retard progress.

The process or the timing of the parent's responses is determined, in part, by the parents' perceptions of the event. This cognitive-mediational approach suggests that parental knowledge, expectations, and labeling must be assessed and understood if the nurse is to monitor the parents' behavioral responses (Parke, Tinsley, 1982).

The birth of a chronically ill infant has outcomes that further increase familial stress. First, the infant frequently requires special medical and nursing support procedures. Such procedures may lead to the separation of the infant from the mother, transport to a high-risk nursery, infant intubation, extensive use of medical support equipment, and surgery; these procedures affect early parent–infant relationships. This shift of the usual and expected hospital procedure reminds us of the importance of considering the institutional environment in which the infant and family are embedded (Richards, 1979). Separation of the infant from the family may last for months.

Second, the birth of a chronically ill infant violates many parental and societal expectations. Most parents have a set of expectations about the events and procedures that will occur, and they expect the pregnancy to culminate in the delivery of a healthy baby. The birth of a sick infant interrupts the natural progression of events and often postpones the establishment of a relationship with the infant (Waechter, 1977). In addition, society rituals surrounding the birth are upset. Religious services may be cancelled. The network of family and friends may stay away because of uncertainty or embarrassment. As Richardson (1969) points out, there are no well-known guidelines of behavior for family or friends of the newborn chronically ill child.

Third, the postpartum period is often a time of high anxiety for the parents because the full extent of the problem may not be known. Parents are often unsure if their infant will survive. They may not know the etiology of the illness or what the chronic illness means in terms of their child's future development. Problems in communicating with health care professionals often occur as the parents try to make sense of the child's problem (Darling, 1979). In addition, the lack of a specific diagnosis and prognosis may lead parents to deny that there is a problem, to postpone telling relatives and friends about the illness, to withdraw from the infant, or to fail to establish a relationship with the infant until they are sure of survival (Drotar et al, 1975; Holaday, 1978; Roskies, 1972).

The way in which professionals share the diagnosis will be a source of stress regardless of the nature of the child's chronic illness. Some parents have related that the diagnosis was not shared with compassion, and others felt that professionals lacked respect for the child as well as the parents. Professionals were frequently viewed as unresponsive to the parents' need to talk and to ask many questions (Bernheimer, Young, 1983; Darling, 1979).

Fourth, the infant's appearance and behavioral characteristics can cause parental anxiety. The infant may be small, listless, or cyanotic or have an atypical-sounding cry, atypical facies, or a visible defect. Research indicates that these attributes influence maternal expectations of infant endowment (Cohen, 1966); lead to parental perceptions of their infant as vulnerable (Green, Solnit, 1964); influence caregiving responses (Holaday, 1981); lead to differences in parental perceptions of their infants that affect the attachment process and the family adaptation process (Mercer, 1974; Richards, 1986); and lead to inappropriate expectations and demands of the infant that may be one source for the genesis of child abuse (Steele, Pollack, 1974). Thus, it seems probable to conclude that the process of adaptation to the infant is complex and challenging for the parents.

Clearly a variety of both individual and environmental characteristics conspire in the parental adaptation process and in the developmental progress of the chronically ill infant. At the individual level, the behavioral and physical characteristics and the medical status of the infant merit consideration. At the environmental level, both the physical environment of the hospital and the societal context (for example, parent expectations, causal attributions, and parent–infant interaction patterns) into which the infant is born are important.

Implications for Nursing Intervention

There is good reason to believe that the detrimental effects of chronic illness are exacerbated in nonsupportive environments and ameliorated in supportive postnatal caregiving environments (Sameroff, Chandler, 1975). One important area, therefore, for nursing intervention is the modification of traditional practices of hospitals. Klaus and Kennell (1976) have shown that concern for the attachment process may be applied to mothers of hospitalized infants with congenital malformations. This approach is supported by psychoanalytic, social learning, and ethological theories. All of these theories point to the centrality of mother–infant attachment or bond as an essential process for normal development. By allowing the mother and father more opportunity for prolonged contact with the infant, the parents' expectations can be revised, and the parents' attachment to the infant can be fostered.

It is an accepted principle of development that the parents are an important early source of stimulation for the infant and in this way promote social and cognitive development. Because research demonstrates that chronically ill newborns are at risk for later parent–infant interaction problems, it is an important area for nursing action (Barnard, Bee, Hammond, 1984; Field, 1979). The parents' visits can represent a time for meaningful interactions with the infant and the staff. However, planning and organization are required if an effective program is to be established. Simply letting the parents visit as desired is not sufficient.

A multidisciplinary team approach is useful in determining what to include in the family's individual program. The goals of the program can range from global (such as providing support for the parents as they adapt to the infant's illness) to the relatively discrete (such as teaching parents a special feeding technique). In planning the intervention program, time should be spent in developing satisfactory responses to the following questions:

1. What will the nature of the interventions be?
2. Why was that particular intervention chosen?
3. How will it be accomplished?

A carefully considered intervention program should be preliminary to the selection of the staff to work with parents.

Finally, family adjustment is aided by the educational and supportive activities of the caregivers. The health professional working with the chronically ill child and family can provide a blend of emotional support and practical suggestions that can be incorporated into the habilitative program. This notion of providing for the emotional support of family members as part of a habilitative session is amplified by Featherstone (1980), who is a parent of a multiply handicapped child:

> . . . if professional training has failed to equip doctors and teachers with specific counseling skills,

why should they put aside time for this sort of thing instead of simply referring parents to a psychiatrist or social worker? Most obviously, because parents will talk about their problems and concerns without much of an invitation anyway. Since doctors and teachers have to listen anyway, they might as well learn to listen well. Second, and more important, because careful, curious listening allows them to grow professionally, even humanly, and to solve some of the problems that hamper their work with disabled children (p. 212).

The Impact of Chronic Illness during Infancy

This section examines the social world of the chronically ill infant—the mother–infant dyad, the father–infant dyad, and the family triad. One of the fundamental keys to the understanding ingingingingof family dynamics is to grasp the essence of the continuing and sequential effects of parent–infant interactions. Infants, including chronically ill infants, profoundly affect their parents, and nurses need to consider not only the effect of the parents' behavior on the child but also the effect of the child's behavior on the parents. The theoretical base for this approach is derived from Bell's (1968, 1971) formulation of an interactional model.

Mother–Infant and Father–Infant Dyads

Chronically ill infants are often deficient in the behaviors that facilitate mother–infant interaction and attachment. In a literature review of the effect of chronically ill infants on parents (Ramey, Bell, Gowen, 1980), the authors found that these infants may differ from normal peers in the rate of development; temperament, including quality and duration of crying, irritability, consolability, and adaptability; social responsiveness, including smiling, eye contact, responsiveness to holding, and nonverbal communication; repetitive behaviors; and caregiving demands. The data suggest that these deficits affect both the quality and quantity of interactions between parents and their chronically ill infants.

Research studies are consistently documenting that the at-risk or handicapped status of the infant will have an influence on patterns of mother–infant interaction (Blacher, 1984; Field, 1979; Holaday, 1981, 1987). Mothers of handicapped infants are described as more controlling or interruptive during interactions, and it is shown they take the initiative in interaction sequences more than mothers of normal infants (Vietze, Abernathy, Ashe, 1977). Chronically ill infants are frequently described as inattentive and unresponsive and as providing unclear behavioral cues (DiVitto, Goldberg, 1979; Henggler, Cooper, 1983). Thus, it appears that behaviors of both the mother and the infant make it more difficult for the pair to develop a synchronous relationship.

Goldberg (1977) proposes a model that focuses on the contingencies that each member of the parent–infant dyad provides for the other. That is, the contingency of experiencing an infant's response is critical in developing an "expectation of effectiveness" in the mother. Thus, when the infant with a chronic illness does not respond contingently to the parent, it contributes to the parental feeling of ineffectiveness or helplessness. This may eventually lead to unresponsive caregiving by the parent.

Additional support for Goldberg's model comes from the work of Prechtl (1963). Prechtl found that mothers of hyperkinetic or hypokinetic babies were anxious about whether or not they treated their babies correctly because they assumed that the source of the problem was not the baby but themselves. There also appeared to be a relationship between the baby's not meeting the mother's expectations and the mother's overprotective or rejecting attitude and behavior.

In summary, the infant's personal characteristics, as seen in the "signaling" aspects of the infant's behavioral repertoire (gazing, smiling, crying, and vocalizing) and in the "executive" aspects (clinging, approaching, and following), initiate and maintain close contact with the mother. Through these behaviors, the infant signals needs to the parent, communicates that the parent has special meaning to the child, and reinforces the parent for initiating some exchange or responding to the infant's overtures. Deficiencies in these behaviors can hamper the development of the affectional bond.

In recent years, the father's important role in infancy has been acknowledged (Lamb, 1981). Fathers are active and interested participants in early infancy and are competent caretakers. Although the majority of studies have involved fathers with their healthy infants, a number of researchers have examined the role that the father plays in the family when an infant is born prematurely or with a chronic illness.

Fathers differ in both the amount of caregiving and the style of play with premature and term infants. Two recent studies confirm that fathers of premature infants are more involved in caretaking than fathers of term infants (Marton, Minde, Perrotta, 1981; Yogman, 1982). When an infant is born prematurely, there is no mother–father difference in play style (Tinsley et al, 1982). Possibly fathers assume that the premature infant is fragile and is unable to withstand intense physical play. In addition, these researchers found that fathers treat premature male and female infants in a similar fashion.

Research on families shows that the father is affected by the chronically ill infant. In a review by Price–Borham and Addison (1978), the authors report major sources of stress for fathers include financial strain, emotional tension, and limitations in social activities. They also found evidence that fathers determine the pattern for rejection or acceptance of the child in the family. Cummings (1976) studied 240 fathers of mentally retarded, chronically ill, and healthy children and found that fathers reported more stress than mothers of similar children. He also found that fathers have few constructive outlets for such stress.

Research on fathers of chronically ill infants suggests that fathers have few constructive ways in which they contribute to the welfare of the child, few opportunities to share their stress with other fathers of chronically ill children, and few opportunities to work through the mourning process, the sense of loss, and the frustration and anger related to having a chronically ill child (Gallagher, 1981; McKeever, 1981). Their contact with the child is often indirect, through bill paying or serving as an arbitrator for problems between the siblings and the ill child.

The Family Triad

Models that limit examination of the effects of interaction patterns to only the mother–infant and father–infant dyads and the direct effects of one individual on the other are inadequate for understanding the impact of social interaction patterns in families and especially in families with a chronically ill infant (Parke, Tinsley, 1982). Triadic contexts (father, mother, and infant interacting together) as well as indirect paths of mutual influence merit attention as the family adapts to the ill infant during the first year. Patterns of interaction with one parent may alter interaction patterns with another caregiver. For example, irritable infant patterns induced by an impatient mother may make it more difficult for the father to pacify the baby.

Parents have been shown to behave differently when alone with their infant than when interacting with the infant in the presence of the other parent. When both parents were with the at-risk infant, each expressed more positive affect and showed a higher level of exploration (Parke, Tinsley, 1982). These results indicate that parent–infant interaction cannot be understood by focusing solely on parent–infant dyads.

Other researchers emphasize the importance of studying the family triad in terms of the impact of the husband–wife relationship on the parent–infant interaction process and the influence of a chronically ill infant on the cohesiveness of the family. Waisbren (1980) found that families with a developmentally delayed infant viewed themselves more negatively and expressed more negative feelings about the infant. However, support from parents and friends helped parents who were able to relate to the infants in a positive way. Blumberg (1980) studied 100 mothers of at-risk infants and found that higher levels of neonatal risk were related to higher levels of maternal depression and anxiety and to a more negative perception of the newborn.

Minde et al (1980) reported that the frequency with which mothers visited their hospitalized premature infants was related to the quality of the husband–wife relationship. Visitation was less frequent in the distressed marriages than in the nondistressed families. Low frequencies in visitation by mothers may contribute to later problems because of the lack of opportunity for the development of a strong mother–infant relationship. It is possible that the poor husband–wife relationship may be a factor in both low visitation and subsequent parenting disorders. In addition, a husband in a poor marriage may not share in the caretaking, which may increase the likelihood of stress in mothers. Further support for this premise also comes from Friedrich's (1979) study of maternal adjustment to a handicapped child. Marital satisfaction was found to be the best prediction of maternal coping behavior.

It is reported that family stress, marital disruption, and divorce increases in families with a chronically ill child (Drotar, 1981; Murphy, 1982). Clinical observations suggest that the stresses of the illness alone may lead to a deterioration in the marital relationship; more often, it is observed that troublesome marriages may succumb under the stresses of illness (Gath, 1978). Arguments may erupt about the cause of the illness, how to best manage the child, or the division of labor. Parents may also be unable to communicate their feelings about the child to one another (Darling, Darling, 1982). When marriages have preexisting problems, the child's illness may simply replace other problems as the focus of disagreement.

Clinical studies also report that some families are successful in coping with a chronically ill infant. These families are characterized by open communication between family members, a willingness to share responsibilities, and a source of accurate information about what the child could and could not do (Anderson, 1981; Power, 1985). Many also engaged in outward-directed activities such as joining parent groups or advocacy groups.

These findings indicate that in order to understand the mother–infant or the father–infant relationship, the nurse needs to assess the total set of relationships among the family members. Interviews will be useful, but these need to be supplemented with direct observation of both mother and father alone with their infants, as well as with the mother, father, and the infant together.

Implications for Nursing Interventions

The central roles parents play in their infant's lives make a partnership between parents and professionals of critical importance. The type and level of that involvement, however, should vary depending on the individual needs of the family. Working together, nurses and family members need to develop individualized family plans (IFPs) that consider assessment, intervention, and evaluation in the broader context of family development. Some efforts have been made in this regard. Bricker and Casuso (1979) describe an individualized parent program calling for assessment of family needs, determination of objectives, and development of an individualized family plan. The National Collaborative Infant Project has also developed a set of objectives and evaluation criteria for programs working with parents (Meisel, 1977).

The activities developed to meet these goals must be, in part, based on an assessment of parent needs, parent coping abilities, and parent perceptions of the illness. Wiegerin et al (1980),

have developed a Parents' Need and Expectations Questionnaire that assesses parents' expectations and priorities for involvement in 36 different activities and support services. Hymovich (1981) has also developed an assessment tool that considers family developmental tasks and the family's ability to cope with chronic childhood illness, and Bromwich (1981) has developed an assessment tool that considers aspects of parenting and parent–child interaction measures.

Family resources, cohesion, and sources of social support must also be considered in the assessment. The Coping Health Inventory for Parents (CHIP) (McCubbin, Patterson, 1983) provides information about the specific coping responses parents use in managing the stress of having a chronically ill child. The Definition Scale (Bristol, 1980) can also be used to assess parental perceptions of the subjective definition of having a chronically ill child. The Holroyd Questionnaire on Resources and Stress (QRS) (1974) provides information about sources of support and the amount of stress the parents are experiencing.

Before the family is enrolled in any kind of an intervention program, the infant must also be evaluated. In large centers, evaluation is frequently conducted by a team of specialists including a physician, clinical nurse specialist, psychologist, physical therapist, and others. The parents should always be included as a part of the evaluation team. Parents should be told why certain tests are being given to their child, how the tests will be administered, and what role, if any, parents will have in the test.

Several measures are available for initial infant screening. These include the Denver Developmental Screening Test (Frankenburg et al, 1970), the Washington Guide to Promoting Development in the Young Child (Barnard, Erikson, 1976), the Developmental Profile (Alpern, Boll, 1972), and the Developmental Screening Inventory (Knobloch, 1980). Along with these general developmental screening measures, most children are also evaluated with other, more specific, tools. Procedures for evaluating infant behavior include examining reactivity to perceptual–cognitive events (Zelazo, 1979), play behavior (Westby, 1980), temperament (Simmeonson, Huntington, Parse, 1980), cognitive development (Mehrolian, Williams, 1971) and feeding (Barnard, 1979).

The information from the assessment of the child and family is used to develop an individualized program. In most cases the intervention program will be carried out in the home by the family. In some cases a nurse may visit the home to help carry out the program or to evaluate progress. Infants with severe problems or delays may have to be brought to the clinic or regional center for special services. However, in both cases the needs and abilities of the family members and the exact nature of the roles of the parents must be clarified.

This can be accomplished by (1) identifying the priority in which the child's and family's needs will be addressed; (2) setting specific goals and objectives in relation to each agreed need; (3) identifying the methods and procedures by which agreed on goals and objectives will be met; and (4) identifying the roles of the professionals and parents for each of these needs. Taken together, these four steps help to build a parent–professional partnership in the intervention program.

The specific types of interventions in the program will vary depending on the child's and family's needs. Many of the programs will include medical management of the infant at home. Other programs will stress the ill child's cognitive, social, and emotional development. The program may also include interventions in these areas. Guidelines for developing infant and parent intervention programs can be found in Garwood and Fewell (1983) and from the PEERS (Parents are Effective Early Education Resources) project (Rossetti, 1986).

In summary, when parents of chronically ill children are asked to state their greatest need, the need for information is mentioned first (Darling, Darling, 1982). They want a truthful explanation of their child's problem and its implications for the future. Once they know and understand, they are ready to act. They need information about services, parent groups, and intervention programs. They want to be and should be actively involved in their child's care. Finally, they need to talk to someone who understands their needs and feelings and wants to help. This supportive-counseling intervention needs to be a part of all programs.

The Influence of Chronic Illness during Early Childhood

As the young child grows out of infancy, different pressures and stresses develop for the parents and for the child. The interactional perspective allows us to consider person–environment interaction in the context of the family as a setting for development. Parents and children change one another, so the environment an individual has at a later time is a function of that individual's characteristics at an earlier time. For example, Field's (1979) research demonstrates that at-risk infants' atypical patterns of interaction during infancy influence the pattern of maternal–child interaction at 24 months. Circular processes of this kind undoubtedly abound in the formation and development of interpersonal relationships within the family, so in a sense individuals are creating their own interpersonal environment at the same time that they are being shaped by this environment. With this in mind, we now turn to some studies that describe the developmental patterns of young chronically ill children. Few of these studies directly address the impact on the parents, so the reader must consider the ways in which the child is influencing the environment now and what this may mean in the future.

Wasserman, Allen, and Soloman (1985a, b) have conducted one of the few longitudinal studies of the development of physically handicapped toddlers. Forty-two mother–child pairs were followed from 9 through 24 months. The researchers found that these infants were less likely to use social skills in the early months and less likely to demonstrate positive affect in the later months. They were behind healthy controls in standardized measures of cognitive–linguistic functioning. The handicapped 2-year-olds were also more passive with respect to exploration and separation. The authors believed that the mothers' interactive behavior could best be understood as an attempted compensatory response rather than as a contribution to patterns of disability in the child. Battle (1974) also found that young chronically ill children may not experience the socialization pressures of a healthy child. The young chronically ill child may be perceived as dependent and requiring protection from danger. There may be delay in achieving locomotion, which is associated with many chronic illnesses. The acquisition of walking is associated with the beginning of toddlerhood and a period of increasing independence and socialization. When a child cannot walk, societal and parental expectations may be for immature socialization. These delays in normal development can also lead to chronic sorrow over the loss of a normal child (Young, 1977).

The dependency associated with physical disability can often create a crisis in childrearing. The usual pattern of development leads to a decrease in the care provided as the child grows. However, the intensity of the care of the physically disabled child often increases during this period. Moving and caring for a 10- to 20 lb infant poses few problems for most parents. However, moving and carrying a 30 lb 3-year-old is more difficult and tiring. The type of crisis created for the parent is what Farber (1960) termed a "role organization crisis." It stems from an inability to cope with the child over long periods of time.

Perrin and Gerrity (1984) note that frequently chronically ill toddlers show increased dependency, difficulty with separation, a poor self-image, and poor impulse control. They tend to be more tentative in their approach to new situations and to require more adult reassurance than do their able-bodied peers. This excessive dependency may also retard their emerging verbal and cognitive abilities.

Chronic illness during the preschool period may limit the child's ability to achieve motor and social competence. Physical restrictions, limited strengths, and repeated episodes of painful experiences associated with illness may limit their enthusiasm for goal-directed play. This limits the child's sense of mastery and may result in a child who is fearful and passive and has a poor self-image (Parker, 1979).

Stinson (1978) notes that many parents have problems in finding the right balance between autonomy and protection. Some children with chronic illnesses such as cerebral palsy or deafness must explore the world in ways that are different from the ways of the healthy child. Just when does protection become overprotection and, conversely, how can parents help to provide the chronically ill child with the kinds of experiences with the physical and social world that foster development?

These studies all suggest that the individual characteristics of the chronically ill child are of contextual significance. The nurse should consider the relation between the child and the context in the assessment. For example, what types of problems may occur in a family that views the chronically ill child as fragile and provides a protective environment? What problems of adaptation might occur when the ill child, who has highly irregular biologic functions (for example, eating, sleep–work cycles, toileting behaviors), interacts in a family setting composed of highly regular and behaviorally scheduled parents and siblings? An interactional viewpoint allows us to understand adequately how human individuality contributes to development.

Siblings

Children encounter most of the significant social experiences to be faced as they progress through life in the sibling relationship. Siblings usually share a common background as well as their parents' time and love. Within the sibling relationship, loyalty, companionship, rivalry, love, hate, jealousy, and envy may all be present in varying degrees at different times (Craft, 1979).

Many studies suggest that the normal sibling of the chronically ill child is at risk for emotional and behavioral disorders. Gath (1973) compared the siblings of 143 children with Down syndrome to 143 matched siblings of normal children. Significant differences were found between the percentage of siblings of Down syndrome children (20%) rated deviant by parents and teachers and that of siblings of normal children (10%). In another study of the families of physically handicapped children (McMichael, 1971), 35% of the mothers reported signs of jealousy on the part of the well siblings. Similar results have been reported by investigators of siblings of children with spina bifida (Tew, Laurence, 1973). Lavigne and Ryan (1979) also found that siblings of children with chronic illness were more likely to experience adjustment or behavioral problems. The siblings of the ill children tended to be more withdrawn socially and more irritable than children in families without chronically ill children. McKeever (1983) found that siblings were poorly informed about the child's illness and therefore kept their thoughts and feelings to themselves. This led to feelings of isolation from the parents.

Investigators have attempted to delineate those factors associated with the apparent adverse effect of the chronically ill child on the normal sibling. Farber (1960) emphasized the importance of age, birth order, and sex roles in the family. Younger retarded children affected the adjustment of siblings more than older retarded children. Another study (Lavigne, Ryan, 1979) found that siblings between the ages of 3 and 6 years were more likely to show evidence of psychopathology. Among siblings between the ages of 7 and 13 years, male siblings were more likely to have problems than females. Among siblings younger than the disabled child, Breslau, Weitzman, and Messenger (1981) found that males evidenced greater impairment than females; the reverse was found for older siblings. These results indicate the complexity of the relationship between age, birth order, and sex roles and show that much more research is needed.

Other studies have concluded that most siblings adjust well to their chronically ill brothers and sisters. McMichael (1971) found that 79% of siblings of physically handicapped children were normal or had only slight adjustment problems. Grossman (1972) discussed the integrative effects of the presence of a handicapped child on the family and specifically on the normal sibling. The siblings in Cleveland and Miller's (1977) study reported mainly positive experiences with their retarded sibling, and Barsch (1961) also noted that siblings did not seem to have any significant problems.

It is difficult to generalize about the impact of a chronically ill child on siblings because the studies have used different populations and different methods. Perhaps the most important factor contributing to the contradiction in results is the age of the sample of siblings, which ranges from preschool to adults. The studies often failed to use valid instruments but instead used interviews or maternal ratings of behavior. There is little information about the siblings' relationship in the total family constellation (Drotar, Crawford, 1985). In addition, most of the studies are unidimensional, considering only the relationship of the ill child on the normal siblings.

Implications for Nursing Intervention

The research just presented is relevant to the interactional approach in a number of ways. First, the work suggests that a nonsupportive or insensitive social environment can create or enhance a problem (Rose, 1961). The parents' perception of a health threat can result in psychosocial disturbance. Rose suggested use of a primary prevention approach, using the life span perspective to assess the effect of the period of crisis on a later period. Because the maternal perception of the viability of the child can be manipulated more effectively during the crisis,

Rose suggested that health professionals consider the long-term effect of how they tell parents about their child's illness.

The work of Perrin and Gerrity (1984) emphasizes the importance of examining the constant changes that are a part of development. As chronically ill children grow, their care requires adaptation on the part of their families, communities, and society. Thus, it is not enough for nurses to evaluate adjustment of the family at birth or at the time of diagnosis. The long-term changes of the child at every level of the social environment must be evaluated.

Two intervention programs may serve as examples. Bromwich (1981) used a developmental sequence of interaction to deal with the developing child. Rather than teaching the parents to teach the child skills, Bromwich suggested that positive parent–child interaction be taught and that this would carry over to skill training and to later developmental periods. She suggested six steps for the sequence of positive parent–child interaction, starting with the parents enjoying being with the child, and ending with the parents generating activities appropriate for the child's developmental level. This program is based on the assumptions that parent–child interaction is a reciprocal process with each changing the other, that the affective aspect of the interaction is important, and that the ultimate goal of intervention should be that of effective, independent parent functioning.

The PEERS project also focused on parent–child interaction. The program was for infants and young children with developmental delays from any type of handicapping condition. The center-based program met once a week on Saturday mornings. During this time, the parents worked with counselors who discussed needs and concerns identified by the parents, basic concepts of child development, and community resources. The sessions also reviewed activities the parents were to carry out at home. Evaluation indicated that the children's developmental functioning improved as did the parents' knowledge about their children's ability.

Both of these programs had a dual focus: (1) to view development as a successive mastery of milestones and (2) to foster the child's development through interaction with the parents. Other programs that have this dual focus and also provide specific content information are Developmental Programming for Infants and Young Children (Schafer, Morensch, 1981), Facilitating Children's Development (Meier, Malone, 1979), and Small Wonder (Karnes, 1979).

Parents of chronically ill children often express concern about the effect of the chronically ill child on siblings. Parents need to have the opportunity to discuss their problems and concerns. Nurses can counsel parents about sibling rivalry, the need for honest communication, sibling participation in care, dealing with feelings of guilt and fear, and symptoms of adjustment problems (Craft, 1979). Nurses can also caution parents against expecting older siblings to assume caretaking responsibilities for the chronically ill brother or sister that exceed their level of maturity and their own needs as children.

Siblings may have fears that they, too, will become ill. Nurses can help siblings deal with these expressed and unexpressed fears. Cransler, Martin, and Valand (1975) have developed a model for a week-long workshop that also includes an agenda and evaluation instrument.

One of the best contributions the nurse can make to sibling welfare is to assist the parents in obtaining adequate support services. Parents with access to reliable babysitting and respite care are more likely to have the time and energy for their other children. If no assistance is available, the parents may be too emotionally drained to respond to the needs of the siblings.

Influences of Chronic Illness during Middle Childhood

fluences on the lives of children change. They gain access to new settings and encounter pressures that present them with distinctive developmental challenges. The widening world of childhood is marked especially by entry into school. Entry into school signifies a new set of social contacts including teachers and peers as well as a wider variety of settings than those that characterize early childhood. Because of this, the family of the chronically ill child must now cope and adapt to changes brought about by the increased number of socialization agents and rearing environments. As a result the family will experience periods of growth and integration, periods of stability, and periods of disorder and disintegration.

Child and Family

During the middle childhood period, the chronically ill child, like all school-age children, is working to shape his or her self-concept. At the most general level, this involves an increasing differentiation of what is "me" from what is "not me," an understanding in Goffman's (1959) terms of what the territories of the self are. Contributing to this understanding are parents, peers, other significant adults, and the recognition the child gains by being successful and productive.

A number of studies have explored the developmental impact of chronic disease. Sperling (1978) noted that deficits in ability or diminished physical attractiveness caused threats to self-esteem and increased levels of stress. A higher incidence of behavioral disorders among chronically ill children has been reported by many investigators (Hobbs, Perrin, Ireys, 1985; Perrin, Genity, 1984; Rogers, Hillemeis, O'Neill, 1981). Conversely, other studies have failed to document higher rates of disturbance (Bedell, 1977; Martin, 1975). Sex, age of diagnosis, severity of illness, visibility, coping styles, the quality of the parent–child relationship, and socioeconomic status are some of the many variables that have been correlated with overall adjustment.

The literature on family impact is also equivocal. Increased stress, problems of diminished parental self-esteem, anxiety, depression, and marital disruption have been reported repeatedly (Holroyd, Guthrie, 1979; Phillips, Bohannon, 1985; Shapiro, 1983). Other studies have noted more adaptive outcomes (Gayton, 1977; Vance et al, 1980). In a review of more than 50 reports on the impact of a chronically ill child, Murphy (1982) found only 16 controlled analytical studies. Vance also noted problems with the development of interview questions. Despite these limitations, the data indicate that a chronically ill school-age child is a stressor to which different families adapt with varying degrees of success.

School

The educational process is a major socializing force in our society. During middle childhood, teachers and peers become major influences in the social environments of children. Dreeben (1968) contends that schools provide children with the psychologic capacities needed for participation in societal institutions by fostering independence, achievement, universalisms, and specificity. However, the school experience of chronically ill children may be very different from that of their healthy peers.

Research indicates that among children at increased risk for school dysfunction and absenteeism are those with a chronic illness or handicap (Fowler, Johnson, Atkinson, 1985; Hall, Porter, 1983; Hobbs, Perrin, Ireys, 1985). They are at risk not only because of the medical aspects of the chronic illness but also from the secondary effects of the illness on their self-concept and on how the family is functioning. Their educational problems usually fall into one of three groups. The first includes children who have severe cognitive or perceptual deficits in addition to or as a result of the illness. Some children with spina bifida or cerebral palsy may be members of this group. A second group includes children who have physical impairments without any associated deficits in cognitive or intellectual functioning. Some children with arthritis or hemophilia would fall into this group. The third and largest group includes children who have no intellectual or physical impairment directly attributable to the illness but who fall behind in school as a consequence of th e illness or its treatment. Children with asthma, diabetes, and leukemia are typical members of this group.

These three groups of children have different educational needs. However, many needed educational services often remain unavailable because the children fit poorly into existing educational categories. Under the rules of Public Law 94–142, chronically ill children may be placed in special education on the basis of an existing learning disability, developmental delay, perceptual handicap, or some other learning problem. Lacking any of these problems, they may qualify for special educational services by falling into a category named "other health impaired." However, determination of special educational services is often dictated by services available in the school system rather than by the specific needs of the child. Thus, for many parents, obtaining proper educational services is an ongoing, frustrating experience (Hobbs, Perrin, 1985).

In addition to obtaining the proper educational programs, parents of chronically ill children have identified other problems that influence the children's experiences at school. One of the most common problems is that the health care team fails to fully explain to the school the ramifications of the illness and its treatment. As a consequence, the school does not provide the proper special educational services or fails to incorporate all the medical aspects of care into the individual educational program (Hobbs, Perrin, Ireys, 1985). For example, the teacher may not understand that a child's limited alertness, lack of stamina, and inability to concentrate may result from the illness or from medications required for treatment and may misinterpret the child's behavior as willful resistance or laziness. As a result, parents must go to the school and explain their child's health problems and negotiate

on behalf of the child for the needed services. Some parents are able to do this, and others are not.

Other research studies have identified additional parental concerns about school. These include absenteeism and the pressure of always having to catch up (Gliedman, Roth, 1980; Fowler, Johnson, Atkinson, 1985); problems of access in the school (Walker, 1984); the teacher's inability to cope with orthotic and other adaptive equipment (Holland, Porter, 1983); underexpectation on the part of teachers (Richman, 1978); and inappropriate peer attitudes (Voelz, 1980; Weitzman, 1984). Thus, even though the "mainstream" placement may clearly be in the interest of the child, it may also increase the stress felt by the parents and other members of the family.

Parents of children with a chronic illness may also experience difficulties when the child starts school. For the first time they must relinquish some of the responsibility for the child's care and development to others. They may worry that the school setting lacks the appropriate support services. Other parents may be reluctant to collaborate with school personnel because of previous painful experiences with human service providers (Weitzman, 1984). They may also fear that disclosing the details of their child's illness will result in discriminating treatment, and therefore they might not inform the school of the illness (Fowler, Johnson, Atkinson, 1985). Some parents may also experience shock when they first visit a mainstreamed classroom and see the discrepancy between their child and the normal children around them. Parents who have not fully accepted the illness may be unreasonably insistent that their child be taught a task beyond his or her physical or intellectual abilities.

Peers

School-age children spend a substantial amount of time with other school-age children in school, in the neighborhood, and in organized activities. For children in this age group, the peer exerts a powerful influence, and contemporary evidence stresses the importance of peer relationships on future development (Mueller, Cooper, 1985).

A study of chronically ill school-age children's use of time out of school (Holaday, Turner–Henson, 1987) found that 80% of these children usually played with children other than their siblings after school and on weekends. The median number of friends listed by the children was two. The number of friends influenced the nature of the activities the children pursued. The more friends the child had the more likely they were to pursue physically active activities and to participate in organizations. Twenty percent of the children in this study could not list a friend. Most of the children in this group were physically handicapped.

Other studies have examined the social acceptability of handicapped youngsters. Richardson's (1961) classic study found a uniformity of rankings for pictures of children with physical disabilities. The ranking (from most to least preferred) was (1) child with no handicap; (2) child with crutches and leg brace; (3) child in a wheelchair with a blanket covering the legs; (4) child with left hand missing; (5) child with facial disfigurement; and (6) obese child. This ranking was uniform across sex, presence of handicap, race, socioeconomic status, and urban–rural settings. Almost a decade later, Alessi and Anthony (1969) replicated the findings. Later studies of physically handicapped and learning disabled children continued to find these children to be lower in sociometric status than their nonhandicapped peers (Asher, Taylor, 1981; Siperstein, Bopp, Bak, 1978). However, Asher and Taylor suggest that research studies need to make a distinction between friendship and acceptance. They found that although handicapped children had no best friends in class, they were generally liked by the group.

The proponents of mainstreaming believed that the physical placement of handicapped children in regular classrooms would result in an increase in social interaction between handicapped and nonhandicapped children (Johnson, Johnson, 1980). There is, however, an accumulating body of data indicating that nonhandicapped children interact very little with mainstreamed handicapped children when there is no planned intervention (Ray, 1985; Strain, 1982; Voeltz, 1980). In general, these studies show that social interaction patterns between nonhandicapped and handicapped children occur at extremely low rates and are generally negative in nature. These studies also note that many handicapped children are deficient in social skills that would lead to peer acceptance. Gresham (1982) states that mainstreaming efforts are likely to continue to result in increased social isolation and more restrictive social environments unless provisions are made to train handicapped children in the social skills necessary for effective social interaction and peer acceptance.

Fortunately, several research studies indicate that positive interaction and acceptance between handicapped and nonhandicapped students can develop if the teacher structures the initial encounters (Martino, Johnson, 1979; Stainback, Stainback, Hatcher, 1984). This is best accomplished through activities that place students in small, heterogeneous learning or play groups.

Implications for Nursing Intervention

The evidence that has been brought together identifies some of the challenges that parents and chronically ill children face as they interact with new physical environments and new social contexts. The parents now must facilitate their children's interaction with these physical and interpersonal environments. The children need to develop new cognitive and social competencies to cope with these new environments. Nursing interventions can be beneficial for both parent and child and for family stability.

The nurse who works with families with school-age chronically ill children needs to be familiar with the laws relating to the education of the handicapped (Schultz, Turnbull, 1983). The law stipulates that all children are to be educated in the least restrictive environment; however, the realities of school budgets and architectural barriers may lead the school to design a program that is unacceptable to the parents. In a case of conflict with the school system, the nurse can help the parents understand the school's position and can direct them toward legal aid if they feel their rights have been violated. The nurse can also teach the parents assertive techniques that can be used in conferences with the school system. Referral to advocacy organizations that are active in the community or on a state or national level is also useful.

Other concerns that arise during middle childhood result from the child's awareness of their own "differentness." Group sessions involving the family and other sessions for the children only can be helpful. Some of the issues that can be discussed by both groups are rejection by peers, independence, inability to participate in certain activities, compliance with the medical regimen, embarrassment, and being surpassed in some skills by younger siblings. The mainstreamed child is more likely to experience these problems.

The nurse can facilitate the chronically ill child's interaction with the interpersonal environment by educating teachers and nonhandicapped children about individual differences. The content of these sessions centers on the general differences and similarities among all students. This information is then related specifically to children with different types of chronic illnesses (Bookbinder, 1978; Stainback, Stainback, 1981). Lecture, discussion, games, role playing, and free-play sessions are all effective teaching methods. These programs can be conducted in special workshops, schools, or clinic settings.

Social skills training for chronically ill children is another important area for nursing intervention. Social skills training techniques derived from the social learning theory literature (Ban-

dura, 1977) can be categorized under three major headings: (1) manipulation of antecedents; (2) manipulation of consequences; and (3) modeling. The reader interested in details about these techniques should consult the following articles (Coombs, Slaby, 1978; Van Hassette, Hersen, Whitehill, 1979).

The rationale for antecendent manipulation is based on the notion that some chronically ill children have low rates of social interaction or are poorly accepted because the social environment does not set the occasion for positive social exchanges between chronically ill children and their peers. The typical procedure in this approach is to involve peer confederates in giving social initiations to chronically ill children (for example, "Let's play a game") or to arrange game-playing activities or tasks to increase social interaction. Both approaches facilitate peer interaction and acceptance.

Strategies involving manipulation of consequences include contingent social reinforcement, token reinforcement, and differential reinforcement of low rates of responding. The general procedure in contingent social reinforcement involves having a teacher socially reinforce (hug, praise) healthy children whenever they approach and interact positively with mainstreamed children. Token-based reinforcement procedures can be used with either group and typically involve having the teacher administer points or tokens to either group or both groups contingent on appropriate social behavior (such as sharing, cooperation, or positive interaction). Differential reinforcement of low rates of responding (DRL) has been used to decrease inappropriate social behavior (such as interrupting) in chronically ill children. For example, a child could earn reinforcement (two pieces of candy) if he interrupted four or fewer times in a 50-minute period. DRL schedules are successful in eliminating undesirable behavior without using punishment.

Modeling can be presented in either live or film formats. Both have been used to demonstrate how to interact positively with others (for example, how to greet someone, join in a game). To be successful, both films and live formats must be carefully planned and sequenced. Live modeling is perhaps the most workable technique because it is less expensive than film.

There is currently enough empirical evidence to suggest that social skills training with chronically ill children may be a means to help these children interact more positively and to become better-accepted by their healthy peers. Also, recent research in social learning theory suggests that chronically ill children can imitate appropriate social behavior as long as the modeling is carefully planned and sequenced.

Community Support and the Family with a Chronically Ill Child

A further extension of the theoretical framework is needed to understand the environment and the development of a chronically ill child. Families are dependent on other social organizations within society. Thus, families need to be viewed within their social context; and the recognition of the role of the community as a modifier of family modes of interaction is necessary.

There are support systems of special relevance to chronically ill children and their families. Two kinds of support systems operate: formal (such as health-care facilities, churches, social service agencies) and informal (such as extended families, neighbors, and coworkers). The formal support programs serve both the educational function of providing childcare information and the mental-health function of alleviating stress associated with chronically ill children. Support systems that serve an educational function include hospital-based courses in childcare; visiting nurse programs; speciality clinics; and parent discussion groups. Some other supportive programs that offer stress relief are community recreation or camping programs; homemaker services; drop-off centers; and hot

lines. Unfortunately, evidence in support of the role of informal and formal support systems in regulating the family's ability to cope with chronically ill children is limited.

A few studies have suggested that there is a positive relationship between informal social networks and a family's adaptation to stress. Specifically, interaction patterns among family members are influenced by the availability and use of informal social networks (Cochran, Brassard, 1979). Interestingly, Crockenberg (1981) found that the extent to which mothers used social support networks was related to the infants' pattern of attachment to the mother. Especially in the case of irritable babies (a characteristic common in many chronically ill infants), use of social support was associated with secure attachment. This study provides an excellent example of the interplay of individual characteristics (infant temperament) and the role of the social environment (social support networks) on later patterns of infant–mother attachment.

Additional evidence of the importance of social support is provided by the study by Bristol (1979) of factors relating to the stress reported by the mothers of autistic children. Bristol found that, in addition to specific characteristics of the child, the lack of informal supports was a major contributor to the amount of stress the mothers reported.

Kazak and Wilcox (1984) examined the structure and function of social support networks in 56 families with handicapped children. The results indicated that the social networks of families with handicapped children tended to be smaller than networks of families with healthy children. This was particularly true with regard to the mother's social and friendship network. However, the networks of families with handicapped children were more dense. This meant that members of their social networks were more likely to know and interact with each other. In another report on this project, the authors noted that the families with handicapped children were able to develop successful coping strategies by using their closely knit social network (Kazak, Marvin, 1984).

Although informal and formal support systems can make independent contributions to family functioning, a number of recent studies have shown that these two types of support systems can work together in supporting families. Links between formal and informal support systems can assume a variety of forms, such as strengthening the informal network through formal intervention (Powell, 1979) and using informal network members to help individuals use formal support services (Olds, 1981). These types of programs need to be developed for families with chronically ill children. The recognition of the embeddedness of the family in formal and informal social networks and of the direct and indirect ways in which these extrafamilial social systems can alter family functioning is necessary to improve our knowledge concerning the interplay between the individual, the family, and the environment.

Summary

The basic components of the person–environment perspective were discussed in this chapter. This interactional framework for the analysis of behavior makes the basic assumption that the development of a chronically ill child cannot be explained by considering person factors or situation factors alone. Instead, we must consider the ill child, the family, and the extrafamilial environments to gain an understanding of the ill child's and the family's functioning.

It was also stressed that the person–environment interactions are a continuous and reciprocal process in which the family environment influences the chronically ill child, and, at the same time, the ill child influences the family environment. Thus, interaction is a dynamic process that should be conceived of as a continuous spiral in which both the person and the environment are being changed as a consequence

of interaction. Attention was also devoted to specific developmental issues that can be examined by using the interactional perspective. It is with this kind of approach that we may begin to understand the impact of a chronic illness on the child and on the family so that we are able to effectively intervene with both the family and the child.

Issues for Further Investigation

1. What is the capacity of urban American environments to serve as support systems to parents involved in the care, upbringing, and education of chronically ill children?

2. To what extent does the development of a relationship over time with a nurse facilitate the family's management of a chronically ill child's health problems? To what extent does it prevent the emergence of developmental problems?

3. What adjustments or arrangements do families with chronically ill children make to balance parenting and employment responsibilities?

References

Alessi DF, Anthony WA (1969): The uniformity of children's attitudes toward disabilities. *Except Child*, 35: 543–545.

Alpern GD, Boll TJ (1972): *Developmental Profile Manual*. Aspen, CO: Psychological Development Publications.

Anderson JM (1981): The social constructions of illness experience: Families with a chronically ill child. *J Adv Nurs*, 6: 427–434.

Asher SR, Taylor AR (1981): Social outcomes of mainstreaming: Sociometric assessment and beyond. *Exceptional Education Quarterly*, 1(4): 13–130.

Bandura A (1977): *Social Learning Theory*. Englewood Cliffs, NJ: Prentice-Hall.

Barnard K (1979): *Teaching and Feeding Scales*. Seattle: University of Washington School of Nursing.

Barnard K, Bee, H, Hammond M (1984): Developmental changes in maternal interactions with term and preterm infants. *Inf Behav Devel, 7:* 101–113.

Barnard K, Erikson M (1976): *Teaching Children with Developmental Problems: A Family Care Approach*. St. Louis: Mosby.

Barsch RH (1961): Explanations offered by parents of brain-damaged children. *Except Child, 27:* 286–291.

Battle CV (1974): Disruptions in the socialization of a young, severely handicapped child. *Rehabil Lit, 35:* 135–140.

Bedell J (1977): Life stress and the psychological and medical adjustment of chronically ill children. *J Psychosom Res, 21:* 237–243.

Bell RQ (1968): A reinterpretation of the direction of effects in studies of socialization. *Psychol Rev, 75*(2): 81–95.

Bell RQ (1971): Stimulus control of parent or caretaker behavior by offspring. *Dev Psychol, 4:* 63–72.

Bell RQ (1979): Parent, child and reciprocal influences. *Am Psychologist, 34:* 821–826.

Bernheimer LP, Young MS (1983): Stress overtime: Parents with young handicapped children. *J Dev Behav Pediatr, 4:* 177–181.

Blacher J (1984): Attachment and severely handicapped children: Implications for intervention. *J Dev Behav Pediatr, 5:* 178–183.

Blumberg NL (1980): Effects of neonatal risk, maternal attitude, and cognitive style on early postpartum adjustment. *J Abn Psychol, 89:* 139–150.

Bookbinder S (1978): Mainstreaming: What every child needs to know about disabilities. The Meeting Street school curriculum for grades 1–4. Providence: Rhode Island Easter Seal Society.

Breslau N, Weitzman M, Messenger K (1981): Psychologic functioning of siblings of disabled children, *Pediatrics, 67:* 344–353.

Bricker D, Casuso V (1979): Family involvement: A critical component of early intervention. *Except Child, 46:* 108–117.

Bristol MM (1979): Maternal coping with autistic children: Adequacy of interpersonal support and effect of child's characteristics. Unpublished doctoral dissertation, University of North Carolina.

Bristol MM, DeVellis R (1980): The Definition Scale: The subjective meaning of having a handicapped child. Unpublished assessment tool. Chapel Hill: University of North Carolina.

Bromwich R (1981): *Working with Parents and Infants: An Interactional Approach*. Baltimore: University Park Press.

Cleveland DW, Miller NB (1977): Attitudes and life commitments of older siblings of mentally retarded adults: An exploratory study. *Ment Retard, 15*(3): 38–41.

Cochran MM, Brassard JA (1979): Child development and personal social networks. *Child Dev, 50:* 601–616.

Coda EJ, Lubin GI (1973): Some special problems and guidance needs of families with handicapped children. In: *Family Roots of School Learning and Behavior Disorders*, Friedman R (ed.). Springfield, IL: Charles C Thomas.

Cohen RL (1966) Pregnancy, stress and maternal perceptions of infant endowment. *J Ment Subnormality, 12*(27): 18–23.

Coombs TP, Slaby DA (1977): Social skills training with children. In: *Advances in Clinical Child Psychology*, Vol 1, Lahey B, Kazdin AE (eds.). New York: Plenum.

Craft MJ (1979): Help for the family's neglected "other" child. *Am J Mat Child Nurs, 4,* 297–300.

Cransler DP, Martins G, Valand MC (1975): *Working With Families*. Winston-Salem: Kaplan.

Crockenberg SB (1981): Infant irritability, mother responsiveness, and social support influences on the security of infant-mother attachment. *Child Dev, 52:* 857–865.

Cummings ST (1976) The impact of the child's deficiency on the father: A study of fathers of mentally retarded and chronically ill children. *Am J Orthopsychiatry, 46:* 246–255.

Darling RB (1979): *Families Against Society: A Study of Reactions to Children With Birth Defects*. Beverly Hills: Sage.

Darling RB, Darling J (1982): *Children Who Are Different*. St. Louis: Mosby.

DiVitto B, Goldberg S (1979): The effects of newborn medical status on early parent-infant interactions. In: *Infants Born at Risk,* Field T et al (eds.). New York: Spectrum.

Dreeben R (1968): *On What Is Learned in School.* Reading, MA: Addison-Wesley.

Drotar D (1981): Psychological perspectives in chronic childhood illness. *J Pediatr Psychol, 6:* 211–228.

Drotar D et al (1975): The adaptation of parents to the birth of an infant with a congenital malformation: A hypothetical model. *Pediatrics, 56:* 710–717.

Drotar D, Crawford P (1985): Psychological adaptation of siblings of chronically ill children: Research and practice implications. *J Dev Behav Pediatr, 6:* 355–362.

Farber B (1960): Perceptions of crisis and related variables in the impact of a retarded child on the mother. *J Health Hum Behav, 1:* 108–118.

Featherstone H (1980): *A Difference In the Family: Life with a Disabled Child.* New York: Basic Books.

Field T (1979): Interaction patterns of high-risk and normal infants. In: *Infants Born at Risk.* Field T et al (eds.). New York: Spectrum.

Fowler MG, Johnson MP, Atkinson SS (1985): School achievement and absence in children with chronic health conditions. *J Pediatr, 106:* 683–687.

Frankenburg W, Dodds J, Fandal AW (1970): *Denver Developmental Screening Test Manual.* Denver: University of Colorado Medical Center.

Friedrich WN (1979): Predictors of the coping behavior of mothers of handicapped children. *J Consult Clin Psychol, 47:* 1140–1141.

Gallagher JJ (1981): Parental adaptation to a young handicapped child: The father's role. *J Div Early Childhood, 3:* 3–14.

Garwood SG, Fewell RR (1983): *Educating Handicapped Infants.* Rockville, MD: Aspen.

Gath A (1973): The school age siblings of mongol children. *Br J Psychiatry, 123:* 161–167.

Gath A (1978): *Down's Syndrome and the Family.* London: Academic Press.

Gayton W (1977): Children with cystic fibrosis. 1. Psychological test findings of patients, siblings, and parents. *Pediatrics, 59:* 888–894.

Gliedman J, Roth W (1980): *The Unexpected Minority: Handicapped Children in America.* New York: Harcourt Brace Jovanovich.

Goffman E (1959): *The Presentation of Self in Everyday Life.* New York: Doubleday.

Goldberg S (1977): Social competency in infancy: A model of parent-infant interaction. *Merrill-Palmer Quarterly, 23:* 162–177.

Green M, Solnit AJ (1964): Reactions to the threatened loss of child: A vulnerable child syndrome. *Pediatrics, 34:* 58–66.

Gresham F (1982): Misguided mainstreaming: The case for social skills training with handicapped children. *Exceptional Children, 48:* 422–433.

Grossman FK (1972): *Brothers and Sisters of Retarded Children: An Exploratory Study.* Syracuse, NY: Syracuse University Press.

Hall CD, Porter P (1983): School intervention for the neuromuscularly handicapped child. *J Pediatr, 102:* 210–214.

Henggler SW, Cooper PF (1983): Deaf child-hearing mother interaction: Extensiveness and reciprocity. *J Pediatr Psychol, 8:* 83–95.

Hobbs N, Perrin JM (1985): *Issues in the Care of Children with Chronic Illness.* San Francisco: Jossey-Bass.

Hobbs N, Perrin JM, Ireys HT (1985): *Chronically Ill Children and their Families.* San Francisco: Jossey-Bass.

Holaday B (1978): Parenting the chronically ill child. In: *Current Practice in Pediatric Nursing:* Vol 2, Brandt P et al (eds.). St. Louis: Mosby.

Holaday B (1981): Maternal response to their chronically ill infants' attachment behavior of crying. *Nurs Res, 30:* 343–348.

Holaday B, Turner-Henson A (1987): Chronically ill school age children's use of time. *Pediatr Nurs, 13:* 410–414.

Holaday B (1987): Patterns of interaction between mothers and their chronically ill infants. *Maternal-Child Nurs J, 16:* 29–45.

Holroyd J (1974): The questionnaire on resources and stress: An instrument to measure family response to a handicapped member. *Am J Community Psychol, 2:* 92–94.

Holroyd J, Guthrie D (1979): Stress in families of children with neuromuscular disease. *J Clin Psychol, 35:* 734–739.

Horan ML (1982): Parental reaction to the birth of an infant with a defect: An attributional approach. *ANS, 5:* 57–68.

Hymovich DP (1981): Assessing the impact of chronic childhood illness on the family and parent coping. *Image, 13;* 71–74.

Johnson D, Johnson R (1980): Integrating handicapped students into the mainstream. *Except Child, 47:* 90–98.

Karnes MB (1979): *Small Wonder.* Circle Pines, MN: American Guidance Service.

Kazak AE, Marvin RS (1984): Differences, difficulties and adaptation: Stress and social networks in families with a handicapped child. *Fam Relations, 33:* 67–77.

Kazak AE, Wilcox BL (1984): The structure and function of social support networks in families with handicapped children. *Am J Community Psychol, 12:* 645–661.

Klaus M, Kennell J (1976): *Maternal–Infant Bonding.* St. Louis: Mosby.

Knobloch H (1980): *Manual of Developmental Programs.* New York: Harper & Row.

Lamb ME (1981): *The Role of the Father in Child Development.* New York: Wiley.

Lavigne JV, Ryan M (1979): Psychologic adjustment of siblings of children with chronic illness. *Pediatrics, 63:* 616–627.

Magnusson D, Endler NS (1977): Interactional psychology: Present status and future prospects. In: *Personality at the Crossroads: Current Issues in Interactional Psychology,* Magnusson D, Endler NS (eds.). Hillsdale, IL: Erlbaum.

Martino L, Johnson DW (1979): Effects of cooperation versus individualistic instruction or interaction between normal progress and learning-disabled students. *J Soc Psychol, 110:* 177–183.

Marton P, Minde K, Perrotta M (1981): The role of the father for the infant at risk. *Am J Orthopsychiatry, 51:* 672–679.

McCubbin HI, McCubbin MA, Patterson JM (1983): CHIP—Coping health inventory for parents: An assessment of parental coping patterns in the care of the chronically ill child. *Fam Relations, 45:* 359–370.

McKeever PT (1981): Fathering the chronically ill child. *Am J Mat Child Nurs, 6:* 124–128.

McKeever PT (1983): Siblings of chronically ill children. *Am J Orthopsychiatry, 53:* 209–218.

McMichael JK (1971): *Handicap: A Study of Physically Handicapped Children and their Families.* London: Staples.

Martin P (1975): Marital breakdown in families of patients with spina bifida cystica. *Dev Med Child Neurol, 17:* 757–763.

Meier JH, Malone PJ (1979): *Facilitating Children's Development.* Baltimore: University Park Press.

Meisel J (1977): *Programming for Atypical Infants and their Families: Guidelines for Program Evaluation.* Monograph no. 5 of the nationally organized collaborative project to provide comprehensive services for atypical infants and their families. New York: United Cerebral Palsy.

Mercer RT (1974): Mothers responses to their infants with defects. *Nurs Res, 23(2):* 133–137.

Minde KK et al (1980): Some determinants of mother-infant interaction in the premature nursery. *Am Acad Child Psychiatry J, 19:* 1–21.

Mueller E, Cooper C (eds.) (1985): *Process and Outcome in Peer Relationships.* New York: Academic Press.

Murphy MA (1982): The family with a handicapped child: A review of the literature. *J Dev Behav Pediatr, 3:* 73–82.

Olds DL (1981): The prenatal/early infant project: An ecological approach to prevention. In: *In the Beginning: Readings in Infancy,* Belsky J (ed.). New York: Columbia University Press.

Parke RD, Tinsley BR (1982): The early environment of the at-risk infant: Expanding the social context. In: *Intervention with At Risk and Handicapped Infants: From Research to Application,* Bricker D (ed.). Baltimore: University Park Press.

Parker H (1979): Children and youth with physical and health disabilities. In: *Understanding Exceptional Children and Youth,* Swanson B, Willis D (eds.) Chicago: Rand McNally.

Perrin EC, Gerrity PS (1984): Development of children with a chronic illness. *Pediatr Clin North Am, 31(1):* 19–31.

Phillips S, Bohannon WE (1985): Parent interview findings regarding the impact of cystic fibrosis on families. *J Dev Behav Pediatr, 6:* 122–127.

Powell DR (1979): Family–environment relations and early childrearing: The role of social networks and neighborhoods. *J Res Dev Educ, 13:* 1–11.

Power PW (1985): Family coping behaviors in chronic illness: A rehabilitation perspective. *Rehabil Lit, 46:* 78–83.

Prechtl HF (1963): The mother–child interaction in babies with minimal brain dysfunction. In: *Determinants of Infant Behavior: Vol II,* Foss BM (ed.). New York: Wiley.

Price-Bonham S, Addison S (1978): Families and mentally retarded children: Emphasis on the family. *Fam Coordinator, 27:* 3, 221–230.

Ray BM (1985): Measuring social position of the mainstreamed handicapped child. *Except Child, 52:* 57–62.

Ramey CT, Bell PB, Gowen JW (1980): Parents as educators during infancy: Implications from research for handicapped infants. In: *New Directions in Exceptional Children,* Gallagher JJ (ed.). San Francisco: Jossey-Bass.

Richard N (1986): Interaction between mothers and infants with Down syndrome: Infant characteristics. *Top Early Special Educ,* 6(3): 54–71.

Richards MP (1979): Effects on development of medical interventions and the separation of newborns from their parents. In: *The First Year of Life,* Schaeffer D, Durin J (eds.). New York: Wiley.

Richardson SA (1969): The effect of physical disability on the socialization of a child. In: *Handbook of Socialization, Theory and Research,* Goslin D (ed.). Chicago: Rand McNally.

Richardson SA et al (1961): Cultural uniformity in reaction to physical disabilities. *Am Soc Rev, 26:* 241–247.

Richman LC (1978): The effects of facial disfigurement on teachers' perceptions of ability in cleft palate children. *Cleft Palate J, 15:* 155–160.

Rogers BM, Hillemeier MM, O'Neill E (1981): Depression in the chronically ill or handicapped school-aged child. *Am J Mat Child Nurs, 6:* 266–273.

Rose JA (1961): The prevention of mothering breakdown associated with physical abnormalities in the infant. In: *Prevention of Mental Disorders in Children,* Caplan G (ed.). New York: Basic Books.

Roskies E (1972): *Abnormality and Normality: The Mothering of Thalidomide Children.* Ithaca: Cornell University Press.

Rossetti L (1986): *High Risk Infants.* Boston: College Hill Press.

Sameroff A, Chandler MJ (1975): Reproductive risk and the continuum of caretaking casualty. In: *Review of Child Development Research:* Vol 4, Horowitz RD (ed.). Chicago: University of Chicago Press.

Schafer DS, Moersch MS (eds.) (1981): *Developmental Programming for Infants and Young Children.* Ann Arbor: University of Michigan Press.

Schulz J, Turnbull A (1983): *Mainstreaming Handicapped Students.* Boston: Allyn & Bacon.

Shapiro J (1983): Family reactions and coping strategies in response to the physically ill or handicapped child: A review. *Soc Sci Med, 17:* 913–931.

Siperstein GN, Bopp MJ, Bak JJ (1978): Social status of learning disabled children. *J Learn Disabil, 11:* 98–102.

Solnit A, Starck M (1961): Mourning and the birth of a defective child. *Psychoanal Study Child, 16:* 523–537.

Sperling E (1978) Psychological issues in chronic illness and handicap. In: *Psychosocial Aspects of Pediatric Care,* Gellert E (ed.). New York: Grune & Stratton.

Stainback S, Stainback W (1981): Educating nonhandicapped students about severely handicapped students: A human difference training model. *Educ Unlim, 3:* 17–19.

Stainback W, Stainback S, Hatcher C (1984): Teaching nonhandicapped students about individual differences: A pilot study. *Behav Disorders, 9:* 196–206.

Steele BF, Pollack CB (1974): A psychiatric study of parents who abuse infants and small children. In: *The Battered Child,* 2nd ed, Helfer R, Kempe C (eds.). Chicago: University of Chicago Press.

Stinson M (1978): Effects of deafness on maternal expectations about child development. *J Spec Educ, 12:* 75–81.

Strain P (1982): *Social Development of Exceptional Children.* Rockville, MD: Aspen.

Tew BJ, Laurence KM (1973): Mothers, brothers and sisters of patients with spina bifida. *Dev Med Child Neurol,* 15(29): Suppl. 69–76.

Tinsley BR et al (1982): Reconceptualizing the social environment of the high-risk infant: Fathers and settings. Paper presented at the International Conference on Infant Studies, Austin, Texas.

Vance J et al (1980): Effects of nephrotic syndrome on the family: A controlled study. *Pediatrics, 65:* 948–955.

Van Hassette VB, Hersen M, Whitehill MB (1979): Social skill assessment and training for children: An evaluation review. *Behav Res Ther, 17:* 413–437.

Vietze P, Abernathy S, Ashe M (1977): Contingent interaction between mothers and their developmentally delayed infants. In: Observing behavior: Vol 1, Sackett C (ed.). Baltimore: University Park Press.

Voeltz LM (1980): Children's attitudes towards handicapped peers. *J Ment Defic Res, 84:* 455–464.

Waechter E (1977): Bonding problems of infants with congenital anomalies. *Nurs Forum, 13:* 298–319.

Waisbren SE (1980): Parents' reaction after birth of a developmentally disabled child. *Am J Ment Defic Res, 84:* 345–351.

Walker D (1984): Care of chronically ill children in school. *Pediatr Clin North Am, 31:* 221–234.

Wasserman GA, Allen R, Solomon CR (1985a): The behavioral development of physically handicapped children in the second year. *J Dev Behav Pediatr, 6:* 27–31.

Wasserman GA, Allen R, Solomon CR (1985b): At-risk toddlers and their mothers: The special case of physical handicap. *Child Devel, 56:* 363–389.

Weitzman M (1984): School and peer relations. *Pediatr Clin North Am, 31*(1): 59–69.

Westby C (1980): Assessment of cognitive and language abilities through play. *Lang, Speech Hear Serv Schools, 11:* 154–168.

Wiegerin K et al (1980): Parents needs and expectations questionnaire: Experimental edition. Chapel Hill: University of North Carolina.

Yogman MW (1982): Development of the father-infant relationship. In: *Theory and Research in Behavioral Pediatrics:* Vol 1, Fitzgerald H, Lester B, Yogman M (eds.). New York: Plenum.

Young RK (1977): Chronic sorrow: Parents' response to the birth of a child with a defect. *Am J Mat Child Nurs* 2(1): 38–42.

Zelazo PR (1979): Reactivity to perceptual-cognitive events: Application for infant assessment. In: *Infants at Risk: Assessment of Cognitive Functioning,* Kearsley RB, Sigel IE (eds.). Hillsdale, IL: Erlbaum.

20

THE FAMILY WITH A CHRONICALLY ILL ADOLESCENT

Marilyn C. Savedra, RN, DNSc

Suzanne L. Dibble, RN, DNSc

Parents with adolescent children are faced with the task of helping their children through the often difficult transitions to young adulthood. When an adolescent is chronically ill, the entire family must play a more prominent role in this transitional phase. This chapter describes how chronic illness in an adolescent affects the lives of individual family members as well as the family unit. It also discusses the factors that influence the family's responses to a chronically ill member and suggests ways for helping families cope with the challenge.

Marilyn Savedra is an Associate Professor in the Department of Family Health Care Nursing at the University of California at San Francisco. She has established a research program in the areas of pain and coping strategies for children and adolescents.

Suzanne Dibble, a Nurse Researcher at the Stanford University Hospital, is responsible for the development of clinical research proposals and works with staff nurses to facilitate the development and implementation of research projects. Her own research has focused on adolescents with cystic fibrosis.

Introduction

Families with an adolescent face the task of helping the young person to master the final steps to achieve adult independence. When the adolescent has a chronic illness, the difficulty of the task is compounded. Parents often feel overwhelmed by the enormity of the demands as the adolescent struggles to break away while dealing with the realities of a chronic disease. Although the adolescent and parents are usually the principal players, other individuals, including brothers, sisters, grandparents, stepparents, aunts, uncles, family friends, and peers, play a role in helping adolescents to cope with the stresses of physical and sexual development or the lack of it; to achieve intimacy; to select a career; and to assume responsibility for his or her life as well as to cope with the disease.

Effects of Chronic Illness on Family Members

If the health needs of families with a chronically ill adolescent are to be met, it is critical to recognize that each member is at a specific point in the developmental sequence of tasks (Erikson, 1963; Havighurst, 1948). Transition points—the moving from one stage to another, as from latency to adolescence, adolescence to adulthood, and early adulthood to middle adulthood—produce crises that place special demands on the individual. Transition points signify physical changes, changes in roles and relationships, and changes in responsibilities. When a situational crisis, such as the diagnosis of a chronic disease, the exacerbation of a chronic condition, prolonged hospitalization, or the institution of a rigorous treatment protocol, is superimposed on a developmental crisis, not only does the individual member experience added stress but all family members feel the effects.

Effects on the Adolescent

Adolescence brings major bodily changes in size, proportion, and contour. Not all adolescents experience these changes at the same chronologic age, and the end result varies from one individual to another. For all, however, there is an expected spurt in height and weight and changes in body contours; that is, there is a broadening of the shoulders and increase in muscle mass for boys and a curving of the hips and rounding of the breasts for girls.

More dramatic than the height and weight changes and the growth spurt of internal organs are changes related to sexual development that prepare the adolescent for a reproductive role. Pubic and later axillary hair appears in both sexes, and boys develop the downy facial hair that will eventually develop into a full beard. In girls, breasts bud, menstruation begins, and ovulation is established. In boys, the increase in testes and penis size accompanies the ability to produce sperm and ejaculate. For most, if not all, adolescents, the overriding concern of the early adolescent period is "Am I normal?" In part, this stems from the variability in timing, if not in sequence, of events. For instance, portions of the face may grow at uneven rates, which may produce a nose that dominates the face. For many adolescents, accurate knowledge and understanding of these bodily changes is minimal. This concern accounts in part for the adolescent's engrossment in his or her body and the need to spend hours in front of a mirror examining the body, combing the hair, and, for girls, applying makeup to achieve the look that is "in."

Although becoming comfortable with one's body is a major task of early adolescence, also important is the need to achieve new and more mature relations with age mates and the need to achieve a masculine or feminine social role (Havighurst, 1948). Middle and late adolescents are focused on achieving emotional independence from parents and on selecting and preparing for a career that will provide economic independence. For some, these tasks are accomplished in stages. The adolescents may move to an apartment while attending school yet still rely on the family for financial support. Again, the young person may obtain a job with a family member that is tailored to his or her needs.

Many of the behaviors of adolescents that are so frustrating to other family members—occupying the bathroom for hours on end, excluding parents and siblings from private space, wearing sexually provocative clothing that reflects what every other teen is wearing, monopolizing the telephone during endless conversations with friends, refusing to participate in family events that interfere with peer events, and spending countless hours doing nothing—are the direct result of a need to accomplish the aforementioned tasks. The sense of invulnerability common to adolescents is a factor in much of the risk-taking behavior characteristic of the teenage years (Senft et al, 1981).

Because the need to be the same as peers is so high during adolescence, a chronic condition can be devastating. Many chronic diseases delay or prevent the physical changes characteristic of adolescence (Woodhead, Murph, 1985). Growth spurts fail to occur, and the adolescent appears childlike well after the time peers have achieved more mature bodies. Although the petite girl may not be as much at risk for appearing different, the short or underweight boy not only looks different but may be shunned by classmates as well. The athletic figure, if not athletic ability, is often what attracts friends.

Adolescents whose sexual development lags may be embarrassed and anxious. Boys who must appear naked in the locker room are more at risk than girls, who have greater opportunities to avoid public exposure. For both sexes, however, the ongoing monitoring of their physical condition by nurses and doctors and the constant comparison with "normal" or healthy peers make physical flaws painfully obvious. Treatment protocols often produce bodily changes that add to the pressure of becoming comfortable with bodily changes and the task of developing a positive body image. The obesity associated with steroids and the hair loss that follows chemotherapy are prime examples. At a time when the adolescent agonizes over being normal, it is clear that he or she is different from peers. When adolescents look different, cannot eat the teen food favorites, are physically unable to participate in activities, and are frequently absent from school, developing relationships with peers, particularly special, intimate friendships, is enormously difficult.

Chronic illness often increases the anxieties associated with experimenting with adult sexual behavior (Frauman, Sypert, 1979). How will your date respond if he or she knows you have cancer? Will you have a coughing spasm during your first kiss if you have cystic fibrosis? What would happen should a seizure occur when you are having sex? If you have a cardiac condition, could you die during sex? How do you handle your insulin injections on a school trip? In a culture where parents are eager to have their child popular and socially involved, conditions that hinder this are equally difficult for parents.

Chronic illness often makes the adolescent's struggle to become independent from family more difficult, if not impossible (McAnarney, 1985). The need for assistance with treatments and transportation to health care facilities, hospitalization, and the lack of strength or energy to manage personal care all contribute to the dilemma. These same factors are also responsible for problems in finding or holding a job. Most older adolescents grapple with career decisions and the possibilities of relationships or marriage that will produce children of their own. Chronic illness may limit these options. Some occupations, for example, airline pilot for the epileptic or winetaster for the diabetic, are inappropriate. Pregnancy may produce greater risks than average for both mother and fetus, or the uncertainty of life expectancy may make long-term commitments more tenuous.

Although the accomplishment of adolescent developmental tasks is affected by chronic or life-threatening illness, the outcomes are not as negative as might be expected. The research data of Zeltzer et al (1980), comparing 345 healthy adolescents and 168 adolescents with renal, rheumatologic, or cardiac diseases, cancer, cystic fibrosis, or diabetes mellitus, indicate that adolescent concerns are not dissimilar, regardless of pathology or lack of it. Restriction of freedom was identified, however, as the major disruption brought about by a chronic illness. The data nevertheless support the resiliency and coping strategies of chronically ill adolescents. Hope and denial appear to be healthy strategies that enable these adolescents to manage their lives.

Effects on Parents

Parents, too, have developmental tasks. Some tasks, including physical maintenance, protection, education, socialization, recreation, and affection, are directly related to the parenting role. Other tasks are more individual in nature and depend on the stage in the adult cycle—early, middle, or late adulthood—as well as being influenced by the age of each child in the family. Parental age in families with an adolescent has a wide variance, depending on biologic and societal factors. Some parents may be in their thirties, and other parents may be in their fifties or sixties.

Although much is yet to be learned about developmental tasks during mid-life, Levinson (1977), building on Erikson's concept of stage-specific tasks, speaks to the developmental tasks of men moving from early to middle adulthood, the age of many fathers with an adolescent child. Levinson (1977) describes the settling down period (ages 32 or 33 to 39 or 40) when the major tasks for the man are:

(a) To establish a niche in society: to dig in, anchor his life more firmly, develop competence in a chosen craft, become a valued member of a valued world. (b) To work at making it, planning, striving to advance, progressing along a timetable. (p. 104)

In the late thirties, the man may enter a period where the desire to achieve a greater measure of authority and to follow personal desires may run counter to the demands of his situation. Levinson has named this period "becoming one's own man." The act of achieving a more senior role with the accompanying rewards also brings greater responsibility and increased pressure. Valliant's (1977) record, although less age specific, supports the view that mid-life for men is a time for self-evaluation and inward reflection.

For other developmentalists, timing of events related to bodily changes, work career, and family role (father of preschooler versus father of adolescent or young adult) is the critical issue (Neugarten, 1979). For example, the mother experiencing menopause at the time of puberty for her daughter may also be grappling with concerns regarding bodily changes and sexuality. Fears of diminishing sexual attractiveness come at a time when her daughter is beginning her reproductive role. Rossi (1980) reports from her study of 68 women, 33 to 56 years old with at least one child in early adolescence, that childrearing was viewed as more difficult when the family size was large and the child was older. Economic pressure related to family size and the needs of adolescents may be an influencing factor. Better-educated mothers reported less difficulty in rearing adolescents than mothers with lower levels of education. Rossi's data suggest older women see the adolescent years as more difficult, raising the possibility that mothers may be emotionally less accessible to their children as they cope with growing older.

When the adolescent child has a chronic illness or chronic disease strikes in the teen years, parents experience added conflict as they seek to meet the needs of their child as well as those of their own. Personal dreams may have to remain only that as time and energy are channeled into treatment schedules, physician visits, and hospitalizations. Decisions may need to be made regarding stopping one career in order to care for the ill adolescent. Parents may feel locked into jobs that provide little satisfaction but provide finances to meet the drain of medical care. A second job may be necessary. With the added demands, less time is available to spend with personal interests, family, or friends. In cases where the illness is life threatening or severe, it may be unrealistic to hope that the adolescent will achieve complete independence.

Effects on Grandparents

Although grandparents in families with a chronically ill adolescent have received little attention in the literature, their lives, too, are affected. If they live close by or in the same household, they may be involved in caring for other children while parents meet the needs of the adolescent. This may have a positive or a negative effect on the grandparent. For those who no longer have the stimulus of a job or professional involvement, the role in the family associated with the adolescent may provide a meaningful dimension to their lives. On the other hand, if freedom from job activities and the time to pursue personal interests were eagerly anticipated, responsibilities related to grandchildren may be viewed as demanding and disruptive. The health of the grandparents influences their level of involvement; they may need more from the family than they can give. A grandparent who is putting his or her life in order and proceeding with dignity toward death can, however, provide special support for a terminally ill grandchild who also must prepare for death. Although grandparents may attenuate family stresses by their supportive help, counsel, and financial assistance, they also may increase family tensions when their view of how

the chronic illness should be managed differs from that of their child or grandchild or when they also need care and financial assistance.

Effects on Siblings

Siblings may or may not be in the same developmental stage as the chronically ill adolescent. Although some years appear to be smoother and less troubled for a given child, each phase of development brings a struggle for growth and is accompanied by special needs. Ferrari's (1984) study failed to support the hypothesis that siblings of chronically ill children are at greater risk for psychosocial distress; however, when developmental transition points in siblings coincide with changing health problems, with demanding treatment regimens, or with hospitalizations for the ill child, siblings' needs may be neglected or ignored. More often, however, needs are recognized, but parental time is justifiably limited. Trips to the hospital supersede trips to the park with a young child or the chauffeuring of older children to music lessons, sports activities, and school events. Because of heavy financial responsibilities for the ill member, there is less money to meet the needs or wants of other children. Younger children in particular may feel the loss of individual time with parents, especially when the chronic illness in their sibling is a new diagnosis. Preschoolers in the stage of preconventional thinking see themselves to blame for changes in the family with shifts in parental attention away from them. Older siblings, although cognitively able to understand what is happening, may come to resent the special attention, favors, and leniency bestowed on the child who is ill (Kramer, 1980).

Effects on the Family Unit

A major effect of a chronically ill adolescent on the family unit is related to family cohesiveness. Whether the family is a nuclear family, a stepfamily, a gay or lesbian family, or a single-parent family, many of the issues—such as adolescent development, time commitments, financial burden, and energy expenditure—are similar. Differences are the direct result of available support systems, financial resources, coping strategies, and ethnic and cultural behaviors.

Factors Affecting Family Responses

How families will respond when an adolescent member has a chronic illness is dependent on several factors. Responses vary in relation to the time of onset (Gode, Smith, 1983). When the chronic condition has been present since birth, the adolescent and other family members incorporate the effects of the disease with its accompanying symptomatology into their daily activities. When, however, the chronic disease has its onset in adolescence, when being different is a catastrophe, the impact on the adolescent causes major upheavals in the family. Closely related to the age of onset is the type of illness, or the nature of the disease. Is the condition potentially life-threatening (cancer, cystic fibrosis)? Is there an expected time limitation (acne, scoliosis)? Is the disease acquired or congenital (arthritis versus hemophilia)? Are normal activities impeded by the disease (end stage renal disease, scoliosis)? Is pain associated with the disease or its treatment (arthritis, cancer)? Is the condition visible or nonvisible (amputation versus diabetes)? Conditions that have a poor prognosis (for example, muscular dystrophy), that interfere with usual adolescent activities, that have pain as a major component of pathology or treatment, and that alter appearance increase the level of stress. In some illnesses, there is a relentless increase in the quality and quantity of the symptoms. The nature and number of symptoms influence how the adolescent and family will respond to changes in the disease process. The anticipation of possible death at a time when life is seen as just beginning is particularly stressful for all family members.

The treatment protocol may present more stress than the disease itself. The side effects of the treatment regimen may be seen as an intolerable assault on the body and may cause the adolescent to reject therapy. Family conflict may result. Treatments, trips to health care providers, and hospitalization may place time demands on all family members and cause disruption to family life in general.

The health, physical or emotional, of other family members is a major factor in how families will deal with a chronically ill adolescent. The factors that must be considered are (1) number of ill members and the percent of the total family that is ill; (2) the extensiveness of each treatment regimen; (3) the similarity of the various diagnoses; (4) the genetic component of the conditions; and (5) the individual prognosis. The fiscal impact of a chronic illness, although difficult to assess, also has a major impact on the functioning of families.

Responses of Family Members

Responses of the Adolescent

Because each adolescent is a unique individual and because for each individual the conditions surrounding the illness vary, no one pattern of behavior can be predicted. If the illness is a new diagnosis and if other major stressors have been part of the life experience, the adolescent is likely to use coping strategies that have worked in the past. The magnitude of stress may render past ways of dealing with crisis situations ineffective, and new strategies must be developed. Denial is often used effectively and, contrary to the belief of some, is not inappropriate. An adolescent may choose not to acknowledge that he or she has a particular disease. More common, however, is a refusal to acknowledge the seriousness of the condition. Although adolescents have an understanding of the meaning of death, they also view themselves as infallible. Death may come to others but not to them. Denial becomes a dangerous way of coping when it leads to a discontinuation or refusal to take needed medications, to follow a required diet, or to perform needed treatments.

Some adolescents cope by learning all that they can about their illness. Information is sought from a variety of sources, including health care providers, written materials, and the media. This strategy, known as intellectualization, is possible because of the ability of adolescents to comprehend and think on an abstract level.

As opposed to denial and intellectualization, the response of anger is unacceptable. Anger manifests itself in verbal or physical behaviors that are annoying and frustrating for those who interact with the adolescent. Adolescents who have lived with a chronic disease for a long time may become expert in using the disease to manipulate others. For some adolescents, withdrawal, or pulling away from peers and activities, is the preferred coping strategy. Depression is often a component of this isolation from friends and school. Normal developmental tasks may be delayed or avoided.

Because adolescents can be sensitive to the effects of their disease on the family, they may experience enormous guilt for the disruption in daily activities, for the care demands placed on others, and for the financial drain on parents. For many adolescents with a chronic disease, acceptance and adaptation to the existing condition is achieved. Strengths are discovered and developed. Involvement with the health team and hospital may open new career possibilities and provide them with a new and expanded support system. Relationships with same-and opposite-sex peers are developed. Independence to the degree possible is mastered.

Parents' Responses

Parental responses are not dissimilar to those of the adolescent and vary with changing circumstances. For the most part, parents have a genuine concern for the adolescent's well-being, and their responses are directed to providing the best possible care. When diagnosis is made during adolescence—particularly if the disease is potentially life-threatening—shock, disbelief, anger, and sadness may be evident. Parents often feel overwhelmed by the enormity of the demands placed on them. If power struggles already exist between parent and child, the responsibility of carrying out necessary treatment protocols is seen as an impossible task. It is not unusual for overprotection and overindulgence to accompany conscientious caring. Although these responses flow from a real concern for the good of the child, they often impede rather than help the adolescent's struggle for autonomy and independence. Irrational guilt may accompany the parents' search for the cause of the disease when none is known. Guilt may resurface for parents whose child has an inherited disease as awareness of the impact of the disease on achieving life goals becomes more obvious during adolescence. Although rejection of the adolescent is rare, resentment and frustration can accompany caring involvement. As is true of the adolescent, parents, too, adapt to the demands of the disease, relate to their child in a supportive manner, and manage their own needs as well as the needs of other members of the family. Faith in God and involvement in church or organizations related to the disease often provide a source of strength and meaning. However, divorce is a frequent occurrence in parents of a chronically ill child.

Siblings' Responses

Sibling behaviors, although affected by a number of variables, are profoundly influenced by age, by the attention they receive from their parents, and by the way their ill sibling is treated. Very young children may be sad and lonely during periods when parents are involved with the ill brother or sister. Preschoolers often share the parental guilt for the cause of what is happening. Older children, although capable of understanding the situation, also may respond to the decreased parental attention, to the increased role responsibilities, and to the indulgence of the ill adolescent by acting out. The extra attention and privileges are seen as unfair. What can be accepted for a brief time, during a hospitalization for instance, becomes more difficult when the period is extended. Siblings may worry that they too will develop the disease. However, siblings often cope effectively with the stress of having a chronically ill brother or sister.

Nursing Management

Nursing plays an important role in the care of families with a chronically ill adolescent. Although the focus in terms of the health care system is on the adolescent, care can only be effectively delivered if attention is paid to the effect of the adolescent's health problems on the family unit as well as on individual members. In addition to management of a specific disease, the health care team should be concerned for the developmental tasks of all family members.

Regardless of the disease and irrespective of whether a nurse is providing primary care management in outpatient settings or direct patient care in the hospital, there are aspects of care that nurses manage. The following case illustrates an example of nursing management when an adolescent is chronically ill.

> Alice is a 16-year-old admitted to the adolescent unit for shortness of breath—an acute exacerbation of her cystic fibrosis. Although diagnosed in infancy, this was only the third hospitalization for Alice. She was in acute distress on arrival, with cyanotic nailbeds and lips. After starting her on oxygen in the hall, room placement was an issue. The only bed available was that in which her older brother Joe had died two weeks previously. The staff was well aware that Alice was the last of five children who had cystic

fibrosis. Four other siblings were free of this disease. Alice was accompanied by both of her parents, who were obviously very concerned yet supportive.

The primary nurse set up an interdisciplinary care conference for the following day with the physician, the social worker, the nutritionist, the respiratory therapist, and nurses from different shifts. Critical questions addressed were:

- What is the current medical status and prognosis of this hospitalization?
- What is the meaning of this hospitalization to Alice?
- What is the meaning of the oxygen therapy to Alice and other family members?
- Will her treatment regimen be increased in frequency? How will this time commitment affect her peer relationships, schooling, and outside activities?
- Will the parents need help in performing the treatments? What other family members or peers are available?
- What kind of nutritional support is Alice willing to accept?
- What concerns does Alice have about her physical development? What are her educational needs in this area?
- What realistically are her career options?
- What impact does this hospitalization have on family functioning?
- Can the family support Alice while grieving for Joe?
- Is religion an important family support? If so, would the family desire to speak with a member of the clergy?
- What agencies are appropriate for the support of the family's outpatient care of Alice?

The answers to these and other questions were critical for planning, implementation, and evaluation of Alice's care. Questions not only addressed Alice's needs or concerns but focused on the family members and their interrelationships.

Future Directions

Directions for nursing management of adolescents with chronic illness are dependent on research of the psychosocial implications of living with a chronic disease both from the individual as well as the family perspective. Appropriate psychosocial studies are currently rare in the literature. Two groups of researchers (Orr et al, 1984; Zeltzer et al, 1980) have provided us with some beginning data from which to understand the chronically ill adolescent. Most of our assumptions and interventions are based on clinical impressions and theories. Realistically, studies will most likely continue to focus on specific disease entities such as anorexia nervosa (Braisted et al, 1985), renal disease (De-Nour, 1979), and cystic fibrosis (Smith, Gad, O'Grady, 1983). Exploratory questions must be addressed prior to future intervention studies. Meta-analytic procedures could be useful in the future once a large enough number of studies of families with chronically ill adolescents has been completed and reported. An ultimate goal of nursing research is to improve the understanding as well as the care of the family with a chronically ill adolescent.

Summary

Chronic illness occurring in an adolescent has specific effects on other family members. The specific response of the family as a unit and of the individual family members is a function of the character of the particular family. Nursing care must consider carefully the developmental needs of all family members.

Issues for Further Investigation

1. What is the role of social support, that is, grandparents, peers, and church groups, in relationship to social development of the chronically ill adolescent?

2. What is the impact on family functioning of a chronically ill adolescent?

3. What factors influence the transition of care from parent to adolescent?

References

Braisted JR et al (1985): The adolescent ballet dancer: Nutritional practices and characteristics associated with anorexia nervosa. *J Adolesc Health Care,* 6(5): 365–371.

De-Nour AK (1979): Adolescents' adjustment to chronic hemodialysis. *Am J Psychiatry,* 136(4A): 430–433.

Erikson EH (1963): *Childhood and Society.* New York: W.W. Norton.

Ferrari M (1984): Chronic illness: Psychosocial effects on sibling. 1. Chronically ill boys, *J Child Psychol Psychiatry,* 25(3): 459–476.

Frauman AC, Sypert NS (1979): Sexuality in adolescents with chronic illness. *Am J Mat Child Nurs,* 4(6): 371–375.

Gode RO, Smith MS (1983): Effects of chronic disorders on adolescent development: Self, family friends, and school. In: *Chronic Disorders in Adolescence,* Smith MS (ed.) Boston: John Wright.

Havighurst RJ (1948): *Developmental Tasks and Education.* New York: David McKay.

Kramer RF (1980): Living with childhood cancer: The healthy siblings' perspective. *Issues Compr Pediatr Nurs, 5:* 155–165.

Levinson DJ (1977): The mid-life transition: A period in adult psychosocial development. *Psychiatry,* 40(5): 99–112.

McAnarney ER (1985): Social maturation: A challenge for handicapped and chronically ill adolescents. *J Adolesc Health Care*, 6(2): 90–101.

Neugarten BL (1979): Time age, and the life cycle. *Am J Psychiatry*, 136(7): 887–894.

Orr DP et al (1984): Psychosocial implications of chronic disease in adolescence. *J Pediatr*, 104(1): 152–157.

Rossi AS (1980): Life-span theories and women's lives. *Signs*, 6(1): 4–32.

Senft KR et al (1981): Risk-taking and the adolescent hemophiliac. *J Adolesc Health Care*, 2(2): 87–91.

Smith MS, Gad MT, O'Grady L (1983): Psychosocial functioning, life change, and clinical status in adolescents with cystic fibrosis. *J Adolesc Health Care*, 4(4): 230–234.

Vaillant GE (1977): *Adaptation to Life*. Boston: Little Brown.

Woodhead JC, Murph JR (1985): Influence of chronic illness and disability on adolescent sexual development. *Seminars in Adolescent Medicine*, 1(3): 171–176.

Zeltzer L et al (1980). Psychological effects of illness in adolescence: Part II. Impact of illness in adolescents—crucial issues and coping styles. *J Pediatr*, 97(1): 132–138.

21

THE FAMILY AND CANCER

Kay B. Tiblier, PhD

The American Cancer Society (1983) estimates that 30% of Americans now living will contract one or more forms of cancer, and that three out of four families will have a family member diagnosed with cancer. This chapter discusses the impact of cancer on the family from diagnosis through death and family reorganization, and explores associated research and clinical issues.

Kay Tiblier, Associate Clinical Professor in the Department of Family Health Care Nursing at the University of California at San Francisco, is also a Lecturer in Sociology at San Francisco State University. Known for her study of the sociology of life-threatening illness, the majority of her clinical work is with families responding to the demands of cancer and AIDS.

Introduction

The American Cancer Society (1983) estimates that about 30% of Americans now living will contract one or more forms of cancer. Three out of four families will have a family member diagnosed as having cancer. Thoughts of this illness arouse images associated with pain, isolation, mutilation, hopelessness, and death (Burns, 1982).

Psychosocial Dimensions

Effective social support is a crucial factor in psychologic adaptation during terminal illness (Revenson, Wollman, Felton, 1983; Bloom, 1982). The ability of persons to maintain or to develop psychologic comfort depends not only on their intrapsychic resources but more importantly on the social supports available (or absent) in the environment (Mechanic, 1974). Weisman and Worden (1975) suggest that patients who maintain cooperative and sustaining relationships tend to live significantly longer than expected. Patients who are depressed or apathetic, who wish to die, and who are in mutually destructive relationships survive for shorter periods of time. Thus, nurses who become skilled with psychosocial interventions may be facilitating adaptation and contributing to a more favorable prognosis.

The Impact of Cancer on the Family

Family reactions in coping with the experience of cancer are worthy of emphasis because the family is in a position to mediate the stress of its members (Kaplan et al, 1973). The family has many alternative forms, which may include a lover or friends rather than, or in addition to, the family of origin. This expanded sociologic definition of the family is adopted in this chapter and is helpful to those who work with the significant others of the cancer patient. Nurses and other caregivers benefit all concerned by extending their concern beyond the patient to the immediate family and perhaps to other close relatives and friends and by offering, as appropriate, help to resolve specific stressful problems (Burns, 1982).

As the patient's illness progresses, latent family conflict may emerge. Old issues may be brought forth, including faulty communication patterns and family roles. Or the patient and family caregivers may owe allegiance to two systems—one to the family of origin and another to the family of procreation. Frequently, family members find themselves in conflict. They may be helped to move beyond their differences by attending to the patient or by dividing tasks. They work together to provide resources.

Recent perspectives on cancer and the family regard the family not only as the principal source of support for the sick but also as the unit that faces the disease (Giaquinta, 1977). The family system's integrity and function are threatened. Each family member is personally affected by the diagnosis and its consequences. Within the family, dynamics are altered, communication patterns change, roles shift, and expected sources of support may collapse (Burns, 1982). Bowen (1976) refers to an "emotional shock wave," in which after shocks can occur anywhere in the extended family system in the months or years following a serious emotional event.

Hill and Hansen (1964) identify four factors that influence the family's ability to cope with an illness. These include characteristics of the event (nature of illness or disability, prognosis, and perception of the illness); perceived threat to the family (relationship, status, and roles); available resources; and past experience. The diagnosis of cancer, considering this analytic framework, can be devastating.

Many cancer patients and their families adapt fairly well without professional psychosocial intervention. As with other forms of crisis, coping and adaptation may evolve in a myriad of shapes and forms, using friends or other family members or spiritual or comic relief (Tiblier, 1978). Other family members who want to be supportive may not know how to provide emotional reassurance or may have great difficulty providing support, especially when the patient is dying (Olsen, 1970; Spiegal, Bloom, Gottheil, 1983). In many cases family members may themselves feel a need for psychosocial support.

In this chapter, the author's concern is with protecting and using the family's strength when one of its members develops cancer. The task of helping the family understand cancer while allowing them to continue functioning has traditionally been undertaken by the family physician, but nurses will frequently take this role or share it with physicians and other caregivers.

Staging Models

In attempting to systematically address the psychosocial demands of cancer on the patient and family, various stages and phases of illness have been identified by scholars in the fields of sociology, psychology, psychiatry, and nursing. Three examples of staging are those by Kubler-Ross (1969), Giaquinta (1977), and Mailick (1979).

In a pioneering effort to identify a progressive pattern from the time of diagnosis of cancer until death, Kubler-Ross, in *On Death and Dying* (1969), reported the results of 200 interviews. She identified five stages of adaptation to a terminal diagnosis: (1) denial and isolation; (2) anger; (3) bargaining; (4) depression; and (5) acceptance.

Giaquinta (1977) proposed a model of four stages and ten accompanying phases for the systematic description of the functioning of families facing cancer. Her model includes (1) living with cancer, with the five phases of shock and strain,

and with functional disruption; searching for meaning; informing others; and engaging emotions; (2) restructuring in the living–dying interval, with phases of reorganization, and framing memories; (3) experiencing bereavement, with separation, mourning, and grief; and (4) reestablishing through expansion of the social network.

Mailick (1979) identifies three stages with delineated tasks for coping and adaptation: (1) the diagnostic phase connected with the onset of the illness; (2) the adaptation to the long-term or disabling nature of the illness; and (3) the ending of the illness episode through cure, remission, or death.

There are several weaknesses in these staging models. First, such patterns often have been interpreted as literal and sequential, despite the authors' insistence that such sequencing has not been intended. As a result, some educators have taught a "correct" ordering of such stages. This in turn has led to expectations of a "correct" response on the part of the patient. Second, such models suggest a linearity and completeness that is not found in the complexity facing those who are experiencing cancer. Staging models are therefore most useful to place emphasis on a series of critical junctions confronting the patient with cancer.

Sociologic and Psychologic Crises Precipitated by Cancer

The family with a member with cancer faces a series of sociologic and psychologic crises associated with crucial periods during the course of the disease. Although order may be implied by this discussion, delineation of points is not intended as a literal order. Each patient has a unique physical and psychologic response to disease. In addition, the family, both as an aggregate and as individual members, will experience the course of the disease in its own manner. For some, any given period or adaptation to the period may be brief, but for others, the process will take many shapes and turns.

A diagnosis of cancer shatters the orderly and predictable unfolding of time. The type and severity of stress experienced by the family often depends on what point the patient has reached in the life cycle and on the ages of family members. A feeling of loss and sadness develops with the threat of death of any family member, and the cliché that an elderly person "has lived a full life" does not mitigate such feelings. If the patient is young or of middle age, there may be feelings of injustice at the timing of events. For a parent, the death of a child of any age can be particularly disturbing as a tragic and absurd reversal of the expected timing of life events.

Nurses and other researchers may observe any or all of the following periods of crisis experienced by the family of the cancer patient. Although it may be argued that each point represents an intrapersonal, psychologic difficulty, people are primarily social and interactive. Therefore, these hurdles are interpersonal and social–psychologic.

Suspicion and Uncertainty

For some length of time before one receives a specific diagnosis, a series of disturbing changes or symptoms occur. Whether or when one decides to seek medical treatment may depend on sociologic and psychologic variables more than on the extent of the physical changes experienced. Mechanic (1962, p. 189) refers to "illness behavior" as the ways in which given symptoms may be differentially perceived, evaluated, and acted (or not acted) on by different persons.

The Prediagnostic Phase

An initial crisis is reached during the period of uncertainty, during which the symptoms of cancer have been noted but not definitively diagnosed. The patient and family must handle the anxiety of the unknown, the guilt, and the physical and emotional strain of tests, perhaps involving strange machines and painful procedures (Mailick, 1979). Reactions of the patient and family may alternate between acceptance and denial of the potentially devastating diagnosis (Nordlicht, 1982).

Diagnosis of Life-Threatening Disease

One of the more difficult and critical tasks of health professionals is that of informing the patient of the diagnosis. Optimally, the family and patient are informed together. Trust in the caregivers is developed when the truth is imparted with empathy, concern, confidence, and a willingness to support the patient and family along the course of the disease.

Privacy is needed when bad news is given so that feelings such as fear and anger may be expressed. Ideally, a comfortable and private room will be available. This special refuge provides a quiet setting for the beginning of what is to be important family work.

Families that understand the essential nature of the illness are better able to begin this work. Educational orientation sessions may be provided by the hospital or within the community. At such a forum, medical questions may be answered, routines are anticipated, and fears may be ventilated. At such times of heightened anxiety, concentration and memory are poor. The family may need to hear the same information repeated gently and clearly several times or to be given simple directives. Some family members may require more assistance in the form of group, individual, or family therapy; immediate referrals may be indicated.

Nordlicht (1982) has proposed brief care in this early period to achieve stabilization and possibly to avoid undergoing a more time-consuming therapy later. Despair is the hurdle to overcome, with intervention geared toward fostering hope and allowing the patient and family to imagine a future. Intervention involves exploring and combating feelings of despair and discussing tendencies to withdraw from one another (Giaquinta, 1977).

Family reactions at this point are essentially those of grief over anticipated catastrophic losses. Grief, which may be experienced for the first time at this stage, will recur at points throughout the course of illness.

It can be comforting to the family to have a supportive nurse present at the onset of grief, especially in those settings where the nurse will be involved with the care given to the patient over the course of therapy and follow-up.

Disclosure

Because of their own anxieties and fears, the family, if they are told first, may request that the patient not be informed of the diagnosis. Their assertion that "the patient cannot deal with it" indicates that the family cannot deal with it. Rigid and dysfunctional families are more apt to respond this way, needing to protect the family system from change. Avoidance and denial are the family's defenses against change. Intervention may help significant others to understand better their own grief and fear, as well as to learn how they can be of support to the patient. Keeping such a family informed allows everyone to feel included and supported and of help to the patient; thus they become a very real part of the care network.

The family may begin informing others before fully understanding the diagnosis or its impact. This may result in an inability to answer questions and to reassure others about the propriety of the diagnosis and impending therapy, thus creating pressure, dissension, and distrust. Intervention fosters communication of feelings and strengthens cohesion, thus overcoming the hurdle of retreat (Giaquinta, 1977).

Treatment Decisions

Ideally, the patient and family, as active members of the therapeutic team, participate in making crucial treatment plans. There may be apprehensions related to treatment modalities such as surgery, chemotherapy, radiotherapy, or a combination of choices. There may be grief reactions to possible loss of a body part or function, or there may be fears of adverse, debilitating, or disfiguring effects of treatment that threaten self-esteem. The nurse addresses the family's apprehensions by providing information. This information includes (1) the extent of disease; (2) expected treatment outcomes; (3) goals and mechanisms of treatment; (4) how treatment is administered; and (5) estimates of pain or discomfort.

At this time the family is receptive to learning and change. Many questions may be asked about diagnosis, treatment, and side effects. Alternatives and options need to be explored.

Much of the treatment will occur in the hospital setting. Caregivers can aid the patient's adaptation to this foreign environment and to concomitant loss of independence by educating the patient and family about routines and expectations.

Within this setting, medical sociologists Strauss et al (1975) have identified types of "work" performed by the family. These include (1) working with a sick relative "psychologically" (the sentimental work); (2) attending to legal–administrative work; (3) engaging in crucial decision-making; (4) being an advocate for the patient; and (5) monitoring comfort.

A central role for the family is to help the patient to endure or to keep composure as well as to handle identity problems accompanying the illness. This "sentimental work" may alleviate the anxiety, fear, and depression accompanying illness. Mere presence or touching and soothing aid in this work. Empathetic caregivers who touch and handle the patient gently and with acceptance serve as role models and set the pace for cautious relatives.

When the patient with cancer cannot act on his or her own behalf and has no family members present, multiple problems may emerge. Documents must be signed, financial agreements made, and informed consent obtained. It is helpful if someone can be designated to represent the patient in a legitimate manner. In California, it is possible for the patient to grant "durable power of attorney" to empower a significant other to make decisions regarding medical care for the patient.

Decision-making is intellectually and emotionally demanding, difficult to pursue, and fateful of outcome, yet it is little understood by hospital staff. The family possesses unique knowledge that may be used in the decision-making process. Family members can be encouraged to communicate with primary physicians, receive literature or references, and use their accumulated insights to help their loved one make crucial decisions.

The family then serves as advocate for the patient. Successfully negotiating with medical staff and institutions is difficult for the healthy person, and for the patient with cancer, the task may seem insurmountable. The anxiety provoked by tests, reports, and medical opinions can be lessened by a family member accompanying the patient, by taking notes, and by listing additional questions for the next visit. Acknowledging that these family members are interested partners in the patient's medical care can add to the rapport and provide further aid to the family and the patient.

Family members also aid in the provision of comfort for the patient. Music, cards, special foods, or other items may make the surroundings more pleasant. Ensuring silence or screening visitors and telephone calls can add to comfort. Nurses can assist the family and patient in recognizing the ebb and flow of patient energy and in providing stimulation or protection.

Stigma

Stigma involves adjustment to a new and painful identity (Goffman, 1963). The social stigma associated with cancer can be devastating to both patient and family (Winder, Elam, 1978).

Time is needed to cope with public disclosure in the face of potential social stigma. The family may not know what to tell friends, neighbors, or other relatives. They may try to hide the illness or attempt to prevent the diagnosis from being known. The family must decide who to tell and how to cope with others' reactions. It may be helpful for a family to confide in a trusted friend or professional to sort out their feelings.

A search for meaning can be an attempt to gain intellectual mastery over cancer. The family may blame the patient by relating dietary, alcohol, or smoking history to etiology of the malignancy in an attempt to ensure that they are not likely to receive a similar diagnosis. As each family member confronts his or her own mortality, vulnerability must be overcome. Intervention is directed toward supporting the family system and enhancing security by confronting changes in identity.

Caregivers such as nurses and physicians may share the stigma of cancer. Those caregivers who specialize in oncology may be considered strange or may experience social isolation from others in their profession.

Adaptation to Uncertainty of Chronic Disease

The greatest proportion of research attention to the psychosocial impact of cancer has been in the response to critical points in the course. The varying duration of life and the length of time with which one lives with cancer has been neglected. Some forms of cancer, such as early cervical cancer, early breast cancer, and some skin cancer, have a high cure rate. Hodgkin's disease is often cured in early stages by radiotherapy or chemotherapy. In late Hodgkin's disease, cure is possible if there is good patient response to chemotherapy. Adjuvant therapy, combining early treatment by surgery, radiotherapy, chemotherapy, and perhaps immunotherapy, is more frequently used with increasing cure rates for many cancers.

Although one may speak of cure, it is often more accurate to speak of remission, for in many cases, the risk of recurrence may remain high for many years. It may be difficult for the family to adapt to living with such uncertainty. The challenge is to maintain a semblance of normality in the presence of cancer, where the only certainty may be uncertainty.

One difficult matter with which families deal is helping the patient organize personal affairs. Although it is a rational plan for all patients to have their personal and business matters settled, not all do. The timing of suggestions to do so is problematic. Many err by being too eager to approach the issue before a patient has come to terms with impending death or by being reluctant to discuss such issues as wills, bank accounts, or other financial planning at the patient's request. Significant others may be reminded to take their cues from the patient, discussing such items as bank accounts, loans, powers of attorney, and other practical matters when the opportunity exists.

Sexuality

Sexual behavior is simultaneously somatic, psychologic, and interpersonal. Cancer introduces into a sexual relationship the partner's fear of hurting, guilt, and anticipatory grief (Greenberg, 1984).

Anderson (1985) reports that nearly 90% of adult cancer patients may experience sexual problems as a result of surgery, radiotherapy, or chemotherapy. For 44%–79% of women with cervical cancer, sexual function is diminished or completely disrupted; radiotherapy patients may lack lubrication or develop vaginal discharges. After radical hysterectomy, 6%–19% of cancer patients have sex difficulties. Radiation therapy for breast cancer causes sexual disruption in 75% of patients and adjuvant chemotherapy causes disruption in 13%–40%. After surgery for rectal and colon cancers, 28% have less desire, and 21% have genital numbness or dyspareunia (Anderson, 1985).

Sexuality is a central concern within the context of loss of relationship. Physical debilitation or the specific nature of illness may preclude sexual functioning, but psychologic factors are often more important in a couple's abstinence. Some couples may fear contagion, or a spouse may consider the patient too fragile for lovemaking. The meaning of intimacy may be too painful in the context of one person moving toward death and one toward life (Sourkes, 1982).

Caregivers seldom raise the issue of sexuality with the patient. Research is needed to amplify the knowledge and belief systems of physicians and nurses that inhibit their interventions in this crucial area.

Role Conflict

The unique demands and constraints attendant to the role of the cancer patient have been described (Hinton, 1963; Holland, 1976; Haney, 1984). Haney offers four constraints as being particularly problematic: (1) the recurrent need to modify reality; (2) the definition of time; (3) the management of uncertainty; and (4) coping with pain.

Following an initial diagnosis, the patient continues to carry out role obligations by functioning as a family member (Giaquinta, 1977). As the illness progresses, the person with cancer may cease family role performance and become dependent.

Role conflict may be manifest during periods of functional disruption. Specific dilemmas may include changes in the family division of labor or involve the keeping of a hospital vigil to the neglect of household management and childcare. When family members are separated by hospitalization, isolation may occur. Intervention fosters interaction, communication, cooperation, and socioemotional involvement. Needs, priorities, and resources can be identified.

Families that use achieved rather than ascribed role-assignment methods before the onset of cancer, families with older children who can adopt expanded role functions, and families with more interspouse communication have been shown to experience less disruption, less role conflict, and less role strain over time (Vess, Moreland, Schwebel, 1985).

Recurrence

The threat of relapse or recurrence is ever present in the family living with cancer. When hope of cure changes into coping with relapse, grief returns. The family may be torn by the patient's reticence to endure continuing the battle against cancer. The family may again be receptive to nursing intervention that can strengthen its functioning and offer further hope.

Decline

Family dynamics and psychologic techniques for adaptation change again when the patient begins to decline. Volatile emotions surface around changing values, goals, satisfactions, and positions of security. Those who fear loss of control may suppress feelings and withdraw from each other. Weekly conferences among health care personnel to exchange information and to plan strategy for the care of the patient and family allow for change and adaptation. To the extent that it is possible, family and patient may be included in such meetings.

Ending Treatment

At some point, for many patients, there are no remaining conventional treatment options. A choice between cessation versus experimental treatment usually revolves around the quality of life. Once the decision is made, the family may experience great relief. Families need assurance that palliative care is available. The availability of effective pain control may enable the family to care for the patient at home. Other families will require the security of an inpatient hospice program.

The Stress of Home Care

For the most part, information on the emotional situation of patients and families has been collected in hospitals or outpatient clinics, although most cancer patients spend much of their time at home. Several investigators have reported the stress involved in home care. Although there are reduced costs, family members may have to alter their work schedules, which may result in reduced income. Energies once devoted to a job now must be directed toward the ill family member at home. Those who care for the patient have been found to be at risk for physical and mental exhaustion (Rosenbaum, Rosenbaum, 1980), sleep disorders (Rose, 1976), depression, and anxiety. Older families, especially those of men with lung cancer, have been found to be at greater risk of being overwhelmed (Wellisch et al, 1983). Further research is needed to delineate types and stages of cancer as well as family or patient variables that might heighten family management problems or indicate need for additional intervention by the health care team.

Preparation for Death of the Patient

As death appears certain, anticipatory grief may be observed in those close to the patient. In this syndrome, one may go through all of the phases of grief. The emotional stress involved in cancer is intense, and although it often may be shared with another family member or close friend, some feelings may seem too personal to share. The family may be relieved by being made aware that this is a natural response. Some patients may develop primary (organic) or secondary (reactions to the disease process) mental status changes. The nurse can intervene by educating the family in preparation for their experiencing a possible change in the patient's behavior and by referral to preventive interventions for reducing stress, emotional disturbance, and psychologic dysfunction.

The family requires time for framing memories—remembering an individual person with meaningful relationships. Pictures, stories, and scrapbooks may promote the continuity of one's life identity. To direct such an activity is to intervene against the threat of anonymity of the dying family member (Giaquinta, 1977). When all possible has been done, the family may keep conversation with the patient on a social level, in what Glaser and Strauss (1966) describe as "pretense awareness," that is, avoiding the fact that the patient is dying.

Therapeutic intervention can be a crucial factor in facilitating the process of letting go. Significant others must be able to give the patient implicit permission to die. In some unfortunate cases, the family's anticipatory grief will lead to premature disengagement. In "premortem burial" (Hinton, 1963), the family whispers about the patient across the bed, behaving much as one would at a funeral home while viewing the casket. Significant others may need reassurance that wanting it to be over is a normal reaction to the stress of anticipating death. Family members must be reminded to take time for themselves, but their desire to be or not to be with the patient should be supported. Ongoing information about the patient's condition and what to expect may be the most helpful intervention, although there is no adequate way to make the final hours less excruciating.

The Patient's Death

Despite the intellectual recognition that death is inevitable, few people are able to accept the death of one who is loved. Separation begins when the patient's consciousness wanes and awareness of the environment diminishes. Loss and loneliness are experienced, and intervention is aimed toward promoting family intimacy and shared griefwork.

The work of Kubler-Ross (1969) has been popularized for the lay press and has influenced the medical, nursing, and social work scholarship dealing with the dying patient. Following Kubler-Ross's tradition, the literature of these fields often has presented working with the dying as a positive experience of personal growth and enrichment.

Sociologists and psychologists have been less optimistic. Weisman and Kastenbaum (1968) failed to note a pattern of patients following the same sequence toward the acceptance of death, finding instead that people die in different ways, reflecting the spectrum of ways in which people live. Kalish and Reynolds (1976) also emphasize the unique quality of death, which should be viewed in the context of a particular setting, considering the variables of ethnicity, age, gender, education, social status, and religion. Cultural expectations of the professional caregiver (nurse) and the familial caregiver (usually a mother, wife, daughter, or sister) as naturally equipped to serve as death's handmaiden must be illuminated by theory and research.

Bereavement

Bereavement coincides with the imminent dying and death of the patient. Within this stage are the phases of separation and mourning.

The patient's death does not bring an end to a multitude of problems facing the family. The nurse's concern now is assisting remaining family members with griefwork. This process involves a painful reliving and reviewing the joys, sorrows, and misunderstandings of their relationship with the patient. Mourning and grief are personal and unique experiences for each member of the family. Intervention is directed toward alleviating the feelings of guilt, fostering relief, and dealing with uncompleted feelings of previous loss. One goal is the internalization of the deceased into the continued family life (Giaquinta, 1977).

Family Reorganization

Role obligations are redistributed among family members during reorganization and reestablishment. Intervention that fosters a sense of cooperation and compromise may decrease competition. Expansion of the social network is facilitated by successful resolution of grief. The goal of intervention is to overcome alienation by fostering the family's relatedness. Ideally, the family will be open to changing identity and accepting the growth and self-actualization experienced. Readjustment following the loss of the patient may prove a time of extreme stress.

Research and Clinical Issues

Research is needed that would aid in assessment of the psychologic and sociologic impact of cancer on the family.

In employing assessment tools, Weisman et al (1980) express concern that people with cancer may be distinctly different from other medical and psychiatric patients and caution researchers and clinicians not to apply instruments that have not been tailored to the plight of those who are newly diagnosed.

Preventive interventions for those identified at high risk for future psychopathologic or psychosocial problems have been proposed. Using an eight-variable risk index, Parkes and Weiss (1983) have accurately predicted favorable versus poor outcome in 65% of the 131 bereaved spouses studied. Weisman et al (1980) were able to predict subsequent coping problems and vulnerability in over 85% of the patients screened with a psychosocial instrument.

Other methodologic problems seen in cancer research include using one individual as family spokesperson, relying on the subjects' long-term recall, and using only one data-collection-period for multiphase questions (Northouse, 1984).

The interaction between the family system and the health care delivery system lends itself to study by the fieldwork approach, in which data are collected in the participants' natural environment over time with flexible methods and working hypotheses that are tested, refined, restated, and retested in the course of data collection (Geer, 1964; Glaser, Strauss, 1967; Schatzman, Strauss, 1973).

Attention is needed in discovering not only which families are at risk, for what dysfunctional patterns or outcomes, and at what critical points but also to determine the effectiveness of various intervention strategies. An important issue is the scope and intensity of training needed for those who provide social–psychologic care for the families experiencing cancer. Klagsbrun (1983) states the necessity that training and skills in family therapy techniques be included in the qualifications for one who wishes to be an oncotherapist, for this work involves more than a command of the medical aspects of cancer.

Family Support

Weekly supportive psychotherapy sessions have been found to significantly reduce the severity of physical and emotional symptoms in patients undergoing radiotherapy. Those cancer patients who received psychotherapy, as compared with controls who did not, had less nausea, loss of appetite, fatigue, and other physical side effects of radiation therapy. They also felt less depressed, pessimistic, and hopeless. These results indicate that such symptoms are of emotional origin and that the emotional state of the patient influences his or her perceptions of such symptoms or a combination of the two (Kornfeld, Fleiss, 1985).

Of considerable research interest is whether family therapy sessions would yield significant results for those close to the patient with cancer. It is important that someone is available to encourage dialogue between patient, staff, physicians, and family. Following a psychosocial assessment with the patient, and with the patient's permission, a family meeting can be arranged. The goals of this session include acknowledging the family's distress, providing information about the disease process, encouraging open communication, assessing family resources, and providing hospital and community help. Additional sessions are to be arranged as needed throughout the illness. Brief family therapy should be provided if appropriate.

When family intervention is employed, issues are often presented that do not directly relate to cancer. Goldberg and Wool (1985) report that virtually all significant others who agreed to counseling addressing issues related to the patient's cancer used the counseling to deal with issues not directly related to the patient or the illness, such as interpersonal stress, development and difficulties of relationships, and role transitions.

Any effort that attempts to standardize intervention techniques across all people by diagnosis cannot be applied because the individuals involved do not share a single psychosocial diagnosis (Goldberg, Wool, 1985, p. 149). The families of cancer patients represent a wide variety of personality types, developmental stages, interpersonal styles, and life histories, as do the patients themselves.

Who is best trained to provide such specialized care is another question that can benefit from further study. The person who coordinates and/or provides such activities could be from any of a number of disciplines. It is likely that a clinical nurse specialist in oncology would be the appropriate provider in many settings.

Summary

Cancer strikes all ages. Although its course is variable, even during remission the illness does not disappear. In addition to the stigma associated with some cancers, many powerful emotions can result from the patient's loss of control and eventual death. The nurse, who frequently offers care to the patient over the course of the illness, is in a prime position to be facilitative to the family.

Issues for Further Investigation

1. What factors enable families with cancer to function most successfully? How do developmental stages, styles of interaction, and characteristics of the illness affect family functioning?

2. What nursing interventions are most effective in promoting positive family functioning at crucial periods during the course of the disease?

3. Which nursing interventions found effective with families with cancer can be applied to families with other health problems?

4. What are the long-term effects of highly technical treatments on cancer survivors and their families?

5. What are the long-term positive and negative effects of tissue donation on the donor and the family?

References

American Cancer Society. 1983 cancer facts and figures. New York: American Cancer Society, 1983.

Anderson BL (1985): Sexual functioning morbidity among cancer survivors: Current status and future research directions. *Cancer, 55:* 1835.

Bloom JR (1982): Social support systems and cancer: a conceptual view. In: *Psychosocial Aspects of Cancer,* Cohen J, Cullen JW, Martin LR (eds.). New York: Raven.

Bowen M (1976): Theory in the practice of psychotherapy. In: *Family Therapy: Theory and Practice,* Guerin PJ (ed.). New York: Gardner.

Burns N (1982): *Nursing and Cancer.* Philadelphia: W.B. Saunders.

Geer B (1964): First days in the field. In: *Sociologists at Work,* Hammond P (ed.). New York: Basic Books.

Giaquinta B (1977): Helping families face the crisis of cancer. *Am J Nurs, 77:* 1585–1588.

Glaser B, Strauss A (1966): *Awareness of Dying.* Chicago: Aldine.

Glaser B, Strauss A (1967): *Discovery of Grounded Theory: Strategies for Qualitative Research.* Chicago: Aldine.

Goffman E (1963): *Stigma.* Englewood Cliffs, NJ: Prentice-Hall.

Goldberg RJ, Wool MS (1985): Psychotherapy for the spouses of lung cancer patients: Assessment of an intervention. *Psychother Psychosom, 43:* 141–150.

Greenberg DB (1984): The measurement of sexual dysfunction in cancer patients. *Cancer,* May 15, *53* (10 Suppl): 2281–2285.

Haney CA (1984): Psychosocial factors in the management of patients with cancer. In *Psychosocial Stress and Cancer,* Cooper CL (ed.). New York: Wiley.

Hill R, Hansen DA (1964): Families under stress. In: *Handbook of Marriage and the Family,* Christensen HT (ed.). Chicago: Rand-McNally.

Hinton JM (1963): The physical and mental distress of the dying. *J Med, 32:* 1–21.

Holland JCB (1976): Coping with cancer: A challenge to the behavioral sciences. In *Cancer: The Behavioral Dimensions,* Cullen JW, Fox BH, Isom RN (eds.). New York: Raven.

Kalish RA, Reynolds DK (1976): *Death and Ethnicity: A Psychocultural Study.* Los Angeles: Ethel Percy Andrus Gerontology Center.

Kaplan DM et al (1973): Family mediation of stress. *Soc Work, 1:* 60–69.

Klagsbrun D (1983): The making of a cancer psychotherapist. *J Psychosoc Oncology, 1:* 55–60.

Kornfeld DS, Fleiss JL (1985): Psychotherapy during radiotherapy: Effects on emotional and physical distress. *Am J Psychiatry, 142:* 22–27.

Kubler-Ross E (1969): *On Death and Dying.* New York: Macmillan.

Mailick M (1979): The impact of severe illness on the individual and family: An overview. *Soc Work Health Care, 5*(2): 117–128.

Mechanic D (1962): The concept of illness behavior. *J Chronic Dis, 15:* 189.

Nordlicht S (1982): The family of the cancer patient. *N Y State J Med, 82*(13): 1845–1846.

Northouse L (1984): The impact of cancer on the family: An overview. *Int J Psychiatry Med, 14:* 215–241.

Olsen EH (1970): The impact of serious illness in the family system. *Postgrad Med, 47:* 169–174.

Parkes, CM, Weiss RS (1983): *Recovery from Bereavement.* New York: Basic Books.

Revenson TA, Wollman CA, Felton BJ (1983): Social supports as stress buffers for adult cancer patients. *Psychosom Med, 45:* 321–331.

Rose MA (1976): Problems families face in home care. *Am J Nurs, 16*(3): 416–418.

Rosenbaum EH, Rosenbaum JR (1980): Principles of home care for the patient with advanced cancer. *JAMA, 244*(3): 1484–1487.

Schatzman L, Strauss AL (1973): *Field Research: Strategies for a Natural Sociology.* Englewood Cliffs, NJ: Prentice-Hall.

Sourkes BM (1982): *The Deepening Shade: Psychological Aspects of Life-Threatening Disease.* Pittsburgh: University of Pittsburgh Press.

Spiegal D, Bloom JR, Gottheil E (1983): Family environment as a predictor of adjustment to metastatic breast carcinoma. *J Psychosoc Oncology, 1:* 33–44.

Strauss, AL, Glaser BG (1975): *Chronic Illness and the Quality of Life.* St. Louis: Mosby.

Tiblier K (1978): Keepin' on in New Orleans: A study of psychological stress and coping. Unpublished doctoral dissertation, Tulane University.

Vess JD, Moreland JR, Schwebel AI (1985): An empirical assessment of the effects of cancer on family role functioning. *J Psychosoc Oncology, 3*(1): 1–16.

Weisman AD, Kastenbaum R (1968): The psychological autopsy: a study of the terminal phase of life. New York: Community Mental Health Journal.

Weisman AD, Worden JW (1975): Psychosocial analysis of cancer deaths. *Omega, 6:* 61–75.

Weisman AD, Worden JW, Sobel HJ (1980): Psychological screening and intervention with cancer patients: Research report. Boston: Harvard Medical School.

Wellisch DK et al (1983): Evaluation of psychosocial problems of the home-bound cancer patient: The relationship of disease and the sociodemographic variables of patients to family problems. *J Psychosoc Oncology, 1*(3): 1–15.

Winder AE, Elam JR (1978): Therapist for the cancer patient's family: A new role for the nurse. *J Psychiatr Nurs, 16:* 22–27.

The author wishes to acknowledge the loving support of the late Barbara Rosenblum, PhD.

22

THE FAMILY AND CARDIAC ILLNESS

Catherine L. Gilliss, RNC, DNSc

As the leading cause of premature death in adults, heart disease is an important threat to the health of middle-aged families. This chapter reviews what is already known about the role of the family in three areas: (1) prevention of cardiovascular disease; (2) the impact of a cardiac event on the family in the acute phase of illness; and (3) family behavior and concerns during the rehabilitative stages of illness. The chapter concludes with a discussion of nursing care designed to improve the health of the individual and the family group.

Introduction

The social unit of the family is significant to the prevention and treatment of cardiovascular disease. Though it is tempting to view the critically ill cardiac patient in isolation from the family, the family unit must be understood to effectively intervene in changing lifestyle behaviors such as diet, stress management, and exercise patterns. These behaviors are initially learned in the family, and in adult life they are coordinated within the family. Nurses can promote the heart health of individuals by working with family members. When illness is evident, the nurse works to reduce the risk of family disruption. Employing the strengths of the family and its members, the nurse assists the family to make changes that are necessary to manage illness or recovery of individual members.

In a review of the cardiovascular nursing research presented between 1972 and 1983 at the scientific sessions of the American Heart Association and abstracted in *Circulation,* Kinney (1985) noted that individuals, families, and communities were represented as the objects of nursing care and study; however, of 132 referenced abstracts, only 6 referred to the family or other family members (Balda, Cohen, 1980; Becker, Levine, 1983; Dracup, 1982; Gilliss, 1983a; Howe, 1972; Larter, Sechrist, 1975) and of those 6, 3 concerned themselves with family members rather than the family group (Balda, Cohen, 1980; Becker, Levine, 1983; Larter, Sechrist, 1975). In nursing research, there have been surprisingly few investigations into the relationships between cardiac illness, the family, and the family members.

Preventing Cardiac Disease

Reducing Risk by Changing Lifestyle Behaviors

Nurses are generally well aware of the identified risk factors for coronary artery disease (CAD) and often counsel patients about changing lifestyle behaviors, including (1) altering diets to reduce sugars, fats, and sodium; (2) seeking regular exercise; (3) reducing stress or becoming more competent in stress management; and (4) ceasing to smoke. Each of these lifestyle behaviors that pose cardiac risk could be initially reduced or extinguished in the home through the education of young children about diet, exercise, and behavior. Yet the family group has been largely overlooked as a unit of intervention to promote heart-healthy behavior.

In a comprehensive review of family life and cardiovascular risk, Venters (1986) called for the use of a family systems approach for understanding cardiovascular risk behavior. She pointed out that cardiovascular risk behaviors are learned in early childhood and that risk factors are remarkably similar among family members. Further, she proposed that prevention and risk reduction interventions must be aimed at children and their families, and in the case of adults, interventions must be considerate of the particular marital lifestyle.

The Family Health Project (Nader, 1986) aims to test the effectiveness of a family-based intervention program to initiate and maintain heart-healthy diet and exercise behaviors in two ethnic groups (Anglos and Mexican–Americans). This study has enrolled 206 families to follow prospectively for two years. Current reports suggest that the experimental and control groups are comparable and that Anglo children consume less dietary fat and fewer saturated fats. Pilot data (Baranowski et al, 1982; Nader et al, 1983) published on 24 families suggest that diet and exercise behaviors were significantly changed for up to two months following an intervention that included family education and support.

Reducing Risk by Changing Type A Behavior

The Type A behavior pattern—characterized by achievement strivings, aggression, and time urgency—has been identified as an important independent risk factor for CAD. Recently Smith and Anderson (1986) proposed that Type A behavior actually persists through a behavioral pattern in which the subject actively pursues demanding and challenging experiences that keep the subject in a desired and heightened state of arousal. The physiologic effects of this arousal put the subject at risk for CAD. This interactional approach acknowledges both the subjects' role in seeking stimulating experiences and the continuous nature of feedback to maintain the cycle of challenges within the immediate environment. Social learning in early childhood may play a role in the development of these behaviors.

Children have been the subject of investigations into the development of Type A behavior pattern (Matthews, 1977). There is evidence to support that childrearing practices may influence the future development of Type A behavior in children. In such cases, the parental behavior has been characterized by frequent use of approval and disapproval, contingent on the improvement of performance or the standards of other evaluators (Matthews, Glass, 1977; Krantz, Glass, Synder, 1974; Matthews, 1977). Mothers of Type A children less often appraised positively the performances of their children than did the mothers of Type B children (Matthews, Glass, Richins, 1977). Ironically, in these homes children were punished for aggressive acts with aggressive punishment. Although the precise mechanism of learning Type A behavior is unknown, the family as the basic unit of socialization must be examined as a possible contributor.

Gillum et al (1985), in a report on the Minneapolis Children's Blood Pressure Study, found a positive relationship between social status and risk for hypertension but no relationship between family environment and hypertension risk in the sample of 1505 7- to 10-year-old children. In this study, family environment was measured by the Family Environment Scale (Moos, 1974), administered to mothers, fathers, or other adults. It is unlikely that large surveys

of this sort will reveal the complex relationships that exist between family behavior and individual health. Methods required to detect the desired level of subtlety will, no doubt, require observations and dialogue with subjects.

In adult populations, research reports of risk behavior modification are often context free and are not considerate of the family or marital lifestyle. A notable exception exists. Hoebel (1976) reported using five hourly treatment sessions with wives to significantly change high-risk behavior in seven of nine "difficult" cardiac patients. This was accomplished by educating these wives on how their own behavior was reinforcing their husbands' high-risk behavior.

Changing Type A behavior has been the recent focus of Friedman et al (1984). A dramatic reduction in the rate of cardiac recurrence was demonstrated in the treatment group of 592 subjects who received both cardiologic counseling and Type A behavioral counseling when compared to the control group (n=270), which received only cardiologic counseling (p.>005). This suggests that Type A behavior, known to be a significant independent predictor of CAD, can be learned and unlearned. A related question is the role of the family of origin's contribution to the development of the behavior pattern. But then, how is the pattern further developed and reinforced by the adult family, or family of procreation? These represent important, unanswered questions in this area.

McCance et al (1985) conducted a clinical trial of specific preventive nursing education to 59 first-degree relatives of young victims of sudden cardiac death (ages 30–55). Three to five months after the death, she administered an assessment of health history and health behaviors and a health education class on coronary heart disease (CHD) risk and risk reduction to all experimental subjects. Seven months after the intervention, she demonstrated reductions in alcohol intake among the experimental group (sibling subset), reduction in red meat consumption, and an increased frequency in obtaining blood pressure and cholesterol screening.

Reducing Risk Through Environmental Manipulation

Reducing risk can also be accomplished through environmental manipulation. Victims of sudden cardiac illness often survive when cardiopulmonary resuscitation is begun by bystanders. Dracup et al (1986) used a controlled trial to evaluate the effect of teaching cardiopulmonary resuscitation (CPR) to the families of high-risk cardiac patients. Although no differences were seen in family members' depression or anxiety across groups, patients (who had been excluded from the trial) in the two treatment groups appeared more anxious than controls at three and six months after the family intervention. Although patient anxiety may have been related to changes in behavior of family members, exclusion from the program may also have contributed to anxiety and depression. Dracup's findings were unexpected and raise concerns about the impact of family education on the patient.

Given that particular patterns of behavior have been shaped in the family of origin, who, then, do the victims of coronary artery disease marry? In a report on mate selection among those with CAD, ten Kate et al (1984) compared spouses (n=126) of male myocardial infarction (MI) survivors to an age-matched control for frequency of MI and CAD in first-degree relatives. Significantly more spouses' relatives had MIs or CAD, as compared with controls. The authors suggest that familial aggregation of CAD is not limited to the patient's relatives but also affects the wife's family. This may be explained by selection of marriage partners who choose to lead similar lifestyles and experience, as a result, similar risks.

Apart from the genetic or behavioral contributions to risk made by the family is the question of the buffering effect of spousal or familial love and support on the development of cardiac disease. In the Israeli Heart Study (Medalie, Goldbourt, 1976; Medalie et al, 1973), family problems were strong predictors of the develop-

ment of angina in 10,000 healthy male civil servants over 40 years old. Spousal support buffered the effects of anxiety reported. When anxiety was high, subjects who did not have the love and support of their spouses were 1.8 times as likely to develop angina than those who reported spousal love and support (Berkman, 1984). With respect to the buffering aspects of family support, this work suggests that family support may offer some protection against future cardiac illness.

The Family and Acute Cardiac Illness

Most of what is known regarding the family's response to the immediate impact of cardiac illness results from the study of adult families after MI or cardiac surgery. Reports of these two situations are remarkably similar. Because children's cardiac illness is often the result of a congenital abnormality, studies of family responses are often generalized as examples of coping with a "defective" infant rather than coping with an illness experience. Reviews of these reports have been omitted from this chapter. With the increasing number of cardiac transplantations being undertaken, a new area of investigation and clinical practice has developed in nursing the family in preparation for and following cardiac transplantation (Murdaugh, 1986).

As the rapid onset of infarction leading to surgery varies from the planned entry to cardiac surgery, these two situations might be contrasted. Gilliss et al (1985) compared the events leading to treatment for bypass patients and families to a contrast group of medically controlled coronary heart disease patients and families. They reported that considerably more disruption of family patterns was seen in the bypass group and concluded that the bypass cohort, in contrast to their medically controlled counterparts, viewed the surgery as a crisis. Given the magnitude of difference between a planned surgery and surgery after a myocardial infarction, the MI families might be expected to report an even greater degree of disruption to family life. This, however, has not been demonstrated.

Seeking Care

Even before an illness is diagnosed, family members become involved in identifying and naming the problem and seeking help. Alonzo (1986) interviewed 1102 subjects hospitalized with a suspected MI to review their process of deciding to seek care. He reported that 60% of his large sample experienced a personal evaluation stage in which they alone wrestled with how they were feeling and whether to seek help. This phase was followed by a lay evaluation phase in which those with the victim observed or were informed of the symptoms and offered advice regarding appropriate action. The lay evaluation phase was experienced by 92% of the sample. Mean length for this phase was 30 minutes. Although the spouse was most often the participant in the lay evaluation phase (51%), the spouses took 16 minutes longer to act than did nonrelated lay evaluators (35 minutes for spouses versus 19 minutes for unrelated others). These observations dramatize the powerful effect that family relations, specifically, patterns regarding communication and symptom recognition, can have on illness experiences before they reach the health care system.

Patient–Spouse Differences

Speedling (1982) has written a descriptive account of the events surrounding the diagnosis, treatment, and rehabilitation from a heart attack in eight stable, lower-middle-class families. In his work he described the experience of the family group in the diagnosis of the event, care-seeking, and rehabilitative stages. He noted that patients and family members have different experiences, or differential exposures, during the illness experience. Therefore, patients and spouses often have differing perspectives.

Patients' views of their conditions were more positive, and they were aware of the daily gains they made while in ICU. Spouses were fearful of the future and tended not to see the gradual improvements made in ICU. There were additional discrepancies between patient and family over what activities were viewed as healing or appropriate. Wives supported nonaction; patients tried to move about. During hospitalization, according to Speedling, these discrepancies were not discussed.

Brown, Glazer, and Higgins (1984) observed that cardiac surgeries triggered fear and apprehension in patients and families. In response, Brown et al established group sessions for patients and family members to review some of the usual emotional, behavioral, and physical responses to surgery. They found that relatives and patients did not have the same concerns as they approached discharge from the hospital. Patients were focused on pain management and specific physical problems, but family members had begun to think of the long-range issues of recovery. Ultimately two groups were set up: one for patients and another for families. Within the family sessions it became clear that relatives generally viewed themselves as having to monitor the patient's activities, as they were responsible for the successful recovery. "Monitoring," however, has been reported to be associated with family conflict during recovery (Gilliss, 1983b; Jenkins et al, 1983).

Dhooper (1983) has described the trajectory of spouse experience after MI. During the hospitalization, anxiety was very high. Reports of reduced social activities were high; but there were few if any reports of reactive illness. Within the first month after hospitalization, anxiety reports fell, but there was a reported increase in illness episodes experienced by the nonpatient spouse. Within three months, most MI families reported a return to normal. Surgical families have been studied by Gilliss et al (1987) for the first six months of recovery. Reports of family satisfaction dropped significantly for patients and spouses between hospitalization and the three-month data collection interval. Although patient scores returned to baseline by six months, spouse scores remained significantly lower than baseline scores. This suggests that patients and spouses may respond differently because they do not experience the same event from their independent perspectives.

A competing hypothesis would suggest that patients and spouses see things differently because their personalities are different. Though not reporting on the period of acute illness, Swan, Carmelli, and Rosenman (1986) reported the findings of an evaluation of 45 males with CHD and their wives and 50 noncase males and their wives using the California Psychological Inventory (CPI). Though all subjects fell into the well-functioning ranges of the CPI, interesting patterns emerged. Case wives were significantly more dominant and less flexible than noncase wives; case husbands were significantly more dominant than noncase husbands. Case couples demonstrated nonconcordant profiles, in which only the depression measures were correlated. In contrast, noncase couples were more similar, or concordant. The investigators propose three possible interpretations of these findings: (1) that the effects of the disease have affected spouse–pair concordance; (2) that the effect of the spouse–pair dissimilarity has affected the disease; or (3) that there is a developmental and interacting relationship between the dissimilarity in the pair, the disease, and the continuing dissimilarity.

Needs for Specific Information

During the period of acute illness, usually during hospitalization, families have specific and focused needs. From care providers they need information about care and treatment choices, about the patient's condition, about how to behave, about resources, and about what is going to happen in the near future. Although family members may be anxious about the future and may need information or validation about these feelings, a greater need drives most family members in search of concrete information about the situation and assurances of technical competence in those delivering patient care. These needs tend to reinforce the focus on the individual patient, again limiting provider involvement with the family. Unwittingly, the nurse can contribute to the familial disorganization that has been described during early recovery by focusing on the patient and ignoring the family. This disorganization appears to have its roots in the period of hospitalization, when families are under stress and at risk.

With respect to the need for information, Rodgers (1983) reported the results of a small descriptive sampling of 20 relatives of 11 patients. The family members she questioned overwhelmingly wanted to be assured that they would be notified by the nurses if there was a change in the patient's condition. Lovvorn (1982) wrote of the need to help patients and families cope with the routine postoperative bypass problems by giving more information to patients and families in anticipation of these events. She provided suggestions for including detailed information on possible problems, side effects, and expectations. However, she omitted from her discussion any information on resumption of sexual activity or family relations.

Two reports of cardiac patient and family education program evaluations are in the nursing literature. Mills et al (1985) evaluated a program for hospitalized ischemic heart disease patients. The content of the program, as described, included disease pathology, diet, medications, symptoms and appropriate responses, exercise, stress and the heart, and risk factors. The investigators accounted for 28% variance in one-month compliance behavior; however, from information in the published report, it is not clear why the program was described as patient/family education. Family members were not included or appraised in the evaluation; no content about family relationships appears to have been included in the classes. Scalzi, Burke, and Greenland (1980) reported the results of a similar program in which post-infarction patients and family members (optional) were invited to classes covering disease pathology, emergency treatment, physical activity, diet, smoking, psychologic factors, resumption of sexual activity, and problems of returning to work or home. Over a two-year period, only 32 of 40 subjects remained in this controlled trial. Unfortunately, this probably contributed to the no-difference result. The authors offered their observation that a lack of instruction is available to patients and families after discharge, despite the fact that patients and their family members have more questions than anticipated during the first six weeks after discharge from the hospital.

Pimm and Feist (1984) evaluated the long-term effect of crisis intervention on postsurgical depression through a controlled trial of 104 men. Treatment was initiated in the hospital and continued for two months afterward. Minimal data were collected from a family member, mostly to validate patient reports of condition. The investigators conclude by urging that more family involvement would be helpful to patients.

Mumford (1982) has published an excellent review and meta-analysis of studies evaluating the impact of psychologic interventions on recovery from surgery and heart attacks. She concluded that, overall, psychologic intervention appeared to reduce hospital stays by approximately two days. The most effective interventions were those that included psychotherapeutic and educational approaches. Inclusion of family members in this preparation might reduce hospital stays even further.

Spousal Distress

The subjective distress reported by the spouses of hospitalized MI patients has been described by Bedsworth and Molen (1982). By and large, the threats described to these investigators were related to losses of husbands, of own life goals, or of mate's health. These stresses are similar to those reported for the spouses of surgical patients described by Gilliss (1984). She reported that spouses' levels of stress were higher than those reported by patients during this acute phase. This finding was sustained even when spouses' scores were adjusted for sex. Contrary to reports of female inflation of stress score reports, in this correlational examination of 71 subjects, it was the *role* of spouse and not the *gender* of spouse that was most closely related to reports of stress.

Preparation for Discharge

Several reports conclude that spouses are either not well prepared for or not comfortable about taking patients home from the hospital. Rudy (1980) interviewed 50 patient–spouse pairs during hospitalization and one to two months after an acute MI. She sought to determine the lay explanation of the illness episode. She found that reports of tension at work, at home, or in general were most often given as causes for the attack. However, over 50% of the subjects changed their minds between hospitalization and recovery, and over 50% of the patients and spouses disagreed with each others' reports of the cause. She concluded that spouses should be included in discharge planning to be better prepared to handle the mood swings, changes, and questions that arise in recovery. Hentinen (1983) surveyed 59 wives of MI patients, who indicated that they were not well prepared for home care of the patient and that they needed instruction prior to discharge from the hospital.

The Family in Recovery

Epidemiologic studies have demonstrated that those married at the time of MI have a greatly decreased risk of death during hospitalization and for 10 years thereafter (Chandra, 1983). Ruberman et al (1984) reported that social isolation and high stress, when taken together, were better predictors of 2- to 4-year survival from infarctions than were any of the physiologic measures. It is not clear whether married individuals are inherently different or whether there is something about the experience of marriage and family life that contributes to the amorbidity. The answer is far from obvious. Most reports of the rehabilitative period describe this phase as extremely difficult for families.

Continued Spousal Distress

A number of reports address the long-term effect of the cardiac event on wives. Stern and Pascale (1979) describe high levels of anxiety and depression in post-MI wives six months after the event. These women described themselves as being in a double bind: They were accused by their recovering husbands as being either nagging and overprotecting or cold and uncaring. The authors proposed providing discussion groups for spouses for purposes of education and support.

Croog and Fitzgerald (1978) have reported high levels of subjective stress for 263 spouses of first-time MI patients. Reports of stress remained stable and elevated throughout one year following the event. Although not clearly correlated with severity of patient illness, spousal stress reports do seem highest for those spouses whose husbands were rehospitalized during the 12-month study. Additionally, a negative correlation existed between reports of marital satisfaction and subjective distress. Similarly, Sikorski (1985) found that the worst spousal relations were reported by those families wherein the patient had experienced postoperative complications.

Lough (1986) has recently reviewed the major issues surrounding quality of life for transplantation patients and noted that family relations continue to be disrupted and labile for six months into recovery; however, by two years they appear to have adjusted.

Family Conflict

Speedling's data (1982) portrayed homegoing after infarction as a time of conflict for families.

He attributed much of this conflict to discrepant expectations related to patient activity. He described three styles employed by these families for the resolution of this conflict: (1) *coercion* (in which the spouse and children forced the patient to comply with their definitions of the situation and their expectations about activity and role performance; (2) *disengagement* (in which no one was particularly involved in directing the home care approach); and (3) *reorganization* (in which the female spouse provided major direction to the plan of care).

Similar observations were made by Gilliss (1983b, 1984) in her study of families after bypass surgery. Families were seen at hospitalization and again six months later in the home. Her reports summarize her observations and family descriptions of a nagging, overprotecting spouse who feels responsible for controlling the behavior of a patient who wants to become more active and defies physician orders in an attempt to determine the limits of his physical abilities. Segev and Schlesinger (1981) described numerous family changes during the period of recovery. These included shifts in role responsibilities; patient–spouse conflicts over dependence—independence; conflicts with young children; and disrupted sexual relations.

Jenkins (1983), in a report on the six-month findings from his study of 318 bypass patients, noted that 28% of the subjects interviewed believed themselves to have been overprotected during recovery. Stanton et al (1984) suggests in another report on this sample that the problem of overprotection was the major problem in family relations after surgery. She suggests that it would be useful to encourage family members not to overprotect the patient.

In contrast, some investigators report improved or stable relations within the family or marital pair (Lough, 1986; Meddin, Brelje, 1983; Sikorski, 1985; Stanton et al, 1984). The characteristics of the family or the illness that might predict which families are strengthened and which are weakened are not yet known. This is another fruitful area for investigation.

Spousal Support of the Patient

Hilbert (1985) sampled 60 couples three months after the male's infarction to learn more about the relationship between the spouses' support and the patients' compliance. She found no relationship. Although this may result from the investigator's use of a nonstandardized instrument, the investigator acknowledges that supportive behaviors are difficult to measure because they are often defined in the context of the marital relationship. For example, although one husband may find it desirable for his wife to pour his medications with the morning orange juice, another might find this to be controlling behavior. Understanding meanings that are associated with marital practices becomes an important key to identifying supportive behaviors. Tyzenhouse (1973) attempted to alter patient behavior by changing spousal behaviors in a study of 20 couples. Her research did not demonstrate any differences, though the work is worthy of replication with a more complete conceptualization of marital interactions.

Altering perceptions of spouses may be an avenue to changing the family dynamics in recovery. This might be accomplished by offering new experiences to spouses or by educating spouses. One of the most innovative approaches to the family problems of rehabilitation has been developed at Stanford's Cardiac Rehabilitation Program. Taylor et al (1985) put wives on the treadmill at a performance level similar to their husbands'. The treadmill wives, in contrast to those who only watched their husbands and those who did not watch, rated their confidence in their husband's condition to be significantly higher than wives in the other groups.

With respect to education in preparation for discharge, the lack of importance given to family-related content or inclusion of family members in classes was noted earlier. Sikorski (1985) interviewed 30 post-bypass female spouses two to three weeks after discharge. The majority had received convalescent preparation, usually by a physician or someone with experiential information. She found that most had insufficient knowledge about (1) their husband's medications and (2) the relationships among coronary artery disease, angina, and surgery. They were often well informed about recommended activities but had little information about the resumption of specific activities, including sexual activity. Sikorski suggests that spouses need guidelines for understanding ingingand participating in recovery, as well as a postdischarge opportunity for discussion and support.

Bramwell and Whall (1986) investigated the development of the support role performance and anxiety in a study of 82 wives of men hospitalized for first MIs. They demonstrated that role performance had a direct negative effect on spousal anxiety. In another report of the same data, Bramwell (1986) described the sources of information offered to wives in anticipation of discharge. Among the 56% who reported to understand the role requirement of supporting their husbands at home, most cited information from written documents or videotapes to be helpful information sources. They also expressed trust in and appreciation of the hospital staff. For those wives who reported unclear role requirements (44%), the lack of information was the dominant complaint. These wives believed they lacked information about diet, physical activity, and the experiences of hospitalization, including preparation for the cardiac care unit. Specifically, some subjects indicated their desire to be prepared for discharge.

Promoting Health of the Family

The literature that describes recovery from a cardiac event generally acknowledges a period of disruption of normal psychologic and social functioning. Long-lasting effects and disruption are confined to a minority of subjects (Doehrman, 1977). What is not well understood is how to limit devastating effects to the minority of families who would experience these and how to hasten recovery for those families who are only temporarily affected. Our developing knowledge base begins to suggest several directions for the development of nursing care programs and for further examination.

1. Clearly, families are at high risk for disruption following a cardiac event. In response to this observation, nursing care must be offered to inform families of their risk. Families need information about the usual nature of the family experiences. Families at especially high risk need to be better identified early in the care. These families may need special services to maintain their integrity during an episode of cardiac illness.

2. Spouses need preparation to perform the roles they are expected to perform after discharge. Role preparation should include information about the disease, the infarct or the surgery, diet, medications, and smoking and specific information about activity, including sexual activity. To reduce the chance for disagreement, this information can be shared with patient and spouse together. A discussion of how the couple believes needed changes can be accomplished may reveal important data about the family to the nurse.

3. Patients and spouses need care, or contact, following hospitalization. Complications and questions arise when families leave the hospital. Often there is no one the couple "wants to bother" with their questions. Contact at this time offers support to anxious and unsure spouses and discovers early problems that require medical attention. Unfortunately, all families cannot, or do not, participate in cardiac rehabilitation programs. Alternative services must be available, such as telephone monitoring of families in early recovery.

Descriptions of several model programs for the care of cardiac families have been published (Dracup et al, 1984; Gilliss, 1984). Evaluation reports from such projects are needed to document the usefulness of family care in minimizing family disruption and in hastening the discharge and recovery of the individual patient.

Summary

Both the family and the patient are affected by the experience of cardiac surgery. Although the particular responses of the family are related to the family's character, a generic pattern of disruption during recovery has been described. Approaches to nursing care for promotion of family health during recovery are in need of systemic testing for efficacy.

Issues for Further Investigation

1. How can nursing care promote the development of heart-healthy behaviors in families?

2. What strategies are effective for changing health-endangering behaviors once these have been enacted in a family?

3. Do families with particular behavioral or interaction styles change and maintain these changes more easily than others?

4. What are the long-term effects of offering family level care to families of cardiac surgery and myocardial infarct patients?

5. What influences the natural pattern of a family's recovery from a cardiac event (such as age, gender of the patient, characteristics of the illness)?

References

Alonzo A (1986): Impact of family and lay others in care seeking during life threatening episodes of CAD. *Soc Sci Med, 22*(12): 1297–1311.

Balda J, Cohen F (1980): Group sessions: Their effect on distress levels of wives of myocardial infarction patients. Circulation 62(4)III, 172.

Baranowski T et al (1982): Family self-help: Promoting changes in health behavior. *J Commun, 32*(3): 161–172.

Becker D, Levine D (1983): Risk behavior in the unaffected brothers and sisters of people with premature ischemic heart disease. Circulation 68 (4)III, 291.

Bedsworth J, Molen M (1982): Psychological Stress in Spouses of Patients with Myocardial Infarction. *Heart Lung, 11*(5): 450–456.

Berkman L (1984): Assessing the physical health effects of social networks and social support. *Annu Rev Public Health* 5: 413–432.

Bramwell (1986): Wives' experience in the support role after husband's first MI. *Heart Lung,* 15 (6): 578–584.

Bramwell L, Whall A (1986): Effect of role clarity and empathy on support role performance and anxiety. *Nurs Res,* 35 (5): 282–287.

Brown D, Glazer H, Higgins M (1984): Group intervention: A psychosocial and educational approach to open heart surgery patients and their families. *Soc Work Health Care,* 9(2): 47–59.

Chandra V, Szklo M, Goldberg R (1983): The impact of marital status on survival after acute myocardial infarction. *Am J Epidemiol, 117:* 320–325.

Croog S, Fitzgerald E (1978): Subjective stress and serious illness of a spouse: Wives of heart patients. *J Health Soc Behav,* 19: 166–178.

Dhooper S (1983): Family coping after heart attack. *Soc Work Health Care,* 9(1): 15–31.

Doehrman S (1977): Psycho-social aspects of recovery from coronary heart disease: A review. *Soc Sci Med,* 11: 199–218.

Dracup K (1982): Influence of a role supplementation program on the psychosocial adaptation of cardiac patients and spouses. Circulation 66(4) II, 280.

Dracup K et al (1986): Cardiopulmonary Resuscitation (CPR) Training: Consequences for family members of high-risk cardiac patients. *Arch Int Med, 146* (9): 1757–1761.

Dracup K et al (1984): Family-focused cardiac rehabilitation. *Nurs Clin North Am,* 19(1): 113–124.

Friedman M et al (1984): Alteration of type A behavior and reduction in cardiac recurrences in post-myocardial infarction patients. *Am Heart J,* 108(2): 237–248.

Gilliss CL (1983a): CABG and the family: A closer look at recovery. Circulation 68(4) III, 37.

Gilliss CL (1983b): Identification of factors contributing to family functioning after coronary artery bypass surgery. Doctoral Dissertation, University of California at San Francisco (Abstr# 83-26, 402, Dissertation Abstracts).

Gilliss CL (1984): Reducing family stress during and after coronary bypass surgery. *Nurs Clin North Am,* 19(1): 103–112.

Gilliss CL et al (1985): Events leading to the treatment of coronary artery disease: Implications for nursing care. *Heart Lung,* 14(4): 350–356.

Gilliss CL et al (1987): Improving family functioning after cardiac surgery. Presented at Sigma Theta Tau, Edinburgh, Scotland, July, 1987.

Gillum R et al (1985): Personality, behavior, family environment, family social status and hypertension risk factors in children. *J Chronic Dis, 38(2):* 187–194.

Hentinen M (1983): Need for instruction and support of the wives of patients with myocardial infarction. *J Adv Nurs,* 8: 519–524.

Hilbert G (1985): Spouse support and myocardial infarction patient compliance. *Nurs Res,* 34(4): 217–220.

Hoebel F (1976): Brief family-interactional therapy in the management of cardiac-related high-risk behavior. *J Fam Pract,* 3: 613–618.

Howe J (1972): Family relationships involving children with congenital heart disease. Circulation 46(4) II, 240.

Jenkins C et al (1983): Coronary artery bypass surgery: Physical, psychological, social and economic outcomes six months later. *JAMA,* 250 (6): 782–788.

Kinney M (1985): Trends in cardiovascular nursing research: 1972–1983. *Cardiovas Nurs,* 21 (5): 25–30.

Krantz D, Glass D, Snyder M (1974): Helplessness, stress level, and the coronary-prone behavior pattern. *J Exp Soc Psychol*, 10: 284–300.

Larter M, Sechrist K (1975): The relationship between life style alteration, manifest anxiety, and demographic variables in wives of men experiencing myocardial infarction. Circulation 52(4)II, 261.

Lough M (1986): Quality of life issues following heart transplantation. *Progress Cardiovas Nurs*, 1 (1): 17–23.

Lovvorn J (1982): Coronary artery bypass surgery: Helping patients cope with postop problems. *Am J Nurs*, 82(7): 1073–7125.

Matthews K (1977): Children's reactions to loss of control and the type A coronary-prone behavior pattern. Unpublished study, Kansas State University, Manhatten, Kansas.

Matthews K, Glass D (1977): Learned helplessness and pattern A behavior in children. In: *Behavior Patterns, Stress, and Coronary Disease*, Glass D (ed.). Hillsdale, NJ: Lawrence Erlbaum.

Matthews K, Glass D, Richins M (1977): Behavioral interactions of mothers and children with the coronary-prone behavior pattern. In: *Behavior Patterns, Stress, and Coronary Disease*, Glass D (ed.) Hillsdale, NJ: Lawrence Erlbaum.

McCance K et al (1985): Preventing coronary heart disease in high-risk families. *Res Nurs Health*, 8: 413–420.

Medalie J, Goldbourt V (1976): Angina predictors among 10,000 men: II psychosocial and other risk factors as evidenced by a multivariate analysis of a five year incidence study. *Am J Med, 60:* 910–921.

Medalie J et al (1973): Angina pectoris among 10,000 men: five year incidence and univariate analysis. *Am J Med, 55:* 583–594.

Meddin J, Brelje M (1983): Unexpected positive effects of myocardial infarction on couples. *Health Soc Work, 8*(2): 143–146.

Mills G et al (1985): An evaluation of an inpatient cardiac patient family education program. *Heart Lung*, 14(4): 400–406.

Moos R (1974): *Family Environment Scale Manual.* Palo Alto, CA: Consulting Psychologist Press.

Mumford E, Schlesinger H, Glass G (1982): The effects of psychological intervention on recovery from surgery and heart attacks: An analysis of the literature. *Am J Public Health, 72*(2): 141–151.

Murdaugh C (1986): Support for families of patients with cardiovascular disease: The transplant family. A paper read before the Council of Cardiovascular Nurses, American Heart Association Scientific Sessions, Dallas, Texas, (November 1986).

Nader P et al (1983): The family health project: Cardiovascular risk reduction education for children and parents. *J Dev Behav Pediatr, 4:* 3–10.

Nader P et al (1986): San Diego family health project: Reaching families through the schools. *J School Health, 56*(6): 227–231.

Pimm J, Feist J (1984): *Psychological Risks of Coronary Bypass Surgery.* New York: Plenum.

Rodgers C (1983): Needs of relatives of cardiac surgery patients during the critical care phase. *Focus Crit Care, 10*(5): 50–55.

Ruberman W et al (1984): Psychosocial influences on mortality after myocardial infarction. *N Engl J Med, 331:* 552–557.

Rudy E (1980): Patients' and spouses' causal explanations of a myocardial infarction. *Nurs Res, 29*(6): 352–356.

Scalzi C, Burke L, Greenland S (1980): Evaluation of an inpatient educational program for coronary patients and families. *Heart Lung, 9*(5): 846–853.

Segev U, Schlesinger Z (1981): Rehabilitation of patients after acute myocardial infarction—an interdisciplinary approach. *Heart Lung, 10*(5): 841–847.

Sikorski J (1985): Knowledge, concerns, and questions of wives of convalescent coronary artery bypass graft surgery patients. *J Cardiac Rehabil, 5:* 74–85.

Smith T, Anderson N (1986): Models of personality and disease: An interactional approach to Type A behavior and cardiovascular risk. *J Pers Soc Psychol, 50*(6): 1166–1173.

Speedling E (1982): *Heart Attack: The Family Response at Home and in the Hospital.* New York: Tavistock.

Stanton B et al (1984): Perceived adequacy of patient education and fears and adjustments after cardiac surgery. *Heart Lung, 13*(5): 525–531.

Stern M, Pascale L (1979): Psychosocial adaptation post-myocardial infarction: The spouses' dilemma. *J Psychosom Res, 23:* 83–87.

Swan G, Carmelli D, Rosenman R (1986): Spouse-pair similarity on the California Psychological Inventory with reference to husband's coronary artery disease. *Psychosom Med, 48*(3/4): 172–186.

Taylor B et al (1985): Exercise testing to enhance wives' confidence in their husbands' cardiac capability soon after clinically uncomplicated acute myocardial infarction. *Am Cardiol, 55:* 635–638.

ten Kate L et al (1984): Increased frequency of coronary heart disease in relatives of wives of myocardial infarct survivors: Assortative mating for lifestyle and risk factors? *Am J Cardiol, 53:* 399–403.

Tyzenhouse P (1973): Myocardial infarction: Its effect on the family. *Am J Nurs, 73*(6): 1012–1013.

Venters M (1986): Family life and cardiovascular risk: Implications for the prevention of chronic disease. *Soc Sci Med, 22*(10): 1067–1074.

23

THE FAMILY AND DIABETES MELLITUS

Jeanne C. Hallburg, RN, PhD

Marilyn J. Little, PhD

Diabetes mellitus is already prevalent in the United States and, because of the genetic factor, the incidence of diabetes will double every fifteen years. By the year 2040, there may be 40 million diabetics in the United States. This chapter presents an extensive review of the scientific literature that addresses the impact of diabetes mellitus on family life. The problems inherent in research incorporating the family are identified, and the need for continued psychosocial, educational, and service-related research is documented. The chapter closes with a three-part photo documentary that touches on such topics as preventative maintenance, self-management, and self-maintenance.

Marilyn Little is an Associate Specialist at the University of California at San Francisco, in the Department of Family and Community Medicine. She is a sociologist with particular interest in the socialization of family practice physicians.

Introduction

Diabetes mellitus is a condition both serious and costly for the individual, the family, and the nation. Approximately 2.43% of the population of the United States reports having diabetes (NCHS, 1981). Another 4.9% with no history of diabetes had "diabetic-like" fasting blood glucose levels when they received oral glucose tolerance tests (Harris, 1982). Because of the genetic factor, the incidence of diabetes will double every 15 years, so that by the year 2010 there could be some 40 million diabetics in the United States alone (Kilo, 1982). Young families frequently struggle with issues related to the genetic factor. Diabetes is the third leading cause of death in this country and often results in chronic and disastrous complications (National Diabetes Advisory Board, 1982). The associated suffering of individuals and loss for families are substantial.

The National Commission on Diabetes (1975) reported that diabetics are 25 times more prone to blindness than nondiabetics, 17 times more prone to kidney disease, and over 5 times more prone to gangrene of the lower extremities, often leading to amputation. The pain of such complications is rarely borne by the individual alone. The statistical reports associated with the complications of diabetes give us information about the aggregate of subjects with diabetes. The dread and actual impact of blindness, renal problems, and circulatory insufficiency on the individual and other members of the family—or on the family as a unit—can only be surmised.

The Commission also estimated the annual cost of diabetes to the American economy at 5 billion dollars. Since 1975, the cost of medical care and the losses due to disability and premature mortality have caused this figure to almost double to 9.5 billion dollars annually. Clearly, the costs for the nation are high. Expenses for the individual and family range from day-to-day supplies to long-term care. It is financially expensive to be a diabetic, and the expenditures of time and energy for the individual and family are also costly.

For chronically ill people, the burdens of symptom and regimen management are intertwined with all of life's other work (Strauss, 1985). This is most certainly true for the diabetic individual and related family members. Diabetes, in fact, is a classic example of a chronic disease as a family affair. The ramifications of the condition on family functioning are multiple. A rigorous regimen involving exercise, diet, testing of blood or urine, manipulation and routinization of schedules, treatment judgments and decisions, possible frequent insulin injections, and maintenance of a high level of awareness of physical and mental status impose difficult demands on day-to-day family functioning. These unusual demands are added to the normal burdens assumed by families in childbearing and parenting. To cope with the diabetic member, families must normalize lifestyles and adapt their living arrangements and shared responsibilities. The organizational requirements of a family, including efforts to assure some kind of stability within the patterns of family living, necessitate considerable attention to communication, negotiation and renegotiation, mutuality in respect and exchange, a special mixture of flexibility and stability and an awareness of self.

The challenge to nurses and other health care professionals is to comprehend the interrelationship of the physiologic, psychologic, sociocultural, and economic impact of diabetes on the individual and the family.

Review of the Literature

The preponderance of scientific literature about diabetes mellitus is in the biomedical arena. Most research is directed toward the search for basic and fundamental information about the etiology and pathogenic mechanisms of diabetes mellitus, with increasing emphasis on the outcomes of various treatment protocols. The literature on the psychosocial implications of diabetes tends to focus on specific concepts or constructs (for example, compliance, control, stress, or manipulation). The consequence of the disease on family life is beginning to receive serious attention, although great concern is repeatedly expressed about methodologic issues (Anderson, Auslander, 1980; Burish, Bradley, 1983). In most research on families, the diabetic member is invariably a child; that is, 95% of the literature concerns 5% of the population of people with diabetes. The review that follows reflects this emphasis on the child in family research.

Families with Diabetic Children

The extensive literature on families with diabetic children can be divided into three major areas. First, some literature describes the powerful role families play in formulating definitions of illness and in moderating consequences of that illness on children. Parents who are diabetic themselves can be negative or positive role models. Second, stage of development can affect the impact of diabetes on the child. Responses to the illness and its treatment change as the child becomes an adolescent and then a young adult. Third, the illness can serve as a central focus within the family. It may become a vehicle for expressing conflict as family members with different definitions of the illness fight over compliance and control. This conflict can create additional stress for the diabetic child and can affect the course of the illness.

Significance of Diabetes for Families

The family is critically involved in implementing the treatment regimen for a diabetic child. Benoliel (1975) notes that the family is expected to assume the role of agent in the diabetic treatment of the child as well as to modify other established roles to accommodate the changed conditions produced by the diabetes, for ex-

ample, "responsibility for being shot-giver, food-fixer, law-enforcer, record-keeper, or supervisor of the child's activities." The adult members in the family form collaborative partnerships around the range of responsibilities for the diabetic youngster and the rest of the family unit. The diabetic regimen of their child can also overlap with and restrict many well-established family routines (Drash, Becker, 1978).

Mattsson (1977) discusses the multitude of emotional stressful situations to which children with long-term physical disorders are subjected. The young diabetic and his or her family are faced with threats of lasting physical impairment of unknown proportions; medical expenses; and interference with schooling, leisure activities, job opportunities, and future adult roles as spouse and parent. Family members may be concerned about episodes of hypoglycemia or acidosis as a result of emotionally charged family interaction. These threats are in addition to the day-to-day concerns.

These difficult life situations can contribute to emotional problems in children. Minuchin's classic study (1978) of young children frequently hospitalized for unexplained episodes of acidosis demonstrated the children's difficulties in handling stress, their immature coping abilities, and their tendencies to internalize anger.

The disease is so threatening that the parent's first response to this diagnosis may be disbelief (Mattsson, 1977). After the initial shock, parents may typically respond with either overprotection or rejection of the youngster. Fisher and Dolger (1946), in one of the first published studies of family's responses to the disease process, found that overprotection and rejection each corresponded to a distinct personality type in the child. The overprotective parent had either a submissive–dependent child or one that was rebellious; the rejecting parent produced resentment and belligerence in the diabetic child. Rejection and neglect of the child are less common responses compared to overprotection.

Parental overconcern or overprotection may result from anxiousness and guilt related to hereditary factors (Mattsson, 1977). Parents must also attend to the needs of healthy siblings who may harbor feelings of anxiety, guilt, and resentment toward a diabetic brother or sister.

Mothers and fathers may have different responses to the diabetic child because they are involved quite differently in the day-to-day care of the child. Fallstrom (1974), one of the first investigators to interview both mothers and fathers, found that mothers assumed principal responsibility for treatment-related tasks. Mothers also knew more about the illness (Etzwiler, Sines, 1962). Because they are more involved and knowledgeable, they appear to be more affected by the diabetic child. Borner and Steinhausen (1977) found that mothers of diabetic children were more reserved and depressed than mothers of nondiabetic children. Fathers of diabetic children did not differ from fathers of nondiabetic children on these measures. Etzwiler and Sines (1962) found that fathers' participation appeared to be greater if the child was male or if the disease was judged by the physician to be particularly difficult to control.

A parent who has diabetes can have a particularly important effect on the diabetic child. Maines (1984) describes the impact of family members with diabetes on two young males who became diabetic. One young man adopted the detrimental attitudes of the family—the "I don't care" attitude of his diabetic grandmother and the family's expectation that he would not live long. He pursued his fatalism. The other young man spent years in self-destructive behavior before deciding to reject the self-defeating behaviors of his diabetic father. This decision led him to search for greater stability and control in his life. The stress, then, of growing up diabetic can be compounded when a diabetic parent or grandparent presents a negative role model either as a diabetic or as a parent.

Normally, one would assume that a child who has a diabetic parent would be more knowledgeable about the illness, but one study demonstrated opposite results. Collier and Etzwiler (1971) found that knowledge scores of diabetic

parents were comparable to scores of all parents in their study, but their adolescents scored well below the mean of other diabetic children. These scores are opposite from what might be predicted. The authors suggest that when the parent is diabetic, certain assumptions about the child's knowledge are made and less interaction regarding education of the child is undertaken.

Diabetes and Stage of Development

In assessing the effect of the illness on the child, Moos (1977) notes that stage of development can profoundly affect changes in self-image, dependency conflicts, and interpersonal relationships. The transition from dependence to self-reliance and independence is important in every child's development. If a chronic illness occurs before independence is established, regression to dependent patterns of behavior may occur. At various stages, the young diabetic may be dependent on parents for insulin injections, blood glucose monitoring, and special food preparation.

As the child grows older, patterns of functioning change, and the family faces new problems. In adolescence, when children are rebelling against parental authority, diabetes can cause many problems. Angry, depressed, and rebellious adolescents may abandon the diabetic regimen as a means to threaten or retaliate against family members (Mattsson, 1977).

Benoliel (1970) studied two interrelated problems: (1) the meaning of diabetes mellitus as a social crisis in the family and (2) the emergence of the identity of the diabetic in the transition from childhood to adolescence. Using a symbolic interactionist perspective, she studied the meaning of being diabetic at different points of maturation; the meaning and management of diabetes by different types of families; and the effects of diabetes and its treatment on the enactment of social roles by the person with diabetes, by his or her friends, and by health care professionals. She interviewed all members of the household to obtain a more valid image of the social meanings of diabetes. This total family interview proved to be a valuable tool in investigating the "tremendous and variable influence of family relationships on the emerging role-identities of children." She found that the attitudes and actions of parents were the most important elements affecting the social environment in which young persons began to understand the personal and social meanings of being diabetic.

Moos (1977) suggests that parents and children must accept the reasonable limits to independence that the diabetic condition creates. At the same time, it is important that parents encourage maximum development within these limits.

Diabetes as a Source for Family Conflict

Diabetes places a severe strain on the family's repertoire of physical, emotional, cognitive, and financial resources. Controversy over the meaning of the individual's therapeutic regimen and the precision with which directions should be followed can occur among family members. Diabetes may become the focus for conflict within a family because family members differ in their definitions of the illness and appropriate treatment. Children may be more willing to engage in risk-taking behaviors than their parents. Siblings may resent roles as protectors or normalizers. Resentment, fear, or guilt may govern behavior and affect attempts to deal with conflict.

The matter of dietary compliance seems to be an especially important target in family conflict. Diabetologists themselves do not agree on the relative merits of "tight control." Most parties may agree that control is necessary for the prevention of ketoacidosis or insulin reactions but may not agree on the long-term effects of control on degenerative changes and complications (Watts, 1980). Knowles et al (1965) found that juvenile diabetics on a free diet fared no worse than those on a regulated diet in terms of metabolic control. The thoroughness and prospective design of this study gives it particular

credibility, but strict dietary control continues to be controversial. If the experts cannot agree, it is not surprising that family members disagree on amount of control they should attempt to place on their children.

Even if family members could theoretically agree on dietary goals, they may experience conflict around compliance to those goals. Watts (1980) maintains that treatment compliance by diabetic individuals is very poor. Haynes and Sackett (1976) found that complicated regimens persisting over a long period of time and requiring substantial degrees of behavioral changes were associated with poor treatment compliance. Treatment for diabetes implies a complicated regimen; as a lifetime condition, it requires considerable change in a wide range of behaviors. It is not surprising, then, that families experience serious conflict over their goals for treatment and their efforts to comply with these treatments.

Conflict can, of course, increase family stress. Crain et al (1966) reported that families with diabetic children experienced more marital conflict, stress, and disruption than control families. Behavioral scientists have been interested in this relationship between stress and the course of the illness. In general, they have found that stress does not cause the onset of diabetes, but it can affect its course. Although studies on the relationship between stressful life events and the course of diabetes have been criticized for their retrospective designs and small sample sizes, it appears that stressful events can have a destabilizing effect on the course of the disease as indicated by an increase in ketones, free fatty acids, and glycosuria. The effect on blood glucose levels is more variable. Bradley (1979) found that although stressful life events were not reflected in blood glucose measures, increases in blood glucose did appear to be registered as glycosuria. Insulin-treated groups scored higher on these disturbance measures than those groups receiving oral hypoglycemia medications.

The Hinkle and Wolf (1952) study on the metabolic effects of stress has become a classic. A series of 64 diabetic patients were seen for regular intervals over a three-year period to examine the relationship between life events and fluctuations in diabetic control. Responses of diabetic and nondiabetic patients to experimentally induced stress were essentially similar, though somewhat more extreme in diabetics. The more unstable the diabetic, the more marked the metabolic reactions.

Metabolic effects of stress continue to be of interest to scientists. Blood sugar levels can be increased or decreased by stress, depending on a number of factors, including the amount of available insulin and the kind of stress experienced. Simonds (1977) reports that children with poorly controlled diabetes have significantly more interpersonal conflicts than those with well-controlled diabetes. Unstable diabetics may be relatively sensitive to all factors affecting control, and emotional stress may have an especially destabilizing effect (Watts, 1980).

Various studies have explored interventions to reduce conflict and stress in families with diabetic members. Minuchin et al (1978) found that individual therapy had no impact. An open-systems model approach, which highlighted the complexities of family interactions and widened the field of observations, was more effective. Therapy became more effective when it viewed the child in the family context rather than as an individual.

Burnish and Bradley (1983) examined three models for providing some understanding of the effect of stress on physiologic functioning. The linear causation model and psychophysiologic models were described respectively as "unsatisfactory" and "incomplete." The authors viewed the third model, the transactional model, as "more encompassing." They perceived this last model as incorporating various stages of cognitive processing, but they did not specifically mention the relevance of the family.

Anderson and Auslander (1980) point out that the focus of research and intervention has now moved to the broader family milieu, with emphasis on patterns of cooperation and conflict among family members around issues of treatment. They state that the linear model of parental influence is now overshadowed by a systems model of family interaction based on the concept of mutual influence among family members. In a study using this systems model, Koski and Kumento (1977) pointed out that satisfactory control of diabetes in one member is only one aspect of a healthy, well-functioning family. Newbrough et al (1985) proposed a family development approach as a way of understanding the stages of management when a child has diabetes. This approach incorporates a long-term view of the individual and family development.

Families with Adult Diabetics

Most research focuses on families with diabetic children. Families with diabetic children, however, constitute only about 5% of all families with diabetic members. The adjustment problems in families with adult diabetics have received very little attention. Even with the recent interest in the caretaking behaviors of family members for their elders, there is a paucity of attention given to older diabetics. A special issue of *The Diabetes Educator* (1983) on the diabetic elderly did carry an article about the psychosocial aspects of aging (Papatheodorou, 1983).

Families with adult diabetics, although seldom the focus of study, face some poignant and difficult problems. A middle-aged woman with a diabetic husband provides a third-person account of a terrifying experience:

> The woman sometimes wondered what it was that warned her, what awoke her out of her deep sleep in the night. Was it the constant lurking unease, a subtle change in the rhythm of the man's breathing, a sixth sense? She didn't know. She only knew that suddenly she would be awake. "Are you all right?" she would whisper, her palm on his forehead. Often he would be all right; she would simply have disturbed him. And if he were incoherent, perspiring, she would adminis-

ter the orange juice, urging him gently, as though he were a child. It frightened her that she didn't know what woke her. What if her built-in indefinable tocsin failed them both? What if she didn't wake in time? Don't panic, she'd tell herself sternly when this fear obtruded.

But, once, she did panic. She did awake too late in the black hours before dawn. The man was in a coma, his breathing stertorous, rasping like a saw in her ears, in her heart; his body twitching, sweat already soaking the mattress. She tried to force the sugar between his teeth; the big man, resisting, was a dead weight in her arms. Her heart pounding, she stumbled across the room for the needle and the tiny vials; she couldn't see, where were her glasses, the needle seemed wrong, where was everything she needed?

Despising herself for her weakness, her helplessness, the woman picked up the telephone with shaking hands and dialed the fire department. Moments later, when the fire engine arrived, and the ambulance, sirens screaming, she was outside the house, nightgown billowing in the cold wind, no memory of her bare feet on the stone steps to the street.

After the man regained consciousness, the woman asked him, "Are you feeling better?" The man looked dazedly at the three firemen, the three paramedics looming in their black uniforms in his bedroom, and he fumbled around in his head and found his sense of irony, his sense of humor. "Better than *what*?" he asked, and managed a small half smile.

He was a strong man, he recovered well after the usual brief aftermath of feeling sick. Later, the doctor said to the woman, "Too bad you had to panic." And it *was* too bad; there is no room for panic here. The woman felt guilt and remorse and sadness. She built another game plan around her glasses, the needle, the vials, the emergency equipment that she had thought was all where it was supposed to be; and she felt a little better. And how, in comparison, did the man feel, the sufferer?

The man was a victim of diabetes, unstabilized; he was what is known as a "brittle" diabetic, frequently out of control. The night the woman panicked he had suffered insulin shock in his sleep, the result of an overdose of insulin in relation to the amount of sugar in his blood (Drewes, 1981).

The family with an elderly member with diabetes mellitus faces special challenges. Davidson (1983) notes that diabetes mellitus in the elderly is a common and often serious problem. As with diabetics in other age groups, when compared to nondiabetics, these older individuals are much more likely to become blind (25 times), develop renal problems (17 times), develop gangrene (20 times), and possibly undergo an amputation (15 times) or suffer a heart attack or stroke (2 times) (National Commission on Diabetes, 1976; Most, Sinnock, 1983). Because these complications are related in large part to the duration of diabetes, older individuals are a preferential target.

Responsibility for observation, assessment, and care of the older diabetic often falls to family members. The elderly are more likely to have noninsulin dependent diabetes than insulin dependent diabetes mellitus. The diagnosis of diabetes superimposed on other chronic problems may increase the sense of anxiety, loss, depression, and guilt of the elderly person. The further loss of physical health may be compounded by diminished self-esteem (Papatheodorou, 1983). The dual problem of diabetes and obesity presents a particularly vexing problem for older people who find it difficult to eat or to prepare food for a small family (spouse and self). Because of an inadequate income, the individual may buy highly refined sweet or starchy foods at more expensive neighborhood stores if they are unable to get to a supermarket. It is not unusual for one partner in an older marriage to be on a special diet; when a diabetic diet is simultaneously necessary, the juggling of the shopping and preparing of food to meet what might be divergent requirements may prove to be very difficult. Getting adequate exercise may present another problem. It is not known whether diabetics exercise more if they live alone or within a family or friend group.

The elderly diabetic living alone needs to be in contact with family or friends in person or by phone on a daily basis. The conversations should be long enough for the family member to determine any change in speech or cognition that may signal complications. In addition, the older individual needs to articulate his or her perception of his or her present status.

The majority of studies and papers presented in this review concern juvenile diabetics and to a lesser extent juvenile diabetics and the family. The impact of diabetes on the young, childbearing-age couple has received some comment. The dearth of studies about the group that constitutes 95% of the diabetic population—that is the middle-aged and older adult and his or her family—precludes the attention that this group deserves.

Current State of Research

The research on diabetes within the family has two major problems. First, it centers almost exclusively on families with diabetic children. Second, most studies assume a biomedical model. The research stems from a medical perspective that:

1. Is individual, care–cure oriented rather than family oriented.
2. Assumes medical definitions of control and compliance.
3. Assumes linear, cause–effect relationships among variables rather than a systems approach.

In this section, we will discuss the implications of this perspective on research, professional education, and health care and suggest alternative ways for viewing families with diabetic members.

Individual, Care–Cure Orientation Versus Family Orientation

Most health care in the United States today is individual and acute care–cure oriented. Not surprisingly, research on illnesses has assumed the same orientation. Approaches to research, education, and service seldom include the family as a critical variable in understanding and treating the person with diabetes.

Health care inpatient and outpatient services are organized around diagnoses and treatment regimens designed to stabilize the diabetic's metabolic status. Most teaching is directed toward assisting the person in following the prescribed regimen. Some educational programs also help the diabetic acquire knowledge, skill, and competency in living with diabetes. Family members are seldom included, except as medical extenders, reinforcers, or monitors. Mothers, for example, are expected to assume responsibility for reinforcing the medical regimen set up for their children. The family, when considered at all, thus becomes an extension of the medical system.

Most scientific literature about diabetes mellitus is also in the biomedical arena, where research moneys have been allocated to the search for basic and fundamental information on the etiologic and pathogenic mechanisms of the disease. Research that does focus on the family falls into the category of psychosocial research or research by behavioral scientists. They have been primarily interested in the causes or mediating factors in the illness, such as stress. Using a biomedical framework similar to that used by physicians, behavioral scientists have investigated the family's role in mediating stress. Thus, when the family is considered, it is studied as a cause or source of a medical problem. Knowledge about families thus seems to be generated primarily to serve the medical system's need for the family's cooperation in extending medical treatment.

Similarly, educational programs for health care professionals are generally based on a biomedical, individual, cure-oriented model. Such a model does not easily accommodate the family, either as an important factor in care of the diabetic individual or as the unit of care. Endocrinologists and diabetologists pursue the level of specialization deemed necessary for treating this complex disease. In recent years, the preparation of family specialists and primary care practitioners in nursing and medicine departs from a general trend toward specialization. Quite possibly, these clinicians may adopt more of an orientation to the family in their treatment of diabetic patients.

The following vignette serves to challenge the individual adequacy of the care–cure orientation:

A young woman with diabetes recalls the experience of being diagnosed at the age of 8. Her physician was a very strict diabetologist; early on she began to "fudge" on her urine tests and gradually gave up on her diet. When she was 12, her 7-year-old sister was diagnosed as having diabetes mellitus. The 12-year-old was expected to be a good example. "Some example! We rarely discussed the matter. I guess she chose to ignore it, too, as I found the yellow food coloring which I added to water to test as urine in front of mom in the bathroom, and I was certain I'd replaced it in the kitchen cabinet earlier that day. I think we both felt guilty that we weren't able to keep sugar out of our urine.

"When I was 30, my sister died at the age of 25. She had been losing her vision and was having a terrible time with reactions. On the advice of a friend, she consulted a doctor who ran tests and told her she was not diabetic but only troubled with a severe food allergy. He prescribed a diet of nuts and berries and took her off insulin. That was that.

"Teri's death was a great shock. People said, 'Well, Teri never took care of herself like you do,' to reassure me. I knew in my heart that Teri and I had treated our diabetes the same way for many years; by ignoring it! I think at the time of Teri's death, she was tired and discouraged and afraid of total blindness. I think she got tired of feeling sick, felt trapped by a regimen she couldn't get herself to believe in again. . . . She wanted to believe she was not diabetic.

"After Teri's death, I began to see myself as a survivor. I began to wonder why I was surviving and I began trying to understand what it takes to survive with diabetes so I could help other diabetics and myself survive" (Wendy Ullman-Duarte, Marriage, Family, and Child Counselor, 1983).

Medical Definitions of Control and Compliance

Because research, education, and service programs are dominated by the biomedical model, it is not surprising that definitions of the illness reveal a medical rather than a social orientation. In particular, attitudes about control and compliance suggest a medically oriented framework.

Most health care personnel interested in teaching diabetes assume that control of this illness is a desirable goal. Diabetes is, in fact, one of the few chronic illnesses that can be controlled quite successfully by specific forms of therapy, and some programs strive to teach patients effective methods for monitoring and controlling their illness. It is precisely this factor of control that makes chronic illness such a problem for most people. Shapiro (1983) maintains that a need for control is a fundamental human drive and that illness becomes particularly threatening when it interferes with control of daily living. Forces beyond one's comprehension or regulation then shape everyday life and create problems of management. Illness thus raises issues of vulnerability and fragility of life. Both the chronically ill person and the family members may then exert much energy to contain the illness and to regain a sense of mastery and control over life.

Because control over diabetes is considered desirable, health care personnel encourage participants to monitor their illness and to make every effort to use new procedures to control their illness. For some people, however, acceptance or compliance may not be that straightforward. For these individuals, the real question may not be whether or not they shall comply but to which system? Professional diagnoses and treatment plans formulated in the context of medical and nursing care may have little relevance to such individuals. There may be little fit between medical definitions and these individuals' perceptions of the illness and its consequences (Schneider, Conrad, 1981). These individuals construct their understanding of illness within the context of family and culture. They may choose to comply with respected family and cultural systems that require behaviors quite different from those recommended by health care practitioners.

Because diabetes is a long-term, incurable illness, the family system assumes a critical role in shaping the diabetic's attitudes and behaviors. The person with diabetes is forced to rely more on family and friends than on professionals. Because it is a chronic and not an acute illness, family members may perceive diabetes as a condition rather than as an illness and may define the diabetic as impaired rather than as sick (Honig–Parnass, 1981). Family perceptions of diabetes as "illness" or as "condition" will affect their responses: How serious is the condition? How will it be treated? What do the symptoms mean and how should they be interpreted? When should the patient return to the doctor? And possibly even more important, who should be responsible for monitoring, making decisions, and treating the illness? Will the diabetic be primarily responsible for his or her own management, or will another family member assume responsibility for monitoring and controlling?

Although control of illness appears to be a desirable objective, it is not advisable to assume that each person with diabetes necessarily *wants* to maintain control of his or her own illness. There are some secondary benefits in retaining an impaired role. Illness offers the adult an opportunity to accept a more passive role, claim more nurturance from spouse or children, and avoid threatening work or student roles. To acquire the more normal life that may come with better control of illness thus involves a trade-off of independence in functioning with the attention and privileges associated with the impaired role. Furthermore, family members may experience some secondary benefits in relating to the diabetic as a dependent person.

It is quite possible, therefore, that although diabetic individuals may understand and even accept a goal of increased control over their own illness, progress toward this goal will be uneven. Families that have become accustomed to functioning with an impaired member for whom they have assumed considerable responsibility may find it difficult to shift their expectations. These families will, of course, have difficulty with the medical system because their definitions of illness and desired objectives in controlling that illness are in conflict with the providers' definitions. More research needs to focus on family definitions and strategies for maintaining their sense of integrity when confronted with diverse biomedical definitions.

Linear and Systems Models

The biomedical model generally assumes linear or cause–effect relationships among variables. Thus, researchers have been interested in investigating causes and cures. This concentration on identifying factors that cause or relieve an illness, including diabetes, has created several problems. First, some aspects of an illness have been studied intensively, but other aspects have been ignored. For example, many studies have focused on the link between control of disease (diabetes) and patient outcomes in terms of hospitalization and complications, but few studies have focused on less directly associated variables, such as family patterns and control of disease. Second, an overall model that takes into consideration a complex array of interacting factors has not been fully elaborated.

A systems approach is more appropriate than a linear, causal relations approach in developing this type of comprehensive model. For example, a comprehensive model for teaching a person with diabetes may take into consideration factors from an education program to patient outcomes, as shown in Figure 23-1.

Thus, an effective diabetes educational program will theoretically increase knowledge, which will increase frequency of self-management behaviors, which, in turn, will establish

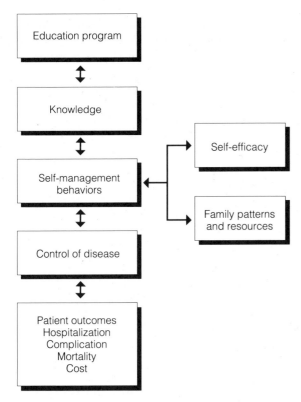

Figure 23–1 A comprehensive model of variables in teaching diabetics.

better control of the disease. Control will lead to reduced hospitalization, lower mortality rates, and reduced costs. Because persons with diabetes often live in a family context, family patterns and resources plus their own feelings of self-efficacy and control will affect their approach to the disease and will profoundly influence attempts to learn new procedures in managing the illness. Two-directional arrows in Figure 23-1 indicate that these relationships resemble "feedback loops" more than linear, cause–effect relationships. For example, obtaining readings of blood sugar in the normal range may serve as a positive reinforcement and may encourage the patient to greater use of self-management behaviors.

A review of the literature indicates that most studies do not consider these intervening variables; instead they attempt direct comparisons between the education program and either the control of the disease, as measured by blood glucose levels, or patient outcomes (hospitalization, complications, mortality, and cost). Comparatively little is known, therefore, about the intervening links. With the model in Figure 23-1 in mind, the following conclusions may be drawn from research on diabetes education and patient outcomes.

First, the studies that have connected education programs directly to either control or patient outcomes have had mixed results. Several studies have demonstrated that education and medical supervision of diabetic patients can reduce mortality rates and costs of medical care (Deckert, Poulsen, Larsen, 1978; Davidson et al, 1981; Isaf, Alogna, 1977). Korhonen et al (1983), however, was not able to establish any relationship between education, whether intensive or short term, and permanent changes in self-management behaviors or control of diabetes.

Second, perhaps the best-documented link in this chain of events is between control and complications. Physiologic condition, as measured by the blood glucose levels, relates quite consistently to onset of complications. Pirart (1978a, 1978b) followed a large group of diabetic patients for 26 years and found that as blood glucose levels rose, the incidence and prevalence of microangiopathies increased. Isaf and Alogna (1977) also reported that improvement in blood glucose levels contributed to lower morbidity rates.

Third, associations among knowledge, performance of self-care tasks, and improved control have not been documented. Most studies do not consider these relationships, and those that do report inconsistent results. In his review of 320 articles on patient education, Mazzuca (1982) found that increasing knowledge did not always lead to self-management behaviors or better control. Watkins et al (1967) reported that greater knowledge was associated with greater frequency of performing self-management tasks, such as urine glucose testing, but they did not find any relationship between the performance of these tasks and diabetes control.

Again, the relationship between education and desirable patient outcomes is by no means well established. Several explanations may be given for this lack of a consistent positive relationship. First, educational programs vary; some are obviously more effective than others. Second, compliance as a desirable patient outcome may fit a medical definition but may not fit the patient or family notion of a means for coping with illness or its consequences (Schneider, Conrad, 1981). Cultural and family definitions of illness will shape the individual patient's responses to a therapeutic regimen (Shapiro, 1983; Quint, 1969). Studies on program effectiveness seldom examine the impact of the patient's social and cultural context on management of illness. Third, methodologic problems may contribute to inconsistency in research findings. Christensen et al (1983) describe the difficulties in finding an adequate method for measuring dietary behavior. Windsor et al (1981) maintain that sophisticated, qualitative analysis of self-care data—cognitive, affective, skill, and behavior—for diabetic patients is keenly needed. Until recently, there was no standardized test for measuring patient knowledge, nor were there reliable technologic methods for patients to measure their blood glucose levels.

A diabetes teaching program may have a direct effect on the diabetic's knowledge, self-management behaviors, subsequent use of health care services, and possibly on family interaction and perceptions of resources. The person's implementation of a new therapeutic routine will depend, however, to a considerable degree on the social and family environment in which he or she lives. Family members' understanding of the illness, their coping responses, and resources available to them and the diabetic may serve as intervening variables in shaping the person's efforts to control the illness.

More research needs to be done to fill in the gaps in this model. This research may be more difficult because it involves examination of areas not easily defined or measured. In some ways the easiest work has been done, as investigators have tackled those areas that lend themselves most readily to quantification and to cause–effect relationships. Assessing interactions among more complex variables will require creative use of a variety of methodologies, qualitative as well as quantitative.

Future Directions

The design of research protocols, professional education programs, and health care services that integrate the family as involved members or as the unit of focus is a major challenge. The call for research to incorporate family challenges the already severe methodologic problems inherent in the study of diabetes.

Research

The trend toward the conduct and support of psychosocial, educational, and service-related research is somewhat encouraging, but much remains to be done. Burish and Bradley (1983) maintain that little attention has been given to how families and diabetic members cope with particular problems of diabetes. Many studies suggest that the majority of families manage very well under considerable stress when a member has diabetes, but very little is known about the characteristics of their coping patterns and how in fact they do manage so successfully. Hopefully the empirical basis for the efficacy of successful approaches to assisting diabetics and families to cope more effectively with diabetes will be reported. There will need to be considerably more study of adult diabetics in a given family. Although many investigators have been interested in the relationship between stress and diabetes, the area merits considerably more research.

Many of the studies on compliance or self-care have been conducted with middle-class, well-educated subjects, which raises serious questions regarding whether such findings can be generalized to groups with other beliefs, values, and attitudes about diet, obesity, and self-management of diabetes. Systematic study, then, needs to be conducted involving people with diabetes mellitus and members of their family who come from a variety of cultures; are in various developmental stages of individual and family life; have insulin dependent or non-insulin dependent diabetes; have particular learning disabilities and needs; and lead risky and unusually complex lives.

Research on pancreatic (beta cell) transplants has begun. Judging from the experiences associated with other kinds of transplants, the introduction of the new cells into a body is but the beginning of challenges that await the patient, the family, nurses and other health care professionals, and scientists.

An exploratory study by May et al (1985) examined how diabetes affects family processes and relationships by focusing on the process of decision-making about childbearing when the diabetic member in the family was the female spouse. Studies regarding genetic issues and childbearing concerns merit attention.

Although much of the biomedical research has successfully met the canons of scientific investigation, less than optimal approaches to research design and data analysis have characterized other research. More attention will need to be paid to sample selection and size, matters of control and comparison groups, the need for longitudinal research designs with the attendant problems of sample and staff stability, confounding variables and costs, and reliability and validity of multiple measures. Sophisticated statistical analyses will be necessary to explicate relationships among many variables.

Efforts will need to be made to tackle the methodologic problems of overreliance on clinical ratings and subjective judgments to measure parental attitudes or family functioning; the lack of independent assessments of family, child, and health variables; and the use of inappropriate indices to determine effectiveness of diabetes management (Anderson, Auslander, 1980). Little is known about the impact of a diabetic child on family relationships involving healthy siblings, and more information is needed about these siblings' participation in the treatment regimen of the diabetic member. The role of fathers of diabetic children is beginning to attract research attention. An unexplored area continues to be the impact on the family of the specific characteristics of a diabetic child. There is a need to better understand the reciprocal influences of the individual child characteristics with family members.

With the emphasis on pathology that has so characterized research of the past and present, the identification of family strengths and successful strategies for coping with a treatment regimen at home will receive considerably more attention in the future. Anderson and Auslander (1985) suggest that with the study of the family with a diabetic child from a behavioral perspective, there will be an increased capability of helping pinpoint family interactions that support adherence to treatment regimens. These authors suggest that the model of the family that is gaining acceptance in research about diabetes is an interactive one in which the child and other family members continually modify each other and influence the course of treatment. Little is known about the influence of outside sources of support and stress on the family's adaptation to diabetes. The personal–social support networks of the child or adult with diabetes and of the members of the family, the treatment setting, and the health care personnel associated with the diabetic's care have a pervasive influence that deserves considerable attention.

Professional Education Programs

Educational programs that prepare nurses and other health care professionals will need to educate generalists and specialists in the care of diabetics to "think family" and to move beyond the biomedical, individual-oriented model of care.

One of the consequences of such a requirement is that the orientation or socialization of the individual to a professional role will need to expand beyond that of "curer" to that of "a partner-in-care" with the diabetic and the family. Because of the complexities of working with a family constellation involved with a serious condition, some of the training of nurses ideally will take place within a multidisciplinary context. Such an experience is invaluable if health care professionals are going to assist families to have access to the resources they need.

Health Care

It seems clear that a multifaceted service program is needed to effect the kinds of beneficial outcomes important for the individual with diabetes and for the family. A growing trend concerns efforts that are directed not just at control of the diabetes, which is important, but at normalizing the life of the diabetic and the family unit. This approach calls for a plan designed to help the diabetic and the family become the principal managers of diabetes in concert with health care professionals and to incorporate the reality of the diabetes and associated requirements into the functioning of the family unit.

A part of a multifaceted service program would include an educational plan for the diabetic and the entire family. The successful program of the future will consider the educational needs common to the vast majority of people with diabetes mellitus and will provide in addition a thorough assessment of the individual's and the family's specific needs, with a program tailored accordingly. Some of the factors that need to be considered include the type and severity of diabetes and associated requirements of the condition, the age and maturity of the person who has diabetes, the cognitive level and emotional stability of the diabetic, and the structure and functioning of the family unit along with its lifestyle, developmental tasks, beliefs, and values.

A description of an educational program for diabetics and their families that might be con-

sidered a model is illustrated in the second part of the photo documentary at the end of this chapter. The Diabetes Teaching Center, which is housed within the Department of Family Health Care Nursing at the University of California at San Francisco, School of Nursing, offers a 30-hour nurse-directed teaching program for diabetics (clients) and their families. The staff of the center consists of two nurses (the principal instructor and a clinical specialist), a dietitian, a counselor, and a supervising physician, all of whom have expertise in the management of diabetes. The director of the program is a nurse. The aim of the Diabetes Teaching Center is to provide a well-organized program in an outpatient setting designed to help diabetics and their families acquire the knowledge, skills, and confidence necessary to live successfully with the condition. The four-day program is intended to give the diabetic client sufficient skills to self-monitor the disease. It provides an ideal setting for clients and their family members to practice diabetes management skills under supervision. Clients are able to interpret blood glucose results from self-monitoring of blood glucose, and to adjust insulin and food intake appropriately when blood glucose is affected by environmental or emotional changes. They are then able to achieve optimum control of blood glucose, minimize complications, and avoid the need for routine medical supervision for purposes of control. Staff members are aware of the increased sense of confidence and mastery experienced by most of the clients and many of their family members. Information about the psychosocial aspects of living with diabetes mellitus is an essential part of the program. Much of the material discussed is tailored to the concerns of the program participants (clients and family members) who have completed relevant questionnaires at the beginning of the program.

Dietary instruction is provided daily in both group and individual formats. Each participant receives a personalized diet that takes into account individual dietary habits and preferences and the family's eating patterns. Diabetics and family members eat lunches and a breakfast together in a cafeteria with the staff, who counsel them in their food selections. On the last day of the program, the staff and group go to a local restaurant to use new information about dietary control in a natural situation.

Subsequent to the course, there are ongoing support services for clients, family members, partners, and significant others. Support groups and individual counseling are available to the diabetic. A variety of support service formats is available to all class members concerned, including a group for parents of youngsters for whom adjusting to the tasks involved in parenting and care of a diabetic child is discussed around a potluck dinner while children play together under supervision in a nearby setting. There is a group for significant others where friends, family members, and partners of people with diabetes have an opportunity to discuss candidly the stresses, strains, and surprises of a relationship with a diabetic. The group looks at common experiences, issues of communication and responsibility, concerns about sexuality, and the general quality of life.

Nurses provide the leadership in the educational programs described above. Nurses in a variety of other roles have an opportunity to utilize a family-oriented approach by incorporating all members in learning to live with diabetes. Nurses practicing in hospitals or long-term care facilities, in ambulatory care settings or in the community, are becoming increasingly aware that the tendency to keep the family peripheral to our caring and teaching of individuals is counterproductive, most particularly when it involves individuals with diabetes. Family members must be active participants by design and not by chance.

Summary

In conclusion, there seems to be a growing realization that the health care needs of people with a chronic disease are different from those who are acutely ill. One of the salient differences is, of course, the involvement of the family. Chronic illness is a family affair and it is difficult to imagine an example more appropriate than the family with a member who has diabetes mellitus. It is also difficult to imagine an opportunity more challenging for nurses than to involve families with diabetic members in their research, education, and service plans.

Issues for Further Investigation

1. How do families and diabetic members cope with the particular problems of diabetes? Are the characteristics of coping patterns related to particular problems or family characteristics?

2. What effect do culture and the various developmental stages of individual and family life have on compliance and self-care?

3. What should be the components of genetic counseling and how can this information best be given to diabetics and their families?

4. What is the personal–social support network and what is its effect on the child or adult with diabetes and members of their families?

5. What influence do the treatment setting and the personnel have on the knowledge and skill acquisition of the diabetic and the family?

References

Anderson BJ, Auslander WF (1980): Research on diabetes management and the family: A critique. *Diabetes Care*, 3(6): 696–702.

Benoliel JQ (1970): The developing diabetic identity: A study of family influence. In: *Communicating*

Nursing Research: Methodological Issues: Vol 3, Batey M (ed.). Boulder, CO: WICHE.

Benoliel JQ (1975): Childhood diabetes: The commonplace in living becomes uncommon. In: *Chronic Illness and the Quality of Life,* Strauss AL, Glaser BG (eds.). St. Louis: Mosby.

Borner S, Steinhausen HC (1977): A psychological study of family characteristics in juvenile diabetes. *Pediatr Adolesc Endocrinol, 3:* 46–51.

Bradley C (1979): Life events and the control of diabetes mellitus. *J Psychosom Res, 23:* 159–162.

Burish TG, Bradley LA (1983): *Coping with Chronic Illness.* New York: Academic Press.

Christensen NK et al (1983): Quantitative assessment of dietary adherence in patients with insulin-dependent diabetes mellitus. *Diabetes Care, 6*(3): 245–250.

Collier B, Etzwiler D (1971): Comparative study of diabetes knowledge among juvenile diabetics and their parents. *Diabetes, 20:* 51–57.

Crain AJ, Sussman MB, Weil WB (1966): Effects of a diabetic child on marital integration and related measures of family functioning. *J Health Hum Behav, 7:* 122–127.

Davidson JK et al (1981): Factors affecting the educational diagnosis of diabetic patients. *Diabetic Care, 4:* 275–278.

Davidson MB (1983): The impact of diabetes in the elderly. Guest editorial. *Diabetic Educator* (special issue on diabetes in the elderly), *9:* 10.

Deckert T, Poulsen JE, Larsen M (1978): Importance of outpatient supervision in the prognosis of juvenile diabetes mellitus: A cost/benefit analysis. *Diabetes Care, 1*(50): 281–284.

Diabetes Educator (1983): Special issue on diabetes in the elderly, *9.*

Drash L, Becker D (1978): Diabetes in the child: Course, special problems, and related disorders. In: *Advances in Modern Nutrition: Vol 2, Part 2,* Katzen H, Mahler R (eds.). Diabetes, obesity, and vascular disease: Metabolic and molecular interrelationships. Washington, DC: Hemisphere.

Drewes C (1981): Learning how to manage diabetes. *San Francisco Examiner,* Scene/Arts section, April 19, p. 1.

Etzwiler D, Sines LK (1962): Juvenile diabetes and its management: Family, social and academic implications. *JAMA, 181:* 304–308.

Fallstrom K (1974): On the personality structure of diabetic school children aged 7–15. *Acta Paediatr Scand (Suppl), 251:* 5–71.

Fischer AE, Dolger H (1946): Behavior and psychological problems of young diabetic patients. *Arch Intern Med, 78:* 711–732.

Harris M (1982): The prevalence of diagnosed diabetes, undiagnosed diabetes, and impaired glucose tolerance in the United States. In: *Genetic Environmental Interaction in Diabetes Mellitus,* Melish JS, Hana J, Baba S (eds.). Amsterdam-Oxford-Princeton: Excerpts Media. Proceedings of the Third Symposium on Diabetes Mellitus in Asia and Oceania. Honolulu, February, 1981.

Haynes DL, Sackett RB (1976): *Compliance with Therapeutic Regimens.* London: Johns Hopkins University Press.

Hinkle LE, Wolf S (1952): Importance of life stress in course and management of diabetes mellitus. *JAMA, 148:* 513–520.

Honig-Parnass T (1981): Lay concepts of the sick role: An examination of the professionalist bias in Parson's Model. *Soc Sci Med, 15A:* 615–623.

Isaf JJ, Alogna MT (1977): Better use of resources equals better health for diabetics. *Am J Nurs, 77:* 1792–1795.

Kilo C (1982): *Educating the Diabetic Patient.* New York: Science and Medicine.

Knowles HC et al (1965): The course of juvenile diabetes treated with unmeasured diet. *Diabetes, 14:* 239–273.

Korhonen T et al (1983): A controlled trial on the effects of patient education in the treatment of insulin-dependent diabetes. *Diabetes Care, 6:* 256–261.

Koski ML, Kumento A (1977): The interrelationship between diabetic control and family life. *Pediatr Adolesc Endocrinol, 3:* 41–45.

Maines D (1984): The social arrangements of diabetic self-help groups. In: *Chronic Illness and the Quality of Life,* (2nd ed.) Strauss A et al (eds.). St. Louis: Mosby.

Mattsson A (1977): Long-term physical illness in childhood: A challenge to psychological adaptation. In: *Coping with Physical Illness,* Moos R (ed.). New York: Plenum.

May K et al (1985): The childbearing decision of diabetic couples. Preliminary Report, Div. of Nursing,

USPH Service, R21 NU00828-05. Washington, DC: US GPO.

Mazzuca SA (1982): Does patient education in chronic disease have therapeutic value? *J Chron Dis*, 35: 521–529.

Minuchin S, Rosman B, Baker L (1978)): *Psychosomatic Families*. Cambridge: Harvard University Press.

Moos RH (ed.) (1977): *Coping with Physical Illness*. New York: Plenum.

Most RS, Sinnock P (1983): The epidemiology of lower extremity amputations in diabetic individuals. *Diabetes Care*, 6: 87–91.

National Center of Health Statistics. (1981, April). Current estimates from the National Health Interview Survey: United States, 1979, series 10, no. 136. DHHS pub. no. (PHS) 81-1564. Washington, DC: US-PHS.

National Commission on Diabetes. (1975, December 10). Report to Congress: Long range plan to combat diabetes. (Response to Public Law 93-354, July 23, 1974).

National Commission on Diabetes (1976): Report to Congress. DHEW, PH Service, NIH, 4 vols. DHEW pub. #NIH 76-1018, 76-1022, 76-1031, 76-1033.

National Diabetes Advisory Board (1982, May): *Diabetes in the 80s*. Washington, DC: US GPO.

Newbrough JR, Simpkins C, Maurer H (1985): A family development approach to studying factors in the management and control of childhood diabetes. *Diabetes Care*, 8: 83–92.

Papatheodorou NH (1983): The psychological aspects of aging in diabetes. *Diabetes Educator* (special issue on diabetes in the elderly), 9: 49–53.

Pirart J (1978a): Diabetes mellitus and its degenerative complications: A prospective study of 4,400 patients observed between 1947 and 1973, part one. *Diabetes Care*, 1(3): 168–188.

Pirart J (1978b): Diabetes mellitus and its degenerative complications: A prospective study of 4,400 patients observed between 1947, part two. *Diabetes Care*, 1(3): 1(4), 252–263.

Quint JC (1969): Becoming diabetic: A study of merging identity. Doctoral dissertation, University of California, San Francisco, 1969. Ann Arbor: University Microfilms.

Schneider J, Conrad P (1981): Medical and sociological typologies: The case of epilepsy. *Soc Sci Med*, 15A: 211–219.

Shapiro J (1983): Family reactions and coping strategies in response to the physically ill or handicapped child: A review. *Soc Sci Med*, 17(14): 913–931.

Simonds JF (1977): Psychiatric status of diabetic youth in good and poor control. *Int J Psychiatry Med*, 7: 133–151.

Strauss AL (1984): *Chronic Illness and the Quality of Life*. St. Louis: Mosby.

Ullman-Duarte W (1983): Psychosocial aspects of diabetes. Unpublished manuscript, San Francisco State University, San Francisco.

Watkins JD et al (1967): A study of diabetic patients at home. *Am J Public Health*, 57: 452–459.

Watts FN (1980): Behavioral aspects of the management of diabetes mellitus: Education, self-care and metabolic control. *Res Therapy*, 18: 171–180.

Windsor RA et al (1981): Qualitative issues in developing educational diagnostic instruments and assessment procedures for diabetic patients. *Diabetes Care*, 4(4): 468–475.

DIABETES
A Trilogy

This year, 600,000 newly diagnosed diabetics will join the ranks of the 10 million diabetics in the United States. Not only is the incidence of diabetes increasing, but the level of sophistication necessary for self-care is advancing and the cost of care associated with complications is escalating.

This three-part series on diabetes mellitus demonstrates the potential uses of photography for education and the promotion of health care. Photographic representation, which mirrors reality, can be both convincing and informative.

Most photographs of health care situations are produced by media professionals trained to capture certain kinds of images, usually the most sensational. Documentary photography at its best is more involved with its subject than is commercial photography. The documentary is investigative rather than illustrative. Its goal is to expose a kind of truth rather than to create a fiction that plays into the commodity goals of the marketplace.

Part 1, The Diabetic Child, promotes preventative maintenance at an early age by showing a child practicing self-maintenance. Part 2, Diabetes Teaching Center, presents a program that prepares children, adults, and their families for self-management. Part 3, The Story of George Estrada, demonstrates the importance of teaching self-maintenance through the presentation of an adult who suffers some of the unfortunate consequences.

THE DIABETIC CHILD

by Gail Garvin

When a child is found diabetic, shifts in priorities and concerns must be made by the entire family. The way in which the family handles this adjustment helps determine the course of the child's acceptance or denial of the diabetes and its management.

This gallery depicts efforts to normalize individual and family life and the environment, and it has been used to teach children about proper self-maintenance. As the child takes her responsibility seriously, these photographs present a positive view of a peer adapting to diabetes. They also present the role of the parent; the mother's involvement in activities associated with the diabetic is an important aspect of self-maintenance.

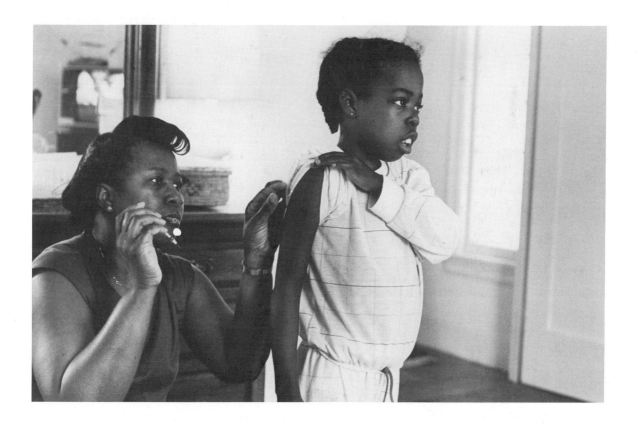

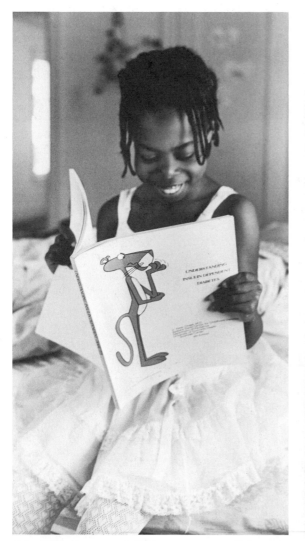 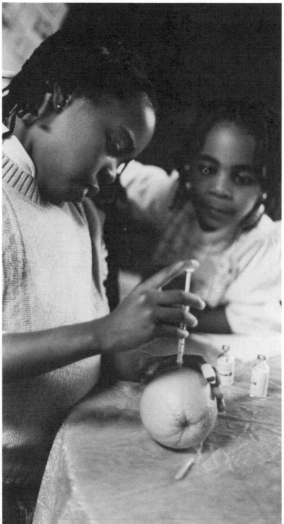

It is difficult to get children to manage diabetes properly. First they must be taught to understand the basic characteristics of the disease, then they can begin practicing the tasks, such as urine testing and blood monitoring.

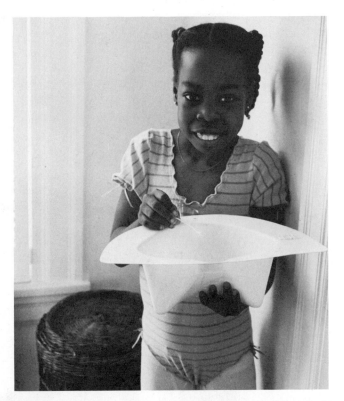

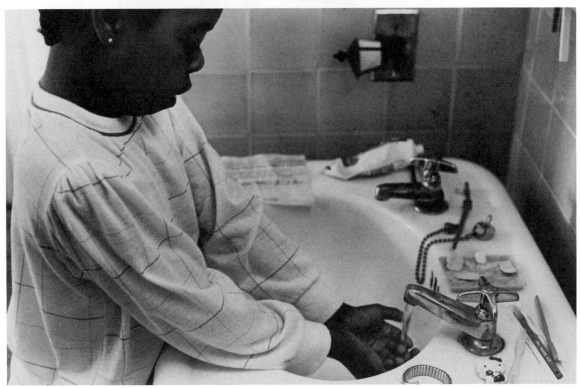

Insulin must be taken every day to maintain good health. Teaching children to inject themselves with insulin and to avoid sugar on a regular basis poses many problems, some of which can be overcome through role modeling.

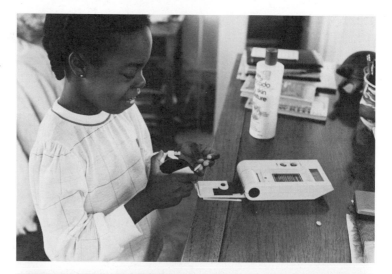

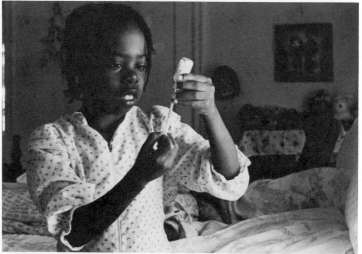

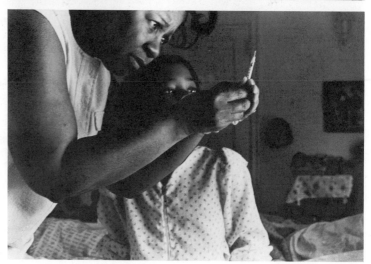

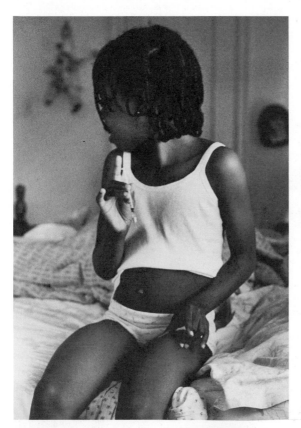

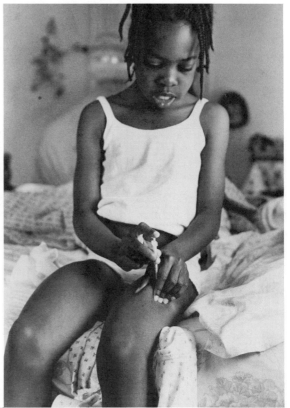

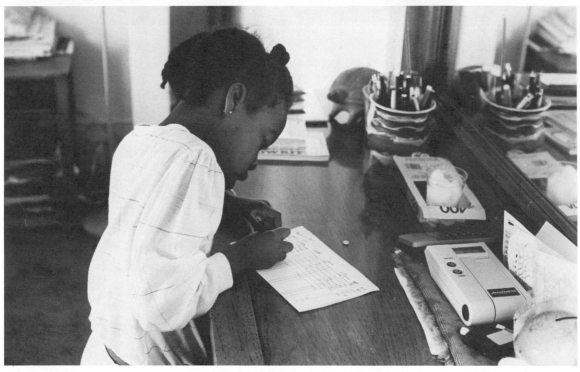

A diabetic child must pay close attention to food intake and exercise. Good nutrition, adequate exercise, play, and rest are essential ingredients for a sound self-maintenance program.

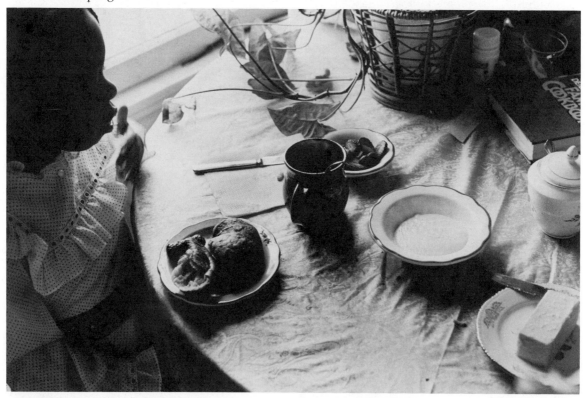

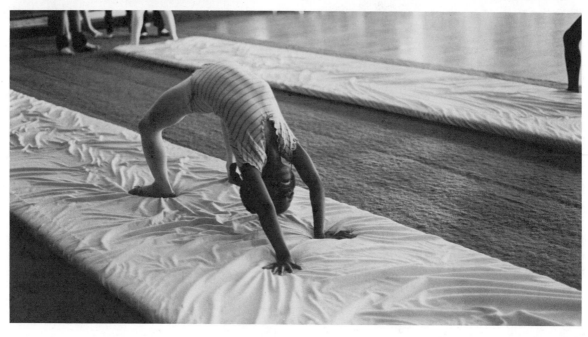

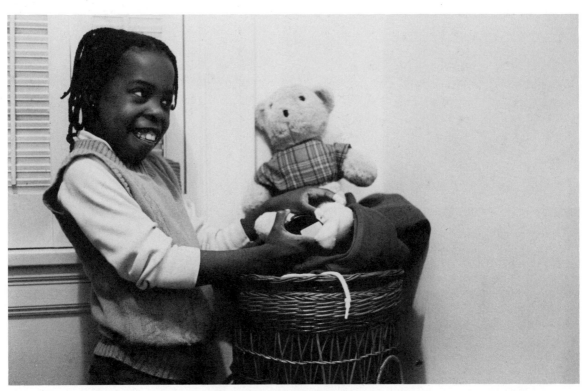

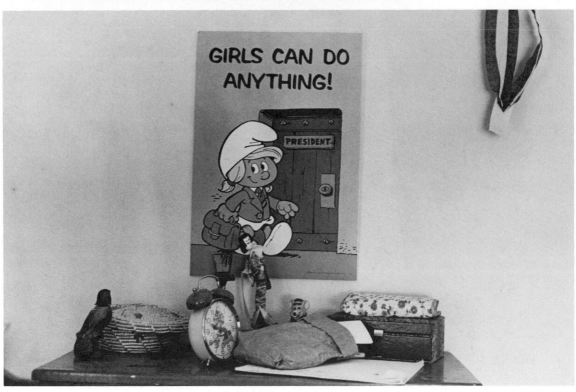

3–9

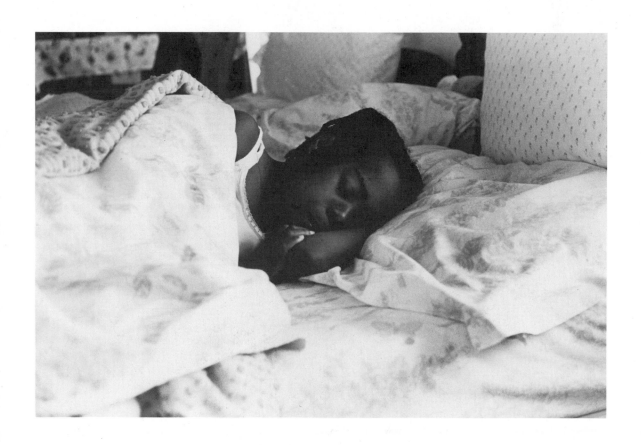

Gail Garvin, RN, MS, was a graduate student at the School of Nursing at the University of California at San Francisco when she produced this photoessay. She is currently a clinical specialist in endocrinology at Children's Hospital in Oakland, California.

DIABETES TEACHING CENTER

by Betty L. Highley

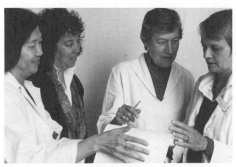

This gallery documents the Diabetes Teaching Center at the University of California at San Francisco. It was established to help people successfully manage diabetes on a day-to-day and long-term basis in partnership with health care professionals. The goal of the center is to make participants feel good physically and mentally, to live full and productive lives, and to reduce the frequency of acute complications requiring hospitalization or emergency care.

The staff of the Diabetes Teaching Center consists of a team of two nurses, a dietitian, a counselor, and a physician within the university facility, all of whom have specialty expertise in the management of diabetes. Clients are referred by physicians in private practice, by health care plans, by self, or by university facilities. The teaching program covers four consecutive days for a total of about 30 hours of instruction.

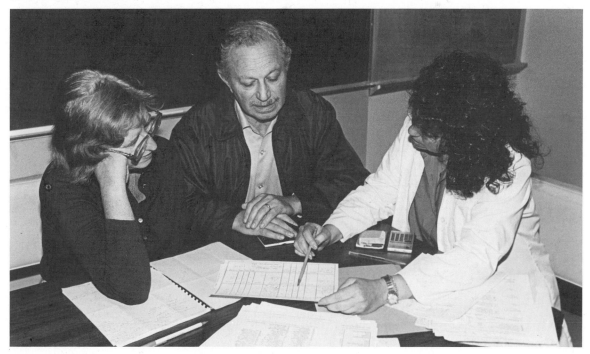

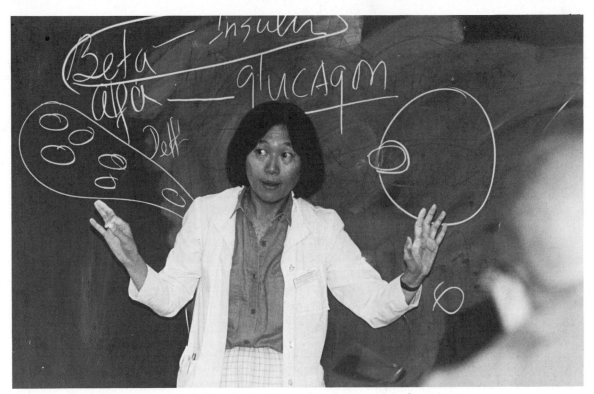

A range of teaching strategies and methods are used in the program: lectures, films, slides, group demonstrations, skills demonstrations by participants, and tutorial conferences.

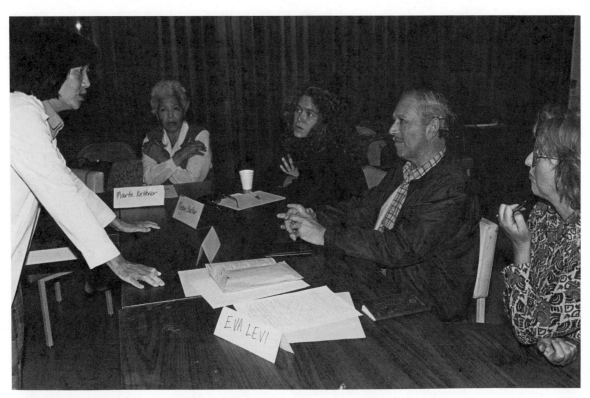

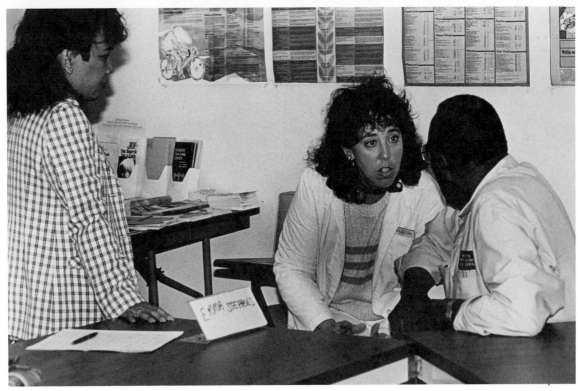

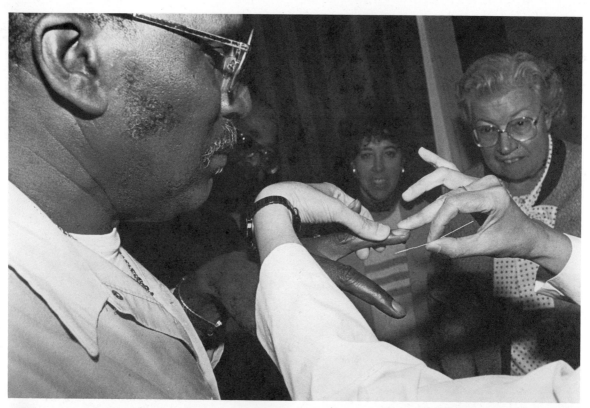

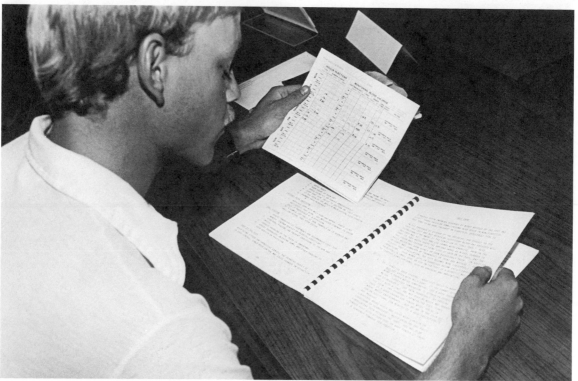

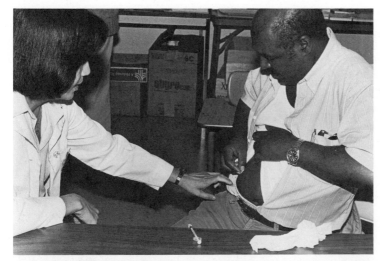

The diabetic is taught different aspects of proper self-care, including administration of diabetic medications, self blood glucose monitoring, urine testing, food selection and preparation, and prevention and management of complications.

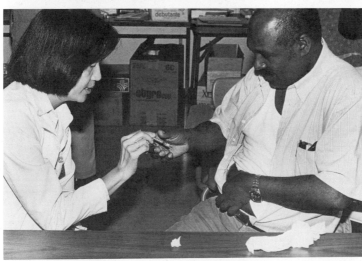

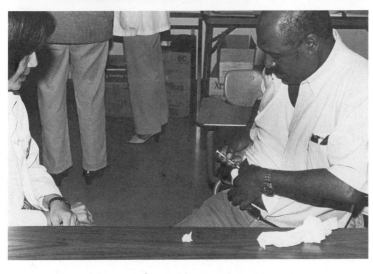

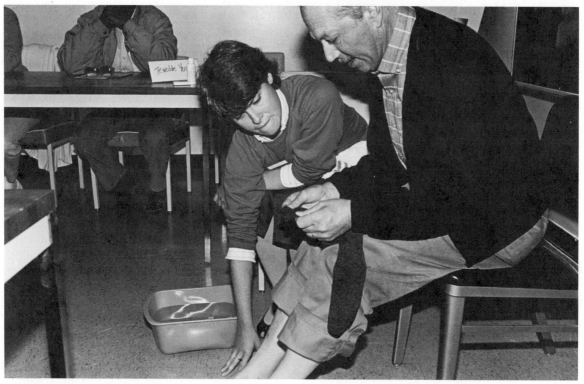

Clients are given an understanding of the diabetic state, including environmental factors that may manifest during work, play, or travel. They are taught that they can eat anywhere with proper attention to food selection; a field trip to a local restaurant provides the teaching medium.

It is a new experience for many diabetics to assume responsibility for their own care. The Diabetes Teaching Center enables them to take that responsibility, through the acquisition of necessary knowledge, skill, confidence, and the courage to try.

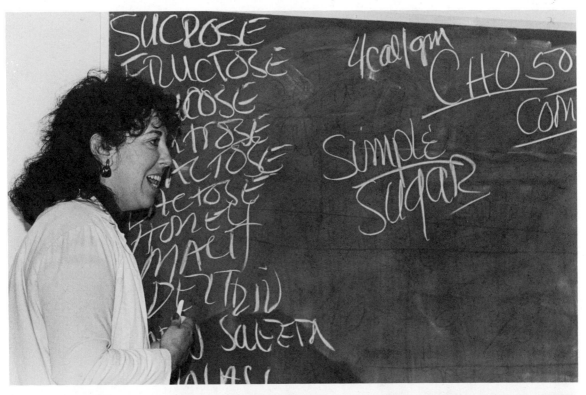

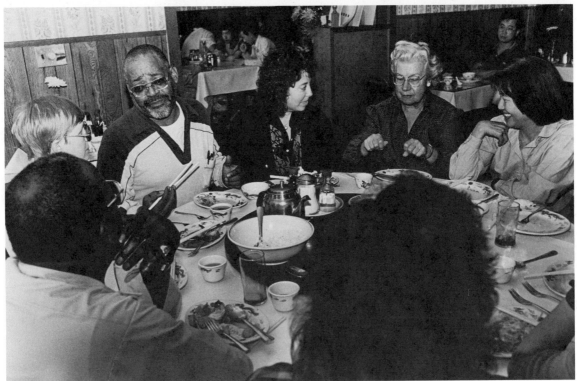

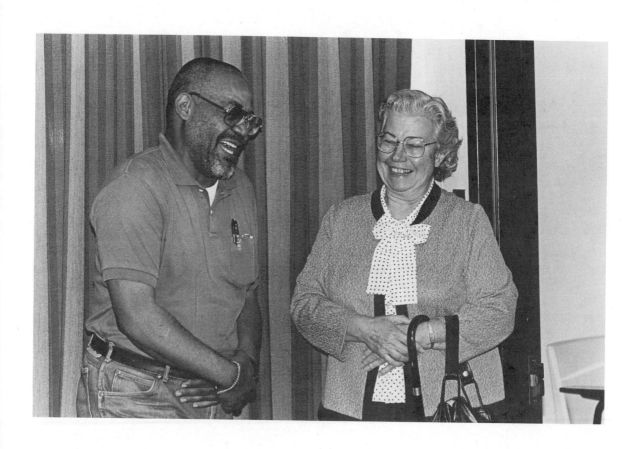

THE STORY OF GEORGE ESTRADA

by Tom Ferentz

This gallery is about George Estrada, a man in his fifties who is experiencing the complications of diabetes. Although he was not an excessive drinker or sugar consumer, he often had a beer or a Mexican sweetbread after work despite his awareness of his diabetic condition. While there is no clear evidence of a causal relationship between sugar and alcohol and complications, George did develop neuropathy and blindness. As a dramatization of the potential consequences of diabetes, this photoessay is meant as a persuasive argument for diabetic self-management.

This is also a story of home care and life with a chronic condition, and it demonstrates the potential for photo-documentary case studies. By giving George a face, a home, a wife, and by showing both his work and his leisure worlds, the study communicates dimensions that a case number and statistical information cannot convey.

Mrs. Estrada takes care of George most of the time. She cooks, manages the house, administers his medication, and attends to his other needs. Following the onset of complications, the Estradas participated in the program at the Diabetes Teaching Center.

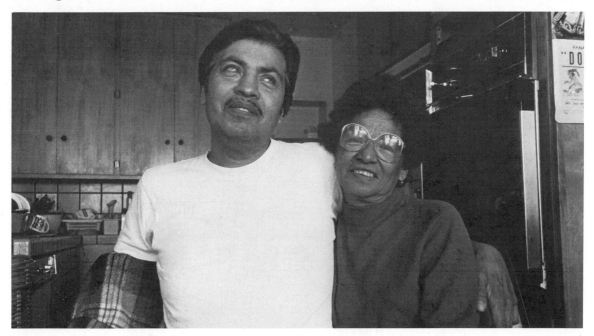

Funding for The Story of George Estrada came from the Evelyn and Walter Haas Foundation in San Francisco.

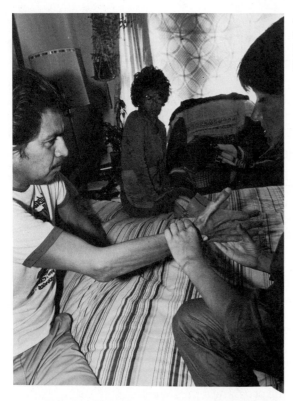

A physical therapist from the VNA visits George to help him maintain his ability to move around his home environment easily.

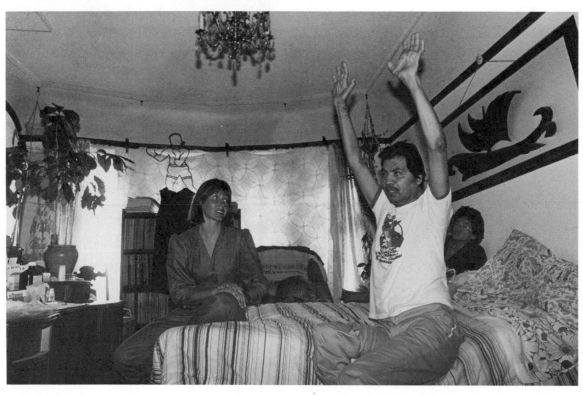

The PT manipulates George's feet periodically to alleviate foot drop.

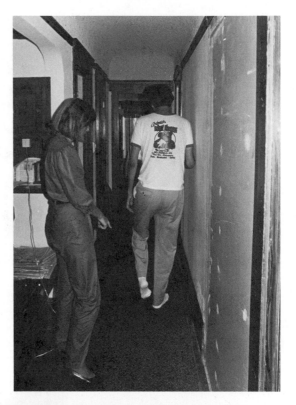

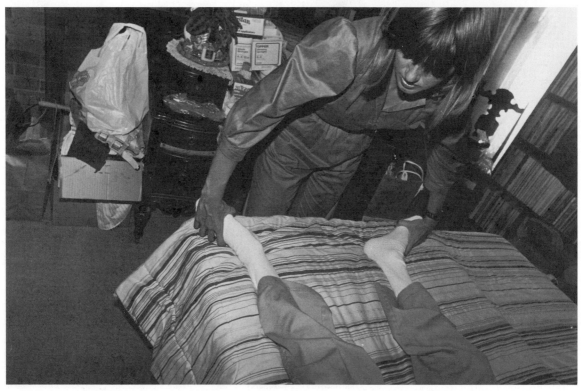

An occupational therapist from the
VNA also visits George.

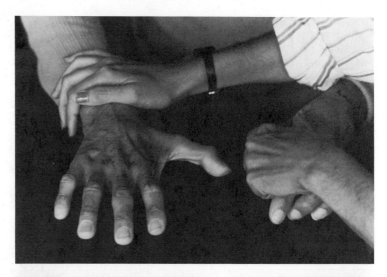

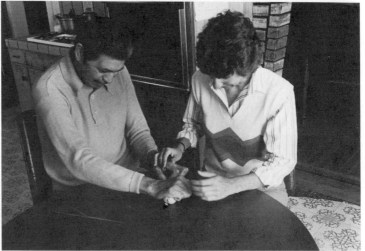

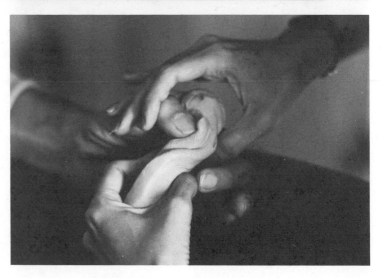

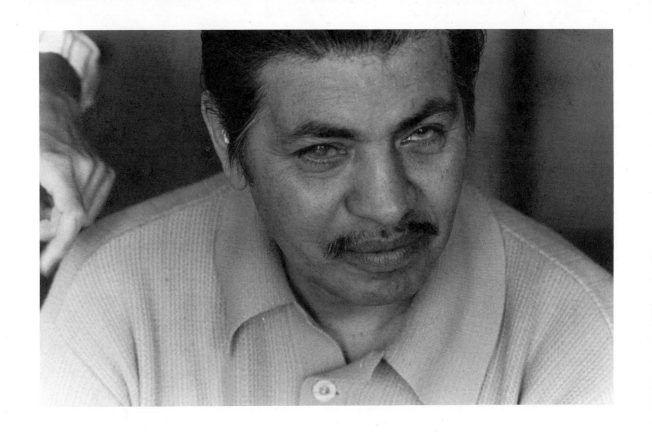

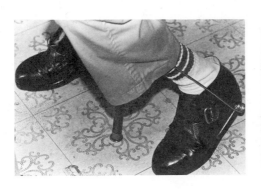

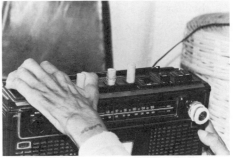

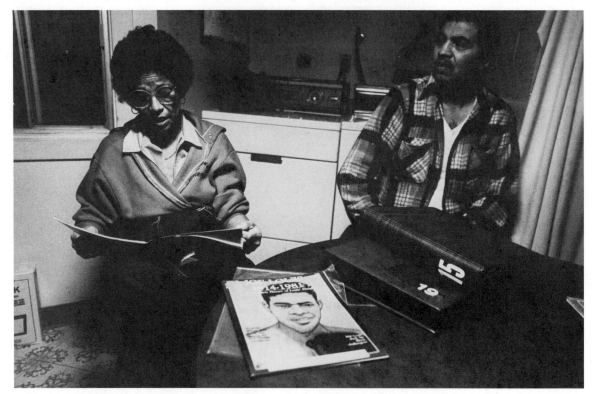

George is a boxing fan. Prior to his blindness, he had started a collection of boxing magazines and articles. After George became blind, Mrs. Estrada took over maintenance of the collection, filing news clippings and fight announcements in numerous binders until she, too, became interested in boxing.

It was evident that the collection had not lost any significance to George merely because he could not see it; Mrs. Estrada's cataloging and verbal descriptions kept it alive for him. He could refer to specific volumes and articles. Their joint enthusiasm for boxing was a bond between them.

George could recount the history of media coverage of boxing, from radio to television. He claimed emphatically that television had destroyed boxing. He spoke of the artistry of live radio broadcasters who could evoke through verbal description alone the intensity of a boxing match. George now hears boxing on a subscription radio service for the blind. Some of these programs are well done, he says, and they recall for him the earlier days of radio.

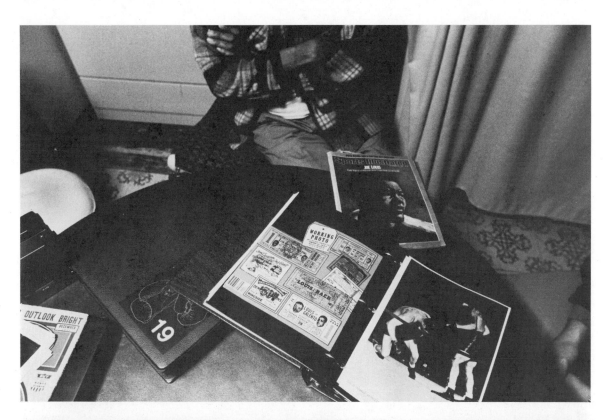

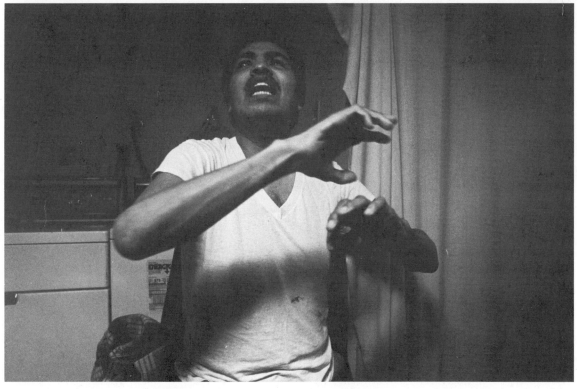

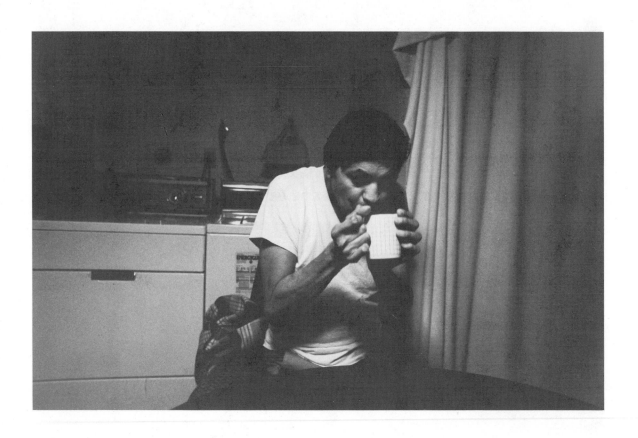

24

MENTAL ILLNESS AND THE FAMILY

Catherine A. Chesla, RN, DNSc

P sychiatric literature has long acknowledged the significance of the family group to the health and illness of family members. As a result, there is much clinical and research literature on which to build a solid base of concepts, theories, measurement strategies, and care approaches to the family unit. This chapter discusses the family and mental illness, particularly schizophrenia, in situations that apply to almost any clinical setting: Family burden, family communication patterns, and family meanings.

Catherine Chesla has practiced psychiatric nursing and family therapy in inpatient and community settings for over ten years. She is currently investigating family care of the chronically mentally ill at the School of Nursing at the University of California at San Francisco, and is interested in interpretative studies of family health and family caregiving relationships.

Introduction

Care for the mentally ill has shifted from the hospital to the community and has established the family as the primary resource for many chronically mentally ill persons (Goldstein, Doane, 1982). Some of these families care for the mentally ill member directly in the home, and others oversee the care from a greater distance, helping the ill member move through complex systems of care, advocating for his or her needs, and filling in gaps that inevitably emerge.

Research on families of the mentally ill has increased in the past five years, in part because scientists saw the family managing care that was previously provided in state institutions and began to wonder how they were doing. Families themselves began to organize and investigate their informational and programmatic needs. In addition, dramatic findings regarding the influence that families can have on the course of the illness emerged, fueling new research and treatment efforts (Goldstein, Doane, 1982; Hatfield, 1979a).

Research on families that care for a mentally ill member can instruct health care providers who work with families in relation to other health problems. Dilemmas are often created because the illness is chronic and debilitating, requires much family attention and support, and is disruptive to family routines. These same dilemmas are faced by any family that must cope with chronic illness of mental or physical origin.

In this chapter, central themes in the research on families of the mentally ill are traced. Five themes are highlighted:

1. What are the burdens for families that provide care for a mentally ill member?

2. How do families respond, in their attitudes and actions, to living closely with a mentally ill member?

3. What do these families need to help them with their situations?

4. What evidence do we have that the family contributes to the onset of mental illness?

5. How does the family influence the course of mental illness?

Within each section, the research addressing the central question is reviewed, and central problems with that research are discussed. In the final section, family intervention programs are reviewed, and implications for future care of families of the mentally ill are discussed.

Most research on mental illness and the family has focused on families whose ill member has schizophrenia. Although families that cope with major affective disorders, personality disorders, and neuroses also present important problems to the family practitioner, more information is available about families that cope with schizophrenia. This chapter reflects this bias in the literature as well as the author's interest in the impact of schizophrenia on the family.

Scope

Estimating the numbers of families that live with a mentally ill member is difficult. National counts are unavailable, thus figures are based on state or county population-based studies. Goldman (1982) estimates that 65% of the 1.5 million mental patients discharged to the community each year return to the family. Approximately half of these return to spouses, and the other half live with parents or other relatives. The chronically mentally ill, those with severe or persistent psychiatric disorders that inhibit their ability to function in the community, comprise about one-fourth of the total number of all mentally ill who live with relatives (Goldman, Gattozzi, Taube, 1981).

Family Burden

Family burden research describes some of the difficulties experienced by families that live with a mentally ill member. *Objective burden* is the disruption of family routine, employment, social and leisure activities, and relations with those outside of the family. Some studies additionally include financial costs and assessment of family members' physical and mental health (Creer, Sturt, Wykes, 1982; Grad, Sainsbury, 1963; Pai, Kapur, 1981; Thompson, Doll, 1982). *Subjective burden* is the family's assessment of the problems it has living with a mentally ill member. Dimensions of subjective burden include feelings of distress, embarrassment, and resentment and loss of control resulting from the ongoing responsibility of caring for an ill member.

Burden Levels in Alternate Forms of Treatment

The central puzzle of family burden research has been the policy question of how much family burden results from different forms of care. Alternatives to traditional hospital care have been compared to normal inpatient care for their relative impact.

In the earliest reported burden study, Grad and Sainsbury (1963), during two years of study, found that families served by community services had significantly less relief of burden than families served by hospital-based care. Two elements of burden that contributed significantly in discriminating the two forms of care were mental health of the family and financial costs. In families that started out severely burdened, relief was almost equal in the two programs.

Subsequent studies that compared brief versus long-term hospitalization (Hertz, Edicott, Spitzer, 1976; Platt, Hirsch, 1981) failed to find differences in degree of burden placed on families by different treatment programs. In randomized, controlled clinical trials, discharge of the patient to the home within 8 days of admission did not result in greater subjective or objective burden to the families than did standard hospitalization over periods of 14 weeks (Platt,

Hirsch, 1981) to 24 weeks (Hertz et al, 1976). These findings contradict Grad and Sainsbury's results in that no additional burden was imposed by a greater percentage of care occurring in the community.

In more recent studies, families of patients treated in the community are significantly less burdened than those treated in hospital programs (Pai, Kapur, 1981; Reynolds, Hoult, 1984). Grad and Sainsbury's finding has never been duplicated and may have been due to the patient population used in their study (they included elderly with dementia) or to the unique nature of the treatments studied (both were a mix of hospital and community treatment).

Reynolds and Hoult (1984) found that a multifaceted community program modeled on Stein and Test's Training in Community Living program (1980) resulted in significantly less subjective burden and in better coping for families than did traditional hospital care and follow-up. The 60 families randomly assigned to community treatment also reported less objective burden, but the differences were not significant. Superior outcomes in community care were attributed to the constant availability of a multidisciplinary staff and to better communication of program information and support to families. Interestingly, nearly all of the families from both treatment groups felt that future hospitalization could be avoided if professional consultation similar to that offered in the community-based program were available on a 24-hour basis.

Home visits and consistent support and education of families by nurses compared favorably with hospital care in terms of family burden and level of patient social function in a study conducted in India (Pai, Kapur, 1981). Patients presenting for admission who both lived with families and were diagnosed for the first time as schizophrenic were alternately assigned to one of the two programs. Fifty-four patients and families were followed for six months. Although burden decreased and social functioning improved in both groups, families receiving home care showed consistently better results. The authors concluded that home care relieved family anxiety and allowed them to learn how to care for their family member through direct teaching and modeling.

Reductions in burden caused by patient symptoms, odd behaviors, physical strains of the family, and disruptions to household routine and family members' personal lives were achieved in a home-care program directed at family needs at the time of hospital discharge (Smith, 1969). Significantly fewer burdens were reported by families that participated in this program than by families that had only normal follow-up care. This study underlines the consistent finding that flexible, home-based care reduces burden in a way that traditional care and outpatient follow-up does not.

Levels of Family Burden

Questions about family burden that are more relevant to clinicians include: How burdened are these families? How does their assessment of problems match with objective measures? Do patient characteristics, such as age, diagnosis, or duration of illness, influence the family's level of burden? Intervention programs and purely descriptive studies of family burden will be used to answer these questions. Five descriptive studies of family burden are summarized in Table 24-1. All five studies examine varying concepts of burden in large samples of families that take primary responsibility for a mentally ill member.

Substantial numbers of families report burden related to the care of their mentally ill member: 70% to 80% of families report some objective burden. Hoening and Hamilton (1966) found 76% reported adverse effects on finances, health, or general well-being in the household, and 60% found patient behaviors disturbing. Similarly, in families studied by Creer et al (1982), more were burdened by caring for the ill members' self-

care, social, and recreational needs than by the patients' difficult or embarrassing behaviors.

In intervention programs, family objective burden at intake was similar to that reported previously, but it dropped substantially by the conclusion of treatment or by the time of follow-up. For example, the percentage of families burdened decreased from 75% at intake to 25% for the community treatment group and 38% for the hospital treatment group (Reynolds, Hoult, 1984). Similar reductions in burden were achieved in all treatment programs (Pai, Kapur, 1981; Grad, Sainsbury, 1966; Platt, Hirsch, 1981).

Subjective burden, the family's evaluation of its feelings about its situation, or the emotional cost of caring for an ill member, was less prevalent than objective burden. The percentage of families that felt they experienced no burden because of living with a mentally ill relative ranged from 23% (Thompson, Doll, 1982) to 60% (Creer et al, 1982). Disparity of reports of subjective and objective burden may have been due to the family's denial of discomfort or to reluctance to report distress that was acknowledged privately.

Correlates of Family Burden

Extensive evaluation of the correlates of burden remains to be completed. Two factors—the prevalence of symptomatology and behavior problems in the ill member—consistently demark the highly burdened family (Creer et al, 1982; Grad, Sainsbury, 1966; Hertz et al, 1976; Thompson, Doll, 1982). Most projects combined measures of patient symptoms and functioning, making a separate examination of these distinct concepts impossible. The general point remains, however, that symptomatology and/or behavior problems in patients increase the disruption in family routines and in individual members' personal lives.

Few other patient characteristics correlate with measures of burden. Patient age has been

Table 24–1 Descriptive Studies of Family Burden

Author	Families of	Sample Size	Objective (O) and Subjective (S) Burden Dimensions		Period Studied
Hoening and Hamilton, 1966	Chronic schizophrenics	62	O:	a. Adverse effects on household: finances, health, children b. Patient disturbing behaviors	Past four years
			S:	Global rating of S	
Robin, Copas, and Freeman-Browne, 1979	Formerly hospitalized schizophrenic, neurotic, and depressed patients	154	O:	a. Problem patient behaviors b. Family health c. Family need for help	Discharge and five to eight years postdischarge
Creer, Sturt, and Wykes, 1982	Long-term mental health patients	52	O&S:	a. Patient self-care needs b. Symptoms c. Problem behaviors	Present (variable time postdischarge)
			S:	a. Attitudes about patient	
Thompson and Doll, 1982	Discharged state hospital patients	125	O:	a. Family finances b. Disruption to family routine c. Patient supervision problems	six months postdischarge
			S:	Family: a. Embarrassment b. Resentment c. Feeling trapped d. Feeling overloaded e. Extruding patient	
Runions and Prudo, 1982	Mental health support group	70	O:	a. Problem patient behaviors b. Degree of difficulty managing patient behaviors	Time of survey

positively related (Grad, Sainsbury, 1968), negatively related (Hoening, Hamilton, 1966), and unrelated (Thompson, Doll, 1982) to burden measures. Burden levels were consistently found to be independent of patient gender, marital status, and diagnosis (Grad, Sainsbury, 1968; Robin, Copas, Freeman-Browne, 1979).

More central to this review is the question of what is most burdensome to these families? The issue is difficult to characterize adequately because each project approached the question in a unique way. A fair summary is that disruption in family routine and financial losses were the major contributors to objective burden. Subjective burdens mentioned most often were concern about the future and feelings of being overloaded.

Issues in Burden Research

Questions that have not been addressed in relation to family burden are what it means for the family to care for its ill member and how the family manages this responsibility over time. Researchers have formulated questions in a negative fashion, assuming burdens, problems, and troubles accompany family caregiving. Neither the positive aspects of caring for a loved one nor the ways families cope with the situation have received adequate attention. Some recognition of the positive aspects of care are evident in the work of Creer et al (1982), who label family care "support" rather than burden. They make explicit their observation that families describe the care of a loved one in terms of concern rather than in economic, exchange, or suffering terms. Other authors provide adequate descriptive data to back up the observations of Creer et al (Hoening, Hamilton, 1966; Robin, Copas, Freeman-Browne, 1979; Thompson, Doll, 1982).

Family burden literature fails to examine how the burden reported by families affects the well-being of the family as a unit or the members individually. Investigation of family outcomes is needed to validate that families identified as burdened are in some way different from those that are not so identified.

Family Attitudes and Behavioral Response

Kreisman and Joy's (1974) comprehensive review of the literature of family response to the mental illness of a relative summarized the attitudinal and behavioral responses of families to the diagnosis and treatment of the mentally ill relative and the effects that family attitudes had on patient outcomes. Their review remains current because so few investigations of family attitudes have been completed since their review.

Shame and social rejection of the patient were the two most common themes investigated in family attitude research (Kreisman, Joy, 1974). Descriptive reports suggest that most felt sympathy and understanding; many were confused or puzzled by their member's behavior; and only a minority felt anger, fear, guilt, or shame. In addition, few families reported that they acted in ways that might indicate shame or rejection, such as isolating the patient or misrepresenting the patient's problem to people outside the family.

Social rejection, a second major theme, was examined in reports of social distance, visiting patterns, and the family's willingness to care for the patient at home. Although no firm conclusions could be drawn, association with the mentally ill increased willingness for closeness with the patient. In a number of studies, education was positively correlated and age was negatively correlated with acceptance of close physical relations with the ill member. Visiting patterns, a sign of family attachment, were maintained by all but one-fifth of families studied, even when hospitalization lasted for years. Willingness to accept the patient back into the home after hospitalization was generally high: 65% to 95% of families welcomed their members home.

To summarize, although researchers selected themes of shame and rejection to guide their work on families of the mentally ill, these themes were not prominent in the families themselves. In general, more positive attitudes were expressed, and accepting behaviors indicative of these attitudes were demonstrated.

The influence of family attitudes on patient outcomes was less frequently studied. A positive accepting stance on the part of the family was generally associated with lower rates of rehospitalization, although not consistently so (Kreisman, Joy, 1974). Expectations placed on the patient to perform social roles were positively associated with higher social functioning but had no impact on readmission rates. Kreisman and Joy criticize attempts to find simple relationships between family attitudes and outcomes because many reality factors, such as family income and social resources, play important roles in determining outcomes.

Classic Studies of Family Response

Two classic studies of family response to the mental illness of a relative deserve special mention. Clausen and Yarrow (1955) documented the natural history of wives' discovery and acceptance of mental illness in their spouses. Creer and Wing (1975) examined the day-to-day effects of living with a schizophrenic family member. Both these studies provide methodologic and substantive areas for further research on family responses but have received much less attention and replicative research than they deserve.

Clausen and Yarrow (1955) were the first to attempt to document the meaning that mental illness had for a family member. The study was conducted in the mid-1950s, long before the in-crease in public education about mental illness and before deinstitutionalization was widespread. This may account for the wives' view that mental illness was something to be ignored, grudgingly admitted, hidden from friends, financially accommodated, and eventually, socially accepted into their lives.

Creer and Wing (1975), in a sample of 80 families, studied family practices that accommodate a schizophrenic member. Two behavior patterns were most troublesome to the families: (1) seclusiveness and noncommunicativeness; and (2) extremely active, socially embarrassing behavior. Families coped with these behaviors by trial and error, and although the solutions were quite individual, an indirect, positive approach to the patient seemed most successful. For example, one mother found that criticizing her son's appearance accomplished little, but setting clean clothes in easy reach encouraged him to dress appropriately. Families learned when to ignore unusual behavior and when to try to shape it to a more acceptable form. Creer and Wing found families felt guilty, anxious, depressed, and frustrated with their situations. They also discovered that families generally coped in ways that allowed them to minimize the patient's handicaps and to achieve a quality of life that included both pleasures and disappointments.

Current Research on Family Attitudes

Remarkably little research on family attitudes has been conducted since Kreisman and Joy's review. Two notable exceptions are Rose's (1983) investigation of family understandings of the initial treatment episode and Goldstein's (1979) reexamination of the relationship between attitudes and patient outcomes.

Rose documents the reluctance of families to identify their member as mentally ill. In her in-depth study of seven families from the point of diagnosis through hospitalization, she found families tolerated, sometimes angrily and impatiently, bizarre and inappropriate behavior for long periods of time before seeking help. Diagnosis of mental illness was a turning point for many of these families, allowing them to recognize the member as seriously ill. Hospitalization brought with it self-evaluation and a search for past behaviors that may have contributed to the patient's condition. These families found major differences in psychiatric as opposed to medical treatment. The intangibility of the illness and the treatment made families reluctant to communicate the problem to friends and neighbors, from whom they feared misunderstanding. Their hopes for the future were for the patient to return to normal. As hospitalization progressed and dramatic changes in the patient were not seen, thoughts about the future became more guarded. Previous beliefs about mental illness, notions of cause and cure, fear of stigma, and caution about the future influenced how these families defined their current situation. Rose's study is an excellent example of one way to increase understanding of the family experience in the early phases of the mental illness of a relative.

Goldstein (1979), in a study of 30 schizophrenic and borderline patients, discovered several family attitudinal variables related to improved patient outcomes in an inpatient setting. The degree of parental help-seeking prior to hospitalization and willingness to be involved with treatment positively correlated with improved outcomes. In addition, a positive attitude toward hospitalization, realistic expectations about outcome, and a good relationship between parent and patient—variables measured at completion of treatment—correlated with improved outcomes. The aut..or admits that positive attitudes at completion may, in fact, have been caused by the improved patient status. The significance of the study lies in the fact that family attitudes changed during the course of treatment and may have been influenced by social work interventions during the course of their family member's inpatient treatment.

Research on Family Needs

The needs of families of schizophrenics have been documented through systematic study (Hatfield, 1979a, 1979b; Kint, 1977; Platman, 1983), through the impressions of clinicians who have worked with these families (Bernheim, Lewine, Beale, 1982), and through the experiential reports of families themselves (Weschler, 1972; Wilson, 1968; Hibler, 1978; Walsh, 1985). There is surprising consistency in the different sources of information on what these families feel they need.

Among families surveyed systematically, most wanted information on how to cope with specific patient problems and how to understand patient symptoms (Creer et al, 1982; Hatfield, 1979a; Kint, 1977). Families feel information needs most acutely because these needs are poorly addressed by systems of care. For example, Creer and Wing (1975) learned that none of the families in their study received advice from health professionals about actions they could take to inhibit problem patient behaviors.

Several explanations can be offered for why the information needs of these families go unmet. Most obvious is the bias against any kind of family involvement in care because of the family's presumed etiologic role in the onset of schizophrenia (Lamb, Oliphant, 1978). Many training programs continue to use theories that implicate the family, although research supporting these theories is far from conclusive. Another reason for the lack of information exchange is the fact that professionals lack the knowledge themselves on how to cope with day-to-day problems. Only one systematic study has attempted to document the in-home practices that are helpful to families and patients alike (Creer, Wing, 1975). Professionals have documented the practices that families in their care have found helpful (Bernheim et al, 1982), but these limited resources are not widely known or applied (Creer et al, 1982). Finally, given the current state of knowledge, many of the questions posed by families regarding symptoms and behavior expectations cannot be answered (Torrey, 1983).

The secondary needs of families are more varied. Leading the list are (1) financial relief; (2) someone to talk to who understands the disorder; and (3) respite care for brief periods of time (Creer et al, 1982; Hatfield, 1979b; Kint, 1977). These financial, emotional, and social relief needs match the aspects of care that families felt to be most burdensome, that is, upset in daily routine and finances.

From practitioners' clinical impressions and from families' personal accounts, the need for recognition and respect for the family as primary caregiver is expressed. Dramatic examples of disrespect for the family's feelings are given by Weschler (1972) and Wilson (1968). The families were, at one point in their child's illness, directly blamed for the disorder. This practice, according to more recent accounts (Lamb, Oliphant, 1978; Torrey, 1982), has not changed. The most typical stance for mental health professionals to take is to encourage separation of the schizophrenic member and the family (Hibler, 1978). This stance is disrespectful of the commitment families feel for their members and provides them with untenable options.

Families, as primary caregivers, ask for participation in all aspects of the ill member's treatment. They see stark differences in the ways families of the mentally ill as opposed to families of the physically ill are treated (Kint, 1977). For example, next of kin are the first to be notified in the case of physical illness, but in cases of psychiatric illness, any information regarding patient status is considered confidential. Even in instances where permission has been granted to release information, nondisclosure is the rule (Torrey, 1982). Although the responsibility for care often falls to the family after the patient is released from the hospital, families are seldom involved in the planning for discharge and sometimes are not even notified of impending discharge (Leavitt, 1975). Families ask, in increasingly more organized ways (Hatfield, 1979b), for a legitimate role in the care of their

family member, regardless of the system of care he or she enters.

The research on the needs of families of schizophrenics is fairly sketchy and unsystematic. All of the surveys have been done with families that already participate in support groups. The families surveyed may differ dramatically from those that do not choose to join such groups. The needs, at least for this subset of families, are for increased information, involvement, respect, and occasional respite.

The Family and Schizophrenia

Onset

Early efforts to prevent schizophrenia led researchers to examine family traits and interactions that potentially caused the illness. Four major family theorists, Bowen (1960), Bateson (1968), Lidz (1965), and Wynne (1981), provided theoretical justification for this research. Each suggested that a particular pattern of family relations might cause schizophrenia in a family member. Although many family factors, such as patterns of power, role relationships, and family structure, were thought to contribute to the disorder, only disordered family communication has been consistently linked to schizophrenia in a family member.

Several reviews conclude that communication in families of schizophrenics is unclear, disordered, or identifiably different from that in normal families or in families who have members with other psychiatric disorders (Falloon et al, 1984; Goldstein, Doane, 1982; Goldstein, Rodnick, 1975; Liem, 1980). Families observed during activities such as problem-solving, storytelling, decision-making, and therapy have been consistently discriminated as schizophrenic or nonschizophrenic families based on the adequacy and clarity of their communication. Although researchers often assume that the unclear communication found in these families causes the illness, the reverse may be the case.

Families living with a schizophrenic member may develop communication problems.

The most consistent line of research has been that of Singer and Wynne on family "communication deviance" (Wynne, Singer, 1963a, b; Singer, Wynne, 1965a, b; Wynne, 1981). *Communication deviance* is the unclear or incomplete communication of ideas and perceptions. Families with communication deviance cannot focus on one subject, and they have interactions filled with distractions and incomplete ideas. The communication deviance model suggests that genetic makeup predisposes the individual to schizophrenia, and family factors influence its expression. Factors proposed as increasing the risk of schizophrenia in offspring are family styles of communicating, styles of relating, affective tone, and family structure. Research on this paradigm has focused exclusively on styles of communicating.

In an early project, Singer and Wynne (1965a, b) attempted to predict the diagnosis, degree, and type of thought disorder in a group of 35 psychiatrically disordered young adults. Predictions were based on observations of parents' and siblings' performances on projective tests. Investigators were blind to patient diagnosis. Family communication style proved to be an accurate predictor of the offspring's diagnosis, the severity of symptomatic ego disorganization, and the form of disordered thinking.

In a second study, the investigators blindly rated communication in parents of normal, neurotic, borderline, and schizophrenic patients and confirmed their central hypothesis that the severity of communication disorder in parents is significantly related to the severity of psychiatric disorder in offspring (Wynne, 1981). The sample consisted of 114 families composed of a father, mother, index offspring aged 15 to 45, and one sibling. Families completed a battery of tests, including individual projective tests from which communication deviance was rated. Scores for parents of normal and neurotic offspring differed significantly from those for parents of schizophrenics. The range of scores for parents of borderline patients overlapped the other two groups. These data suggest a continuous, direct relationship between parental communication deviance and severity of illness in offspring.

Problems in Communication Research

Three major problems in communication deviance research urge caution in accepting the conclusions: (1) study design; (2) sample description; and (3) method of data collection. The studies conducted by Wynne and Singer examined previously diagnosed schizophrenics. Although the raters were blind to the diagnoses, families were not. Patterns of communication may be reflective of living with the disease rather than of causing the disease. Prospective studies of families at risk for schizophrenia are needed.

A second problem is that families tested are poorly described. Largely ignored are the patient and family characteristics that correlate with levels of communication deviance and give a more balanced picture of who these families are. Patient age and premorbid status, which have been shown to influence family interaction (Goldstein, Rodnick, 1975; Lieber, 1977), are not examined. Family structure or stage of development are equally ignored. Clear descriptions of these samples are needed.

Finally, it is difficult to judge whether laboratory ratings of the family members' communication with an individual tester reflect the way they actually communicate in everyday life. Two studies of family interaction suggest that face-to-face communication between members can be used to discriminate schizophrenic from nonschizophrenic families (Wild, Shapiro, Goldenberg, 1975; Behrens, Rosenthal, Chodoff, 1968). In contrast, Lieber (1977) found that ratings of family interaction data did not discriminate between members with a high, medium, or low risk for schizophrenia. The latter study suggests that concern about the generalizability of communication deviance ratings across situations and relationships is warranted.

Course of Illness

While American researchers were engaged in communication deviance research, a group of British researchers were investigating the impact of the family's effect on the course of a member's schizophrenia. It is striking that these two parallel lines of research remained distinct, separated by their differing foci, that is, etiology as opposed to course of the disorder, and communication structure as opposed to emotional quality of communication. Only in the descriptive and intervention research has both the nature of the communication and the quality of the emotional overtones in the interaction been examined together (Doane et al, 1981; Doane et al, 1985; Falloon, Boyd, McGill, 1984).

Families that are highly critical, hostile, and overinvolved with their schizophrenic member have been designated as "high expressed emotion" families. Schizophrenics who live with high expressed emotion families are at greater risk for a worsened course of the illness than those who come from families with low expressed emotion (Brown, Birley, Wing, 1972; Vaughn, Leff, 1976; Vaughn et al, 1984). A brief review of this research follows.

In a prospective study of 101 schizophrenic patients and their families, Brown, Birley, and Wing (1972) found that the best single predictor of relapse in a nine-month postdischarge period was a measure of expressed emotion in the family at the time of discharge. Numerous factors—such as being male, unemployed prior to hospitalization, more disturbed in behavior or symptoms, or nonaccepting of hospitalization—also independently correlated with relapse at significant levels. The relationship between the family's expressed emotion and relapse remained when any other single correlate of relapse was controlled. Medications and limited contact between the patient and family protected the patient from relapse in high expressed emotion homes.

In two replications of the expressed emotion research, the relationship between family emotion and the course of the illness has held. Relapse rates for schizophrenics from high expressed emotion families were two to three times higher than their counterparts from low expressed emotion homes (Vaughn, Leff, 1981; Vaughn et al, 1984). In all cases, patients had an improved relapse rate if they spent less than 35 hours per week with the family and if they took medications regularly. In one instance, both a low amount of contact and regular medication were required to reduce relapse rates below 70% in high expressed emotion homes (Vaughn et al, 1984).

Descriptive research on family emotion consistently shows that high levels of criticism, hostility, and emotional overinvolvement place a patient at greater risk of relapse. Patient groups that appear most vulnerable are unmarried males with poor work histories. The protective effects of little interaction with the family and regular medication correlate uniformly with lowered relapse rates, yet these factors seem least influential in the most vulnerable group.

Issues in Expressed Emotion Research

A major criticism of this work is its focus on relapse as the key outcome variable. Although relapse or rehospitalization in schizophrenia is a significant event, psychologically, socially, and economically, the quality of life and the levels of social functioning during periods of remission are also important factors. Past research indicates that symptom level and functioning are not always parallel. Environments that foster high levels of social functioning are not always associated with the lowest rates of relapse (Platman, 1983); thus both factors must be examined if the true impact of an environment is to be known. In addition, low contact between the patient and the family may not be a protective factor against relapse but merely a distance that makes the family less aware of periods of symptomatology in the patient. In most studies, relapse was defined as rehospitalization, therefore patients who denied symptoms or withdrew from the family during symptomatic periods were not counted as relapses.

Risk of Illness

Prospective research on families at risk for schizophrenia in an offspring addresses the question of whether family interaction patterns precede the development of the disorder. The primary goal is to identify factors that allow for early identification and preventive intervention with those at risk of developing psychiatric disorders, including schizophrenia. Theoretical models employed in risk research include genetic, sociocultural, and interactional models (Goodman, 1984). The smaller body of research on interactional variables is focused on here. The reader is referred to reviews of the genetic and sociocultural research (Goodman, 1984; Garmezy, 1979a, b).

In a prospective study of schizophrenia, adolescents exhibiting behaviors similar to those found in histories of schizophrenics were considered to be at risk (Garmezy, 1979b). Families with adolescents who displayed patterns of aggressive, antisocial, conflictual, passively negative, or withdrawn behaviors were followed prospectively for five years. Follow-up data on these families provides beginning evidence that both expressed emotion and communication deviance patterns are predictive of schizophrenic onset.

Fifty-two of the 65 families originally inducted in a UCLA family study completed the five-year follow-up (Doane et al, 1981). At intake, individual psychologic assessments of the index child (age 15–18) and each parent, as well as family interactional assessments, were made. Family communication deviance and emotional style were statistically significant predictors of schizophrenia spectrum disorders in offspring five years later (Doane et al, 1981). The investigators noted a substantial number of "false positives"—parents who scored high on either expressed emotion or communication deviance and whose offspring were not diagnosed with schizophrenia.

Prediction of the schizophrenic spectrum outcome was substantially improved when measures of communication and emotion were combined. Outcome was correctly predicted 100% of the time when the two extremes of the two measures, poor communication and emotional style or good communication and benign affect, were considered. All of the children from the former and none from the latter group exhibited schizophrenia spectrum disorders. Offspring from families with only one risk factor had low rates of illness, suggesting that the two factors in combination create the substantial risk (Doane et al, 1981).

Issues in Risk Research

The UCLA project gives solid evidence that communication and affective patterns in families, long correlated with schizophrenic onset and relapse, do precede the onset of schizophrenic spectrum disorders in one sample of families. A number of qualifications must be attached to this finding. First, true schizophrenic outcome was noted in only one case; the remaining diagnoses were within the schizophrenia spectrum , which ma y or may not represent a continuum with schizophrenia. Second, the temporal priorit y of family patterns with illness onset must be questioned. Parental style of communication and affective tone may have been reactive to adolescent behavioral disturbance in this sample. Also, one must question whether communication disturbances and affective styles that have been labeled as expressed emotion are unique to families of schizophrenics. Families with other forms of mental illness or without psychopathology have not been sufficiently studied. Some believe these patterns of communication and affect are more indicative of chronic illness in general than of schizophrenia (Falloon et al, 1984). Further comparative research is needed to resolve this issue.

Family and Affective Disorders

Family factors influencing the onset and course of affective disorders have received much less attention than family factors in schizophrenia. The reasons for this are not clear but might include the fact that family theories initially evolved with schizophrenics, and therefore research continued to focus on those families. Additionally, the study of affective disorders within individual biologic models may have been so productive (NIMH, 1983) that the impetus to shift the focus to the larger social system of the family has been lacking.

Risk of Illness

Studies of vulnerability to depression in the offspring of depressed parents are beginning to reach completion (Strauss, Harding, Weissman, 1984). In a recent comprehensive review of research on children of parents with major affective disorders, several conclusions were reached. First, children of depressive adults show a high rate of impairment in several realms: behavior problems, school problems, and clinical status. The rate of psychiatric diagnosis in these children was found to be approximately 40% (Beardslee et al, 1983).

Although 11 cross-sectional studies and 5 longitudinal studies of children of depressed adults demonstrate fairly consistently that children are significantly impaired and that the nature of their problems is wide ranging, one must question what these impairments mean. Are they long lasting, and do children with psychiatric illness experience disability as adults? Answers to these questions are not available, and follow-up studies of these children into adulthood are needed (Beardslee et al, 1983). Genetic, neurochemical, neurophysiologic, and clinical studies begin to suggest that there are continuities between childhood and adult depression (NIMH, 1983). The findings are far from conclusive, and thus additional research must be com-

pleted before children of depressed parents can be considered at risk for adult psychiatric disorders.

Childhood Relations of Depressed Adults

Retrospective studies of adults diagnosed with major affective disorders can provide clues to family influences in the onset of depression. In general, these studies suggest that the childhood family relations of depressed adults differ from those of nondepressed controls. Depressed adults recall their relations as being less satisfactory and rate their parents as less caring and more overprotective. A summary of retrospective studies can be found in Table 24-2.

A study of the childhood experiences of depressed women showed results largely consistent with the general findings (Jacobsen, Fasman, DiMascio, 1975). Depressed women and one family member were recruited from inpatient rolls and outpatient clinics and asked about their childhood experiences. They were found to have poorer quality childhood relations than a comparable sample of nondepressed women. Depressed women reported more abusive, shaming, rejecting, and overprotective experiences and also received less tolerance and affection from their parents.

Parker (1979) concludes from three separate studies that depressed adults recall their parental care in a characteristic fashion. Outpatients diagnosed with neurotic depression, when compared with a matched, nondepressed group, recalled their parents as significantly less caring and more overprotective. In a second study, parental ratings of outpatients diagnosed with bipolar affective disorder were not significantly different from a matched, nondepressed group. Parker (1979) and others (Abrahams, Whitlock, 1969; NIMH, 1983) note the importance of differentiating subclassifications of depressed groups in research because their clinical and family features differ. In this third study, Parker asked a normal population of graduate students to rate parental behavior and correlated this rating with self-reports of depression. He found that depression in this nonclinical group was associated with parental overprotection and recollections of parents who were less caring.

Raskin et al (1971) found that normal adults had more positive memories of their parents' childrearing practices and attitudes than did depressed inpatients. Depressed adults' memories of childrearing were clearly discriminated by reports of (1) less positive involvement, and interest in the child's life; (2) negative control, or parents' efforts to control their child in ways that were potentially psychologically harmful, such as control through hostility, intrusiveness, guilt, and anxiety; and (3) lax discipline, or parents who ignored misbehavior and failed to establish clear limits or rules in the family. A second project found similar patterns of parenting were recalled by depressed adults, but in this instance the findings were validated by an independent rating of parenting practices documented in records and by siblings and spouses (Crook, Raskin, Eliot, 1981).

Issues in Retrospective Research

The limitations of retrospective studies of depression must be noted. Depressed persons, as a symptom of their illness, may tend to emphasize the negative aspects of their experiences and relationships (Parker, 1979). Attempts to control for this bias were made by assessing patients after they had been in treatment for a period of time (Parker, 1979; Raskin et al, 1971; Crook et al, 1981) or by using an independent observer's rating of the childhood experience, based on information from sources other than the depressed individual (Crook et al, 1981; Jacobsen et al, 1975). A second limitation of this research is that although negative parent–child experiences are implied as etiologic in depression, parents of the depressed adults may in fact have

Table 24–2   Descriptive Research on Adult Depressives: Childhood Relations with Parents

Author	Subjects	Sample Size	Dimension of Relations Measured
Abrahams and Whitlock, 1969	Depressed inpatients	152	Interview: self-report of quality of childhood relations with parents
	Matched, medical outpatients	152	
Jacobson, Fasman, and DiMascio, 1975	Depressed women		Interview with patient and family: negative and positive parental attitudes and behaviors
	Inpatient	347	
	Outpatient	114	
	Comparison group	198	
Parker, 1979	Bipolar manic-depressives	70	Parental bonding instrument (Parker et al, 1978)/ Parental caring and protectiveness
	Matched controls	70	
	"Neurotic" depressives	52	
	Matched controls	52	
	Normal sample	242	
Raskin et al, 1971	Depressed inpatients	548	Child Report of Parental Behaviors Inventory (CRPBI)/ Parental involvement, control, strategies, discipline
	Normal adults	254	
Crook, Raskin and Elliot, 1981	Depressed inpatients	714	CRPBI
	Normal adults	387	

been responding to a child who was already negative, or depressed.

Family Treatment Programs

Model Family Intervention Programs

Interventions with families of the mentally ill have focused primarily on families of schizophrenics. These family-focused treatment programs have repeatedly produced better results when compared with individual treatment programs in controlled clinical trials. These positive results argue for the expansion of family-based care to additional types of mental illnesses. Family programs targeted for other mental illnesses were not located. Interventions with families of schizophrenics can serve as models for programs to be developed for families coping with other mental disorders.

Four family intervention programs for families of schizophrenics are described here. Basic program parameters are described for each, and information on the relative effectiveness in preventing relapse and helping the family is described.

One of the earliest family intervention programs tested variable doses of phenothiazine injections in combination with six weeks of family crisis intervention counseling. Families of 104 schizophrenics were randomly assigned to one of four groups, who received high or low doses of prolixin and family or no psychosocial intervention. The goals of counseling were recognizing the event as psychosis, recognizing precipitants of the event, and planning for future stresses that might precipitate further psychosis (Goldstein et al, 1978).

Significantly lower relapse rates were found in the high dose family treatment group as compared with the low dose no treatment group. Relapse rates were 0% and 50% respectively. Examination of the data by type of treatment showed there was a significant (high dose) drug effect and a nonsignificant but positive effect from family therapy (Goldstein et al, 1978).

A British family intervention program addressed the risk factors that had been discovered in expressed emotion research (Leff et al, 1982). The aim was to reduce family expressed emotion or decrease the amount of contact between the schizophrenic patient and relatives. The program combined medication for the index patient with education, multiple family groups, and family therapy sessions.

Twenty-four families of schizophrenics were randomly assigned to the family intervention or to no treatment group. All schizophrenic members continued to receive their usual individual care. Participants in the family intervention program had significantly reduced relapse rates (Leff et al, 1982). Criticism was significantly reduced in the experimental group but not in the control group, and reduction in face-to-face contact was more successful in the experimental group.

The psychoeducational program designed by Anderson, Hogarty, and Reiss (1981) attempted to decrease the schizophrenic's vulnerability through medications and improve the stability of the family environment by addressing family anxiety, knowledge deficits, and management needs. This program differed from others because it focused on broad principles for living with a schizophrenic and on the family's response to this process. Direct training in communication or problem-solving skills was minimized.

The program was structured into four phases. First, the treatment team attempted to connect with the family, learn its interpretation of events, and establish a treatment alliance. The second comprised educating families about (1) the nature of the disorder; (2) the kinds of structure and distancing that are most beneficial to families; (3) communication; and (4) how to take care of family needs as well as patient needs. The third phase gave families the opportunity to apply this information to unique family problems in therapy sessions held every two to three weeks for a period of a year. The fourth phase was an additional two years of less intensive, less frequent sessions.

This program was tested with schizophrenics in high-risk homes, who were randomly assigned to family or individual interventions. At one year, 10% of the sample in the family treatment program relapsed as compared with 34% in individual treatment. Anticipated changes in the social functioning of clients were not achieved at the one year follow-up. A substantial number of patients in the family treatment program remained inactive and unemployed (Anderson et al, 1981).

Falloon, Boyd, and McGill (1984) focused on teaching families to manage the rehabilitation of a schizophrenic member. The program comprised communication training and problem-solving. Family treatment was contrasted with individual treatment administered according to an identical schedule: weekly meetings for 3 months, biweekly meetings for the next 6 months, and monthly visits for the last 15 months of the study.

Evaluation of this program with 36 high-risk families demonstrated superior results of the family treatment program as opposed to the individual treatment program (Falloon et al, 1984). At nine months, patients who were treated with family interventions had less symptomatology and substantially lower relapse rates (6%) than those in individual treatment (40%). Patient social adjustment was markedly better in family treatment with significantly fewer cases of behavior disturbance, medication noncompliance, and family distress. Employment rates for the two groups were equal (44%) at nine months, but substantial gains in employment, unparalleled by control patients, were made by the family program patients during the second year.

The family's social functioning and health were altered little by either treatment program. Family burden, however, was significantly reduced in the family treatment group. Seventy-eight percent of these families were burdened at

intake and only 17% were still burdened at nine months. Families receiving individual treatment showed an increase in burden in the same time period (Falloon et al, 1984). Examining the influence that family affective style had on the families' ability to incorporate new patterns, the investigators found that families with negative affective styles, that is, those that demonstrated more guilt induction, criticism, and intrusiveness in direct interaction with their mentally ill member, were less able to absorb the family interventions and had more difficulty coping with day-to-day stresses (Doane et al, 1985).

Implications for Family Treatment

Several components were included in all of the model family treatment programs and seem warranted in interventions with families who cope with mental illnesses:

1. Education about the nature of the disease, the expected symptomatology, and the course.

2. Information on the forms of treatment available, including medications, psychosocial treatments, and vocational rehabilitation.

3. Medication (when appropriate) for management of the patient's symptoms. Printed as well as verbal communication about the intent and side effects of medications should be available to families.

4. Guidance in identifying and managing the problems in daily living that arise when living with a family member who has a mental illness.

Additional interventions with families are suggested by practitioners who have worked with these families and by the families themselves. First, families want respectful treatment from health care providers. Many families must overcome a reluctance to seek help, which is based on past experience with caregivers who have blamed them for their family member's illness. Respectful communication of information and provision of opportunities for families to participate in the treatment decisions are warranted.

Families suggest that what they need most is information on how to handle the day-to-day problems that arise with the ill member. problems of living with a schizophrenic family member as well as strategies for managing these problems are documented to a limited extent and can be shared with families (Bernheim et al, 1982; Torrey, 1983; Walsh, 1985).

Problems with living with family members who have chronic psychiatric disabilities other than schizophrenia are less widely known. Certainly unique kinds of problems arise when the ill member has cycles of overactivity as in bipolar disorders or periods of self-destructiveness characteristic of borderline personality disorders. Unfortunately, the experiences of families living with these persons have not been examined. Professionals can be most helpful by taking a learning stance *with* the family. Helping members identify problems and work out solutions that fit the family's current patterns of living will be helpful in this relatively uncharted territory. In addition, families should be encouraged to participate in mutual support groups where practical knowledge, acquired by living with these mental illnesses, can be shared among families and professionals.

Summary

Chronic mental illness is a significant family concern as mentally ill family members frequently live at home rather than in institutions. The family burdens resulting from this caring have been reviewed along with the responses of families to caring for a mentally ill member. Family needs are appropriately addressed by nurses.

Issues for Further Investigation

1. What aspects of living with and caring for a mentally ill family member are most troublesome to the family?

2. What personal meanings and/or life circumstances influence families to care for a mentally ill family member at home?

3. How does a family care of a mentally ill member influence family health? Individual health? Are there particular individuals, such as spouses or mothers, who are at greater risk for health problems than other family members?

4. How does family care of a mentally ill member influence the family's work, social, and recreational patterns?

5. Which treatment interventions are most beneficial for the mentally ill member's and the family's health over time? Consider family level treatment, individual treatment, and residential care programs.

6. What aspects of the treatment programs for families of schizophrenics can be helpful for families with members who have other mental illnesses?

References

Abrahams MJ, Whitlock FA (1969): Childhood experience and depression. *Br J Psychiatry, 115*: 883–888.

Anderson CM, Hogarty G, Reiss DJ (1981): A psychoeducational program for families. In: *New Directions for Mental Health Services: New Developments in Interventions with Families of Schizophrenics*, Goldstein M (ed.). San Francisco: Jossey-Bass.

Bateson G et al (1968): Toward a theory of schizophrenia. In: *Communication, Family and Marriage*, Jackson D (ed.). Palo Alto, CA: Science and Behavior Books.

Beardslee WR et al (1983): Children of parents of major affective disorders. *Am J Psychiatry, 140*: 825–832.

Behrens ML, Rosenthal AJ, Chodoff P (1968): Communication in lower-class families of schizophrenics: Observations and findings. *Arch Gen Psychol, 18*: 680–696.

Bernheim KF, Lewine RJ, Beale CT (1982): *The Caring Family. Living with Mental Illness.* New York: Random House.

Bowen M (1960): A family concept of schizophrenia. In: *The Etiology of Schizophrenia*, Jackson D (ed.). New York: Basic Books.

Brown GW, Birley JTL, Wing JK (1972): Influence of family life on the course of schizophrenic disorders: A replication. *Br J Psychiatry, 121*: 241–258.

Clausen JA, Yarrow MR (1955): The impact of mental illness on the family. *J Soc Issues, 11*: 1–67.

Creer C, Sturt E, Wykes T (1982): The role of relatives. In: Long term community care: Experience in a London borough. *Psychological Medicine, Monograph Supplement, 2*, Wing SK (ed.).

Creer C, Wing JK (1975): Living with a schizophrenic patient. *Br J Hosp Med, 14*: 73–82.

Crook T, Raskin A, Eliot J (1981): Parent–child relationships and adult depression. *Child Dev, 52*: 950–957.

Doane JA et al (1985): Parental affective style and the treatment of schizophrenia. *Arch Gen Psychiatry, 42*: 34–42.

Doane JA, Goldstein MJ, Rodnick EH (1981): Parental patterns of affective style and the development of schizophrenia spectrum disorders. *Fam Process, 20*: 337–349.

Doane JA et al (1981): Parental communication deviance and affective style: Predictors of subsequent schizophrenia disorders in vulnerable adolescents. *Arch Gen Psychiatry, 38*: 679–685.

Falloon JRH, Boyd JL, McGill CW (1984): *Family Care of Schizophrenia.* New York: Guilford.

Garmezy N (1979a): Children at risk: The search for antecedents of schizophrenia: Part I. Conceptual models and research methods. *Schizophr Bull, 8*: 14–92.

Garmezy N (1979b): Children at risk: The search for antecedents of schizophrenia: Ongoing research programs, issues and interventions: Part II. *Schizophr Bull, 9*: 55–125.

Goldman HH (1982): Mental illness and family burden: A public health perspective. *Hosp Community Psychiatry, 33*(7): 557–560.

Goldman HH, Gattozzi AA, Taube CA (1981): Defining and counting the chronically mentally ill. *Hosp Community Psychiatry, 32*: 22–27.

Goldstein EG (1979): The influence of parental attitudes on psychiatric treatment outcome. *Soc Casework*, 350–359.

Goldstein MJ, Doane JA (1982): Family factors in the onset, course and treatment of schizophrenic disorders. An update on current research. *J Nerv Ment Dis, 170*(1): 692–700.

Goldstein MJ, Rodnick EH (1975): The family's contribution to the etiology of schizophrenia: Current status. *Schizophr Bull, 14*: 48–63.

Goldstein MJ (1978): Drug and family therapy in the after care of acute schizophrenics. *Arch Gen Psychiatry, 35*: 1169–1177.

Goldstein MJ, Rodnick EH, Jones JE (1978): Family precursors of schizophrenia spectrum disorders. In: *The Nature of Schizophrenia: New Approaches to Research and Treatment*, Wynne LC, Cromwell RL, Matthysse S (eds.). New York: Wiley.

Goodman SH (1984): Children of disturbed parents: The interface between research and intervention. *Am J Community Psychol, 12*: 663–687.

Grad J, Sainsbury P (1963): Mental illness and the family. *Lancet, 1*: 544–547.

Hatfield AB (1979a): The family as partner in the treatment of mental illness. *Hosp Community Psychiatry, 30*: 338–340.

Hatfield AB (1979b): Help-seeking behavior in families of schizophrenics. *Am J Community Psychol, 7*: 563–569.

Hertz MI, Endicott J, Spitzer RL (1976): Brief versus standard hospitalization: The families. *Am J Psychiatry, 133*(7): 795–801.

Hibler M (1978): The problems as seen by patients' families. *Hosp Community Psychiatry, 29*: 32–33.

Hoening J, Hamilton MW (1966): The schizophrenic patient in the community and his effect on the household. *Int J Soc Psychiatry, 12*(3): 165–176.

Jacobsen S, Fasman J, DiMascio A (1975): Deprivation in the childhood of depressed women. *J Nerv Ment Dis, 160*: 5–14.

Kint MG (1977): Problems for families vs. problem families. *Schizophr Bull, 3*: 355–356.

Kreisman DE, Joy VD (1974): Family response to the mental illness of a relative: A review of the literature. *Schizophr Bull, 10*: 34–57.

Lamb HR, Oliphant E (1978): Schizophrenia through the eyes of the family. *Hosp Community Psychiatry, 29*: 803–806.

Leavitt M (1975): The discharge crisis: The experience of families of psychiatric patients. *Nurs Res, 24*: 33–40.

Leff J et al (1982): A controlled trial in the social intervention in the families of schizophrenic patients. *Br J Psychiatry, 141*: 121–134.

Lidz T, Fleck S, Cornelison A (eds.) (1965): *Schizophrenia and the Family*. New York: International University Press.

Lieber DJ (1978): Parental focus of attention in a videotape feedback task as a function of hypothesized risk for offspring of schizophrenia. *Fam Process, 16*: 467–475.

Liem JH (1980): Family studies of schizophrenia: An update and commentary. *Schizophr Bull, 6*: 429–455.

National Institutes of Mental Health (1983): *Science Reports: Special Report on Depression*. Rockville, MD: US HHS.

Pai S, Kapur RL (1981): Impact of treatment intervention on the relationships between dimensions of clinical psychopathology, social dysfunction, and burden on the family of psychiatric patients. *Psychol Med, 12*: 651–658.

Parker G (1979): Parental characteristics in relation to depressive disorders. *Br J Psychiatry, 134*: 138–147.

Platman SR (1983): Family caretaking and expressed emotion: An evaluation. *Hosp Community Psychiatry, 34*: 921–925.

Platt S, Hirsch S (1981): The effects of brief hospitalization on the psychiatric patient's household. *Acta Psychiatr Scand, 64*: 199–216.

Raskin A et al (1971): Factor analyses of normal and depressed patients' memories of parental behavior. *Psychol Reports, 29*: 871–879.

Reynolds I, Hoult JE (1984): The relatives of the mentally ill. A comparative trial of community and hospital oriented care. *J Nerv Ment Dis, 172*: 480–489.

Robin AA, Copas JB, Freeman-Browne DL (1979): Treatment settings in psychiatry: Long-term family and social findings. *Br J Psychiatry, 135*: 35–41.

Rose LE (1983): Understanding mental illness: The experience of families and psychiatric patients. *J Adv Nurs, 8*: 507–511.

Runions J, Prudo R (1983): Problem behaviors encountered by families living with a schizophrenic member. *Can J Psychiatry, 28*: 382–386.

Singer MT, Wynne LC (1965a): Thought disorder and family relations of schizophrenics. 3. Methodology using projective techniques. *Arch Gen Psychiatry, 12*: 187–200.

Singer MT, Wynne LC (1965b): Thought disorder and family relations of schizophrenics. 4. Results and implications. *Arch Gen Psychiatry, 12*: 201–212.

Smith CM (1969): Measuring the effects of mental illness on the home. *Can Psychiatr Assoc J, 14*: 97–104.

Stein LI, Test MA (1980): Alternatives to mental hospital treatment. 1. Conceptual model, treatment program and clinical evaluation. *Arch Gen Psychiatry, 37*: 392–397.

Strauss JS, Harding CM, Weissman MM (1984): Vulnerability to depressive and schizophrenic disorders. Conference report. *Schizophr Bull, 10*: 460–465.

Thompson EH, Doll W (1982): The burden of families coping with the mentally ill: An invisible crisis. *Fam Relations, 31*: 379–388.

Torrey EF (1983): *Surviving Schizophrenia. A Family Manual*. New York: Harper & Row.

Vaughn CE, Leff JP (1976): The influence of family and social factors on the course of psychiatric illness. A comparison of schizophrenic and depressed neurotic patients. *Br J Psychiatry, 129*: 125–137.

Vaughn CE, Leff JP (1981): Patterns of emotional response in relatives of schizophrenic patients. *Schizophr Bull, 7*: 43–44.

Vaughn CE et al (1984): Family factors in schizophrenic relapse: A California replication of British research on expressed emotion. *Arch Gen Psychiatry, 41*: 1169–1177.

Walsh M (1985): *Schizophrenia: Straight Talk for Family and Friends.* New York: Warner.

Weschler JA (1972): *In a Darkness.* New York: Norton.

Wild CM, Shapiro LN, Goldenberg L (1975): Transactional communication disturbances in families of male schizophrenics. *Fam Process, 14:* 131–160.

Wilson L (1968): *This Stranger, My Son. A Mother's Story.* New York: Putnam.

Wynne LC (1981): Current concepts about schizophrenics and family relationships. *J Nerv Ment Dis, 169:* 82–89.

Wynne LC, Singer MT (1963a): Thought disorder and family relations of schizophrenics. 1. A research strategy. *Arch Gen Psychiatry, 9:* 25–32.

Wynne LC, Singer MT (1963b): Thought disorder and family relations of schizophrenics. 2. A classification of forms of thinking. *Arch Gen Psychiatry, 9:* 33–40.

25

ABUSIVE BEHAVIOR IN FAMILIES

Janice Humphreys, RNC, MS

Jacquelyn C. Campbell, RN, PhD

Family violence is a serious health problem in the United States, and nursing care of abusive families is currently a major area of research and scholarly interest. This chapter discusses the nature and scope of abusive behavior in families, and presents several explanatory models. Nursing diagnosis and treatment of the response to abusive behavior are discussed in terms of theory application.

Janice Humphreys is a doctoral candidate at the College of Nursing at Wayne State University. She and Dr. Campbell have an impressive record of practice, research, and publication in the field of family violence. They are coeditors of Nursing Care of Family Violence.

Jacquelyn Campbell, Interim Chair of the Community Health Nursing Program at Wayne State University, is also on the Board of Directors of the Women's Justice Center in Detroit. She and Ms. Humphreys were invited participants in the Surgeon General's Workshop on Family Violence and Public Health.

Introduction

Abuse in families has been identified as a major health problem in the United States (Campbell, Humphreys, 1984). However, only recently has it been given widespread attention in the literature. Abuse in families has been addressed primarily in terms of establishing incidence, describing the characteristics of perpetrators, or explaining the behavior of victims (Gelles, 1980).

Nursing has identified the family as a focus of care. However, relatively little attention has been given by nurses, either in terms of research or education, to the problem of family violence. According to the ANA Social Policy Statement, "Nursing is the diagnosis and treatment of human responses to actual or potential health problems" (American Nurses' Association, 1980, p. 7). Certainly abusive behavior within families fits within the scope of this definition.

The Nature of the Problem

A discussion of abuse within families involves several different conceptual issues. There is a need to define what is meant by abuse, the different kinds of violence that occur between family members, and who is affected by the abuse.

Abuse is defined most easily as maltreatment, which can be physical, emotional, sexual, or financial in nature. Legal definitions have been formulated for child abuse and neglect, with *child abuse* referring to actual physical violence or the threat of such toward children by a caretaker. *Child sexual abuse* is considered a specific form of child abuse, because of the belief that no child under the age of 18 is capable of consenting to sexual activity with an adult. Therefore, a form of violence or violation occurs in cases of sexual abuse even without physical force. *Child neglect* generally includes harm to a child's health or welfare from negligent treatment by a caretaker (Humphreys, 1984a). *Elder*

abuse and *neglect* have been conceptualized along similar parameters, with financial abuse and neglect added (Sengstock, Barrett, 1984). The *battering of female partners* has been defined as a process within which an adult woman has been the recipient of perceived intentional acts of physical violence resulting in physical pain or injury by an adult man with whom she has or had an ongoing intimate relationship (Campbell, 1984). Although mutual violence does occur between marital partners and the phenomenon of husband abuse has been documented, it is well established that all but a tiny minority of spouse abuse is actually wife abuse.

Emotional abuse has proved very difficult to define, whether directed toward children, marital partners, or elderly family members. As described by Sengstock and Barrett (1984), *emotional* or *psychologic abuse* "involves assault or the infliction of pain through verbal or emotional means" (p. 147). Because of the difficulty of operationalizing such abuse, almost all the research in the area of family violence has been restricted to physical abuse.

No matter what form of abuse is occurring within a family, all family members are affected, and there is overlap in types of abuse. The children of battered women have been the peripheral group most frequently studied. Westra and Martin (1981) found similar developmental delays in a sample of these children to those of abused children. Furthermore, the children of battered women are at risk to be abused themselves or to become unintended victims of men who batter the children's mothers (Appleton, 1980; Giles–Sims, 1985; Nelson, 1984). Battered women are frequently sexually abused as well as physically beaten (Russell, 1982; Walker, 1984). One form of adolescent abuse is an extension of abuse from childhood, and abuse of elderly members may be a form of spouse abuse or a reversal of early child abuse within the same parent–child dyad (Blum, Runyon, 1980; Sengstock, Barrett, 1984).

Straus, Steinmetz, and Gelles (1980) found significant intercorrelations between severity of spousal violence, the violence against children, and the violence between siblings. In a longitudinal study, Steinmetz (1977) reported intergenerational consistency in how much physical aggres- sion families use in the resolution of conflicts. Several studies have supported the finding that husbands who batter their wives are likely either to have been abused as children or to have witnessed the abuse of their mothers (Carroll, 1977; Gelles, 1980). Child-abusing mothers have frequently been victims of incest or suffered serious personal violence (Burgess, 1984). The evidence strongly suggests that whatever the form of abuse, violence between family members can best be conceptualized as a family problem. It affects all members as actual and potential victims, as actual and potential perpetrators, and as involved bystanders who respond emotionally, physically, and behaviorally to the violence around them.

Incidence

Although many estimates about the extent of abuse within families have been advanced, the only study that can be generalized nationally was conducted by Straus, Steinmetz, and Gelles (1980). According to statistics from this study, approximately 28% of cohabiting couples have at some time used some form of physical aggression against each other. One in 20 have had a "beating up" episode during their cohabitation, and 3.6% of the parents in the study admitted to using a violent act against a child that had a high probability of injuring the child. These statistics translate into at least 1.8 million battered women and between 1.4 and 1.9 million abused children each year in this country.

The Straus, Steinmetz, and Gelles study did not measure abuse of elderly family members or sexual abuse in families. Sengstock and Barrett (1984) cite possible incidence of elder abuse from 2.5 per one thousand aged persons to 6 or 7 per thousand. Russell's (1982) landmark study of

rape in marriage suggests that 12% of wives have been sexually assaulted by their husbands. Summit (1981) estimates that approximately 5 million women in this country have been sexually abused by a male relative. These estimates are considered to be conservative because of the general underreporting and lack of recognition of these forms of abuse within families.

The extensive injuries and risk of homicide from family violence is well documented (Campbell, 1981, 1986a). Evidence from child and wife abuse research suggests that abuse within families tends to escalate in severity and frequency over time and to spread to other forms of violence. The need for primary and secondary forms of prevention of this major health problem is acute. In order to formulate nursing interventions for prevention, it is necessary to examine theories of causation.

Causation Theories and Implications for Intervention

The major theories of causation of abuse within families can be grouped under four major headings: (1) individual psychopathology, with the connection with alcohol as a subset of these theories; (2) systems theory, which subsumes the ecological model and Millor's nursing model; (3) social learning theory, of which exchange theory can be considered a part; and (4) feminist theories. Each theory and the research concerning each model will be critically analyzed in this section of the chapter. Along with each model, the nursing interventions that have been derived from that model are briefly presented.

Individual Psychopathology

Much of the early research on child and wife abuse focused on individual psychopathology of the abuser, and in the case of abuse of female partners, on the victim. In spite of the instinctive reaction that abusers of loved ones must be crazy, neither wife-batterers nor child-abusers have been diagnosed as mentally ill more frequently than the rest of the population (Campbell, Humphreys, 1984). In addition, the evidence supports that psychologic difficulties specific to battered women are the result of their abuse rather than occurring previous to it.

Several authors have raised concern over the role that alcohol and other substance abuse may play in family violence (Cork, 1969; Dobash, Dobash, 1979; Gelles, 1972). Victims of violence frequently report the concurrent existence of substance abuse by the abuser. In at least three studies, more serious injuries to a female partner were associated with alcohol intoxication by the man (Coleman, 1980; Eberle, 1982; Snyder, Fruchtman, 1981).

Compelling evidence, however, questions the validity of using alcohol abuse as a causative factor in family violence. The majority of known alcoholics are not abusive toward family members, and the majority of abusers are not diagnosed alcoholics (Dobash, Dobash, 1979; Scott, 1974). Variable amounts of alcohol use are associated with wife-battering incidents. Even known batterers who are problem drinkers are not necessarily drunk when violent nor violent when drunk (Eberle, 1982). Careful review of the evidence has led researchers to conclude that alcohol abuse is probably a spurious rather than a directly causative factor (Berk et al, 1983). Downey and Howell (1976) concluded that abusers may drink in order to have a socially acceptable excuse for the violent behavior.

In spite of the questionable status of the individual psychopathology theories in connection with abuse within families, there are several nursing implications to be derived. Populations exhibiting substance abuse or other major psychologic difficulties need to be assessed carefully, along with their families, for the possibility of family violence. Abuse in the family of childhood may be an important factor in the etiology of the person's emotional difficulties. Perhaps more important, these clients may be continuing to experience or perpetrate violence in their present families.

It is also important to recognize that the successful treatment of a problem such as alcohol abuse will not necessarily improve the problem with violence. Because it is probable that neither alcohol abuse nor other psychopathology causes family violence, resolution of these difficulties is not enough. Separate treatment for the abuse is also necessary.

Systems Theory and Related Frameworks

Systems Theory

Straus (1973) conceptualizes the family as a goal-directed social system with violence as a possible system product. His model is multifactorial in nature and seeks to explain all of family violence. It emphasizes the societal tolerance for violence, the influence of learning violence in childhood through exposure to physical aggression, and the effects of stress on families. The model proposes negative and positive feedback loops that discourage or facilitate family violence. A similar kind of model has been described by Foley (1983) and Millor (1981). Millor's model is described later in this chapter.

Various aspects of Straus's model have been tested by research and received support in those studies (Straus, Gelles, Steinmetz, 1980; Giles-Sims, 1983). Phillips (1983), however, did not find abused elders and their caregivers to have experienced more stressful events than other families with elderly members. In addition, the Straus model as a whole has yet to be examined by a multivariate theory-testing analysis. The research conducted thus far based on the Straus model has provided an explanation of very little of the total variance in family violence. An additional problem has been that the large number of variables present in this model has made designing multivariate research prohibitive.

In spite of a lack of full testing of the systems framework, the evidence of applicability, at least for wife and child abuse, warrants prevention intervention measures based on the model. Nursing implications include primary prevention work at the societal level to decrease the acceptance of violence in all forms. In order to decrease the exposure to violence in childhood, issues such as the glorification of aggression on television and in our national policy need to be addressed. Secondary and tertiary prevention interventions with families already violent or tending toward aggressive conflict resolution will act as primary prevention measures with the children of those families.

In addition, interventions with families to decrease the amount of stress in their lives and to increase their ability to cope with unavoidable stressors are important according to the systems framework. One research study identified that even small, immediate stress-reducing interventions could successfully eliminate the need for larger, agency action later in the case of child-abusive and neglectful families (Horowitz, Wintermute, 1978). These kinds of interventions are well described by Pender (1982).

The Ecological Model

The ecological model, which can be considered a form of systems theory, has been applied to family violence mainly in terms of child abuse and neglect (Garbarino, 1977; Garbarino, Gilliam, 1980). It is also possible, however, to apply an ecological model to family violence as a whole. The ecological model is discussed briefly, with specific attention to family violence.

The ecological model is founded in the study of interrelations of organisms and the environment and is based on the concept of ecosystem, the interactions system of living things with their habitat or the environment that surrounds them (Bubolz, Whiren, 1984). Such an approach emphasizes the biologic and physical dimensions of the organism and environment as well as their psychosocial characteristics and interactions. In an ecological model, the physical resource base of the family and its transactions with other systems in the environment are very important (Andrews, Bubolz, Paolucci, 1980). The basic premise of the ecological models is that a change in any part of the system affects the system as a whole.

Frey (1985) describes the Family Ecological Framework, which views the family holistically. In this framework the family is viewed as existing within its environment, which is composed of physical, biologic, and social components. The family itself serves as the environment for the individual. The environment of the family provides the essential resources necessary to facilitate coping and adjusting to changing internal and external conditions (Hogan, Buehler, 1983). At various points in time, subsystems of the family may be growing and developing, causing the other subsystems to change as well. Such changes call for reintegration of the subsystems within the family and require an increase in energy expenditure on the part of the family as a whole.

Various authors have looked at the family within the ecological model (Auerswald, 1980; Bubolz, Eicher, Sontag, 1979; Frey, 1985). As previously stated, however, the area of family violence that has received the most attention within this model is child abuse and neglect.

Garbarino (1977, 1980) incorporates the major components identified by many to be involved in child abuse and neglect—culture, family, parents, child, and stress. He views child abuse and neglect as being part of the much larger problem of maltreatment, which includes neglect, sexual abuse, and a variety of unhealthy patterns of parent–child interactions. Belsky (1980) suggests that

> since the parent–child system (the crucible of child maltreatment) is nested within the spousal relationship, what happens between husbands wives—from an ecological point of view—has implications for what happens between parents and the children (p. 326).

The ecological framework suggests that abuse in families is created by a confluence of forces that lead to a pathologic adaptation between members. Other family members also contribute to the existence of abuse. There is not just one malfunctioning dyad but rather multiple interacting systems containing more than two people (Garbarino, 1977). The family can be viewed as a system, with patterns of abuse described as system dysfunction.

Garbarino (1977) weakens his model by separating out abusive parents who are psychologically ill from all other abusive parents. It has been documented that less than five percent of all abusive parents are psychotic (Justice, Justice, 1976). It would seem better to consider psychotic abusive parents as any others and to view their psychoses as another aspect of the environment that the family is forced to deal with.

Applied to abusive families as a group, the ecological model suggests that families may experience situationally defined incompetence in their functioning (McClelland, 1973). Various family members may experience situationally defined low levels of skill, and/or the demands on the family may be too great. Within this context, abusive families are experiencing role dysfunction.

The ecological framework suggests that all family members contribute to the abusive situation. This is not to say that a child is abused by one parent and the other parent is collusive. Rather, it proposes that every family member brings something to the family, and that abuse occurs when a family experiences dysfunction.

From the ecological model, certain interventions can be identified for nursing practice. At the level of primary prevention, the ecological model of family violence suggests that social policies or plans that are designed for true prevention of family violence should be directed toward the family as a whole. It is not enough to educate the parents about family abuse; education should be directed toward all family members. Appropriate support and services must be provided to the total family unit. Community support and services can be resources that prevent a family from becoming dysfunctional. These services increase the family's total energy input so that resources become greater than the demands placed on the family. Furthermore, information about these resources needs to be accessible to potentially abusive families.

At the secondary level of prevention, families that have already become abusive also need to have easy access to information and resources. The design and implementation of delivery systems for community programs for abusive families should consider the entire family, not just the abuser and the victim. One method of identifying all the subsystems of any family can be the use of a genogram. This technique allows the nurse to identify each member of the family, including people who are not blood relatives and who do not have legal responsibilities to any other member but are considered family. In addition, the access each member has to every other member and the strength and direction of relationships are diagrammed.

Finally, at the level of tertiary prevention, planning for foster or institutional care should consider the ecological model. According to a study of 370 abused children in a variety of institutional placements, the majority of institutions operated on the basis that the children, rather than the families, had problems and were in need of treatment (Bush, 1980). In addition, Bush reported that the environment and activities were organized primarily to facilitate the running of the institution. The ecological model suggests other operating principles in the case of institutional care.

The Millor Framework

Millor (1981) has proposed a conceptual framework that follows a systems approach for examining child abuse and neglect. In a later, unpublished paper, she and Campbell (1984) applied the same framework to abusive families. The framework arises from theories of the symbolic interaction, stress, and temperament theories of personality. The interaction of concepts in Millor's framework is depicted in Figure 25-1.

Millor (1981) presents family violence as a multifactorial phenomenon with an environment (cultural tolerance for physical conflict resolution) that fosters family tolerance for physical violence and establishes the framework for family transactions. The family tolerance for physical conflict resolution is further determined by the childrearing history of each member of the family. Parents' experiences when children direct the parents' own characteristics later and, in turn, parent role expectations.

According to Millor (1981), each member of the family plays a role in family violence. This is not to say that some members "deserve to be hit" but rather that each member brings to the family certain self-characteristics that interrelate with their own role behavior (acceptable and unacceptable).

Within this framework, stress is interrelated with the characteristics of all the family members. Abusive parents have long been identified as subject to the effect of stress, and the role of stress in wife abuse has been recognized as well (Berger, 1980; Carlson, 1977; Friedrick, Boriskin, 1976; Helfer, Kemp, 1976). Millor (1981) asserts that stress has its impact on all family members, not just the abused and abuser.

The behavioral outcome of the complex interaction of culture, family, individual members, stress falls on a continuum, from normative/ nurturance, to normative conflict resolution to neglectful and abusive families. The healthy family that uses occasional physical discipline of its children need not automatically be labeled "high risk" in this schema. The nurse may, by detailed assessment of all contributing factors of the framework, more clearly understand the strengths and resources of specific families.

Several nursing interventions are suggested by Millor's framework. At the societal level, this framework proposed changes in the value placed on women, children, and the elderly. The existing cultural tolerance for violence is iden-

tified within the framework as influencing both the family transactional environment and the family's tolerance for violent conflict resolution. Decreased societal tolerance for violence, according to Millor, would decrease the likelihood of violence in families.

As well as the stress and stressor reduction interventions previously discussed, the Millor framework suggests that family members' characteristics and expectations influence family outcomes. Individuals who have knowledge and understanding of the behavior of other family members would likely be more tolerant of such behavior. Family nursing interventions that help members understand what can be expected at various developmental stages are indicated from this model. Enhancing the clarity of family communications would also be useful in decreasing misperceptions that can set the stage for violent interactions.

Social Learning Theory and Exchange Theory

Social Learning

Social learning theory has been used by Bandura (1973) to explain aggressive behavior in a more generalized sense than abuse within families. This theory explains aggression as reinforcement-based behavior. The initial modeling and reinforcement for violence toward family members can be from either being the victim of or witnessing physical aggression as a child. Both descriptive and controlled research has supported a connection between abusive family members and their own experience of childhood aggression, including physical punishment (Carroll, 1977; Straus, Steinmetz, Gelles, 1980).

Some authors also linked social learning theory to women being victimized by abusive husbands. The prediction was that the more frequently a woman was hit by her parents or

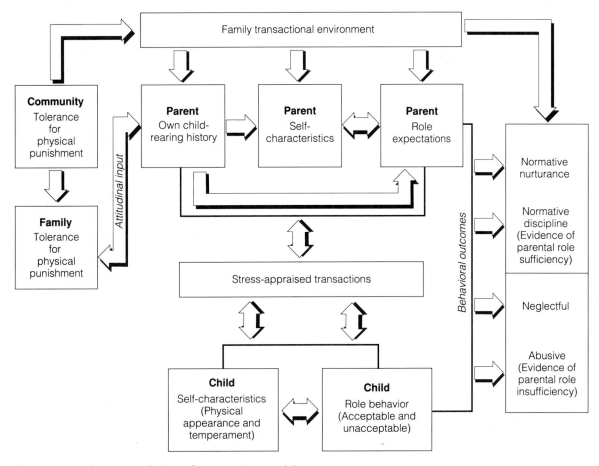

Figure 25–1 Self-role definition of the situation model.

saw her mother being hit, the more conditioned she was to becoming the victim of marital abuse. Peterson found support for this contention in a random sample of women in Maryland, but the majority of descriptive studies consistently indicated a significantly lower percentage of abused women who were beaten or witnessed abuse as children than the batterers (Dobash, Dobash, 1979; Peterson, 1980). Controlled studies by Carroll (1977) and Star (1978) did not support childhood exposure to violence as a risk factor for battering for women.

The social learning model has, therefore, explanatory power for abusive family members but not necessarily for the victims of abuse. It

also needs to be kept in mind that the association of childhood violence and later abusive behavior was generally fairly modest across the research (Gelles, 1980). The majority of abusers in most samples were neither victims of child abuse nor witnesses of violence between parents. Yet the amount of violence modeled and reinforced from other sources, such as violent television, participation in violent sports, and physical punishment, generally has not been considered.

Perhaps the most important nursing intervention to be derived from social learning theory is the primary prevention measure of teaching parents other means of discipline than physical punishment. The use of corporal punishment, at home and in schools, teaches a lesson that violence is condoned, which may be far louder than the lesson of right and wrong intended. The person who uses physical aggression easily maintains power and is thus reinforced for the violence. These lessons are being modeled for the child in a particularly memorable fashion. Nursing can break into this cycle by dealing seriously and carefully with perhaps the most frequently expressed concern of parenting, how to discipline a child.

Exchange Theory

Exchange theory originated in the discipline of sociology, where it has been used to look at interactions between individuals and groups (Gelles, 1976, 1983; Homans, 1966; Nye, 1978, 1979). According to Nye (1979), the strategic concepts of exchange theory (choice theory) are rewards, costs, and profit.

Rewards refer to pleasures, satisfactions, and gratifications a person enjoys (Thibaut, Kelly, 1959). These include statuses, relationships, interactions, experiences other than interactions, and feelings that provide gratification (Nye, 1979).

Costs refer to any status, relationship, interaction, milieu, or feeling disliked by an individual (Nye, 1979). Thibaut and Kelly (1959) state that costs also include factors that deter an activity. There are two distinct types of costs: punishments, or things disliked, and rewards foregone. Certain statuses, such as being known as a child molester, could be included in this group. In the second category of costs are various desirable positions, relationships, interactions, feelings, or milieu that are foregone because an alternative was taken. An example of this is forgoing the position and feelings associated with being a husband as a result of the decision to be abusive to one's wife and subsequently being arrested.

The third concept in exchange theory is profit. A profit is determined in terms of greater magnitude of rewards than costs. The major premise of exchange theory is that interaction is guided by the pursuit of profit—the desire to gain rewards and avoid costs. If reciprocal exchange of rewards occurs, the interaction will continue, but if reciprocity is not achieved, exchange theorists argue that the interaction will not continue.

It is within these assumptions that problems arise. Exchange theory assumes that all individuals have equal opportunity to rewards and costs and therefore equal opportunity to experience profit. This unfortunately does not always reflect the real world. It has been well documented that women have had subordinate status to that of men throughout almost all of recorded history (Chodorow, 1974). Children have had and continue to have a subordinate status to adults (Humphreys, Humphreys, 1985). Evidence of this can be found in court rulings that allow corporal punishment in schools (Ingraham vs. White, 1976). Should the same violent acts be directed toward an adult, charges of assault could be filed. Exchange theory, at times, fails to consider the context of such realities.

Gelles and Straus (1979) offer another criticism of exchange theory. They identify that intrafamilial relations are more complex than those in simply dyadic relations or in less permanent and less normatively structured groups. For at least two reasons, therefore, the lack of reciprocity does not automatically mean that family relations will be broken off. This is supported by the work of Thibaut and Kelley (1959). They report that satisfaction–dissatisfaction with relationships is also influenced by the alternatives available to the individuals. Thus, a woman who experiences violence at the hands of her significant male partner may stay in the relationship because she lacks the resources to go elsewhere. Recent research in the area of wife abuse has reported this to be the case (Strube, Barbour, 1983).

Gelles and Straus (1979) refer to what Homans (1966) called "distributive justice." According to Homans, it is not maximizing rewards minus costs in the absolute that the individual seeks but "justice" in the distribution of outcomes. Therefore, a person stays in a relationship as long as they perceive that they are receiving rewards in correspondingly the same proportion as they deserve. This phenomenon can be seen in battered women who remain in violent relationships through the misconception, perpetuated by much of society and the literature alike, that they are in some way to blame for the violence inflicted on them.

Exchange theory, then, is one theory that has been proposed to explain abuse in families. Although inadequate in explaining the totality of abusive relationships, it does suggest some direction for nursing care of families experiencing abuse.

Within exchange theory, social changes can be identified that alter what is considered a reward and raise the costs of abusive behavior, thus changing the likelihood of profit for abusers. These social changes are varied.

Law enforcement and the criminal justice system have long used the right to privacy as an excuse for treating victims of family violence differently from other assault victims. Humphreys (1984) states that this thinking has haunted battered women's, and conceivably abused elders', attempts to obtain assistance from the police and courts.

Violence against women is considered by many as acceptable and as an indication of masculinity (Toby, 1966). Campbell (1984) has conceptualized this kind of thinking as "machismo." To be a known woman or elder beater may actually increase a man's perceived status. Some men may even brag about the abuse of their female partners (McNulty, 1980).

The very structure of relationships within families has been identified as unequal, with males dominating over females, adults over children, and young adults over the elderly (Beneria, 1979; Chodorow, 1974; Humphreys, 1984b; Ortner, 1974; Phillips, 1983; Young, 1978). Each of these aspects of our society heavily weight potential profits in abusive families in favor of the abuser. This is reflected in the statis-

tics that indicate that women, children, and the elderly are primarily the victims of abuse, and the abuser is usually a man. These facts suggest the need for major societal changes that make the system more egalitarian and less patriarchal (Hoff, 1983).

Another intervention suggested by exchange theory is the incorporation of family life classes as part of secondary school curricula. Students in these classes would have the opportunity to learn about how to deal with the cost and reward realities of intimate relationships. Such classes would be hard-pressed to overcome some of the misconceptions promoted in movies and television, but they might be an initial step.

Finally, Humphreys and Humphreys (1985) propose mandatory arrest laws as a way of decreasing the rewards and increasing the costs, thereby eliminating most of the profit to men who abuse women. Such arrest laws convey a clear message to the potential abuser that battering will not be tolerated and will be followed by the filing of a protection order. It serves as a form of primary prevention of abuse of female partners. The existence of mandatory arrest laws makes it clear that society disapproves of such behavior. Research results support the position that mandatory arrest of abusers serves as a form of secondary prevention as well (Sherman, Berk, 1983).

Feminist Model

The feminist model has been used to explain abuse within families that is directed especially toward women, that is, wife abuse and incest. Dobash and Dobash (1979) propose that the single underlying causative factor in the battering of women is the patriarchal societal organization. Stark–Adamec and Adamec (1982) place wife abuse and incest within the context of all violence against women, which is theorized to be nourished by patriarchy and to arise from men's unconscious fear of women. These theorists maintain that abuse of women, even if within the confines of the family, is a separate issue from other forms of family violence. Kelly (1984) maintains that rape, incest, and wife abuse are all forms of sexual violence. The feminist analysis posits that to subsume wife abuse and incest under the general rubric of family violence is to obscure the political forces that are operating.

The feminist theory has been supported by historical research (Davidson, 1978; May, 1978) and by qualitative studies such as those by Hoff (1983) and Dobash and Dobash (1979). Additional research from the feminist model is the emergency room study by Stark, Flitcraft, and Frazier (1979). These researchers analyzed the medical records of women using an urban hospital's emergency department facilities over a one-month period for evidence of battering. Their finding that battering was seldom diagnosed in spite of clear indication of its presence has been supported by other research (Appleton, 1980). Their contention, however, that the battered women were prescribed tranquilizers and analgesics to an unwarranted extent was not replicated in a different emergency room sample (Goldberg, Tomlanovich, 1984).

Other data supportive of the feminist model were the findings that batterers were generally traditionalists in their insistence on dominance and control in the marital relationship (Bernard, Bernard, Bernard, 1985; Coleman, 1980; Gondolf, 1985; Walker, 1984). Straus et al (1980) reported a significant correlation between a batterer's insistence on the final say in family conflicts and the severity of wife abuse.

The major weakness of the feminist model is its failure to provide explanation for other forms of family violence. Even though the political and social forces of patriarchy and sexism need to be recognized when exploring abuse within families, the interconnectedness of the various forms of family violence also must be taken into account.

The feminist model indicates several important nursing interventions that might otherwise be considered less important. Growing up male in this society is frequently associated with the necessity to keep feelings inside, to control, and to be aggressive. These attitudes are conducive to using violence to maintain status as head of household, even if they may not actually cause abuse within families (Campbell, 1984; Gondolf, 1985). Primary prevention measures for nursing involve both helping parents raise boys who do not so fiercely need to control and working with couples to establish more egalitarian families.

On the treatment level, abusive men need not only to learn other ways of dealing with anger but also to restructure their values about women and families (Gondolf, 1985). Battered women can learn to use assertiveness skills and to recognize the part that social forces play in their victimization. All family members can be helped to realize that conflict resolution does not have to mean that someone in the family wins. Family communication that denigrates the traditionally less powerful females and children or threatens the already shaky self-esteem of abusers is a further important area for assessment and intervention in abusive families (Goldsmith, Rosenbaum, 1985).

Response Theories and Interventions

The following four theoretical frameworks have been chosen as useful orientations for explaining the response to abusive family behavior: (1) learned helplessness; (2) traumatic stress syndrome (including the rape trauma syndrome); (3) crisis theory; and (4) attachment and loss or grieving theory. Each theoretical framework and research supporting that framework will be described. Nursing interventions based on each framework will also be suggested.

Learned Helplessness

Walker (1979) used the theoretical framework of learned helplessness to explain the psychologic responses she saw in her qualitative study of battered women. Walker worked from Seligman's (1975) theory based on observations that in situations of response–outcome noncontingency people may learn that purposive action is unrewarded, and therefore they stop trying. Walker postulated that learned helplessness occurred because battered women perceived that no matter what they did, their husbands beat them and effectively controlled their lives economically, socially, and sexually.

Learned helplessness has been shown to have three major components: motivational, cognitive, and affective (depression) (Abramson, Seligman, Teasdale, 1978). As applied to battered women, the model has received some independent support. Samples of abused women have been reported as less effective at problem-solving and as more depressed and apathetic than nonbattered groups of women (Claerhout, Elder, Janes, 1982; Hilberman, Munson, 1978; Rounsaville, 1978). However, other research using normative measurement instruments has not found battered women to be more depressed (Arndt, 1981; Star, 1978).

Learned helplessness theory has not been applied to abused children or elders. However, there is theoretical congruence with the situations of other abused family members as well as of abused wives. Abused children were reported as depressed and as having low self-esteem (Kinard, 1982; Martin, 1979). The reformulated view of learned helplessness considers low self-concept to be part of the depressive syndrome (Abramson, Seligman, Teasdale, 1978).

The Walker (1979, 1984) application of learned helplessness to battered women was tested in subsequent research using a large (N=403), diverse sample. Some aspects of the model were supported, but others were not. For example, path analysis supported the relationship between childhood learned helplessness, noncontingency in the battering relationship, and a measure of the current state of learned helplessness. In addition, the battered women who were employed were considerably less depressed than those who were unemployed. This result suggested that employed women perceived themselves to have more control in their lives, thereby experiencing less noncontingency.

Nonsupportive of the model were Walker's (1979) findings of higher scores of battered women than controls on measures of self-esteem, attitudes toward women, and internal locus of control. Walker had predicted that battered women who were still in the relationship would experience more noncontingency and therefore would exhibit more learned helplessness than those who had left the relationship, but her measures failed to differentiate the two groups. Although the battered women as a total group were at higher risk for depression than the norms on a depression scale, the abused women who had left the batterer were more depressed than those remaining. This finding was actually more consistent with the grieving model than with a learned helplessness framework. In a multivariate model comparison, Campbell (1986a) found support for both grief and learned helplessness theoretical explanations of responses to battering.

Nursing Interventions

The learned helplessness framework is promising as at least a partial explanation for responses to abuse, but it may not account for the responses of all women to battering. Further research is needed to test the model in other abused family members and to refine the model as it may apply to battered women. There is enough support, however, for the theory of learned helplessness in general and for its application to abused family members to assess for the presence of learned helplessness in cases of family violence and to design nursing interventions based on the theory when signs of this syndrome appear.

These nursing interventions would be centered around increasing control for victims and reducing noncontingency. Nurses can assist the victim to regain a sense of control through a variety of techniques. First, the nurse can discuss with the abused family members all the things they have done to avoid the abuse. Burgess and Holmstrum (1974) state that this is especially important in the case of survivors of rape. They urge helping the women see that they were not passive victims in the situation but rather took a variety of steps to escape or minimize the violence. Clinical experience with battered women has revealed the amazing creativity of their actions. Yet, until it was brought to their attention, they did not see how they deliberately and continuously took self-protective action.

Second, nurses should never underestimate how concrete material resources can increase a person's sense of control. Research supports that the majority of battered women state that a major reason for staying in an abusive relationship is economic dependency and lack of a place to go (Strube, Barbour, 1983). Knowledge of community resources, local and state laws, and agency procedures can give control back to the victim.

Individual therapy would also be indicated for family members experiencing significant depression from learned helplessness. The Beck (1972) model of cognitive therapy for depression offers an appropriate therapeutic regimen for this form of depression.

Traumatic Stress Syndrome

The rape trauma syndrome, first identified by Burgess and Holmstrum (1974), has also been used to explain the response of battered women. The more general theoretical framework, characterized as a stress response or traumatic stress syndrome, has been explored by researchers in the general area of victimization. It has been postulated that victims of violence experienced similar psychologic responses whether the violence was experienced as a rape or as an assault from a family member or someone outside the family (Janoff–Bulman, Frieze, 1983; Symonds, 1975). Symptoms similar to those experienced by rape victims have been identified in populations of battered women, abused children, and incest victims (Brunngraber, 1986; Conte, 1985; Hilberman, Munson, 1978). Responses reported across studies included anxiety, somatic symptoms, guilt, shame, anger, and despair.

The attributions about the cause of the victimization have been postulated as an important determinant of eventual outcome of the traumatic stress syndrome (Janoff–Bulman, Frieze, 1983). Attributions have also been used to make the learned helplessness model more explanatory. The reformulated model of learned helplessness postulated that depression was more likely to occur and was more enduring if the person made internal, personal, and stable attributions for failure (Abramson, Seligman, Teasdale, 1978). Research in social psychology has supported this inclusion of attributions as a part of learned helplessness theory (Peterson, Schwartz, Seligman, 1981).

The application of these tenets about attributions have been explored in research with both battered women and rape victims. Frieze (1979) found that abused women who made external attributions of blame for the violence in their relationships were more likely to have tried a wider variety of solutions. She also reported that the attributions of battered women tended to change over time from internal to external blame, a finding supported in the longitudinal research of Giles–Sims (1983). Miller and Porter (1983) found that the battered women in their sample blamed themselves less for causing the abuse as time passed but more for allowing the abuse to continue.

Other aspects of the postulations made about the effect of attributions on the traumatic stress syndrome were either not supported or not clearly tested in the Frieze (1979) study. Miller and Porter (1983) found that attributions of battered women were difficult to classify as stable or unstable. They also argued that internal attributions (self-blame) gave victims a way of maintaining control over their lives and would therefore be *less* predictive of depression and other long-term problems. In fact, studies suggested that other victims of violence or disasters coped more successfully if they blamed themselves (Baum, Fleming, Singer, 1983; Bulman, Wortman, 1977).

Nursing Interventions

It is unclear, therefore, if interventions with abused individuals should include encouragement of internal or external attributions. Desire to alleviate the guilt frequently seen as part of the traumatic stress syndrome has resulted in general suggestions in practice literature to encourage the victim to blame the abuser rather than themselves, but this approach may not be supported by existing research. The key may be the issue of control rather than of internal attributions. If what is blamed in oneself for the violence is controllable (or behavioral versus characterological), this may enhance healthy eventual outcomes (Damrosch, 1985; Peterson, Schwartz, Seligman, 1981). Other research suggests that a combination of self-blame and other blame is the least predictive of problem outcomes (Campbell, 1986a; Langer, 1983).

The role of attributions has not been directly studied in other populations of survivors of family violence. Conte (1985) argued that the findings in the child abuse literature are consistent with the premise that attributions play an important part in the response of abused children. The low self-esteem that has been identified in several studies of members of violent families can be theorized to be a result of characterological self-blame. Implications for interventions include encouraging a sense of control as described previously and generalized measures to enhance self-esteem. Support groups for victims have been used successfully with survivors of battering and incest to work through resultant attributions (Campbell, 1986b; Coates, Winston, 1983).

Crisis Theory

The crisis theory of response to family violence is closely related to the stress response syndrome. Hoff (1983) and Burgess and Holmstrum (1974) have used a crisis theory as the basis of nursing research and interventions for battered and sexually abused women. The Hoff model, as applied to battered women, took into account social and cultural influences as well as situational stressors. Her qualitative research demonstrated a lack of mental or emotional disturbances in battered women prior to their experience of a violent intimate relationship. These findings have been supported in prior research with battered women (Arndt, 1981; Dobash, Dobash, 1979). The Hoff sample also reported severe stress during the battering phase of their lives, but both pre- and postbattering-relationship stress scores were definitely lower.

The Hoff (1983) crisis model allowed for growth and development as an outcome of the crisis stage as well as for negative outcomes such as emotional disturbances, violence against others, and self-destructive behaviors (such as substance abuse). Kelly (1984) also identified positive as well as negative long-term effects in survivors of both incest and wife abuse. Approximately one-third of her sample felt more independent and stronger and closer to other women as a result of the experience. Brunngraber's (1986) nursing research with incest survivors corroborated these findings.

The crisis theory of response to stress as developed and investigated by Hoff (1983) also demonstrated the importance of support systems in optimally resolving the crisis of family violence. Researchers in the area of child abuse have also postulated that support systems can buffer the effects of stress and thus serve as a means of primary prevention of child abuse and neglect (Howze, Kotch, 1984; MacElveen–Hoehn, 1984).

In spite of the frequently stated contention that violent families are generally socially isolated, McKenna (1985) found that her sample of battered women had social networks that were equal in size and frequency of contact to a comparison (nonbattered) group. Similarly, Phillips (1983) found no significant difference in support network variables between abused and non-abused elders. These important nursing research findings suggest that social isolation should not be assumed when working with violent families but that existing support networks need to be explored and facilitated.

Natural support systems (family and friends) of abused women in Hoff's (1983) sample generally tried to be helpful, but their attempts were inadequate. This finding was supported in Bowker's (1983) study of battered women who had successfully ended the violence in their lives. For these women, there was a progression from use of informal support systems to formal agencies and professionals who were more effective in helping to end the battering.

Nursing Interventions

One implied intervention is the need to have more and better formal support systems for victims of family violence. It has only been since 1962 that child abuse was formally identified in the literature (Kempe et al, 1962). Wife abuse was recognized as a serious problem somewhat later, and elder abuse has received the least attention of all. Services to these groups also have been slow to develop, and services for abused elders are absent in most communities (Sengstock, Barrett, 1984). There is a clear need for more formal supports for victims of abuse and education of the public with regard to these systems. Both victims and sources of informal support would be better able to use the formal support systems.

Hoff (1983) identified that both the abused women and their natural network of social support seemed minimally aware of the relationship between the violence inflicted on women and the larger public issues regarding women. This finding suggests the need for consciousness raising and widespread political action on behalf of disempowered groups such as abused women, children, and the elderly.

Gottlieb (1983) suggests strategies for marshaling sources of support to enhance morale and health. These interventions fall into two categories. The first involves the restructuring of existing social networks or the optimization of their helping capabilities so that they reach more people and more adequately fulfill people's requirements for support. Gottlieb describes one such program that attempted to help local residents understand and take advantage of existing mental health facilities. Nurses in all practice areas, if familiar with agency and community resources, can provide this kind of intervention to abusive families.

The second category of intervention involves the development of "event-centered support groups" that can be organized and tailored to the specific needs of the group. Johnson and Jacobs, in a chapter by Burgess (1984), describe one nurse-facilitated group designed for individuals who had been incest victims. The women in the group are reported to have benefited from the intimacy, sharing, and acceptance of the group. This resulted in an increase in self-esteem and feelings of self-worth. Such groups conceivably also could assist families experiencing abuse.

Attachment and Loss

Classic research and theory concerning attachment, loss, and grieving has been used as the basis for examination of the response of adult humans when they were faced with the death or impending death of a spouse (Bowlby, 1980; Glick, Weiss, Parkes, 1974; Hoagland, 1983; Lindemann, 1979; Marris, 1974). Research such as that by Marris (1974), Parkes (1972), and Weiss

(1975) supported the contention that a similar grief reaction or separation anxiety was elicited with similar losses, including the loss or impending loss of a spouse by divorce or separation.

There appear to be many conceptual similarities between the responses to abuse in the family and to other forms of bereavement in family members. The abused family member faces many losses: loss of the ideal parent, spouse, or child; loss of security; loss of body image from physical injury; loss to self-esteem from the degrading nonverbal message inherent in battering; and possible actual loss of the abusing family member if legal action is taken. The family as a whole suffers similar losses. It is theoretically congruent to expect both abused and other family members to experience similar patterns of response and specific effects to loss as have been identified by research in other situations of grieving. There is indirect evidence from research on abuse to support these inferences. In addition, a nursing study of battered women supported both a grief and a learned helplessness model (Campbell, 1986a).

Attachment in human beings, once firmly established, has been found to be "extraordinarily resistive to dissipation," no matter what the relationship entails (Weiss, 1975, p. 45). The majority of divorced spouses were found still to feel attachment to their ex-spouses, even when it was recognized that the marriage needed to be ended (Kitson, 1982; Weiss, 1975). The most common reason women have given for staying in a battering relationship in many studies is that they still love the man. Abused children are known to continue to express love and yearning for their parents in spite of their victimization (Gelles, Cornell, 1985).

Grief is usually considered to be a process with somewhat identifiable stages. The amount of time required to complete the process of grieving varied in the bereavement literature from six months to four years, and the determinants of variations in time were not firmly identified. The

descriptions from Bowlby (1980) of normal stages of response to the loss of an attachment figure can be considered conceptually similar to those found in research on other forms of loss and anticipatory grief (Hackney, Ribordy, 1980; Hamen, 1982; Marris, 1974; Weiss, 1975). Bowlby (1980) characterized his first stage as a period of numbness or disbelief. A similar first response to wife abuse has been described in the literature, but a pattern of response has not been identified in the research on other forms of family violence (Dobash, Dobash, 1979; Ferraro, Johnson, 1983; Walker, 1979).

The behaviors described by Bowlby (1980) as part of a phase of yearning and search may be accentuated when loss is by death, but can be considered conceptually similar to the efforts of divorcing couples and wives of alcoholics and batterers to normalize their situation (Ferraro, Johnson, 1983; Weiss, 1975). In divorcing spouses, the process also included frequent attempted reconciliations, which are considered normal in this group (Weiss, 1975). This facet of the bereavement process may explain the behavior of battered women, who often leave and return to their spouses, much to the chagrin of caretakers and the puzzlement of researchers (Giles–Sims, 1983; Strube, Barbour, 1983).

The phases of disorganization (and despair) and reorganization are comparable both in title and in characteristics to those described by researchers in the other areas (Bowlby, 1980). The frequently noted depression of battered women may be part of the normal despairing stage of grieving. Nurse scholars and others have explored this possibility theoretically, but it has not been the subject of research (Campbell, 1984; Flynn, Whitcomb, 1981; Silverman, 1981; Weinfourt, 1979). Depression has also been noted in abused children, abused elders, and the children of battered women (Phillips, 1983; Westra, Martin, 1981).

As well as a process of grieving, other specific psychologic, behavioral, and physical effects of actual or impending loss have been identified in research. Anxiety; depression; hostility; problem-solving difficulties; loss of identity, self-esteem, and roles; health problems; psychosomatic symptoms; and behavioral expressions of these reactions were consistently reported in the literature concerning widows, wives of alcoholics, children experiencing the death of a parent, and divorcing spouses (Berman, Turk, 1981; Bloom, White, Asher, 1979; Glick et al, 1981; Paolino, McCrady, Kogan, 1978). These responses were generally considered to be situational in origin rather than existing previously. Similar responses have been identified in battered women, incest victims, and abused children (Burgess, 1984; George, Main, 1979; Walker, 1979, 1984).

Many recent research efforts into the various forms of bereavement were directed toward identification of factors predicting healthy long-term outcomes. There was little agreement about causal modeling or the relative strength of various contributing factors. Many of the same variables were tested across the bodies of literature and received at least some empirical support in multivariate analysis. Those factors supported as significant in positively influencing long-term outcomes include social support, effective individual coping mechanisms, autonomy, and a sense of identity (Berman, Turk, 1981; Kohen, 1981; Hancock, 1980; Vachon et al, 1982). Negative outcomes were associated with the poor quality of previous attachment relationships, poverty, other stressors, and ambivalence or anger toward the lost or to-be-lost attachment figure. In abusive families, it can be inferred that similar variables would be important to consider in predicting outcomes and choosing interventions. However, in research on alcoholic husbands and separated and divorced spouses, the behavior of the attachment figure was more important in terms of outcomes for the bereaved individual than the other variables examined (Berman, Turk, 1981; Orford et al, 1975). This is an important consideration to keep in mind when applying the grieving theoretical framework to abusive family situations.

In summary, the basic theoretical framework for grieving and the research exploring the responses to actual or threatened loss of major attachment figures suggest useful concepts on which to base nursing care of abusive families. The pattern of response, specific responses to loss or impending loss, and factors supported as predictive of healthy outcomes are important in both identification and treatment of a grieving response to family violence.

Individuals who experience abuse, just as those who experience any other loss, should not be left to work through their feelings on their own. Grieving victims need support from their family, friends, and others. Unfortunately, it has been well documented that the people who should be a source of support, including health care providers, frequently fail to provide this resource (Appleton, 1980; Dobash, Dobash, 1979; Stark, Flitcraft, Frazier, 1979). It may well be that family members and friends are also experiencing a grief reaction when they too become aware of the abuse. Nurses will need to keep this possibility in mind as they provide care.

Abuse victims, when confronted with the reality of their situation, frequently deny it. Unfortunately, when faced with the abuse victim's denial, some persons react with anger. Consider this same situation with a person who denies that they have a terminal disease. Nurses have been taught to react to such a situation by listening and providing support. The same is true with victims of abuse. Denial is just one step in a process of grieving. It should be understood, not dealt with by anger.

Children also may deny that they are abused. They may be experiencing a grief reaction or they also may be trying to protect their abusers. There are several reasons why this may occur. First, if the abuser is a parent or close relative, the child may still feel emotionally tied to this person and may be afraid of the loss of this relationship. They may feel that they are somehow responsible for the abuse they experience. This can be especially true in the case of sexual abuse. The child may feel tremendous guilt if they experienced any pleasure from the intimacy of the relationship, or they may have been told time and time again that they were "seductive" and brought the sexual acts on themselves (Blum, Runyan, 1980).

Adult victims who deny abuse may fear reprisals or social disapproval. The nurse who presents a nonjudgmental, caring attitude will best be able to deal with this situation. It is also especially important that the nurse ensure the patient's privacy during any discussion of abuse. Only the most desperate victim will admit to being abused in the presence of their abuser or other family members of whose reaction the abused family member is unsure.

Interventions for abused family members who are grieving include the same kinds of interventions that have been found to be useful with other bereaved individuals. These include support groups, promotion of grief work, mobilization of natural support systems, and assessment and referral for pathologic grieving responses (Carpenito, 1983).

Future Directions

Throughout this chapter, theory has been used to give guidance to understand and care for families experiencing abuse. Little research exists that answers all the questions raised by nurses who care for abusive families. Some of the areas in particular need of the development of nursing theory and research are briefly addressed.

Several authors have raised concern over the role that alcohol and other substance abuse may play in family violence. The holistic focus of nursing would facilitate an avenue of scientific investigation into this question, which would include the physiologic, psychologic, sociologic and cultural forces involved. The lack of a holistic framework in previous research has resulted in "camps" that disagree about causation in terms of substance abuse and other factors as-

sociated with family violence and that sometimes neglect the interplay of these factors.

Some services within the health care system and the community at large currently exist for victims of violence. Other services are still needed, however. Child abuse and neglect teams (sometimes called Suspected Child Abuse and Neglect teams, or SCAN teams) are now common in children's hospitals. Adult and general health care facilities are in need of suspected victimization teams. The need for such is made apparent by the nursing research of Phillips and Rempusheski (1985), which documents the dilemmas associated with the nursing diagnosis of elder abuse. A screening instrument is now available for elder abuse, which could be used by such teams and by nurses in all settings (Sengstock, Hwalek, 1985).

Multidisciplinary suspected victimization teams could be used to develop policies and procedures for dealing with suspected victims of family violence. The team and its members can also serve as coordinators of care of victims and function as consultants as needed. A multidisciplinary team can be most effective in dealing with the variety of professionals who function within a health care setting. Nurses are in an excellent position to contribute to suspected victimization teams and are encouraged to become involved in such groups.

The majority of suggestions for professional interventions in all disciplines have been based on philosophy and the boundaries of the discipline involved rather than on theory and research that explains the response of family members experiencing violence. According to the definition of nursing, this response is an area of nursing inquiry. The development of nursing theory and research about the response to abuse, in conjunction with application of findings from the research of other concerned disciplines, will result in a firmer theoretical base from which to design family nursing interventions. Existing nursing conceptual frameworks can also be applied in family violence situations for intervention formulations (Campbell, 1986; Humphreys,

1986; Limandri, 1986). These interventions can then be tested in experimental research.

Finally, nursing education must prepare nurses to care for families experiencing violence by incorporating appropriate content into the curriculum. Content on abuse and victimization can be included throughout the undergraduate and graduate curricula or presented as part of a specialized course or courses that address these areas. Humphreys (1984a) has described one such undergraduate senior year elective that focused specifically on family violence. The course included both classroom and clinical experience with abusive or potentially abusive families for generic and registered nurse students. The incorporation of clinical contact with victims of violence has been shown to have impact on later nurse attitudes toward victims (Alexander, 1980). Nurse subjects who had previous exposure to victims of violence were significantly less likely to blame the victim for the violence the victim experienced. The need for early clinical contact with abuse victims is particularly important in light of earlier reported poor attitudinal and care responses of health care providers to victims of violence (Davis, Carlson, 1981; Damrosch, 1981; Shipley, Sylvester, 1982).

Summary

Abuse in families is a serious health problem that is in need of nursing attention in terms of practice with families, nursing education, theory development, and research. Beginning empirical support currently exists that can be used to direct the nursing care of abusive families. There has been a recent increase in nursing research and scholarly activity in the area of family violence. Much nursing theory development and research is needed, however.

Throughout this chapter, several major theories have been presented that attempt to explain the causes of family violence. In addition, theories of victim and family response to abuse have been described as a beginning framework for the development of nursing interventions. Finally, four areas in need of further nursing consideration were presented. Of particular concern is the need for nursing education in the care of abusive families, a need this text seeks to address.

Issues for Further Investigation

1. What is the applicability of nursing theories (conceptual frameworks) in the explanation of individual family member and total family responses to violence?

2. What are the similarities and differences of the responses to violence of different family members (for example, abused children, wives, elders)?

3. What are the effects of abuse within the family on total family functioning?

4. What kinds of nursing interventions at all three levels of prevention are most effective with families experiencing violence?

References

Abramson L, Seligman M, Teasdale J (1978): Learned helplessness in humans: Critique and reformulation. *J Abnormal Psychology, 87*: 49–74.

Alexander C (1980): The responsible victim: Nurses' perceptions of victims of rape. *J Health Soc Behav, 21*: 22–23.

American Nurses' Association (1980): Nursing: A social policy statement. Kansas City: American Nurses' Association.

Andrews M, Bubolz M, Paolucci B (1980): An ecological approach to study of the family. *Marr Fam Rev, 3*: 29–49.

Appleton W (1980): The battered woman syndrome. *Ann Emerg Med, 9*: 84–91.

Arndt N (1981): Domestic violence: Psychological aspects of the battered woman. *Dissertation Abstracts, International.* (University Microfilms International no. 8129553).

Auerswald E (1980): Interdisciplinary versus ecological approach. *Fam Process, 7*(2): 202–15.

Bandura A (1973): *Aggression: A Social Learning Analysis.* Englewood Cliffs, NJ: Prentice-Hall.

Baum A, Fleming R, Singer J (1983): Coping with victimization by technological disaster. *J Soc Iss, 39*(2): 119–140.

Beck A (1972): *Depression: Causes and Treatment* (rev ed). Philadelphia: University of Pennsylvania Press.

Belsky J (1980): Child maltreatment: An ecological integration. *Am Psychol, 35*(4): 320–335.

Beneria L (1979): Production and the sexual division of labor. *Cambridge Journal of Economics, 3*: 103–125.

Berger A (1980): The child abusing family: Part 2. *Am J Fam Ther, 8*: 52–68.

Berk R et al (1983): Mutual combat and other family violence myths. In: *The Dark Side of Families,* Finkelhor R et al (eds.). Beverly Hills, CA: Sage.

Berman W, Turk D (1981): Adaptation to divorce: Problems and coping strategies. *J Marr Fam, 43*: 179–189.

Bloom B, White S, Asher S (1979): Marital disruption as a stressful life event. In: *Divorce and Separation,* Levinger G, Moles O (eds.). New York: Basic Books.

Blum R, Runyan C (1980): Adolescent abuse: The dimension of the problem. *J Adolesc Health Care, 1*(2): 121–126.

Bowker LH (1983): *Beating Wife-Beating.* Lexington, MA: Lexington Books.

Bowlby J (1980): *Attachment and Loss: Vol. 3.* New York: Basic Books.

Brunngraber LS (1986): Father-daughter incest: Immediate and long-term effects of sexual abuse. *ANS, 8*(4): 15–35.

Bubolz M, Eicher J, Sontag S (1979): The human ecosystem: A model. *J Home Econ, 71*(1): 28–31.

Bubolz M, Whiren A (1984): The family of the handicapped: An ecological model for policy and practice. *Fam Relations, 33*: 5–12.

Bulman R, Wortman C (1977): Attributions of blame and coping in the "real world": Severe accident victims react to their lot. *J Pers Soc Psychol, 35*: 351–363.

Burgess A (1984): Intrafamilial sexual abuse. In: *Nursing Care of Victims of Family Violence,* Campbell J, Humphreys J (eds). Reston, VA: Reston Publishing Company.

Burgess A, Holmstrum L (1974): Rape trauma syndrome. *Am J Psychiatry, 134*: 69–72.

Bush M (1980): Institutions for dependent and neglected children: Therapeutic option of choice or last resort? *Am J Orthopsychiatry, 50*: 239–255.

Campbell J (1981): Misogyny and homicide of women. *ANS 3*: 67–85.

Campbell J (1984): Abuse of female partners. In: *Nursing Care of Victims of Family Violence,* Campbell J, Humphreys J (eds.). Reston, VA: Reston Publishing Company.

Campbell J (1986): A nursing study of two explanatory models of women's responses to battering. Unpublished doctoral dissertation, University of Rochester.

Campbell J (1986b): A survival group for battered women. *ANS, 8*(4): 36–51.

Campbell J, Humphreys J (1984): *Nursing Care of Victims of Family Violence.* Reston, VA: Reston Publishing Company.

Carlson B (1977): Battered women and their assailants. *Soc Work, 22*: 455–465.

Carpenito L (1983): *Nursing Diagnosis: Application to Clinical Practice.* Philadelphia: Lippincott.

Carroll J (1977): The intergenerational transmission of family violence. *Aggressive Behavior, 3*(3): 289–299.

Chodorow M (1974): Family structure and feminine personality. In: *Woman, Culture and Society,* Rosaldo M, Lamphere L (eds). Palo Alto, CA: Stanford University Press.

Claerhout S, Elder J, Janes C (1982): Problem-solving skills of rural battered women. *Am J Community Psychol, 10*: 605–612.

Coates D, Winston T (1983): Counteracting the deviance of depression: Peer support for victims. *J Soc Issues, 39*(2): 171–196.

Coleman K (1980): Conjugal violence: What 33 men report. *J Marr Fam, 6*(2): 207–213.

Conte J (1985): The impact of sexual abuse on children. *Victimology: An International Journal, 10*(1–4): 110–130.

Cork M (1969): *The Forgotten Child.* Toronto: Paperbacks in association with Addition Research Foundation.

Damrosch S (1981): How nursing students' reactions to rape victims are affected by a perceived act of carelessness. *Nurs Res, 30:* 168–170.

Damrosch S (1985): Nursing students' assessment of behaviorally self-blaming rape victims. *Nurs Res, 34:* 221–224.

Davidson T (1978): *Conjugal Crime: Understanding and Changing the Wifebeating Problem.* New York: Hawthorn.

Davis L, Carlson B (1981): Attitudes of service providers toward domestic violence. *Soc Work Res Abstr, 81:* 34–39.

Dobash RE, Dobash R (1979): *Violence Against Wives.* New York: Free Press.

Downey J, Howell J (1976): *Wife Battering.* Vancouver: United Way of Greater Vancouver.

Eberle P (1982): Alcohol abusers and non-users: A discriminant analysis of differences between two subgroups of batterers. *J Health Soc Behav, 23:* 260–271.

Fawcett J (1978b): The "what" of theory development. In: *Theory Development: What, Why, How?* New York: National League for Nursing, pp. 17–34.

Ferraro K, Johnson J (1983): How women experience battering: The process of victimization. *Soc Prob, 30:* 325–339.

Flynn J, Whitcomb J (1981): Unresolved grief in battered women. *JEN, 7*(6): 250–254.

Foley T (1983): Nursing interventions in family abuse and violence. In: *Principles and Practice of Psychiatric Nursing,* Stuart G, Sundeen S (eds.). St. Louis: Mosby.

Frey M (1985): An ecological framework for examining the relationship between social support, family health and child health in families with a diabetic child. Beatrice Paolucci Symposium: Shaping destiny through everyday life. Michigan State University, East Lansing.

Friedrich W, Boriskin J (1976): The role of the child in abuse: A review of the literature. *Am J Orthopsychiatry, 46*(4): 580–590.

Frieze I (1979): Perceptions of battered wives. In: *New Approaches to Social Problems,* Frieze I, Bar-Tal D, Carroll J (eds.). San Francisco: Jossey-Bass, pp. 79–108.

Garbarino J (1977): The human ecology of child maltreatment. *J Marr Fam, 39:* 721–735.

Garbarino J, Gilliam G (1980): *Understanding Abusive Families.* Lexington, MA: D. C. Heath.

Gelles R (1972): *The Violent Home.* Beverly Hills, CA: Sage.

Gelles R (1976): Abused wives: Why do they stay? *J Marr Fam, 38:* 659–668.

Gelles R (1980): Violence in the family: A review of research in the seventies. *J Marr Fam, 42:* 873–885.

Gelles R (1983): An exchange/social control theory. In: *The Dark Side of Families,* Finkelhor D et al (eds.). Beverly Hills: Sage, pp. 252–265.

Gelles R, Cornell C (1985): *Intimate Violence in Families.* Beverly Hills, CA: Sage.

Gelles R, Straus M (1979): Determinants of violence in the family: Toward a theoretical integration. In: *Contemporary Theories About the Family: General Theories/Theoretical Orientations: Vol 2,* Burr W et al (eds.). New York: Free Press, pp. 549–581.

George C, Main M (1979): Social interactions of young abused children: Approach, avoidance and aggression. *Child Dev, 50:* 306–318.

Giles-Sims J (1983): *Wife Battering: A Systems Approach.* New York: Guilford.

Giles-Sims J (1985): A longitudinal study of battered children of battered wives. *Fam Relations, 34:* 205–210.

Glick I, Weiss R, Parkes C (1974): *The First Year of Bereavement.* New York: Wiley.

Goldberg W, Carey A (1982): Domestic violence victims in the emergency setting. *Top Emerg Med, 3:* 65–75.

Goldberg WG, Tomlanovich MC (1984): Domestic violence in the emergency department. *JAMA, 251:* 3259–3264.

Goldsmith D, Rosenbaum A (1985): An evaluation of the self-esteem of maritally violent men. *Fam Rel, 34:* 425–437.

Gondolf E (1985): *Men Who Batter.* Holmes Beach, FL: Learning Publications.

Gottlieb B (1983): *Social Support Strategies: Guidelines for Mental Health Practice.* Beverly Hills, CA: Sage.

Hackney G, Ribordy S (1980): An empirical investigation of emotional reactions to divorce. *J Clin Psychol, 36*: 105–110.

Hamen L (1982): *Separated and Divorced Women.* Westport, CT: Greenwood.

Hancock E (1980): The dimensions of meaning and belonging in the process of divorce. *Am J Orthopsychiatry, 50*(1): 18–27.

Helfer R, Kempe CH (1976): *Child Abuse and Neglect.* Cambridge, MA: Ballinger.

Hilberman E, Munson K (1978): Sixty battered women. *Victimology: Int J, 2*: 460–470.

Hoagland A (1983): Bereavement and personal constructs: Old theories and new concepts. *Death Education, 7*: 175–193.

Hoff L (1983): Violence against women: A socialcultural network analysis. Paper presented at the 1983 Sigma Theta Tau biennial convention research conference, Boston.

Hogan MJ, Buehler CA (1983, October): The concept of resources: Definition issues. Proceedings of the theory construction and research methodology workshop, National Council of Family Relations.

Homans G (1966): Fundamental social processes. In: *Sociology: An introduction,* Smelser N (ed.). New York: Wiley, pp. 29–78.

Horowitz B, Wintermute W (1978): Use of an emergency fund in protective services casework, *Child Welfare, 57*: 608–617.

Howze D, Kotch J (1984): Disentangling life events, stress and social support: Implications for the primary prevention of child abuse and neglect. *Child Abuse Negl, 8*: 401–409.

Humphreys J (1984a): Child abuse. In: *Nursing Care of Victims of Family Violence,* Campbell J, Humphreys J (eds.). Reston, VA: Reston, pp. 119–144.

Humphreys J (1984b): Implications for nursing. In: *Nursing Care of Victims of Family Violence,* Campbell J, Humphreys J (eds.). Reston, VA: Reston, pp. 403–418.

Humphreys J (1984c): The nurse and the legal system: Dealing with battered women. In: *Nursing Care of Victims of Family Violence,* Campbell J, Humphreys J (eds.). Reston, VA: Reston, pp. 370–383.

Humphreys J (1986): Dependent-care agency and dependent-care in mothers and their children who have experienced family violence. Unpublished manuscript.

Humphreys J, Humphreys W (1985): Mandatory arrest: A means of primary and secondary prevention of abuse of female partners. *Victimology: Int J, 10*(1–4): 267–280.

Ingraham vs. Wright (1976): 97 S.Ct. 1401–1406, citing 525F.2d 909, 917.

Janoff-Bulman R, Frieze I (1983): A theoretical perspective for understanding reactions to victimization. *J Soc Issues, 39*: 1–17.

Justice B, Justice R (1976): *The Abusing Family.* New York: Human Sciences.

Kelly L (1984, August): Effects or survival strategies? The long-term consequences of experiences of sexual violence. Paper presented at the second national conference for family violence researchers, Durham, NH.

Kempe CH et al (1962): Battered child syndrome. *JAMA, 181*(1): 17–24.

Kitson G (1982): Attachment to the spouse in divorce: A scale and its application. *J Marr Fam, 44*: 379–393.

Kohen J (1981): From wife to family head: Transitions in self-identity. *Psychiatry, 44*: 230–240.

Langer E (1983): *The Psychology of Control.* Beverly Hills, CA: Sage.

Lichtenstein V (1981): The battered woman: Guideline for effective nursing intervention. *Iss Ment Health Nurs, 3*: 237–250.

Limandri B (1986): Research and practice with abused women: Use of the Roy adaptation model as an explanatory framework. *ANS, 8*(4): 52–61.

Lindemann E (1979): *Beyond Grief.* New York: Jason Aronson.

McClelland D (1973): Testing competence rather than intelligence. *Am Psychol, 28*: 1–14.

MacElveen-Hoehn P, Eyres S (1984): Social support and vulnerability: State of the art in relation to families and children. In: *Social Support and Families and Vulnerable Infants,* Raff B (ed.). White Plains, NY: March of Dimes Birth Defects Foundation.

McKenna L (1985): Social support systems of battered women: Influence of psychological adaptation. Unpublished doctoral dissertation, University of California, San Francisco.

McNulty F (1980): *The Burning Bed.* New York: Harcourt Brace Jovanovich.

Marris P (1974): *Loss and Change*. London: Routledge & Kegan Paul.

Martin H (1979): Child abuse and child development. *Child Abuse Negl, 3*(2): 415–422.

May M (1978): Violence in the family: An historical perspective. In: *Violence and the family*, Martin J (ed.). Chichester, England: Wiley, pp. 135–163.

Miller D, Porter C (1983): Self-blame in victims of violence. *J Soc Issues, 39*: 139–152.

Millor G (1981): Theoretical framework for nursing research in child abuse and neglect. *Nurs Res, 30*: 78–83.

Millor G, Campbell J (1984): Family violence: Nursing roles in intervention and formulation of health policy. Proceedings of the American Nurses' Association convention, New Orleans.

Nelson K (1984): The innocent bystander: The child as unintended victim of domestic violence involving deadly weapons. *Pediatrics, 73*(2): 119–267.

Nye F (1978): Is choice and exchange theory the key? *J Marr Fam, 40*: 219–231.

Nye F (1979): Choice, exchange, and the family. In: *Contemporary Theories about the Family: General theories/Theoretical Orientations: Vol 2*, Burr W et al (eds.). New York: Free Press, pp. 1–41.

Orford J (1975): Self-reported coping behavior of wives of alcoholics and its association with drinking outcome. *J Stud Alcohol, 36*: 1254–1267.

Paolino R, McCrady B, Kogan K (1978): Alcoholic marriages: A longitudinal empirical assessment of alternative theories. *Br J Addiction, 73*: 129–138.

Parkes C (1972): *Bereavement: Studies of Grief in Adult Life*. New York: International Universities Press.

Pender N (1982): *Health Promotion in Nursing Practice*. East Norwalk, CT: Appleton-Century-Crofts.

Peterson C, Schwartz S, Seligman M (1981): Self-blame and depressive symptoms. *J Per Soc Psychol, 41*: 253–259.

Peterson R (1980): Social class, social learning and wife abuse. *Soc Serv Rev, 54*(3): 390–406.

Phillips L (1983): Abuse and neglect of the frail elderly at home: An exploration of theoretical relationships. *J Adv Nurs, 8*: 379–392.

Phillips L, Rempusheski V (1985): A decision-making model for diagnosing and intervening in elder abuse and neglect. *Nurs Res, 34*: 134–139.

Rounsaville B (1978): Theories in marital violence: Evidence from a study of battered women. *Victimology: Int J, 3*(1–2): 11–31.

Russell D (1982): *Rape in Marriage*. New York: Macmillan.

Scott P (1974): Battered wives. *Br J Psychiatry, 125*: 433–44.

Seligman M (1975): *Helplessness: On Depression and Death*. San Francisco: W. H. Freeman.

Sengstock M, Barrett S (1984): Domestic abuse of the elderly. In: *Nursing Care of Victims of Family Violence*, Campbell J, Humphreys J (eds.). Reston, VA: Reston, pp. 145–188.

Sengstock MC, Hwalek M (1985): *Comprehensive Index of Elder Abuse*. Detroit: Wayne State University Press.

Sherman L, Berk R (1983): *Police Responses to Domestic Assault: Preliminary Findings*. Washington, DC: Police Foundation.

Shipley S, Sylvester D (1982): Professionals attitudes toward violence in close relationships. *JEN, 8*: 88–91.

Silverman P (1981): *Helping Women Cope with Grief*. Beverly Hills, CA: Sage.

Snyder DK, Fruchtman LA (1981): Differential patterns of wife abuse: A data-based typology. *J Cons Clin Psychol, 49*: 878–885.

Steinmetz S (1977): *The Cycle of Violence: Assertive, Aggressive and Abusive Family Interaction*. New York: Praeger.

Star B (1978): Comparing battered and non-battered women. *Victimology, 3*(1–2): 32–44.

Stark E, Flitcraft A, Frazier W (1979): Medicine and patriarchal violence: The social construction of a "private" event. *Int J Health Serv, 9*(3): 461–493.

Stark-Adamec C, Adamec R (1982): Aggression by men against women: Adaptation or aberration? *Int J Wom Stud, 5*: 1–21.

Straus M (1973): A general systems approach to a theory of violence between family members. *Soc Sci Inform, 12*(3): 105–125.

Straus M, Gelles R, Steinmetz S (1980): *Behind Closed Doors: Violence in the American Family*. Garden City, NY: Anchor.

Strube M, Barbour L (1983): The decision to leave an abusive relationship: Economic dependence and psychological commitment. *J Marr Fam, 45*: 785–793.

Summit R (1981): Recognition and treatment of child sexual abuse. In: *Providing for the Emotional Health of the Pediatric Patient*, Hollingsworth CE (ed.). New York: Spectrum.

Symonds M (1975): Victims of violence: Psychological effects and aftereffects. *Am J Psychoanal, 35*: 19–26.

Thibaut J, Kelly J (1959): *The Social Psychology of Groups.* New York: Wiley.

Toby J (1966): Violence and the masculine ideal: Some qualitative data. *Ann Am Acad Polit Soc Sci, 364*: 19–28.

Vachon M et al (1982): Predictors and occelates of adaptation to conjugal bereavement. *Am J Psychiatry, 139*: 998–1002.

Walker L (1979): *The Battered Woman.* New York: Harper & Row.

Walker L (1984): *The Battered Woman Syndrome.* New York: Springer-Verlag.

Weinfourt R (1979): Battered women: The grieving process. *J Psychiatr Nurs Ment Health Serv, 17*(4): 40–47.

Weiss R (1975): *Marital Separation.* New York: Basic Books.

Westra B, Martin H (1981): Children of battered women. *Mat Child Nurs J, 10*: 41–54.

Young K (1978): Modes of appropriation and the sexual division of labor. In: *Feminism and Materialism,* Kuhn A, Wolpe A (eds.). Boston: Routledge and Kegan Paul, pp. 124–154.

26

ALZHEIMER'S DISEASE AND THE FAMILY

Mary Lou Muwaswes, RN, MS

Catherine L. Gilliss, RNC, DNSc

Ida M. Martinson, RN, PhD, FAAN

Glen Caspers Doyle, RN, EdD

Catherine A. Chesla, RN, DNSc

Joycelyn King, RNC, MS

Alzheimer's disease is the most common cause of severe dementia in this country; a conservative estimate suggests that 1.5 to 2 million Americans are currently suffering from the disease. This chapter provides an in-depth examination of Alzheimer's disease and its effects on the patient and the family. The prevalence and incidence of the disease, as well as descriptions of physiologic and behavioral aspects are discussed. Introduction to the nursing management of the symptoms is illustrated with a case study.

Mary Lou Muwaswes, an Assistant Clinical Professor in the Physiological Nursing Department at the University of California at San Francisco, is a specialist in neurological nursing and in the care of demented patients and their families.

Glen Doyle is Associate Professor and Director of the Interdisciplinary Gerontology Program at the School of Health and Social Work at California State University, Fresno. She is an expert gerontological nurse practitioner whose practice and teaching have emphasized care of Alzheimer's patients and their families.

Joycelyn King is a Clinical Nurse Specialist in Gerontology and the Family at the Veteran's Administration Hospital in Palo Alto, California, as well as an Assistant Clinical Professor in the departments of Family Health Care Nursing and Physiological Nursing at the University of California at San Francisco. In her clinical specialist's role, she has been successful in initiating programs for patients, family, and staff in long-term care of the elderly.

Introduction

In the United States, the prevalence of severe dementia changes from less than 1% at ages 65 to 70 to over 15% by age 85 (Gurland, 1984). Alzheimer's disease is the most common cause of severe dementia in the United States (Terry, Katzman, 1983). A conservative estimate suggests that 1.5 to 2 million Americans are currently suffering from Alzheimer's disease and that 100,000 die each year from its consequences (United States Publication, 1984). The annual cost of this disease in the United States exceeds $10 billion in nursing home care alone. The devastating nature of Alzheimer's disease and its financial and social impact led the popular science writer Lewis Thomas (1981) to characterize Alzheimer's disease as the "disease of the century."

Alzheimer's disease occurs most commonly in elderly individuals over age 70 but may occur less commonly in adults as young as 40. The development of Alzheimer's disease currently appears to be sporadic, but it is estimated that between 10% and 20% of cases are familial (Jarvik, 1978). The familial pattern of incidence is not clear, and the nature of transmission suggests an autosomal dominant pattern of transmission (Terry, Katzman, 1983; Prusiner, 1984b). There is evidence of a higher incidence of Down syndrome in the relatives of individuals with Alzheimer's disease. It has been demonstrated that Down syndrome adults develop dementia that histologically resembles Alzheimer's disease, although clinically not all of these cases develop manifestations of dementia (Creasey, Rapoport, 1985).

Description of Alzheimer's Disease

Morphologic and Biochemical Changes

The morphologic changes that develop in the brain with Alzheimer's disease also occur to a lesser degree and with different distribution in nondemented aged brains (Cote, 1981; Lauter, 1985). The neuropathologic features found in the brains of individuals with Alzheimer's disease are characterized by neuronal degeneration and by the presence of neurofibrillary tangles and neuritic or amyloid plaques found widely distributed in the cerebral cortex (Prusiner, 1984a; Perry, Perry, 1985). In addition, granulovascular changes have been found in the Hirano bodies in the hippocampus (Coyle, Price, DeLong, 1983). Recent findings (Hyman et al, 1984) suggest a specific pattern of cellular pathology that involves the major projection neurons of the hippocampal formation, which isolates the association cortices, basal forebrain, thalamus, and hypothalamus from the hippocampus.

Since the initial work of Tomlinson, Blessed, and Roth (1970), which correlated the degree and severity of the morphologic changes (neurofibrillary tangles and neuritic plaques) with the occurrence of dementia, the severity and degree of clinical presentation of dementia in Alzheimer's disease is believed to be strongly correlated with the extent of neuroanatomic abnormalities, specifically the number of amyloid plaques (Prusiner, 1984a; Perry et al, 1978). Although a correlation between these variables has been found, a causal relationship has not been established.

A reduced concentration of the enzyme choline acetyltransferase (ChAT) in the neocortex and paleocortex is the biochemical abnormality confirmed most often in brain tissue of individuals affected by Alzheimer's disease (Wurtman, 1985). This enzyme catalyzes the acetylation of choline to the neurotransmitter acetylcholine and is present in small quantities in cholinergic cells. Muscarinic cholinergic receptors are present in normal amounts in the brain tissue (Terry, Katzman, 1983). The reduction of ChAT and therefore of acetylcholine in the cortex may be related to the reductions of neurons in the basal forebrain nuclei. The relationship of these cellular abnormalities to the clinical manifestations of

Alzheimer's disease is based on the finding that the neuroanatomic pathways involved with maintenance of memory are cholinergic pathways and that cells of the hippocampus involved with memory are innervated by cholinergic pathways (Hyman et al, 1984). In fact, the degree of reduction of ChAT has been correlated positively with the density of neurofibrillary tangles, senile plaques, and the degree of dementia. The cholinergic deficiencies found in Alzheimer's disease may be only one of many interacting biochemical abnormalities of synaptic transmission (Terry, Katzman, 1983; Perry, Perry, 1985). The current theoretical hypotheses of the cause of Alzheimer's disease are presented in Table 26-1. There is strong scientific evidence to support the acetylcholine model, although this model does preclude the operation of other pathogenic mechanisms in Alzheimer's disease.

Behavioral Manifestations

Currently, there is no definitive clinical marker to detect the presence of Alzheimer's disease. The diagnosis of Alzheimer's disease during life is based on clinical criteria to evaluate the presence of dementia and diagnostic testing to rule out other clinical conditions that may resemble the dementia of Alzheimer's disease. A definitive diagnosis is made with pathologic confirmation postmortem that identifies the specific neuroanatomic abnormalities found in the brain of the individual with Alzheimer's disease (McKhann et al, 1984; Muwaswes, 1986).

The central feature, and usually the earliest manifestation, in the clinical presentation of Alzheimer's disease is an impairment of recent memory. A progressive and irreversible decline in cognitive function subsequently develops and abilities that involve reasoning, abstraction, and thinking are impaired (Terry, Katzman, 1983). Other salient features, perhaps resulting from these primary impairments, include changes in personality and manifestations of affective disturbances (Seltzer, Sherwin, 1983). Disturbances

associated with higher cortical function appear in some individuals, most often later in the course of the disease, and include aphasia, agnosia, and apraxia.

There is no unique behavioral pattern of dysfunction in individuals with Alzheimer's disease. The clinical course demonstrates individual differences and patterns of progression. Once symptoms are detected, individuals will be severely demented within 3 to 10 years (Barclay et al, 1985; Wurtman, 1985). At this time the inevitable consequence of Alzheimer's disease in the individual is progressive, irreversible loss of functional ability to a state of total dependence.

The Significance of Alzheimer's Disease to the Family

Since the 1970s, the health care and social science literature has recognized the significance of the role of the family in caring for a member with an illness that causes the symptoms of dementia. It is estimated that for every institutionalized individual with dementia, two reside in the community (Wilder, Teresi, Bennett, 1983). The family (nuclear or extended) remains the primary caregiver for individuals with dementia and provides day-to-day assistance as well as emotional, social, and financial support (Gurland, 1983; Wilder et al, 1983; Sainsbury, Grad de Alercon, 1970). This finding concurs with that of other investigators who have reported on family responsibility for a dependent family member (Brody, 1985; Johnson, Catalano, 1983; Lowenthal, 1964; Shana, 1978). Brody (1985) estimates that families provide 80% to 90% of medically related personal care, household help, transportation, and financial assistance for elderly family members. Additionally, it is the family that links the dependent member to the formal support systems (Aronson, Lipkowitz, 1981).

Table 26-1 Summary of Current Models of the Causes of Alzheimer's Disease (Principal investigator listed; see reference list for complete citation)

Model	Major Findings(s)	Investigators
Acetylcholine	The consistent postmortem biochemical abnormality identified in the brains of Alzheimer's patients found to be a reduction in the level of choline acetyltransferase	Davies, Maloney, 1976; Bowen et al, 1976; Coyle, 1983; Perry et al, 1978; White et al, 1977
Genetic	Identification of a high incidence of Alzheimer's disease within certain families	Heston, White, 1980; Jarvik, 1978
Abnormal protein	Presence of morphologic abnormalities of neurofibrillary tangles within neurons, amyloid surrounding and invading blood vessels, and amyloid plaques that replace degenerating nerve terminals	Terry, Wisniewski, 1975; Blessed et al, 1968; Prunsiner, 1984b
Infectious Agent	Identification of abnormal proteins in other models of dementia such as scrapie and Creutzfeldt–Jakob disease	Prunsiner, 1984a; Salazar, 1983
Toxin	Aluminum found in neurons with neurofibrillary tangles; precise role of aluminum in Alzheimer's disease not known	Perl, Brody, 1980; Klatzo et al, 1985; Crapper et al, 1978
Blood Flow	Secondary decline in cerebral blood flow and oxygen consumption in Alzheimer's patients, which may be the result of primary neuronal loss	Frackowiak, 1981; Yamaguchi, 1980; Mahendra, 1984; Ingvar, 1983

If the family member with Alzheimer's disease is at home, management of these patients involves a great deal of personal care, constant surveillance for physical safety, and intense attention to interpersonal interactions necessitated by the change in cognitive function. Established family patterns of communication, role responsibilities, daily activities, and social interactions are disrupted. Financial burden can compound this situation, particularly in view of the limited health care services available for Alzheimer's individuals. The family is forced to face significant legal issues that previously may not have been considered. Inevitably, the question of institutionalization will be addressed, and another set of difficult decisions and consequences arises. Thus, the stress on the family with a member who has Alzheimer's disease is enormous and unrelenting. Recent studies (George, 1983; Gilhooly, 1984; Pratt et al, 1985) have highlighted the fact that even after the family member with dementia has been institutionalized, the family continues its familial responsibilities, provides support and vigilant care, and experiences difficulties.

The diagnosis of Alzheimer's disease is therefore presumed to represent a stressful experience for family members, particularly when it is understood that no curative medical treatment is currently available and that the diagnosis signals a future of progressive deterioration of the mental and ultimately physical capabilities of the afflicted family member.

The diagnosis of Alzheimer's disease is also presumed to establish eventually a new role of a caregiver within a family network. The progressive nature of the symptoms of dementia, loss of mental function, and eventually physical function, are the igniting factors that necessitate that someone must assume responsibility for the individual with Alzheimer's disease.

One goal in research related to the family with a member with Alzheimer's disease is to describe the socioeconomic, psychologic, and physiologic factors that are part of the caregiver situation. The ultimate goal of research is to develop management interventions based on a sound theoretical framework that (1) provide support to the family and individual to maintain integrity and dignity and (2) develop substantive knowledge that can be applied to public policy issues.

Research Review

The purposes of the following review of the research literature related to dementia and Alzheimer's disease are (1) to identify the circumstances of the caregiving situation, (2) to describe the theoretical constructs or concepts that have currently been formulated to explain the impact and the consequences of caregiving on the family and (3) to devise management strategies to support family caregiving. In other words, we will attempt to answer the question "What do we currently know from research literature about the effects on the family who has a member with Alzheimer's disease?"

Although not inclusive of all the work in this area, the three themes chosen for review are (1) description of caregiving problems reported in the research of the last two decades by family and caregivers; (2) contributors to and correlates of caregiver burden; and (3) management of the behaviors that result from dementia.

Problems Experienced by Families and Caregivers

Numerous studies have described the specific behaviors of the demented family member that the family has reported as problematic or troublesome. Sanford (1975), in a British study of 50 elderly dependent subjects presented for hospital admission, examined the reported reasons the caregivers requested admission and the resources needed to alleviate the reported problems. Among the problems most often identified were sleep disturbances; incontinence of urine and feces; accidental falls; limited mobility; caregiver depression and anxiety; and restriction of caregiver social life. Fuller et al (1979) identified similar themes of concern to relatives who care for demented family members. In addition, these researchers identified the inability of the demented individual to recognize family members, changes in sexual behavior, disorientation, and paranoid behavior as problems.

Rabins et al (1982) interviewed the primary family caregivers of 55 demented individuals to determine the frequency and seriousness of problems for which the caregivers sought help. Though the patient's memory disturbances, catastrophic reactions, demanding and critical behaviors, night waking, and hiding things were identified most often, families reported physical violence, memory disturbances, incontinence, and catastrophic reactions to be the most serious problems. In a descriptive study comparing the families', staff's, and patients' evaluations of mental problems and functional impairment, Reifler et al (1982) found that the patients' evaluations of their levels of impairment were consistently underestimated, and the families' and staff's evaluations were consistently similar.

Caregivers also report problems with the role of caregiver. Feelings of anger, resentment, and shame have been reported by caregivers (Fuller et al, 1979; Rabins et al, 1982; Lazarus et al, 1981). Other investigators found that in addition to these emotional expressions to the caregiving situation, family caregivers also reported physical symptoms, interpersonal family problems, and problems adjusting to a new role. Rabins et al (1982) found that the most commonly reported problem of family caregivers was chronic fatigue (87%). Next often reported are loss of friends and family conflict. Lack of time for the caregiver's personal needs, the caregiver's fears for the future, and the excessive dependency of the demented individual were reported by Zarit et al (1980) as the most frequently reported troublesome problems. Seventy-nine percent of 240 family caregivers studied by Pratt et al (1985) reported that caring for an Alzheimer's family member had affected their health in a negative way. George (1983), in a retrospective survey of 502 family caregivers compared to several community samples, reported higher psychotropic drug use, more stress symptoms, less life satisfaction, and less ability to pursue recreational and social activities. Gilhooly (1984) studied 37 family caregivers to describe the factors that influence their psychologic well-being and found an overall low morale in caregivers. A higher morale was reported by those who care for a female rather than male dependent.

These descriptions of the problematic behaviors manifested by the demented individual and the problems experienced by the caregivers provide considerable insight into the difficulties that families may experience when caring for a family member with dementia. Additionally, these descriptive studies emphasize the variability in behaviors that may be manifested by the Alzheimer individual as well as the variability in the caregiver's reaction to the role of caregiver. Several investigators have found that caregivers reported no problems. Unfortunately, use of self-reported problem identification as the only method of quantitative data collection limits the understanding of these findings and comparison with other studies, and limits the ability to draw conclusions about the effects these problems have on family caregivers.

In a number of studies, measures of severity of illness have been examined as a variable that influences the family caregiving situation. The evaluation of dementia has been kept separate from the evaluation of functional and physical ability. Several authors have developed checklists for caregivers to rate patients on these

dimensions. An overview of the instruments used to measure severity of illness is provided in Table 26-2.

Contributors to and Correlates of Caregiver Burden

In order to evaluate the impact and consequences of caregiving on the person responsible for care, the concept of caregiver burden has often been used as an outcome variable in studies of families caring for members with dementia. Wilder et al (1983) point out that development of the concept of burden over the past 30 years arose from concern about the use and costs of long-term care in this country and from efforts to study the variables pertinent to families' decisions to institutionalize dependent family members. Lowenthal (1964) suggested that burden is the cost to the psychologic, physical, and financial resources of a family. Poulschock and Deimling (1984) conceptualized burden as a mediating force between elders' impairments and effects on caregivers.

Zarit et al (1980) measured the functional ability and severity of dementia of the Alzheimer family member, as well as perceived burden, functional ability of the caregiver, duration of illness, and frequency of family visits. They found that the number of family visits a caregiver received each week was negatively correlated to the amount of burden caregivers experienced. The authors suggest that social support may be an intervention strategy for family caregivers.

Wilder et al (1983) conceptualized burden as inconvenience and willingness to continue to provide care to a demented family member. They found that the extent of activity limitations and frequency of abnormal behaviors of the demented individual were the most significant predictors of perceived inconvenience and affected intensified burden. The findings of their study suggest that dementia per se and its severity does not predict the perception of inconvenience of caregivers and supports the findings of previous work (Zarit et al, 1980). Subsequent investigators also found that the severity of dementia was not associated with decision-making or indicators of caregiver well-being (Hirschfeld, 1983; George, 1983; Gilhooly, 1984).

Several other investigators have examined the effects and consequences of caregiving on the family by studying caregiver well-being, coping, and decision-making. The instruments used, variables measured, and major findings are presented in Table 26-3.

Hirschfeld (1983) conducted a study of 30 family caregivers of individuals with senile dementia to examine the factors that influence the decision to continue to care for their relative at home. Over half of the caregivers in this study were wives with the average age of 69, and 64%

of the individuals with dementia were severely demented and demonstrated major functional impairment. In spite of this impairment, no relationship between these variables (age, severity of illness, and so on) and the decision to institutionalize the dependent family member was found.

In addition to quantitative data collection methods, Hirschfeld (1983) conducted in-depth interviews from which she identified several important variables. Mutuality, defined as the ability to find gratification in the relationship with the demented person and meaning from the caregiving situation, was identified as the major variable that influences the decision to continue home care. The less the mutuality, the more likely that institutionalization was considered.

Table 26–2 Severity of Illness: Instruments and Variables Measured in Studies of the Family with a Member with Dementia (Principal investigator listed; see reference list for complete citation)

Variables	Instruments	Investigators
Dementia	Kahn Mental Status Questionnaire	Zarit, 1980; Reifler, 1982 Wilder, 1983
	Face–Hand Test	Zarit, 1980
	Mental Status Exam (Jacobs, 1977)	Zarit, 1980
	Blessed Dementia Scale	Levine, 1983
	Short Portable Mental Status Questionnaire (Pfeiffer, 1975)	Hirschfeld, 1983
	Posts Clinical Sensorium (1965)	Gilhooly, 1984
	Modified Crichton Royal Behavioral Rating Scale	Gilhooly, 1984
Functional ability	Physical and Instrumental Activity of Daily Living Scales (Lawton, 1971)	Zarit, 1980
	Comprehensive Assessment and Referral Evaluation (CARE)	Wilder, 1983
	Older Americans Resources and Services Program Questionnaire (OARS) (Duke University, 1975)	Hirschfeld, 1983 Gilhooly, 1984
Physical ability	Older Americans Resources and Services Questionnaire (OARS) (Duke University, 1975)	Hirschfeld, 1983
Type and frequency of behavior problems	Memory and Behavior Checklist Problem List, Type and Frequency	Zarit, 1980 Rabins, 1982; Reifler, 1983; Levin, 1983; George, 1983; Gilhooly, 1984

Table 26–3 Instruments and Variables Measured to Describe the Effects of Caregiving on the Family

Investigator	Sample	Instrument	Variable
Hirschfeld, 1983	30 caregivers	Older Americans Resources and Services Program Questionnaire (OARS) (Duke University, 1975) (FC*, CR**)	Functional and physical ability
	30 caregivers	Short Portable Mental Status Questionnaire (Pfeiffer, 1975) (CR)	Mental status
		In-depth focused interview Participant Observation	Author-developed scales of morale, tension, management ability, and mutuality
George, 1983	502 caregivers All instruments administered to FC	Questionnaire	Demographic data
		demographic	Subjective physical health
		physical health	Psychiatric symptoms
		mental health (Short Portable Emotional Scale, Pfeiffer, 1979); Langer 22-Item Screening Scale, Langer, 1962)	Psychologic distress
		health behavior	Health behavior
		Affect Balance Scale (Bradburn, 1969)	Subjective well-being
		Single Life Item Satisfaction	Amount of satisfaction with social activity
		Amount of Time in Preferred Activities	Economic resources
		Financial Resources	Use of community resources
		Knowledge of Alzheimer's disease and participation in community support group	Severity of illness
		Demographic data about Alzheimer's disease, frequency of symptoms, length of diagnosis	
Pratt et al, 1985	240 caregivers	Caregivers Burden Scale (Zarit, 1980) (FC)	Subjective response of effect
Wilder et al, 1983		F-Copes (McCubbin, 1981) (FC)	Internal and external coping abilities
		Interview (FC)	Demographic data
			Perception of health status
		Family Support Measures (1600 items) 100 scales developed (FC)	Physical and psychiatric symptoms
			Self-perception of inconvenience
			Extendedness
			Family tradition
			Self-reported behaviors of care receivers
		Kahn–Goldfard Mental Status Examination (CR)	Dementia
		Comprehensive Assessment and Referral Evaluation (FC, CR)	Activity ability

*Family Caregiver = FC
**Carereceiver = CR

Hirschfeld (1983) also found that the higher the management ability and morale the less likely was institutionalization considered. In addition, the more severe the tension of the caregiver, regardless of the level of mental or physical impairment of the demented individual, the more likely was the caregiver ready to consider institutionalization.

Wilder et al (1983) proposed a model of family burden after developing and testing a 1600-item family support instrument. Instrument testing was conducted initially on a cross-national United States–United Kingdom random sample of community-based elderly; a subsample of 200 supporters of community-based elderly were also interviewed for further instrument development. From the original family support questionnaire, 100 scales were developed, and important variables were identified. Socioeconomic data were collected. Caregiver burden was conceptualized as "inconvenience experienced while providing assistance to the impaired relative in personal care, visiting, and helping with the household chores" (p. 245). High internal consistency and interrater reliability was obtained for the scale developed for this variable and subsequent variables. Additional scales were developed for the concepts of:

- Extendedness—the degree to which the older person maintains relationships with kin outside the primary unit

- Family tradition—the family's history of caring for their elderly and other family members

- Behavior—abnormal behavior demonstrated by the impaired person

- Dementia—cognitive impairment

- Activity limitation—functional capacity to perform the self-care activities required for independent living (Wilder et al, 1983)

They found that only activity limitation and behavior ratings were significant predictors (positively related) of inconvenience or burden, with activity limitation the most significant when analysis was completed on all scales. The inability of the analysis to account for the variability of the sample (0.34 for informant scales, 0.38 for the diagnostic ratings, and 0.36 for the scales of activity limitation) suggests that other important measures were not accounted for or that the sample is too small to predict changes. The authors suggest that the operational characteristics of the concept of burden, measured in this study as inconvenience, may need to be expanded to include other manifestations such as morale, stress symptoms, and ill health.

Pratt et al (1985) surveyed 240 family caregivers of Alzheimer's patients to identify the coping strategies they used and the relationship of these strategies to their sense of burden. The majority of the family members with Alzheimer's disease lived in the community (62%) and half of those lived with the caregiver. The remainder lived in their own home (12%) or in an institution (38%). Demographic data were collected with an author-developed instrument that asked questions of the caregiver regarding the relationship to the patient, the patient's place of residence, the duration of illness, and the caregiver's subjective reporting of the caregiver's health status, the perception of how caregiving had affected it, and whether or not the caregivers had a confidant.

Caregiver's burden score, measured by the Caregiver Burden Scale (Zarit et al, 1980), did not vary significantly by patient's residence or by caregiver's age, sex, income, educational level, presence of a confidant, or membership in a support group. Caregiver burden scores were negatively correlated with the caregivers' subjective reporting of their health status, and all the respondents stated that caregiving had had a negative effect on their health status to some degree. Coping was measured in this study with the Family-Crisis Oriented Personal Evaluation. Correlation analysis demonstrated that caregivers' lower burden scores were significantly related to use of internal coping strategies, such as confidence with problem-solving and reframing. Lower burden scores were also positively related to the external coping strategies of seeking spiritual support and feeling supported by the extended family.

The studies by Pratt et al (1985), Wilder et al (1983), and Zarit et al (1980) emphasized the subjective sense of burden experienced by the family caregiver. In a study by George (1983), measures of caregiver burden were conceptualized in reverse—that is, by measures of well-being—to study the relationships between subjective well-being and other self-reports of health and psychologic status, economic and social resources, information about the severity of illness, and knowledge of Alzheimer's disease. Procedures to ensure a diverse sampling frame were used, and the sample included 502 caregivers, over half of whom lived with the carereceiver. Twenty-nine percent of the caregivers cared for family members who had Alzheimer's disease. The five predictive variables that had positive significant effects on well-being, as measured by the Balance Score, were higher levels of education (positive relationship); amount of assistance caregivers received from social supports (positive relationship); lower levels of stress symptoms; higher levels of satisfaction with social activities; and perception of a better economic status.

The findings of these studies suggest that severity of the symptoms of dementia is not the best predictor of the effects of caregiving on caregivers. Comparisons across studies are difficult as measurements of illness severity vary. Some are self-reports and others are clinical evaluation tools to evaluate dementia; these tools have inherent problems such as the difficulty of evaluating mild dementia and lack of instrument sensitivity.

Variation in conceptualization and measurement of burden also makes comparisons across studies difficult. Sample size varies in studies, and most studies use convenience samples. Findings generated by these studies, however, point out that a number of negative effects on the family caregiver's health, subjective well-being, satisfaction with social activities, and financial

resources exist. The lack of consistent findings across studies suggests that certain key variables have not been considered in all studies, such as the prior relationship of the caregiver and carereceiver (Hirschfeld, 1983; Gilhooly, 1984) and the dynamic qualities of this relationship and interactions with other family members.

Management of the Symptoms of Dementia

Research related specifically to assisting the family to manage the symptoms of dementia is scarce. Environmental manipulation, psychologic support measures, and pharmacologic treatment of behavioral symptoms of dementia are the three areas that have received the most attention in recent years. These treatments can be conceptualized as being aimed toward prevention or amelioration of the behavioral symptoms of dementia (Muwaswes, 1986).

Reality orientation is a management technique that illustrates the principle of environmental manipulation. Reality orientation involves (1) development of a structured environ- ment and rehearsal of everyday events at specified times or (2) reorientation of a demented individual with each interaction in a structured environment (Folsom, 1968). Systematic studies to evaluate reality orientation have focused on elderly, institutionalized, confused individuals. Difficulties encountered in interpreting the findings are related to (1) the ability to compare the study groups used; (2) the variety of measurement techniques used to evaluate outcome; and (3) the difficulty in ascertaining the effects of reality orientation on all aspects of functional behavior (Burton, 1982). Additionally, although memory-training techniques have been shown to improve performance in normal subjects, their effects on subjects with severe memory disturbances have not been shown to be successful, except for brief periods (Zarit, Zarit, Reever, 1982).

More recently, Harvath (1988) has described a technique known as "going along," successfully employed by caregivers. In this strategy, the caregiver does *not* attempt to change the patient's perceptions but adjusts the environment to respond to the patient's requests.

Psychologic support measures use the principles of reality orientation in a less formal way and also use the principles of psychotherapeutic techniques (Muwaswes, 1986) to manage aberrant behavior in a demented individual. These intervention techniques include using face-to-face contact during conversation; using continual and repeated interpersonal orientation with all interactions; providing reassurance (Boss, 1983); and using verbal as well as nonverbal cues during conversation.

A number of affective and behavioral changes have been described in association with dementia, distinct from the cognitive impairment that occurs. These include such problems as sleep disturbances, agitation, combativeness, and emotional lability. Although many of these behavioral disturbances can be managed by environmental and psychologic support measures, at times pharmacologic treatment is necessary. The neuroleptics (such as haloperidol) are antipsychotic agents used most frequently for the management of agitation in individuals with dementia (Barnes et al, 1982; Thompson, Moran, Nies, 1983). Because of the increased risk of side effects when administering antipsychotics to an aged population and the limited benefits of the drug on treating specific behavioral symptoms, judicious use of antipsychotics is strongly recommended for management of the aberrant behavioral manifestations of dementia (Ayd, 1978; Helms, 1985). When used, antipsychotic medications should be administered in conjunction with psychotherapeutic techniques.

Case Study of a Family Caregiver

This case study describes an interaction between a nurse and a family caregiver in which the nurse requests the caregiver to describe some of the salient issues of care. The family member with Alzheimer's disease is currently in a board-and-care home.

Mr. H. is a 65-year-old electrician. He and Mrs. H. have been married for 25 years; they have no children and no relatives who live close to them. They own their own home and live in a major metropolitan area. Approximately 2 1/2 years ago, Mr. H. noticed memory problems and a mood change in his 65-year-old wife and brought her to their family physician, who referred them to a neurologist. After a complete medical and neurologic evaluation, the possible diagnosis of Alzheimer's disease was made by the neurologist. Mr. H. states he had little understanding of the diagnosis at that time. His family physician explained the implications to him and referred him to a local chapter of the Alzheimer's Disease and Related Disorders Association (ADRDA). He has been attending their monthly meetings for the past two years. Mr. H. states that he initially did not accept the diagnosis. He describes the most difficult time as when his wife was no longer able to verbally respond to him. He saw this period as a turning point in his realization of the implications of the diagnosis.

> When she couldn't understand, when she could not respond with a straight conversation . . . when that first happened, I think that was one of the worst things that struck me . . . when I experienced this, it was almost like saying this is for real.

The feeling that Mr. H. describes during this period is helplessness, which he states is a hurtful emotion.

> You are really going to have to accept this. There is nothing you can do about it. No medication, no more nothing . . . I have the money to give her the best medical care, but there is nothing the doctors can do . . . all you can do is just spend money and then sit there and watch the person suffer. She doesn't know, she's not hurting, she doesn't even know what's happening to her.

When asked what he does when he feels helpless, Mr. H. avoids a direct answer but laments,

We did everything we wanted to do. We lived a good life. We enjoyed ourselves. The only thing I wish that we'd have done is have more of having a good time.

Mr. H. states that his primary worry for the future is financial. Although he currently does not have financial problems, he states that it is difficult to predict the future. He has contacted his attorney for advice about the legal steps to take to protect his assets and to make decisions about his wife.

In spite of the pervading feelings of sadness and hopelessness that Mr. H. reported, he actively pursued help from several formal and informal channels of assistance. Mr. H. used the monthly meetings of ADRDA as a support and way to gather information about methods of caring for his wife. He tried to keep his knowledge about Alzheimer's disease current and wrote letters to physicians whenever he heard about a new treatment being used for Alzheimer's disease. Although he had no close relatives nearby, he maintained an active network of friends and planned for his and his wife's future by instituting the necessary legal procedures. We hear him simultaneously express hope and worry for his and his wife's future.

The caregiver who cares for the person with Alzheimer's disease at home provides for and must cope with the physical and emotional needs of the afflicted family member. In addition to this unrelenting task, family caregivers are witness to the deterioration of personality that occurs with Alzheimer's disease. The following poem succinctly describes one woman's observations of the changes in cognitive function and functional abilities she noticed while caring for her husband. The poem offers a powerful description of the feelings and emotions that these changes precipitated in her.

Blurred

He slips into depression;
Clinging like a sickly child,
Kissing me over and over,

Pulling up a chair very close,
Closing a book I'm reading,
Covering my writing with a hand.

Cruelly rude to visitors,
Undressing over and over,
Yet unable to redress.
Clothes are put on backward,
Shoes always on wrong feet,
and he pees down the vents.

He looks out and tears the curtains,
Eyes plead
For understanding.
Nights are shattered as he calls
For people long dead,
And makes a pistol sign to his head.

With irregular regularity
He gets lost.
Neighbors bring him home
And look at me accusingly.
Doctors say sedate him
and mention nursing homes.

There is no one but me
To decide his fate.
No one but me to guide him.
So put up the lights
Again this Christmas
To see them blurred by tears.

Betty Morgan, 1984
Reprinted with permission.

Nursing Implications

As an individual practitioner or as a member of an interdisciplinary team, the nurse is in a key position to optimize the care of the person with Alzheimer's disease. Because the nurse has knowledge of the disease process, concern about how the family functions with a demented individual, and knowledge and experience with community health organizations and services, the nurse is the logical coordinator of care for the family with a member with Alzheimer's disease.

The nurse may first come in contact with the person with Alzheimer's disease and the family in a variety of care settings, from the acute-care facility to the community setting to longer-term care facilities. The nurse may interact with the patient with Alzheimer's and the family at any point in the disease course. Knowledge of the physical, behavioral, and emotional symptoms of Alzheimer's disease is essential for any nurse who may care for these individuals and families. In addition, knowledge of the potential cost of caregiving that the family pays related to emotional, financial, and social changes they experience is essential. The impact that caregiving has on the family must be evaluated with awareness that each family has developed a unique fabric of beliefs, patterns of social and interpersonal interactions, and manners of behavior in daily life that define them as a family. During the initial contact with a family, the purpose of nursing can be identified as (1) evaluation of how the family functions, which includes evaluation of the individual with Alzheimer's disease; (2) identification of the family response to the behavioral and emotional symptoms of the individual with Alzheimer's disease; (3) identification of the social, financial, emotional, and spiritual needs of the family; and (4) delineation of the current resources that the family uses to manage, cope, and deal with their situation.

The goals of nursing in this situation are (1) to provide accurate information about the disease to the family; (2) to provide accurate information about resources; (3) to assist the family to develop plans related to daily activities; and (4) to be available for emotional or affective support of the family.

Research Implications and Questions

Data essential to the development of sound theoretical understanding of the effects of Alzheimer's disease on the family and afflicted family member is accumulating. The areas that need further exploration are several: (1) descrip-

tion of the course of Alzheimer's disease; (2) description of the consequences of Alzheimer's disease on the family; and (3) the correlation of Alzheimer's disease characteristics with the effects on the family.

Perhaps because of each individual's unique psychologic and physiologic makeup, individuals with Alzheimer's disease manifest the abnormalities of brain function with a wide variety of behavioral and affective responses. Research evidence is conclusive that Alzheimer's disease disrupts the structural and metabolic function of cortical neurons. This primary dysfunction is translated into disorders in memory, language, and abilities that require thinking, perception, attention, and spatial-motor function. Combined, these disorders are termed dementia. The medical diagnosis of Alzheimer's disease is difficult to make with total accuracy during life because of the problems with evaluating dementia, a process that depends on using behavioral responses to observations and questions to establish its presence. In addition, the symptoms of dementia can be precipitated by a wide variety of etiologic events that directly or indirectly affect the metabolic function of the brain; resemble the symptoms of depression; and occur simultaneously with depression. Mild dementia remains difficult to evaluate with accuracy with current evaluation methods.

For these reasons, reliable, valid, and sensitive instruments that evaluate the presence of dementia need to be used in research studies that measure these symptoms as a variable. Further, because of concern about the lack of consistency in terminology, a Work Group on the Diagnosis of Alzheimer's Disease (McKhann et al, 1984) developed a set of criteria for the clinical diagnosis of Alzheimer's disease (Table 26-4), which provides a basis for definition of terms for practitioners in this area.

Measures of dementia have been used to quantify the variable severity of illness in studies related to dementia and the family. Because of the problems in using mental status tools to predict functional and physical function (Vitaliano et al, 1984), researchers have used instruments that separate these functions as variables. Although Wilder et al (1983) found the degree of activity limitation (a measure of physical and functional ability) predictive of self-perceived caregiver burden, this finding has not been consistently reproduced in other studies of caregiver burden (Worcester, Quayhagen, 1983). The inability to correlate severity of illness with outcome variables, such as caregiver burden, decision-making regarding institutionalization, and stress symptoms, may reflect the lack of specificity and sensitivity of the instruments used to measure severity of illness rather than the importance of this variable in predicting effects on the family caregiver.

In addition to the need to quantify the severity of illness variable with measures of frequencies, such as how much and how often a behavior or symptom occurs, Zarit and Zarit (1982) point out that in predicting a subjective feeling like burden or impact, the "other variables that lie along a subjective dimension have more power than do frequency counts." This statement underscores the importance not only of defining accurately the objective manifestations of the illness but also the subjective response to these manifestations that the family has experienced (Cohen, Kennedy, Eisdorfer, 1984).

Although not conclusive, research evidence suggests that in addition to the subjective responses of caregiving that a family experiences, there are changes that can be measured objectively, in areas of psychologic and physical health, social activity, and economic status. Additional variables have been identified as important by researchers through observations and discussions with family members. These include phenomena such as stress, burden, and coping ability. These more abstract variables have been more elusive to measure than others, and their relationship to the effects on the family remain difficult to define.

Current research related to the family with a member with Alzheimer's disease has evaluated and measured possible effects on the family at one point in time. There are limitations to drawing conclusions and making interpretations about family and caregiver function in response to Alzheimer's disease when variables are measured only once. The care and responsibility of a family member is continuous but varies during the day and night as well as from day to day. The family caregiver's response to providing care is equally variable. The dynamic nature of both the afflicted individual's behavior and symptoms and the caregiver's responses demands appropriate research design to account for these qualities.

Burnside (1983) pleads with nurses to increase their knowledge of the problems associated with Alzheimer's disease and challenges nurse researchers to develop knowledge by studying the clinical problems related to this disease, such as wandering behavior, incontinence, aggressiveness, and nutrition needs.

George and Gwyther (1984) underscore the needs of the family with this compelling statement: "The voice of our findings (from a study of 500 family caregivers) seems small compared to the emotions that simply scream to be heard in the essay data."

Examples of research studies that explore the physical and emotional symptoms of Alzheimer's disease are two proposals funded recently by the Alzheimer's Disease and Related Disorders Association (ADRDA). These studies have been developed and will be conducted by nurses. Wells (personal communication, 1985) will examine the aspects of Alzheimer's patients and of the environment that are associated with urine control. Ryden (personal communication, 1985) will explore the occurrence of aggressive behavior in community-situated demented individuals to identify the contextual, frequency pattern, and course of this behavior, as well as the perceptions of the family and their reaction to aggressive behavior.

Table 26–4   Criteria for Clinical Diagnosis of Alzheimer's Disease

I. The criteria for the clinical diagnosis of *probable* Alzheimer's disease include:

Dementia established by clinical examination and documented by the Mini-Mental Test, Blessed Dementia Scale, or some similar examination, and confirmed by neuropsychological tests;

Deficits in two or more areas of cognition;

Progressive worsening of memory and other cognitive functions;

No disturbance of consciousness;

Onset between ages 40 and 90, most often after age 65; and

Absence of systemic disorders or other brain diseases that in and of themselves could account for the progressive deficits in memory and cognition.

II. The diagnosis of *probable* Alzheimer's disease is supported by:

Progressive deterioration of specific cognitive functions such as language (aphasia), motor skills (apraxia), and perception (agnosia);

Impaired activities of daily living and altered patterns of behavior;

Family history of similar disorders, particularly if confirmed neuropathologically; and

Laboratory results of:
normal lumbar puncture as evaluated by standard techniques,
normal pattern or nonspecific changes in EEG, such as increased slow-wave activity, and
evidence of cerebral atrophy on CT with progression documented by serial observation.

III. Other clinical features consistent with the diagnosis of *probable* Alzheimer's disease, after exclusion of causes of dementia other than Alzheimer's disease include:

Plateaus in the course of progression of the illness;

Associated symptoms of depression, insomnia, incontinence, delusions, illusions, hallucinations, catastrophic verbal, emotional, or physical outbursts, sexual disorders, and weight loss;

Other neurologic abnormalities in some patients, especially with more advanced dis-

---

There are many unanswered questions about the management of behavioral and physical symptoms in Alzheimer's disease. Although Alzheimer's disease dementia shares many similarities with other irreversible, progressive dementias, it is important to study as homogeneous a population as possible (as well as to identify the similarities precisely). Few past studies have done this. Suggestions for future research include (1) replication of well-designed studies; (2) use of more qualitative approaches to data collection; (3) use of prospective longitudinal studies to examine the interaction of the caregiver and patient; (4) concept clarification regarding burden; (5) definition of severity of illness using reliable, accurate, and valid instruments; (6) prospective longitudinal studies that evaluate the effect of caregiving on the health of the caregiver; and (7) studies that test nursing interventions to promote family and caregiver health.

Summary

During the last ten years, there has been a heightened awareness about Alzheimer's disease and including motor signs such as increased muscle tone, myoclonus, or gait disorder;

Seizures in advanced disease; and

CT normal for age.

IV. Features that make the diagnosis of *probable* Alzheimer's disease uncertain or unlikely include:

Sudden, apoplectic onset;

Focal neurologic findings such as hemiparesis, sensory loss, visual field deficits, and incoordination early in the course of the illness; and

Seizures or gait disturbances at the onset or very early in the course of the illness.

V. Clinical diagnosis of *possible* Alzheimer's disease:

May be made on the basis of the dementia syndrome, in the absence of other neurological, psychiatric, or systemic disorders sufficient to cause dementia, and in the presence of variations in the onset, in the presentation, or in the clinical course;

Reprinted with permission from *Neurology*, 1984: 34: 940.

May be made in the presence of a second systemic or brain disorder sufficient to produce dementia, which is not considered to be *the* cause of the dementia; and

Should be used in research studies when a single, gradually progressive severe cognitive deficit is identified in the absence of other identifiable cause.

VI. Criteria for diagnosis of *definite* Alzheimer's disease are:

The clinical criteria for probable Alzheimer's disease and

Histopathologic evidence obtained from a biopsy or autopsy.

VII. Classification of Alzheimer's disease for research purposes should specify features that may differentiate subtypes of the disorder, such as:

Familial occurrence;

Onset before age of 65;

Presence of trisomy-21; and

Coexistence of other relevant conditions such as Parkinson's disease.

ease and other neurologic disorders that cause dementia. This awareness has taken several forms and produced several effects. Increased media exposure, in all forms, has been part of the public awareness campaign sponsored by the organizations that represent families who have a member with Alzheimer's disease or a related disorder. This campaign has been successful in describing the symptoms of Alzheimer's disease to the public, in generating public opinion sympathetic to the plight of individuals with Alzheimer's disease and their families, and in presenting and describing the financial and social burden that families experience.

Significant progress has been made recently in the field of neuroscience that has contributed to the understanding of the pathologic and physiologic mechanisms of Alzheimer's disease. Optimism that this trend will continue was reflected in a recent national conference (Hillhaven Foundation Conference, 1985).

There remain many unanswered questions that cover several areas of concern related to the family with a member with Alzheimer's disease. These questions have been generated from the research findings currently available in the area and from observations reported in the narrative literature by health care workers in this field.

Issues for Further Investigation

1. What are the most troublesome and bothersome symptoms to the family that the Alzheimer's afflicted family member has? Does the effect of these symptoms on family members change over time?

2. What personal meanings and life circumstances influence the family to continue to provide care in the home.?

3. What is the effect of the burden of Alzheimer's on the family member's health and life satisfaction over time?

4. What is the process of bereavement for the family members before and after the death of the Alzheimer's victim?

5. What individual and family interventions would be most useful for the families while providing care for their loved one either in home or in an outside institution?

6. What would be the ideal care system for the Alzheimer's victim and family?

References

Aronson MK, Lipkowitz R (1981): Senile dementia, Alzheimer's type: The family and the health care delivery system. *J Am Geriatr Soc, 29*: 568–571.

Ayd FJ (1978): Haloperidol: Twenty years' clinical experience. *J Clin Psychiatry, 39*: 807–814.

Barclay LL et al (1985): Survival in Alzheimer's disease and vascular dementias. *Neurology, 35*: 834–840.

Barnes R et al (1982): Efficacy of antipsychotic medications in behaviorally disturbed dementia patients. *Am J Psychiatry, 139*: 1170–1174.

Blessed G, Tomlinson BE, Roth M (1968): The association between quantitative measurements of dementia & of senile changes in the cerebral gray matter of elderly subjects. *Br J Psychiatry, 114*: 797.

Boss B (1983): The dementias. *J Neurosurg Nurs, 15*: 87–97.

Brody EM (1985): Parent care as a normative family stress. *Gerontologist, 25*: 19–29.

Burnside IM (1983): If I don't worry, who will? *J Gerontol Nurs, 9*: 2.

Burton M (1982): Reality orientation for the elderly: A critique. *J Adv Nurs, 7*: 427–433.

Cohen D, Kennedy G, Eisdorfer C (1984): Phases of change in the patient with Alzheimer's dementia: A conceptual dimension for defining health care management. *J Am Geriatr Soc, 32*: 11–15.

Cote L (1981): Aging of the brain and dementia. In: *Principals of Neural Science*, Kandel RW, Schwartz JH (eds.). New York: Elsevier.

Coyle JT, Price DL, DeLong MR (1983): Alzheimer's disease: A disorder of cortical cholinergic innervation. *Science, 219*: 1184–1190.

Crapper DR, Karlik S, DeBoni V (1978): Aluminum and other metals in senile (Alzheimer's) dementia. In: Alzheimer's Disease: Senile Dementia and Related Disorders (Aging Series), Katzman R, Terry RD, Bick KL (eds.). New York: Raven.

Creasey H, Rapoport SE (1985): The aging human brain. *Ann Neurology, 17*: 2–10.

Davies P, Maloney AJR (1976): Selective loss of central cholinergic neurons in Alzheimer's disease. *Lancet, 11*: 1403.

Folsom JC (1968): Reality orientation for the elderly mental patient. *J Geriatr Psychiatry, 1*: 291–307.

Frackowiak RSJ et al (1981): Regional cerebral oxygen supply and utilization in dementia. *Brain, 104*: 753–778.

Fuller J et al (1979): Dementia: Supportive groups for relatives. *Br Med J, 1*: 1684–1685.

George LK (1983): Caregiver well-being: Correlates and relationships with participation in community self-help groups. A final report submitted to AARP Andrus Foundation.

George L, Gwyther L (1984, June): Caregiver well-being: Selected findings. Paper presented at Veterans Administration Alzheimer's Conference, San Francisco.

Gilhooly MLM (1984): The impact of care-giving on care-givers: Factors associated with the psychological well-being of people supporting a demented relative in the community. *Br J Med Psychol, 57*: 35–44.

Gurland BJ (1984): Public health aspects of Alzheimer's disease and related disorders. In: *Alzheimer's Disease and Related Disorders*, Kelly WE (ed.). Springfield, IL: Charles C Thomas.

Harvath T (1988): Family caregiving to the cognitively impaired older person. Paper given at "Nursing of Families with Acute or Chronic Illness," Oregon Health Sciences University, Portland (February, 1988).

Helms PM (1985): Efficacy of antipsychotics in the treatment of behavioral complications of dementia: A review of the literature. *J Am Geriatr Soc, 33*: 206–209.

Heston LL, White J (1980): A family study of Alzheimer's disease and senile dementia: An interim report. *Proceedings of the American Psychopathological Association, 69*: 63–73.

Hillhaven Foundation Conference (1985): Alzheimer's disease: A mystery unraveling. San Francisco.

Hirschfeld M (1983): Homecare versus institutionalization: Family caregiving and senile brain disease. *Int J Nurs Stud, 20*: 23–32.

Hyman BT et al (1984): Alzheimer's disease: Cell-specific pathology isolates the hippocampal formation. *Science, 225*: 1168–1170.

Ingvar DH (1983): Cerebral blood flow and cerebral metabolism in Alzheimer's disease. In: *Alzheimer's Disease*, Reisberg B (ed.). New York: Free Press.

Jarvik LF (1978): Genetic factors and chromosomal aberrations in Alzheimer's disease, senile dementia, and related disorders. In: *Alzheimer's Disease: Senile Dementia and Related Disorders* (Aging Series: Vol 7) Katzman R, Terry RD, Bick KL (eds.). New York: Raven.

Johnson CL, Catalano DJ (1983): A longitudinal study of family supports to impaired elderly. *Gerontologist, 23*: 612–618.

Klatzo I, Wisniewski H, Streicher E (1965): Experimental production of neurofibrillary degeneration: Vol 1, Light microscope observations. *J Neuropathol Exp Neurol, 24*: 187.

Lazarus LW et al (1981): A pilot study of an Alzheimer patient-relative discussion group. *Gerontologist, 21*: 353–358.

Levine NB, Dastoor DP, Gendron CE (1983): Coping with dementia: A pilot study. *J Am Geriatr Soc, 31*: 12–18.

Lowenthal MF (1964): *Lives in Distress*. New York: Basic Books.

Mahendra B (1984): *Dementia: A Survey of the Syndrome*. Boston: MTP Press.

McCubbin H et al (1981): Coping-health inventory for parents. St. Paul: University of Minnesota.

McKhann G et al (1984): Clinical diagnosis of Alzheimer's disease. *Neurology, 34*: 939–943.

Muwaswes M (1986): Alterations in consciousness: Delirium and dementia. In: *Pathophysiological Phenomena in Nursing: Human Responses to Illness*, Carrieri V, Lindsey A, West C (eds.). Philadelphia: Saunders.

Perl DP, Brody AR (1980): Alzheimer's disease: X-ray spectrometric evidence of aluminum accumulation in neurofibrillary tangle-bearing neurons. *Science, 208*: 207.

Perry EK, Perry RH (1985): A review of the neuropathological and neurochemical correlates of Alzheimer's disease. *Dan Med Bull, 32*: 27–34.

Perry EK et al (1978): Correlation of cholinergic abnormalities with senile plaques and mental test scores in senile dementia. *Br Med J, 2*: 1457–1459.

Pfeiffer E (1975): A short portable mental status questionnaire for the assessment of organic brain deficit in elderly patients. *J Am Geriatr Soc, 23*: 433–437.

Pfeiffer E (1979): A short psychiatric evaluation schedule: A new 15-item monotonic scale indicative of functional psychiatric disorder. In: Bayer-Symposium, VIII: Brain function in old age Berlin/Heidelberg/New York. Springer-Verlag, pp. 228–236.

Poulshock SW, Deimling GT (1984): Families caring for elders in residence: Issues in the measurement of burden. *J Gerontol, 39*: 230–239.

Pratt CC et al (1985): Burden and coping strategies of caregivers to Alzheimer's patients. *Fam Relations, 34*: 27–33.

Prusiner SB (1984a): Prions. *Scientific American, 252*: 50–59.

Prusiner SB (1984b): Some speculations about prions, amyloid, and Alzheimer's disease. *N Engl J Med, 310*: 661–663.

Rabins PV, Mace NL, Lucas MJ (1982): The impact of dementia on the family. *JAMA, 248*: 333–335.

Reifler BV, Cox GB, Hanley RJ (1981): Problems of the mentally ill elderly as perceived by patients, families, and clinicians. *Gerontologist, 21*: 165–170.

Ryden M (1985): Personal communication.

Sainsbury P, Grad de Alercon J (1970): The effects of community care in the family of the geriatric patient. *J Geriatr Psychiatry, 4*: 23–41.

Salazar AM et al (1983): In: *Alzheimer's Disease*, Reisberg B (ed.). New York: Free Press.

Sanford RA (1975): Tolerance of debility in elderly dependents by supporters at home: Its significance for hospital practice. *Br Med J, 3*: 471–473.

Seltzer B, Sherwin I (1983): A comparison of clinical features in early- and late-onset primary degenerate dementia. *Arch Neurol, 40*: 143–146.

Shana E (1979): The family as a social support system in old age. *Gerontologist, 19*: 169–174.

Terry RD, Katzman R (1983): Senile dementia of the Alzheimer's type: Defining a disease. In: *The Neurology of Aging*, Katzman R, Terry R (eds.). Philadelphia: F. A. Davis.

Terry RD, Wisniewski HM (1970): Ultrastructure of the neurofibrillary tangle and the senile plague. In: *CIBA Foundation Symposium on Alzheimer's Disease and Related Conditions*, Wolstenholme GEW, O'Connor M (eds.). London: J. A. Churchill.

Thomas L (1981): On the problems of dementia. *Discover*, pp. 34–36.

Thompson TL, Moran MG, Nies AS (1983): Psychotropic drug use in the elderly, Part 1. *N Engl J Med, 308*: 134–138.

Tomlinson BE, Blessed G, Roth M (1970): Observations on the brains of demented old people. *J Neurol Sci, 11*: 205–242.

United States Publication (1984): A paper presented for the Subcommittee on Health and Long-term Care of the Select Committee on Aging. House of Representatives 98th Congress, 1st Session.

Vitaliano PP et al (1984): Memory, attention, and functional status in community-residency Alzheimer type dementia patients and optimally healthy aged individuals. *J Gerontol, 39*: 58–64.

Wells T (1985): Personal communication.

White P, Goodhardt MJ, Keet JP (1977): Neocortical neurons in elderly people. *Lancet, 1*: 668.

Wilder DE, Teresi JA, Bennett RG (1983): Family burden and dementia. In: *The Dementias*, Mayeux R, Rosen WG (eds.). New York: Raven.

Worcester MI, Quayhagen MP (1983): Correlates of caregiving satisfaction: Prerequisites to elder home care. *Res Nurs Health, 6*: 61–67.

Wurtman RJ (1985): Alzheimer's disease. *Scientific American, 252*: 62–66.

Yamaguchi F et al (1980): Non-invasive regional cerebral blood flow measurements in dementia. *Arch Neurol, 37*: 410–418.

Zarit JM, Zarit SH (1982): Measuring burden and support in families with Alzheimer's disease elders. Paper presented at the 35th annual scientific meeting of the Gerontological Society of America, Boston.

Zarit SH, Reever KE, Bach-Peterson J (1980): Relatives of impaired elderly: Correlates of feelings of burden. *Gerontologist, 20*: 649–655.

Zarit SH, Zarit JM, Reever KE (1982): Memory training for severe memory loss: Effects on senile dementia patients and their families. *Gerontologist, 22(4)*: 373–377.

27

PALLIATIVE CARE NURSING
Promoting Family Integrity

Jennifer Lillard, RN, MS

Linda Marietta, RN, MS

Increasing longevity and a related rise in chronic illness among Americans has created a great need for traditional nursing skills and competent palliative care. This chapter discusses the unique issues faced by patients with end-stage illness, and reviews selected historical trends, current practice and research. It proposes intervention guidelines that can be used by nurses in a variety of settings to assure maximum quality of patient and family life during end-stage illness.

Jennifer Lillard is Liaison Nurse at the Hospice of Marin in San Rafael, California, as well as Assistant Clinical Professor in the Department of Family Health Care Nursing at the University of California at San Francisco. She is widely recognized for her skill and leadership in hospice and home care.

Linda Marietta, Director of Patient Care Services at Home Hospice of Sonoma County in California, is an experienced hospice nurse now involved in hospice administration. She is also a participant in the certification program for hospices in Western states.

Introduction

During recent decades, nursing has moved away from its traditional care focus to play an expanding and exciting role in the delivery of highly technologic curative services such as organ transplantation, chemotherapy, radiation therapy, dialysis, ventilators, and arterial monitoring. The expertise of caring when there is no hope of cure has almost been lost amidst a proliferation of machines and miraculous technologies that often save patient lives (Lillard, 1984). Increasing longevity and a related rise in the incidence of chronic disease among aging Americans has, however, created a new need for old skills. The illness trajectories people with chronic disease face today often involve protracted end-stage phases, and their need for competent palliative care is immediate and pressing (Strauss, 1975). Consequently, nursing must take a fresh look at its time-honored commitments. Capitalizing on modern medical technology and drawing on philosophical precepts espoused by its early progenitors, the profession is actively defining its responsibilities to end-stage illness patients and their families (Donovan, 1980).

End-Stage Illness as a Family Problem

Every year over 70% of deaths in the United States result directly from cancer, heart disease, cerebrovascular disease, or chronic obstructive lung disease (Silverberg, 1985). The last months of life for people are dramatically affected by the many problems associated with end-stage illness, including pain, severe dyspnea, anorexia, pruritus, infections, skin problems, weakness, immobility, nausea and vomiting, anxiety, fear, depression, confusion, disorientation, hallucinations, and a host of other problems, depending on the nature and extent of the specific pathology involved. Clearly, these symptoms can significantly compromise the mental, emotional, and physical functioning of the patient and those close to the patient. Without adequate health care support, the patient's immediate suffering results in overwhelming discomfort, uncontrolled symptoms, and fear, followed by withdrawal of loved ones and deterioration of family systems.

Most Americans diagnosed with end-stage disease are members of a family group, which is defined here as "a unit of interacting persons related by ties of marriage, birth, adoption, or other strong social bonds whose central purpose is to promote the social, mental, physical, and emotional development of its members" (Moore, 1980). Over time, families develop a homeostasis of relationship and behavioral patterns that are relied on to satisfy family needs and tasks (Hansen, Hill, 1964). If life events disrupt the usual homeostasis, or pattern of coping, all the members of the family group respond in an effort to reestablish a satisfactory balance (Satir, 1968). Thus, each individual end-stage diagnosis actually affects the lives of every person in the given family unit. Based on this understanding, approximately 1 to 7 million Americans are dramatically affected by an end-stage diagnosis annually, even though they do not have the disease themselves. A chronologic review of the narrative literature on families and illness helps document the significance of these effects and their reciprocal influence on the diagnosed patients.

Lowenberg (1970) borrowed Lazarus's stress theory to develop assessment and intervention guidelines for nurses working with fatally ill adolescents and their families. She used a case study to illustrate the negative impact of denial, displaced anger, and related somatic symptoms on family relationships during the illness. Olsen (1970) stated that illness onset is a crisis for any family system and recommended including the family in care planning and activities as a preventive and growth-producing measure. *Families in Crisis*, a sociology reader released late in 1970, contained contributions from several authors addressing the problem of illness onset and the family (Glasser, Glasser, 1970). Richardson (1970) indicted hospitals for isolating patients from family members, causing confusion, anxiety, frustration, and somatic symptoms. Mabrey (1970) pointed out that facilitating family involvement with the patient and the illness allows an easier transition to home care after discharge, and Thomas (1970) discussed the complex family role transitions and potential strains that can follow illness onset. Sanchez–Salazar and Stark (1972), in reporting on their work with head and neck cancer patients, maintained that adjustment begins the moment the patient is told the diagnosis and may ultimately lead to symptoms of anxiety, denial, or confusion. They suggested immediate supportive intervention to facilitate adjustment.

Litman (1974), in a comprehensive review of the literature on the family as the basic unit in health care, reported that there is a relationship between illnesses among spouses, between family understanding of the illness and compliance with treatment regimens, and between the degree of member role clarity and ultimate placement decisions. Adams and Lindemann (1974) reported on two ostensibly identical family case histories of long-term disability that had very different outcomes. They hypothesized that therapeutic intervention with the family may have been one of the variables contributing to the surprisingly positive outcome for one patient and his family. Robinson's (1974) text on liaison nursing underlined the importance of the family in the hospital setting by devoting an entire chapter to the topic and calling for nursing support for the entire family unit. She stated that family needs may be unmet if the family is not included in the patient's care.

Strauss and Glaser's (1975) text on chronic illness presented a brief but succinct chapter focusing on the family that stated: ". . . illness cannot be managed effectively without taking into account the ill person's relationships with his kinsmen—and, I might add, a very sensitive 'taking into account.' " MacVicar and Archbold

(1976) presented an assessment framework for families facing major illness. They believed that adequate nursing intervention can significantly enhance the family unit's coping potential and long-term adjustment.

Giaquinta (1977) described a cancer diagnosis as a tragic family crisis, outlined a 10-phase adjustment process, and offered appropriate nursing actions for each phase. Use of her model requires close and consistent nursing contact with the entire family unit. Bruhn (1977) also described the cancer crisis, adding that it can act as a potent change agency and urging caregivers to facilitate family role transition, reassignment of tasks, and reestablishment of emotional equilibrium. He concluded that dysfunctional families have detrimental effects on the clinical management of the illness.

Burkhalter and Donley (1978) stated that oncology units need to promote intrafamily support but failed to recommend specific policies and procedures toward that end. However, the authors raised several pertinent questions about patient to family accessibility and inconclusively debated the merits of team versus primary nursing as an adjunct to patient and family care.

Mailick (1979) provided an overview of the impact of illness on patients and families that described an initial diagnostic phase accompanied by anxiety, fear, guilt, and physical strain. She urged providers to facilitate patient and family expression of feelings, acquisition of information, involvement in the treatment process, and use of resources. Bell (1979) viewed illness onset in the family in terms of role transitions that occur between husband and wife and believed these transitions are increasingly difficult because of new cultural sex role options.

Soffer (1983) asked nurses to include families in treatment planning, education, and other supportive interventions in order to reduce the stress of separation during hospitalization. Fife (1985) provided a model to identify families at high risk for poor adaptation, based on the assumption that family vulnerability increases dramatically during medical crises. Use of her model may assist in targeting families that need extra consideration and support, but all families should be the focus of care during end-stage illness regardless of preassessed risk.

The Essence of Palliative Care Nursing

Until recently, dying patients were relegated to end-of-the-corridor rooms in nursing homes or hospitals, estranged from family and loved ones, and unintentionally ignored by caregivers who lacked the expertise, psychosocial skill, and time to adequately address their needs (Glaser, 1965). The social, psychologic, and economic ramifications of poorly managed end-stage illness have been significant (Parkes, 1972; Blues, Zerwekh, 1984; Hoyt, 1983; Mailick, 1979; Cantor, 1978). During the mid-1970s, however, hospice care was introduced in the United States, offering an alternative that encourages care at home; supports the acceptance of death as an inevitable, natural part of the life cycle; facilitates family integrity; and promises refinement of symptom control strategies to increase patient comfort. End-stage illness accompanied by death is viewed as a personal and family crisis that can result in either growth or deterioration. With adequate symptom control, skilled nursing care, and facilitation of internal and external resources, the individual and family may strengthen established coping styles and develop new ones. Increased family integrity and personal maturation result, giving a life-enhancing quality to an otherwise devastating experience (Capone et al, 1979; Williams, 1976; Power, 1979; Aguilera, Messick, 1974; Malinak et al, 1979).

Although not yet developed as a specialty, palliative care nursing is most often practiced under a hospice umbrella. Hospice care was first introduced in England in the 1960s by Dame Cicely Saunders, a nurse whose frustration with the constraints of her role led to her becoming a physician. Determined to address the unmet needs of dying patients and their families, she focused on promoting optimal quality of life despite the destructive vicissitudes of end-stage illness (Saunders, Summer, Tuller, 1981). Dame Saunders's model of hospice care, named after hospices of the middle ages that sheltered sick and weary travelers, is built on several concepts. These include identification of the patient and family as the unit of care, excellent symptom control, focus on quality rather than quantity of life, multidisciplinary care tailored to individual patient and family needs, volunteer participation, and bereavement follow-up.

Since the 1974 opening of the first U.S. hospice (in New Haven, Connecticut), an estimated 1300 units have begun care delivery (Mahoney, 1985). This remarkably rapid growth measures the eager adoption of the English model in response to burgeoning need; American patients and families welcomed the alternative.

However, until the 1983 federal medicare legislation, hospice care did not qualify for third-party reimbursement (Medicare Programs, 1983). Whereas the English government built the hospice alternative into its socialized health insurance package, U.S. hospices had to struggle for financial viability through contributions, donations, grants, or limited reimbursement from Medicare through traditional third-party reimbursement channels. Consequently, U.S. hospices use many individually structured models, combining volunteer and employed caregivers as well as unique funding packages. The lack of stable funding resulted in a significant American contribution to hospice care; the particular location of care delivery depends on the changing needs and preferences of the patient and family rather than being site specific, as in England. Most care emanates from nurse-coordinated multidisciplinary teams that offer palliative treatment in a variety of settings, including patient homes, hospitals, inpatient hospice units, and other long-term care settings. Nurses providing palliative care facilitate patient and family decision-making about the location of care by exploring the costs, constraints, and benefits of options. One patient and family may need to select a skilled nursing facility because of limited home care third-party coverage or lack of able caregivers; another patient and family may prefer care at home until the time of death. In any case, the choice is often difficult, complicated by guilt for having to institutionalize a patient or the emotional strain of role changes for the entire family system.

This brief examination of English hospice care and its American counterpart produces several guidelines for palliative care nursing practice with end-stage patients and families:

1. Excellent control of physical symptoms, especially pain, is a priority.

2. The patient and family comprise the identified unit of care.

3. Multidisciplinary care should be offered based on patient and family needs and available resources.

4. Successful palliative care can be offered by nurses in a range of settings.

5. Care efforts focus on quality rather than quantity of life.

The Challenges of Palliative Care Nursing

Nursing is faced with the challenge to promote positive outcomes during end-stage illness. Palliative care opportunities are not limited to hospice settings alone. Nurses plan and directly deliver palliative care in all health care settings, including hospitals, nursing homes, clinics, medical offices, and patients' homes. They have more consistent, instrumental, and direct contact with patients and families than other caregivers, and their assessments are an essential component of the treatment decision-making process. But the challenge is not easily met for a number of reasons.

Role attainment in any setting is affected by the social context in which it occurs, so the variables influencing end-stage nursing need to be acknowledged and addressed before practice can occur without unrecognized pressure and constraints (Lillard, 1982). The unique variables faced by nurses working with end-stage illness are well documented. Our death-denying American culture lacks established traditions for managing the end stage of life and has removed the death event from common experience, rendering it strange, unnatural, and highly uncomfortable. In addition, Americans value youth, materialistic achievement, and instrumental accomplishment, and the expressive activities inherent in the letting go process, which is associated with the end stage of life, are overlooked. The exquisite vulnerability of small families makes the death of one member particularly threatening, and decreasing reliance on religious structures contributes further to the problem (Aries, 1981; Feifel, 1977, Weisman, 1972). In reality, the culture has an almost psychotic denial of death's inevitability, and palliative care is practiced without the benefit of social sanction or prescribed behavioral guidelines.

In addition, palliative care nursing occurs within a delivery system that strives for cure at the risk of neglecting the need for care. The fantastic expansion of effective medical technology has resulted in a concentration on curing illness. The rewards that accompany dramatic life-saving interventions are highly visible and immediately gratifying, and few nurses are attracted to palliative care. Palliative care nurses are often viewed with suspicion and misunderstanding by their professional peers.

Unfortunately, nursing education may exacerbate cultural and professional tendencies by failing to provide the education and clinical experience needed in palliative care. Relevant content may be totally excluded from curricula, placed at the end of other courses, assigned to beginning instructors, or presented with a task-oriented focus (Benoliel, 1967; Bunch, Zahza, 1976). Research suggests that students emerging from nursing education programs do not select positions in long-term care settings where palliative care predominates, and those that do experience significant stress and role strain (Stoller, 1980; Lillard, Bystrowski, 1981; Kayser, Minngerode, 1975). Yet nurses in every setting inevitably confront patients and families facing end-stage illness and death, and as committed professionals they are looking for ways to meet the challenge. Cooperation with enlightened (or at least open-minded and willing to be informed) physicians will be helpful.

Recommendations for Patient and Family Care Emerging from Clinical Practice and Research

Perhaps the most important and simultaneously difficult issues that arise in palliative care nursing centers are within the nurse; personal feelings about death and dying will inevitably arise and must be grappled with so that nursing practice can continue, unfettered by counterproductive emotional constraints (Adams, 1984; Lowenberg, 1976). Until intimate anxieties and unfinished concerns are addressed, there is risk that nurses will need to protect themselves from emotional turmoil by avoiding patient and family needs or by projecting their own expectations (Blues, Zerwekh, 1984). To assist nurses in exploration of relevant issues, the authors have used a supportive, small-group format, asking nurses questions like the following:

1. Recall your earliest experience with death. Was it with a loved one, neighbor, pet, or friend? What happened, how did you see others respond, and how do you remember feeling at the time?

2. Imagine you have just started to care for a patient with end-stage illness in your specific work setting. Is there anything the patient might say that could be difficult to respond to? How might you respond?

Each issue is presented, and nurses are asked to write their responses. After some moments, sharing is invited, and all comments are accepted without judgment. Other authors suggest poetry reading followed by discussion (Blues, Zerwekh, 1984). The particular format may vary, but the goal remains the same—nurses need an open, safe opportunity to sort through past experiences, present concerns, and expectations. The process is analogous to conducting a thorough literature search before designing a research plan. It prevents unnecessary effort as a result of ignorance, helps assure the clarity of the study, and avoids repeating procedural pitfalls made by other researchers. In the case of palliative care nursing, self-awareness and understanding are critically important to effective practice.

Experience with end-stage patients and families has revealed another issue that merits consideration. Patients experience highly individualized, often unpredictable, disease trajectories, depending on actual diagnosis, age, general state of health, and other factors. End-stage respiratory and cardiac disease are marked by frequent exacerbations and remissions, but cancer diagnoses tend to follow more predictable and steadily progressive courses (Saunders, McCorkle, 985). Someone who is close to death because of congestive heart failure may enjoy a welcome but temporary remission following intravenous diuretics, antibiotics, and an increased dose of digitalis. Conversely, a patient with progressive respiratory disease may fear immediate death with every episode of increased shortness of breath. Paralyzing fear can accompany new angina attacks or bouts of respiratory infection, yet they may or may not signify impending death. Clearly, patients and families are faced with an uncharted journey through the illness trajectory that they cannot control. However, with accurate information about changes and an opportunity to explain alternative responses, patients and families can achieve some measure of control over their day-to-day actions. Nurses providing palliative care during end-stage illness must be professionally resilient, accept the vagaries of the disease process as they occur, model that acceptance for the patient and family, and demonstrate a commitment to continuing care.

Another observation emerging from clinical practice pertains to the variety of coping styles patients and families exhibit when they encounter the crisis of a terminal diagnosis (Lillard, 1984). There are as many individual family patterns of responding to this crisis as there are families. One family may respond with direct actions designed to reestablish a sense of balance, and another might present with relatively intact denial of the tragic implications of the diagnosis. In either case, palliative care nurses best promote patient and family coping by respecting the response pattern, supporting the functional aspects of the pattern, and avoiding blatant confrontations that may actually precipitate disintegration. For example, requests for more information should be encouraged and promptly responded to, but information should never be forced on a patient and family who are not ready to receive it.

A brief examination of related research also reveals some palliative care principles that have proven useful in clinical practice. One recommendation emerges as a strong theme from studies of patients with chronic illnesses who may or may not be in the end stage. It is helpful to retain a focus on positive, residual abilities of the patient so that management of increasing symptoms or progressing deterioration does not dominate the patient's activities or nurse–patient contacts. For example, patients who can no longer get out of bed may still be able to nurture children with listening, review of their accomplishments, and exchange of significant feedback. Family members can simultaneously be encouraged to reciprocate with listening and feedback of their own initiation. In this way, expressive family functions will continue even though the patient is no longer able to independently manage his or her own daily care.

Power (1979) studied 74 male multiple sclerosis patients and found that attitude toward the disease was a significant factor in overall patient and family coping. The 21 patients who coped adaptively perceived the illness as a handicap, focused on residual capabilities rather than limitations, and were able to maintain active, vital roles within their family systems by delegating physically demanding tasks and assuming more expressive roles. The other men gave histories of withdrawal and passivity, and their families expressed feelings of guilt combined with a need to protect the father. Another researcher looked at families with chronically ill parent members and also found that positive, productive attitudes were associated with effective coping (Anthony, 1970).

Other papers on the clinical aspects of hospice or palliative care include comments about the relationship between hope and the quality of life during end-stage illness (Weisman, 1972). Hope in this context does not refer to hope that life will not end; rather, it pertains to hope for desired, achievable goals involving a sense of personal control over the disease, such as going on a country picnic with loved ones, having a pain-free hour in the garden, or completing an important conversation with a loved one. A focus on residual capabilities operates in tandem with hope; nurses can foster both by exploring wishes and favorite pastimes with patients and families or by contributing crucial symptom control expertise so that small dreams can become realities.

The goal is to remember that life is still at hand and that known time limits need not obliterate an awareness of daily opportunities for new growth, understanding, or joy. Nursing home staff can arrange for visits with favorite pets, an acute-care clinical nurse specialist might encourage a patient to phone a loved one, or a nurse working with a patient and family at home might suggest they plan a special dinner, selecting the patient's favorite cuisine. The spirit of this Zen parable is worth keeping in mind:

A man traveling across a field encountered a tiger. He fled, the tiger after him. Coming to a precipice, he caught hold of the root of a wild vine and swung himself over the edge. The tiger sniffed at him from above. Trembling, the man looked down to where, far below, another tiger was waiting to eat him. Only the vine sustained him. Two mice, one white and one black, little by little started to gnaw away the vine. The man saw a luscious strawberry near him. Grasping the vine with one hand, he plucked the strawberry with the other. How sweet it tasted! (Reps, n.d., pp. 22–23)

Novice practitioners often express frustration and confusion about offering hope when the patient and family face a terminal prognosis. Yet nurses must encourage and support maximization of living potential without contributing to a sense of false hope that the worst is over, that a cure is forthcoming, or that death is not at hand, especially in the presence of physiologic evidence that it is imminent.

A third suggestion for palliative nursing care emanates from early research concerning the quality of life of incurable cancer patients. There is strong evidence that a sense of personal mastery over daily life contributes to a feeling of well-being despite the ominous reality of a terminal diagnosis (Benoliel, McCorkle, 1978; Lewis, 1981; Campbell, 1978; Bautista, 1976). This finding is consistent with opinions expressed during philosophical quality-of-life discussions and gives credence to the following statement from a cancer patient concerning the meaning of his illness:

When you're told you have cancer and that you may have four months to live, your whole life seems in disarray. All your goals have to be changed. When a cancer patient is told he has a specific time to live, he really doesn't run out and get a four year membership to Jack LaLanne. He feels he has a loss of control of his life. It's very important for the cancer patient to get back in control and feel like he has some control over his destiny (Peters, 1983).

The preceding quotation is followed quickly by a plea for caregiver honesty about diagnosis and prognosis. The writer states that patients must have access to specific information when they request it if they are to make reasonable decisions and regain a sense of control. Individual personality styles vary, of course, and some patients and families choose a more dependent coping pattern, abdicating decision-making and control to friends or trusted caregivers.

Finally, the value of hospice care for patients and families has been well researched and documented. In one study, the effect of multidisciplinary hospice services on 58 families treated at the University of Massachusetts Medical Center was examined (Godkin et al, 1983). Over three-quarters of the families reported feeling prepared for the death, and there was a significant reduction in physical problems experienced by survivors as compared with rates reported by other researchers. The authors conclude that hospice care contributed significantly to overall family adjustment during both terminal illness and bereavement.

Another recent study demonstrates that hospice care and related educational efforts have clearly benefited both patients and their spouses (Parkes, Parkes, 1984). Respondents reported less personal distress and fewer perceived problems with pain when compared with a matched group of respondents whose loved ones had died 10 years earlier. The researchers also report that spouses of patients cared for at St. Christopher's Hospice are less anxious than spouses of patients being treated at general hospitals, and they comment that the hospice movement's emphasis on patient and family support and excellent symptom control has had far-reaching effects on the care of the dying.

Symptom Control

Palliative care is based on the philosophy that even when cure is no longer possible, symptoms can be alleviated or controlled to promote maximum comfort, independence, and quality of life.

Because many symptoms have origins in complex interactions between physical and psychologic factors, a multidisciplinary approach with attention to detail is optimal in providing effective symptom control during palliative care. For example, pain has a physiologic component, but there are also psychoemotional and spiritual overtones that may be best addressed by other disciplines. Nurses who are practicing without the benefit of multidisciplinary teams should be aware of community resources that could assist in the plan of care, and they need to facilitate appropriate patient and family use of those resources.

In the absence of multidisciplinary team support, the nurse can use a number of specific strategies to promote patient and family psychosocial health and integrity. These are outlined in earlier sections of the chapter that present recommendations from clinical practice and research and may be implemented simultaneously with measures to control physical symptoms. However, a crucial principle of end-stage illness nursing care bears stating at this point: The debilitating effects of unmanaged physical symptoms must be aggressively addressed as soon as the patient and family seek nursing assistance with palliative care. During their own professional experiences, the authors have found that this is too often neglected or overlooked at great cost to patient and family coping. Perhaps lack of symptom management information and a traditional reliance on medicine to mastermind the resolution of physical symptoms are to blame. The authors believe that nurses in leadership positions in every clinical setting must have solid familiarity with the most recent symptom management strategies if they are going to dynamically participate in the development of palliative care nursing education, research, planning, and practice. Consequently, this section emphasizes the management of physical symptoms.

Once the noxious distractions of pain, nausea and vomiting, constipation, depression, decubiti, anorexia, and oral dysfunctions are minimized, patients and families can be free to focus on their residual abilities, their relationships with others, and the ongoing functional strength of the family unit.

Skilled professional nursing intervention never operates in the domain of the physical to the exclusion of the psychosocial or vice versa. Ultimately, physical and psychosocial problems often occur in tandem, influencing each other, and the best solutions to either involve approaches from both arenas. In the case of palliative care nursing, however, physical problems are pressing, are often inadequately treated by the health care team, and take initial priority over psychosocial issues.

Symptom control also necessitates that the nurse be aware of the individual disease process as well as the appropriate medical and nursing interventions. New symptoms should be assessed in the context of the known disease progression then discussed with the patient and family to develop a plan of care. A patient who has been ambulatory and then develops pneumonia secondary to plural effusion would, in most instances, wish aggressive antibiotic therapy. Meanwhile, the family of a patient who has been semicomatose for several days and develops pneumonia might, with adequate understanding of the situation, elect supportive care only. Patient and family education is a key component of symptom control because understanding of treatment rationale is essential to successful decision-making, compliance, and sense of control.

Pain

Pain is the most distressing of all physical symptoms commonly associated with end-stage illness, and pain relief is the single most important hope the nurses can offer patients and families.

McCaffery (1979) defines pain as whatever the experiencing person says it is, existing whenever he says it does. With this in mind, the nurse always validates the patient's pain as real, regardless of the degree of evident physical cause. Thorough pain assessment involves the following:

1. Where is it located? (Use a drawing of a body for patient to identify pain sites)

2. What is the quality and type of pain sensation? (Use a pain scale of 1 to 10, with 1 identifying mild pain and 10 excruciating pain)

3. What nonmedical strategies relieve pain and for how long?

4. What increases the pain? (Movement, expectation, anxiety, and so on)

5. What is the etiology of the pain? (Disease process, constipation, muscle spasm, and so on)

6. How effective are current medications?

7. What are the patient's fears regarding pain?

Once the pain is assessed, intervention plans, such as those found in Table 27-1, may be implemented.

Mild to Moderate Pain   Nonnarcotics such as aspirin or acetaminophen (Tylenol) are effective first-line medications for the control of mild to moderate pain. Aspirin 600 mg is usually as effective as codeine 60 mg. As analgesics, acetaminophen and aspirin also act as antipyretics, but only aspirin is a nonsteroidal anti-inflammatory drug (NSAID). Aspirin and other NSAIDs such as ibuprofen (Motrin), naproxen (Naprosyn), and indomethacin (Indocin) have been effective in controlling pain from bone metastasis by inhibiting prostaglandin production (Schofferman, 1986). NSAIDs, because of their tendency to cause gastric intolerance, should be taken with food or liquid. If gastric intolerance persists with conservative treatment, cimetidine (Tagamet) 400 mg b.i.d. could be prescribed. Antacids, although effective, reduce aspirin absorption. All NSAIDs also interfere with the clotting process and should not be used with patients with abnormal platelet counts. Be-

cause a patient's response to a NSAID is not uniform, a patient who cannot tolerate one NSAID may find another acceptable. NSAIDs are also used in conjunction with strong narcotics when bone pain is not controlled with NSAID alone (Twycross, Tack, 1983). Acetaminophen every 6 hours is sometimes effective if aspirin or other NSAIDs are contraindicated (Amadeo, 1984). Both aspirin and acetaminophen are available in suppository form for use when the patient can no longer swallow (1:1 oral to rectal potency ratio). Nonnarcotics are not addictive but do have a plateau of therapeutic effectiveness (Twycross, Tack, 1983).

Propoxyphene hydrochloride (Darvon) is also frequently prescribed for pain. One researcher, however, found that propoxyphene hydrochloride 25 mg with aspirin 650 mg is no more effective than aspirin alone (Moertel et al, 1974).

When nonnarcotic analgesics are no longer effective, aspirin or acetaminophen in combination with codeine (Empirin Compound and Tylenol with Codeine) or with oxycodone (Percodan and Percocet) is often useful. Although codeine and oxycodone are considered narcotics, their combination with aspirin or acetaminophen precludes their use for severe chronic pain. Higher dosages would mean more pills for the patient to swallow and higher doses of aspirin or acetaminophen without a proportionate increase in analgesia compared to side effects.

Severe Chronic Pain   For severe chronic pain, oral morphine sulfate has become the drug of choice. Originally, morphine was used in combination with cocaine, alcohol, and syrup and was called a Brompton Cocktail. In England, diamorphine (heroin) was used initially instead of morphine, but now Brompton mixtures are made with either morphine or diamorphine. Because of side effects attributed to cocaine, Brompton Cocktail is used less, and oral morphine is dispensed with or without alcohol and syrup.

Table 27–1 Intervention Plans for Symptom Control of Pain

Principle	Rationale	Practice
Use oral medications whenever possible.	Patient's level of independence in taking medications is maximized. Inadequate muscle mass in the terminally ill precludes long-term use of injections. Poor peripheral venous access hampers the use of intravenous therapy unless a central line is present.	A Mediset or dosage calendar facilitates accurate dose and timing of pills. A clearly marked medicine cup for measuring liquid pain medications prevents dosage error. In the home, a kitchen teaspoon varies in size and should not be used.
Give pain medication around the clock at regular intervals to maximize blood level consistency.	Longer intervals lessen disruption of daily activities and sleep. Around the clock dosing is necessary to maintain adequate serum levels.	Last dose before bedtime may be increased up to twice the usual amount to allow patient to sleep through the night. If patient awakens in pain, resume scheduled doses throughout the night.
Individualize the pain medication dosage.	Pain threshold can be lowered by insomnia, fatigue, anxiety, fear, anger, sadness, depression, mental isolation, and past experience (Twycross, Tack, 1983). Ongoing assessment and intervention involves adjusting dosage frequency or even medication to achieve optimal pain control.	When starting pain medication, assess effectiveness of each dose and titrate medication until pain is controlled for 3–4 hours. If patient is at home, call the patient during the day and leave guidelines for the family on how to increase pain medication if pain increases and 24-hour nursing on-call is not available. When beginning a new pain medication, ask the physician for titration guidelines so that the patient does not have to be in pain while the physician is being contacted for new dosage orders. For example, start patient on oral morphine 10 mg every 4 hours; then if pain is not controlled, increase dose by 10 mg every 4 hours up to 60 mg. Contact physician for additional orders if pain remains uncontrolled at 60 mg every 4 hours.
Do not view narcotics for pain control as a treatment reserved for the very end of life.	Studies have shown that cancer patients may develop tolerance and physical dependence to narcotics but that psychologic dependence (addiction) is rare (Angell, 1982; Porter, Jeck, 1980). Oral morphine and most narcotics do not have a preestablished therapeutic ceiling. Once a patient has been established on a regular regimen of oral morphine, studies have shown that tolerance usually develops slowly.	If a patient has not achieved a satisfying comfort level with a medication regimen of nonnarcotics (aspirin or acetaminophen) or weak narcotics (codeine, oxycodone, and dextropropoxyphene preparations), the patient then needs to take a strong narcotic such as oral morphine. Patients have been maintained for months on oral morphine with very few side effects other than the need to take medication to prevent constipation.

Oral morphine sulfate (OMS) is available in 2, 5, 10, and 20 mg/mL liquid and as a controlled release tablet (MS Contin). Roxanol Concentrated Oral Solution, a 20 mg/mL morphine liquid, is especially effective for patients who have difficulty swallowing large amounts of liquid. Although the 20 mg/mL concentration of oral morphine is not absorbed through the oral mucosa, anecdotal experience has shown it to be effective for patients who are no longer able to swallow.

MS Contin tablets are effective for 12 hours and are usually initiated after the pain has been controlled on oral morphine. MS Contin dosage is determined by doubling the oral morphine dose and dosing schedule. For example, 15 mg of OMS every four hours is converted to 30 mg of MS Contin every eight hours. Dosage interval is lengthened every 48 hours without increasing the dose until a dosage schedule of every 12 hours is obtained (Holmesley, 1986).

Morphine sulfate has a 1:3 parenteral to oral potency ratio when given on a continuous basis (Walsh, 1984). Oral morphine is generally started at 10 mg every 4 hours with a 50% increase every 4 hours until pain is controlled. Patients who are frail or have hepatic or respiratory involvement may be started on oral morphine at lower doses and increased more slowly. However, medication should always be given at the dosage that controls pain (Twycross, Tack, 1983). The mean dose of oral morphine needed to achieve pain control was shown in one study to be 64 mg every 4 hours (Neuman et al, 1982). Patients have tolerated higher doses, and as much as 180 mg every 4 hours has been reported in the literature (Walsh, 1985).

Morphine can also be administered intravenously and by continuous subcutaneous infusion. Patients may initially experience drowsiness, which should not be an indication to stop or reduce the medication unless it is excessive. Patients who have been in poor pain control sleep very little and are usually exhausted by the time oral morphine is started. Patients and family members should be instructed to expect to see the patient sleeping more but not to be overly concerned as long as the patient is arousable. Generally, the drowsiness will clear in three to five days unless the patient is near the end of life. Respiratory depression is generally not a problem unless the patient has severely impaired respiratory function that can no longer be treated. Achievement of comfort and pain control should take priority over a fear of hastening death with the use of narcotics.

Nausea may be another transitory problem with morphine use and can be controlled with an antiemetic such as prochlorperazine (Compazine) on a regular schedule. A suppository form is available for patients who are actively vomiting. Constipation is almost always a problem with any narcotic, and a stool softener and laxative bowel regimen must be started at the time a narcotic is begun.

Hydromorphone (Dilaudid), a semisynthetic opiate, is available in 1, 2, 3 and 4 mg tablets. A 3 mg suppository form is often used for dysphagic patients. Dilaudid is not appropriate for patients requiring high doses of narcotics because of the large number of pills that would need to be taken.

Methadone is a synthetic narcotic analgesic that is effective for 6–8 hours. It is difficult to titrate because the plasma half-life may extend for 15–30 hours. Practitioners must wait 24 hours to assess the level of effectiveness of each increase to avoid cumulative toxicity. Consequently, methadone is not the drug of choice for elderly, confused patients or for patients with increased intracranial pressure or organ failure (Twycross, Tack, 1983).

Meperidine (Demerol) and pentazocine (Talwin) have been of limited value in palliative care treatment. The analgesic effect of meperidine lasts only 2–4 hours and is about one-eighth as potent as morphine. The high doses that are needed to control moderate pain are often related to a high incidence of unwanted central nervous system effects such as tremors, twitching, agitation, and convulsions. Pentazocine acts as an agonist–antagonist in that if given alone it has agonistic (morphine-like) effects, but it becomes antagonistic in combination with morphine. Therefore, if a patient is on pentazocine and needs to be changed to another narcotic, the starting dose would have to be higher than medically indicated in order to counteract the antagonistic effect of Talwin still in the bloodstream. Psychomimetic side effects such as dysphoria, feelings of unreality and depersonalization, and hallucinations are also common with pentazocine (Twycross, Tack, 1983).

Nausea and Vomiting

The vomiting reflex is a complex process activated by stimulation of the vomiting center in the medulla (Frytak, Moertel, 1981). Afferent input to the center can come from the chemoreceptor trigger zone, the vestibular apparatus, the periphery, or the higher brain stem and cortical structures. The chemoreceptor trigger zone appears to be activated by chemical stimuli from blood or cerebrospinal fluid, such as the biochemical changes occurring with anemia, hepatic failure, hypercalcemia, narcotics, and chemotherapy. The inner ear (vestibular process) supplies input through stimulation from motion.

Peripheral input involves stimulation of the gastrointestinal tract via the vagus and sympathetic nerves. Esophageal obstruction, intestinal obstruction, ascites, and stomach involvement can all cause nausea and vomiting through this process. Finally, it is thought that higher cortical areas can be stimulated by increased intracranial pressure, disagreeable tastes and smells, and psychogenic factors (Zerwekh, 1984; Siegel, Longo, 1981).

In treating nausea and vomiting, it is important to identify and treat the cause in order to select an appropriate palliative antiemetic regimen. Phenothiazines are believed to act on the chemoreceptor trigger zone to directly depress the vomiting center (Frytak, Moertel, 1981). Prochlorperazine (Compazine) is available in 10 mg tablets and a 25 mg suppository form for

patients who are unable to tolerate oral antiemetics; rectal absorption is probably less complete than oral absorption (Moffat, 1978). Timed-release phenothiazines are expensive and have not been found to be any better than oral preparations (Frytak, Moertel, 1981). Haloperidol (Haldol) is a very potent antiemetic that acts on the chemoreceptor trigger zone. Usual dosage is 1–2 mg orally every 3–6 hours and is easily administered in a tablet or liquid form.

Antihistamines such as antivert (Meclizine) and dimenhydrinate (Dramamine) are thought to act on the vomiting center and on the vestibular apparatus. Metoclopramide (Reglan) has both peripheral and central antiemetic actions (Siegel, Longo, 1981). When nausea and vomiting are caused by stimulation from more than one site, a combination of antiemetics may be useful, beginning with a phenothiazine, then adding haloperidol and an antihistamine.

Constipation

Constipation is caused by immobility, narcotics, anticholinergic drugs, reduced intake of fluids and fiber, weakness, and reduced sensory awareness (Zerwekh, 1981). Constipation can also be a direct result of tumor growth. Patients on narcotics without accompanying bowel regimens may become noncompliant in order to prevent constipation. Intervention begins by assessing the patient's previous history of elimination and regimens. Ideally, constipation can be controlled with bulk-forming laxatives (for example, Metamucil) but most patients on regular narcotic schedules should also be started on a stool softener (dioctyl sulfosuccinate sodium) 2–3 times a day, with additional laxatives if they do not have a bowel movement every 3–4 days. Unfortunately, many debilitated end-stage patients are unable to drink enough fluid to accommodate the use of bulk-forming laxatives as a singular constipation prevention measure.

There is very little clinical data on the efficacy of various types of laxatives. One study on use of senna demonstrated that it was more effective than milk of magnesia in the treatment of drug-induced constipation (Izard, Ellison, 1982).

Lubricants (mineral oil) are of limited benefit in end-stage illness patients because they impair absorption of fat-soluble vitamins over time and may irritate the perianal region. For the dysphagic or demented patient, there is a risk of aspiration of mineral oil with lipid pneumonitis resulting. Mineral oil penetrates and softens stool and so may be helpful for the treatment of fecal impaction (Klein, 1982). Castor oil seems to have a rapid onset but causes cramping in many patients.

Suppositories such as glycerin or ducolax (contains bisacodyl) are useful in emptying the lower rectum when there is decreased muscle tone secondary to debilitation. Tap water, saline, or soap suds enemas assist fecal impaction evacuation but should not be necessary once a regimen of stool softener and/or laxative has begun. Lactulose (a semisynthetic disaccharide) is useful as a laxative and for the management of portal–systemic encephalopathy in chronic liver disease. It is available as a sweet-tasting syrup, which may be unpalatable to some patients unless mixed with fruit juice or other food. Lactulose is especially nonirritating to the colon and produces a formed stool within 3–5 days (Crowther, 1978; Fingle, 1984). The fact that patients must take at least 15 cc of Lactulose 1–2 times a day limits its use with many end-stage patients.

Depression

End-stage illness is always accompanied by patient and family depression that includes a reactive response to the terminal diagnosis, feelings about loss of independence and role change, and anticipatory grief (Kubler-Ross, 1965). Somatic symptoms such as dysphoria, crying, constipation, insomnia, and anorexia exacerbate other physiologically based problems (Massie, Holland, 1984). Cachexia and weakness related to disease progression compound the symptom control challenge and make it more difficult to work through feelings of loss, inadequacy, guilt, and lowered self-esteem. As identified earlier, the palliative care nurse must provide adequate control of physical symptoms before the psychosocial issues are readily addressed.

Intervention strategies are based on acceptance, active listening, providing the patient and family with choices to promote a sense of control, and appropriate involvement of other disciplines such as social work, volunteer, or chaplain whenever possible. A here-and-now, day-by-day focus facilitates realistic planning and goal achievement. For example, pain relief that allows the patient to have a decent night of sleep may provide energy for an overdue shampoo that ultimately enhances the patient's personal appearance, pride, and ability to relax.

At times, palliative care of depression in end-stage illness is facilitated by use of psychotropic medication. Tricyclic antidepressants such as doxepin (Sinequan), imipramine (Tofranil), amitriptyline (Elavil), and nortriptyline (Aventyl) are commonly used. Dosage is initiated at 25–75 mg, then titrated upward as tolerated to 75–150 mg a day. Amitriptyline has sedative side effects, so patients are usually advised to take it at night to enhance sleep. Other side effects of tricyclics include dry mouth, constipation, and analgesic potentiating qualities (Massie, Holland, 1984). Patients and families must be advised that the antidepressive benefits of tricyclics usually are not apparent until a two- to three-week blood level has been maintained. Compliance with dose schedule is pivotal to achievement of therapeutic results. One investigation has found that treatment with corticosteroids has improved the end-stage patient's sense of well-being (Bruera, 1985).

Decubiti

Clearly, prevention is the optimal palliative approach to decubiti in bedbound patients. But even with assiduous protection of bony prominences, frequent turning, massage, use of special mattresses, and excellent skin hygiene, decubiti can occur. Specific interventions are required to prevent further breakdown. Once a skin site is reddened, it should be protected with a hydrocolloid occlusive dressing such as Duoderm to reduce friction and encourage healing. Treatment of decubiti is based on the understanding that cutaneous wound healing is more rapid if tissue fluid is held on the wound surface with an appropriate protective covering, pressure on the site is minimized, necrotic tissue is removed, healthy skin is protected, and infection is eradicated. Uncovered wounds develop eschars, creating mechanical barriers to epidermal regeneration (Osment, 1975). Pressure can be reduced with mechanical devices such as wheelchair cushions, but sheepskin should be avoided because it retains moisture (Phipps et al, 1984). Noninfected, nondraining wound healing is enhanced by applying dressings that do not stick to the decubiti, such as Duoderm or Op-sit.

Pressure ulcers that do not require debridement but are infected, or have copious drainage, should not have occlusive dressings. Applications of Debrisan or karaya powder to absorb drainage are helpful if gauze dressing alone does not control the drainage. Once the tissue bed is clean and granulated, the use of karaya powder or Debrisan should be discontinued. Surgical debridement may be occasionally indicated, but many end-stage patients cannot tolerate surgical interventions. In these cases, wound irrigation with normal saline and wet-to-dry dressings is appropriate. Wound irrigation should be done with a forceful spray that can clean the wound of exudate without irritating the wound surface. Removal of a wet-to-dry dressing serves to further debride the wound surface.

Iodine, acetic acid, and normal saline are used to wet the innermost gauze layer on a wound dressing. Enzymatic agents such as Santyl and Travase are effective in debriding necrotic tissue, but they are inactivated by low pH and heavy metals. Consequently, they should not be used in combination with silver, mercury, acetic acid, or aluminum acetate. Heat lamps and antacids are contraindicated in the treatment of decubiti because both treatments dry the wound surface and impede healing.

Anorexia

Most end-stage patients experience significant anorexia accompanied by persistent loss of tissue mass and cachexia. Eventually, patients may take only small amounts of fluid throughout the end-stage trajectory, and palliative care nurses play a crucial role in educating and counseling the patient and family about nutritional choices and concerns. Anxiety about the pending death may be focused on the patient's lack of appetite and weight loss. Family members grappling with their fears can unintentionally and unnecessarily harass the patient about eating, thus creating guilt and emotional distance. The nurse needs to identify the process that is occurring, listen, and encourage interventions that promote adequate nutrition and energy without prolonging the patient's life against his or her wishes.

There are some strategies that can be used with relative ease. Nutritional supplements or the addition of powdered milk in cooking can enhance caloric intake with a minimum of additional bulk for the patient to eat. Although alcohol has no nutritional value, a highball before eating or wine with meals can increase appetite. Glucocorticosteroids such as prednisone or enteric-coated prednisolone 5 mg three times a day may enhance appetite and simultaneously improve the patient's sense of well-being (Baines, 1983). Favorite foods served in small, attractive portions when the patient feels relaxed and comfortable is, of course, the least invasive, most natural way to promote adequate intake.

Complete patient refusal of food and fluids may be indicative of imminent death. At this point, questions about the option of hyperalimentation, nasogastric tube feedings, and intravenous feedings are raised. The final decision should emerge from the patient and family's desire to maintain nutrition in order to prolong life. Their wishes should be honored.

Palliative care nursing experience demonstrates that dehydration as a natural component of the dying process may be beneficial in several ways: There will be fewer pulmonary secretions and suctioning will not be necessary unless the patient needed suctioning previously. Urinary output will be reduced leading to fewer episodes of incontinence and avoiding the need for catheterization (Zerwekh, 1983). Dry mucous membranes are assuaged with ice chips, small sips of fluid, and good mouth care.

Oral Dysfunctions

End-stage illness patients are often unable to maintain adequate mouth care on their own. Family members may decide that infrequent eating and drinking obviates a need for scrupulous mouth care. Denture removal and cleaning may be neglected. However, research demonstrates the pressing need for persistent mouth care and moisturizing. In one study, a healthy, young adult developed dryness of lips and buccal mucosa and mucosal color changes after one hour of mouth breathing, continuous oxygen inhalation, no oral intake, and intermittent oral suctioning (DeWalt, Haines, 1969).

Clearly, end-stage patients are at high risk for such things as oropharyngeal candidiasis, identified by a characteristic white coating of the tongue and mucous membrane. Mycostatin Suspension 500,000 units 3–4 times a day; clotrimazole (Mycelex Troche) 5 times a day; or ketoconazole (Nezoral) once a day are the treatments of choice.

Stomatitis is most common in patients who have received chemotherapy or localized radiation, are immunosuppressed, have nasogastric tubes, or are unable to take anything by mouth. It presents as red, shiny, edematous oral mucosa with or without open areas that may eventually ulcerate. Ulcerated lesions become encrusted, and the tongue swells, taking on a white or

brownish coating (Daeffler, 1981). Head and neck cancer patients may also develop painful oral tumors appearing as red, swollen open lesions.

Palliative mouth care requires frequent use of mouthwash diluted with water (1:5) or saline water (1 teaspoon of salt to 1 pint of water), although patients with painful open lesions may prefer water alone (Daeffler, 1981). Regular oral rinsing mechanically removes debris while moistening and softening the mucosa. If end-stage patients are unable to swish fluid orally, the caregiver can use a soft brush or foam stick dipped in saline water to accomplish the same thing.

Lemon and glycerine swabs have no mechanical or cleansing properties and are irritating to open lesions (Wiley, 1969). Glycerin is alcohol based and actually dries and irritates the mucosa rather than freshening the mouth as is commonly believed (Bruya, Maderia, 1975).

Painful oral lesions can be soothed with 2% viscous xylocaine rinses and avoidance of spicy, acidic, and fried foods (Bruya, Maderia, 1975). Popsicles or other cold foods may be welcome and will not retard healing. Dry mouths can be eased with artificial saliva and high liquid diets, and dry lips should be moisturized with K-Y jelly (Daeffler, 1981).

The Time of Death

Regardless of the setting in which it occurs, the time of death is both difficult and delicate. As a directly involved, informed caregiver, the palliative care nurse's relationship with the patient and family can be a significant therapeutic tool at the time of death. Specific strategies include encouraging the family to be with the patient even when family members can no longer offer task-related physical care, letting families know that the patient may actually die when left alone even though they would like to be present, and pointing out that patients are probably still able to hear even when they are no longer overtly responsive. *Being* with the patient is far more important than *doing*. Other helpful strategies are reassuring the family that Cheyne–Stokes breathing does not mean the patient is in distress and suggesting that supportive significant others be called.

Because most Americans have little direct experience with death, the palliative care nurse needs to alert the family to physical signs of imminent death and help them plan for that moment. In this way, undesired emergency measures including paramedic intervention, resuscitative actions, and Code Blues are not initiated, and unfinished interpersonal issues can be addressed. Often end-stage patients die following a gradual disease progression, culminating in inability to swallow, immobility, organ system failure, somnolence, coma, and peripheral vascular shutdown. Occasionally, actual death is heralded by hemorrhage, fatal clotting, pulmonary emboli, or vena cava syndrome. When death occurs, family members should be allowed an opportunity to have final moments before the body is removed to a mortuary. They may or may not choose to do so, and the nurse should offer to stay with them or to provide complete privacy depending on their wishes. Some family members want to assist in final clean-up and preparation of the body.

Professionals from other disciplines may have special skills or additional time to contribute to patient and family preparation for last goodbyes. Counseling topics may involve a review of past hurts, questions, negative and positive feelings, an array of grief-related concerns, plans for funerals or memorial services, education about self-care during bereavement, and options for coping with problems that may arise after the patient's death. As discussed earlier, some patients and families enjoy more closeness and intimacy at the time of death than they have ever experienced before, and the crisis actually engenders new discoveries and growth.

Case Study

Sarah was a 69-year-old widow of Italian descent who lived in her home with her youngest daughter, Margaret. She was diagnosed with cancer of the pancreas two years ago and had responded well to chemotherapy until her admission to hospice four months prior to her death.

Sarah wished to maintain her independence and, if possible, die at home. At the time of admission she was ambulatory with assistance, although she tired easily. Her weight loss was gradual, and she was concerned about maintaining her weight. Sarah was aware that her tumor had metastasized and had stopped chemotherapy because she no longer felt strong enough to undergo treatment that appeared not to help anymore. Mild pain in the lower abdomen was controlled sporadically by Tylenol with Codeine #3. Bowels were of concern because it seemed Sarah had a small obstruction in the lower rectum that impeded bowel movements, and the codeine also slowed bowel motility.

Margaret had initially called hospice for help because she worked during the day and did not feel she could care for her mother and continue to work. Her two siblings—a brother, Ted, and an older sister, Rose—were busy with family and work responsibilities and offered limited support. Margaret, unmarried and living with her mother, was feeling very isolated.

During the intake process, the nurse learned that Sarah felt that she would be fine alone during the day until Margaret came home. She stated that she did not feel comfortable with a lot of strangers in the home. In talking with Sarah over the phone about the services provided by hospice, it was clear that Sarah, like many people, did not realize that dying is often a gradual process of deterioration with the patient increasingly being unable to care for himself or herself. Sarah assumed she would be fairly independent until the day she died. The intake nurse also talked with Sarah's attending physician, who agreed that Sarah's prognosis was six months or less, an admission requirement for most hospices. After further discussion with Sarah about Margaret's feeling she needed help, she agreed to a visit.

In the initial visit, the nurse listened to Sarah talk about her cancer and the changes it had brought about in her life. She was fearful of dying in pain and of not being able to die at home. It was at this time the nurse learned that Margaret had had a psychotic breakdown two years previously. Although she was working, she was still seeing a psychiatrist weekly. Sarah was concerned about Margaret's ability to care for her. There had been some friction between the mother and the daughter, but the daughter had no other place to live, and, for the moment, both seemed to feel comfortable with the current living situation. Sarah also wished to be closer to her other two children, who did not feel comfortable around Margaret. The nurse suggested a social worker visit might be helpful in facilitating a family discussion.

Initially Sarah, wishing to be independent, denied she needed help. However, as the nurse talked about the reality of Sarah having only so much energy and about allowing herself to accept help with the mundane aspects of life, Sarah came to see that if she accepted some assistance, she could have energy for a walk in her yard or a visit with a friend. A home health aide would come in three times a week to help with the bathing because Sarah found this aspect of her care most tiring.

The nurse completed her visit with a physical examination and noted the following problems:

1. *Pain* Sarah was taking her medicine only when the pain became intolerable and was waking regularly during the night with pain. As they talked, Sarah expressed fear that she would build up tolerance for the medicine and not have adequate pain control in the latter stages of her illness.

   The hospice nurse explained that it was important to take the pain medication on a regular basis around the clock in order to maintain adequate analgesic blood levels. The nurse also reviewed the fact that pain medications are used for months by many patients without a problem, partly because around-the-clock dosing actually decreases the overall amount of medicine needed. Once Sarah's concerns were addressed, she agreed to take her Tylenol with Codeine every four hours throughout the day and night.

2. *Nutrition* The nurse explained that, with progressive tumor growth, it might be difficult to maintain weight and suggested small frequent feedings as well as nutritional supplements. The nurse realized that many patients feel guilty because they have no appetite and thus cannot enhance their capability to fight their disease. Again, information was helpful, allowing Sarah to see that her anorexia was not something she could prevent but that there were strategies she could use to counteract it.

3. *Bowels* Sarah had been taking a laxative when she felt constipated and if there were no results, followed that with an enema given by her daughter. Because prevention of symptoms is the major goal of palliative care, the nurse instituted a bowel regimen of Colace 100 mg t.i.d. with 2 Senokot tablets at bedtime.

4. *Skin* For the moment Sarah's skin was intact but dry and fragile because of her weight loss. The hospice nurse instructed the home health aide to massage Sarah's skin with lotion during her visits to promote skin integrity and advised Sarah to put an eggcrate mattress on the bed.

5. *Equipment* Sarah's bathroom was 20 feet away and, even at night, Sarah preferred to walk to the bathroom rather than have a bedside commode. Sarah had a cane that she used occasionally but, for the most part, was strong enough to walk alone. The nurse made her aware of equipment such as a bedside commode and a quad cane that would

be available if she felt she needed additional support.

6. *Family Dynamics* As Sarah began to trust the nurse more, she talked of her fears for her daughter and the friction that was common between the two. The nurse thought it would be helpful for the social worker to visit to provide support to both mother and daughter.

7. *Spiritual* Sarah had a strong faith and had been active in the church. After identifying this, the nurse asked Sarah about her current spiritual support and found that she was visited weekly by the parish priest.

In a subsequent visit that week, the nurse discovered that the pain medication given every 4 hours was controlling the pain with no breakthroughs. The nurse suggested taking two Tylenol with Codeine #3 at night to see if she could sleep through. Sarah tried this and was able to sleep through the night and to wake without pain. Bowels were still a problem as Sarah had not had a bowel movement in four days. The nurse did a rectal exam, removed a small amount of hard stool, and decided to continue the present bowel regimen for the time being.

That same week the social worker met with Sarah and learned that she had worked in a meat-packing plant to supplement the family income for much of her married life. Her husband, who had died five years ago, was a heavy drinker, and that fact had exacerbated their financial problems. She still missed the home they had to sell ten years ago and felt guilty that Margaret had "problems." The social worker talked with Sarah about her strengths and how she had coped with previous crises. The work of the social worker, as well as the whole team, was to provide support to Sarah, decrease her sense of isolation, and facilitate her grappling with the difficult issues in her life. For instance, because of the stormy relationship between Sarah and Margaret, Sarah would probably need additional help in the home, which could be costly or necessitate asking assistance from her other children. The team did not tell Sarah what she should do but offered support and information on the options available.

The nurse and social worker met with Margaret alone to talk with her about her mother and about her own concerns. Margaret was feeling very burdened although she was no longer doing the bulk of the physical care, and a housekeeper had been hired for once-a-week cleaning. It was obvious that Margaret was very fragile emotionally and felt her mother was critical and expected more from her. This was a surprise to the hospice team because Sarah had voiced a strong desire to do things for herself as much as possible.

Plans were made to have a joint meeting with Margaret and Sarah. At the meeting Sarah heard Margaret's concerns, and a daily routine was established. Margaret would leave cereal and milk on the table for Sarah to have at her leisure for breakfast, the home health aide would prepare lunch and leave it for Sarah to heat, and dinner would be fixed by Margaret. A volunteer would come in two nights a week to prepare dinner and provide company so that Margaret would have time to herself. The meeting was helpful in that both women could see their roles had reversed, and Margaret felt that she had support from the hospice team.

The next few weeks were good for Sarah. She was able to accept the help of the volunteer and the home health aide and felt comfortable with the hospice team support.

The nurse visited one to two times per week, which allowed her to identify problems before a crisis occurred. For instance, when Tylenol with Codeine was no longer effective, the nurse obtained an order for oral morphine. The initial dose was 10 mg every 4 hours, but over the next 24 hours the dose was increased until Sarah achieved pain relief on 15 mg every 4 hours. Doubling the evening dose allowed Sarah to sleep through the night.

Sarah had periodic bouts of diarrhea alternating with constipation. The Senokot was decreased to once a day, and a ducolax suppository every other morning was added. This seemed to work well.

The team continued to support Sarah's grieving with active listening and counseling. It seemed reassuring for her to hear that her daughter was a grown woman, responsible for her own life, and that she could no longer be responsible for it. The team noticed that Margaret seemed more despondent and "on edge" as time went by.

One morning Sarah called the nurse and, sounding frightened, reported that Margaret had been verbally abusive. Margaret was accusing her mother of doing terrible things to her as a child. A family conference with Sarah and the other two adult children was held that afternoon with the nurse and the social worker present. The nurse talked about the advancing disease process and the fact that eventually Sarah would need around-the-clock help. The social worker encouraged all the family members to express their feelings about Margaret and the present situation. It was decided that Margaret would need to move and that the other two children, Rose and Ted, would help out on the weekends, with additional help hired during the day. Sarah insisted that she could still stay alone at night and promised she would call her family or hospice if a problem arose. Sarah's only concession would be that she would use a bedside commode at night.

The social worker talked with Margaret's psychiatrist, who eventually arranged for Margaret to live in a half-way house. Margaret agreed to this solution and later felt in control enough to visit her mother.

As Sarah became weaker, the nurse talked with her about obtaining night help. Her husband's life insurance provided enough to cover expenses. During this time, Rose and Ted spent more time with her, although she was still alone at night. It was only after a fall that Sarah agreed to around-the-clock help supplemented with a home health aide from hospice five times per week.

Nausea became a problem, and Compazine 25 mg every 6 hours was added to Sarah's medication regimen. Compazine suppositories were available when she was unable to tolerate the oral medication.

As Sarah's time in bed increased, the nurse focused on teaching the attendant appropriate care strategies. Although attendants may be experienced, they need reassurance and instruction on skin and mouth care, turning and positioning, transfer techniques, and nutrition. Because Sarah had no family with her at night, the hospice on-call nurse was used frequently by the attendants for supervision with nausea, vomiting, pain, or insomnia problems. Duoderm was applied to the coccyx when the area became reddened. Sarah began to allow herself to be taken care of but tired easily and saw less of her friends.

She talked about not lingering and about hoping her life would end soon. The nurse and the social worker kept in touch with Margaret, Rose, and Ted by phone or with visits at Sarah's house, letting them know about Sarah's condition and what to expect.

Sarah had completed her will and left written instructions about her funeral. Rose and Ted were encouraged to visit the funeral home of Sarah's choice to make preliminary arrangements, and they did so.

Sarah's condition changed very rapidly. Two days before her death she stopped eating and took only sips of water. Urinary retention developed, and the nurse inserted a Foley catheter connected to bedside drainage. Her morphine had to be increased to 40 mg (2 cc), and the family was encouraged to say goodbye as Sarah drifted into a comatose state.

Ted and Rose wondered if more could be done for her in the hospital and talked with the nurse about the options available. They needed to hear that Sarah was receiving good nursing care at home, and they agreed to keep her there. The nurse reviewed the physical changes that would occur as Sarah's death became imminent, such as cold extremities, irregular respiration, and loss of control of bowels. The team listened as the family talked about their Dad's death and other memories of previous losses.

Early one morning Sarah died peacefully. The on-call nurse came out and stayed with the family until the body was taken away. Margaret did well and received a psychiatric follow-up later that day. The nurse listened to the family and the attendants talk about Sarah and her death and performed practical tasks such as notifying the attending physician, coroner, and mortuary of the death and calling the durable medical equipment company to have the equipment removed.

The nurse and the social worker attended the funeral and offered bereavement services to the family in the form of one-to-one volunteer support, family support group, and a monthly pot-luck. Margaret continued her psychiatric support, but Ted and Rose felt they did not need bereavement support.

Sarah was able to die at home with dignity. She received care from individuals who allowed her to maintain her independence and sense of control. The team could not mend relationships rooted in long-standing problems but could offer a nonjudgmental attitude and acknowledgment that Sarah's life had been meaningful to herself, her family, and the hospice team who cared for her.

Summary

The following points regarding palliative nursing care of end-stage illness are discussed in detail throughout the chapter:

1. Primary attention to the patient's and family's needs for quality of life, dignity, and sense of control in the face of diminishing capacities and impending death. Recognition of the normal and inevitable nature of death, often denied in our culture.

2. Attention to symptom prevention through the use of individualized, preferably oral, adjustable medication. Constant awareness of the importance of pain control as well as the avoidance and relief of other physical problems frequently involved in end-stage illness.

3. Attention to psychosocial and spiritual components of the patient's and family's experience.

4. Attention to caregivers' own responses and coordination of interdisciplinary personnel.

Issues for Further Investigation

1. What are the factors involved in the family's decision for providing hospice care in the home?

2. What is the cost of hospice care and how does it benefit families?

3. What are the essential components of successfully managing symptoms at home?

4. What are the predictors of the need to institutionalize a dying patient?

5. What is the long-term outcome of providing care to a family member? Does it help or hinder grief management? Is there a difference between spouse caring for spouse and parent caring for child?

6. What is the impact of providing home care on the functioning and satisfaction of the family?

References

Adams F (1984): Six very good reasons why we react differently to various dying patients, *Nurs 84, 84*: 6:41–43.

Adams JE, Lindemann E (1974): Coping with long-term disability. In: *Coping and Adaptation*, Adams J, Hamburg D, Coelho G (eds.). New York: Basic Books.

Aguilera DC, Messick JM (1974): *Crisis Intervention*. St. Louis: Mosby.

Amadeo P (1984): Peripherally acting agents. *Am J Med, 77*: 17–26.

Angell M (1982): The quality of mercy. *N Eng J Med, 306*: 98–99.

Anthony EJ (1970): The impact of mental and physical illness on family life. *Am J Psychiatry, 127*(2): 56–64.

Aries P (1981): *The Hour of Our Death*. New York: Knopf.

Baines M (1983): Drug control of common symptoms. In: *Hospice Care—Principles and Practice*, Corr CA, Corr DM (eds.). New York: Springer-Verlag.

Bautista DH (1976): Modifying the treatment: Patient compliance, patient control and medical care. *Soc Sci Med*, Vol 10, 233–238.

Bell RR (1979): Family roles and illness. In: *A Sociological Framework for Patient Care*, Folta JR, Deck ES, Bell RR (eds.). New York: Wiley.

Benoliel JQ (1967): *The Nurse and the Dying Patient*. New York: Macmillan.

Benoliel JQ, McCorkle R (1978): A holistic approach to terminal illness. *Cancer Nurs, 1*: 143–149.

Blues AG, Zerwekh JV (1984): *Hospice and Palliative Nursing Care*. Orlando, FL: Grune and Stratton.

Bruera E et al (1985): Action of oral Methylprednisolone in terminal cancer patients: A prospective randomized double-blind study. *Cancer Treat Rep, 69*: 751–754.

Bruhn JG (1977): Effects of chronic illness on the family. *Am J Nurs, 4*(6): 1059.

Bruya M, Maderia N (1975): Stomatitis after chemotherapy. *Am J Nurs, 75*: 1349–1352.

Bunch B, Zahza D (1976): Dealing with death: The unlearned role. *Am J Nurs, 76*(9): 1486–1488.

Burkhalter PK, Donley DL (eds.) (1978): *Dynamics of Oncology Nursing*. New York: McGraw-Hill.

Campbell AV (1978): *Medicine, Health and Justice*. New York: Churchill Livingston.

Cantor R (1978): *And a Time to Live*. San Francisco: Harper & Row.

Capone MA et al (1979): Crisis intervention: A functional model for hospitalized cancer patients. *Am J Orthopsychiatry, 49*(4): 598–607.

Crowther A (1978): Management of constipation in terminally ill patients. *J Int Med, 6*: 348–350.

Daeffler R (1981): Oral hygiene measures for patients with cancer. *Cancer Nurs, 4*: 29–35.

DeWalt E, Haines A (1969): The effects of specified stressors on healthy oral mucosa. *Nurs Res, 18*: 22–27.

Donovan H (1980): The hospice movement: A unifying force? *Nurs Forum, 19*(1): 19–25.

Feifel H (1977): *New Meanings of Death*. San Francisco: McGraw-Hill.

Fife BL (1985): A model for predicting the adaptation of families to medical crisis. *Image, 4*: 108–112.

Fingle E (1984): Laxatives and cathartics. In: *The Pharmacological Basis of Therapeutics*, Gilman A, Goodman LS (eds.). New York: Macmillan.

Foley K (1985): Medical progress—the treatment of cancer pain. *N Engl J Med, 313*: 84–95.

Frytak S, Moertel C (1981): Management of nausea and vomiting in the cancer patient. *JAMA, 245*: 393–396.

Giaquinta B (1977): Helping families face the crisis of cancer. *Am J Nurs, 77*(10): 1587.

Glaser B, Strauss, A (1965): *Awareness of Dying*. Chicago: Aldini.

Glasser PH, Glasser LN (eds.) (1970): *Families in Crisis*. New York: Harper & Row.

Godkin MA, Krant M, Doster N (1983): *International Journal of Psychiatry in Medicine, 13*: 153–165.

Hansen DA, Hill R (1964): Families under stress. In: *Handbook of Marriage and the Family*, Christensen HT (ed.). Chicago: Rand McNally.

Holmesley H (1986): Dosage range study of contolled-release morphine (MS Contin 30 mg tablets) in patient with chronic pain. Prepublication pamphlet from Purdue Frederick Company, Norwalk, Connecticut.

Hoyt MF (1983): Concerning remorse: With special attention to its defensive function, *J Am Acad Psychoanalysis, 11*(3): 435–443.

Izard MW, Ellison FS (1982): Treatment of drug induced constipation with a purified senna derivative. *Conn Med, 26*: 592–598.

Kayser J, Minngerode F (1975): Increasing nursing students' interest in work with aged patients. *Nurs Res, 24*(1): 23–26.

Klein H (1982): Constipation and fecal impaction. *Med Clin North Am, 66*: 1135–1141.

Kubler-Ross E (1969): *On Death and Dying*. New York: Macmillan.

Lewis F (1981): Experienced personal control and quality of life in non-curable cancer patients. Research abstract presented at American Cancer Society's meeting: The Cycle of Research, Seattle, August 17–19.

Lillard J (1982): Ageism and sexism: A double-edged sword. *J Gerontol Nurs, 8*(11): 630–634.

Lillard J (1984): Nuclear responsibility (Letter to the Editor). *Oncol Nurs Forum, 2*(2): 18.

Lillard J, Bystrowski K (1981): Role strain in hospice nursing. *Home Health Quarterly*, Spring: 51–53.

Litman TJ (1974): The family as a basic unit in health and medical care: A social behavioral overview. *Soc Sci Med, 8*: 505.

Lowenberg JS (1970): The coping behaviors of fatally ill adolescents and their parents. *Nurs Forum*, 9(3): 269–287.

Lowenberg JS (1976): Working through feelings around death. In: *The Nurse as Caregiver for the Terminal Patient and His Family*, Earle AM, Argondizzo NT, Kutser AH (eds.). New York: Columbia University Press.

Mabrey JH (1970): Medicine and the family. In: *Families in Crisis*, Glasser PH, Glasser LN (eds.). New York: Harper & Row.

MacVicar MG, Archbold P (1976): A framework for family assessment in chronic illness. *Nurs Forum*, 15(2): 180–194.

Mahoney J (1985): Excerpted from address of President of National Hospice Organization at annual meeting of the Northern California Hospice Association, February 1.

Mailick M (1979): The impact of severe illness on the individual and family, *Soc Work Health Care, 5*(2): 117–129.

Malinak D, Hoyt M, Patterson V (1979): Adults' reactions to the death of a parent. *Am J Psychiatry*, 136(9): 1152–1156.

Massie M, Holland J (1984) Diagnosis and treatment of depression in the cancer patient. *J Clin Psychiatry, 45*: 25–28.

McCaffery M (1979): *Nursing Management of the Patient with Pain*. Philadelphia: J.B. Lippincott.

Medicare Program: Hospice Care (1983): *Federal Register*, 48, Monday, August 22, 38146.

Moertel CG, Ahmann O, Taylor W (1974): Relief of pain by oral medications. *JAMA, 229*: 55–59.

Moffat AC (1978): Absorption of drugs. In: *Drug Metabolism in Man*, Carrod JW, Beckett AH (eds.). London: Taylor and Francis Ltd.

Moore J (1980): Lecture on family dynamics, concepts, and assessment. University of California School of Nursing, January 10.

Neuman PB, Henrickson H, Grosman N (1982): Plasma morphine concentration during chronic oral administration in patients with cancer pain. *Pain*, 13: 247–252.

Olsen EH (1970): The impact of serious illness on the family system. *Postgrad Med J, 47*(2): 170.

Osment L (1975): The skin in wound healing. In: *Biologic Basis of Wound Healing*, Menaker L (ed.). New York: Harper & Row.

Parkes C (1972): *Bereavement Studies of Grief in Adult Life*. New York: International Universities Press.

Parkes C, Parkes J (1984): 'Hospice' versus 'hospital' care: Re-evaluation after 10 years as seen by surviving spouses. *Postgrad Med J, 60*: 120–124.

Phipps M et al (1984): Staging care for pressure sores. *Am J Nurs*, 999–1003.

Porter J, Jeck H (1980): Addiction rare in patients treated with narcotics. *N Engl J Med, 302*: 123.

Power P (1979): The chronically ill husband and father: His role in the family. *Fam Coordinator, 34*(3): 140–145.

Reps P (n.d.) *Zen Flesh, Zen Bones*. New York: Anchor/Doubleday.

Richardson HH (1970): A family as seen in the hospital. In: *Families in Crisis*, Glasser PH, Glasser LN (eds.). New York: Harper & Row.

Robinson L (1974): *Liaison Nursing: Psychological Approach to Patient Care*. Philadelphia: F.A. Davis.

Sanchez-Salazar V, Stark A (1972): The use of crisis intervention in the rehabilitation of laryngectomies. *J Speech Hear Disord, 37*(3): 323–328.

Satir V (1968): *Conjoint Family Therapy*. Palo Alto, CA: Science and Behavior Books.

Saunders C, Summers DH, Tuller N (1981): *Hospice: The Living Idea*. London: W.B. Saunders.

Saunders JM, McCorkle R (1985): Models of care for persons with progressive cancer. *Nurs Clin North Am, 20*(2): 365–377.

Schofferman J (1986): Medical management of the dying patient. *Front Radiat Ther Oncol, 20*: 245–248.

Siegel L, Longo D (1981): The control of chemotherapy-induced emesis. *Ann Int Med, 95*: 352–259.

Silverberg E (1985): Cancer statistics. *CA—A Cancer Journal for Clinicians*, January/February. New York: American Cancer Society.

Soffer R (1983): Coping mechanisms of the chronically ill during family separation. *Home Health Care Nurse, 6*: 52–55.

Stoller EP (1980): Effect of experience on nurses' responses to dying and death in the hospital setting. *Nurs Res, 29*: January/February, 35–38.

Strauss A, Glaser B (1975): *Chronic Illness and the Quality of Life*. St. Louis: Mosby.

Thomas EJ (1970): Problems of disability from the perspective of role theory. In: *Families in Crisis*, Glasser PH, Glasser LN (eds.). New York: Harper & Row.

Twycross RG, Tack S (1983): *Symptom Control in Far Advanced Cancer: Pain Relief*. London: Pitman Books.

Walsh TD (1984): Oral morphine in chronic cancer pain. *Pain, 18*: 1–11.

Walsh TD (1985): Common misunderstandings about the use of morphine for chronic pain in advanced cancer. *CA—A Cancer Journal for Clinicians, 35*(3): 164–169.

Weisman A (1972): *On Dying and Denying*. New York: Behavioral Publications.

Wiley JB (1969): Why glycerol and lemon juice? *Am J Nurs, 69*: 342–344.

Williams SL (1976): The nurse as crisis intervener. In: *The Nurse as Caregiver for the Terminal Patient and His Family*, Earle AM, Argondizzo NT, Kutscher AH (eds.). New York: Columbia University Press.

Wright K, Dyck S (1984): Expressed concerns of adult cancer patients' family members. *Cancer Nurs, 10*: 371–373.

Zerwekh J (1984): Symptom control. In: *Hospice and Palliative Nursing Care*, Blue A, Zerwekh J (eds.). Orlando, FL: Grune & Stratton.

Zerwekh J (1983): The dehydration question. *Nursing 83*, 47–53.

Grateful acknowledgement is made to Jerome Schofferman, MD, and Michael F. Hoyt, PhD, for their helpful comments.

On 17 December 1986 Marcia Lillard, mother of Jennifer Lillard, died at home in Sharon, Massachusetts, in the presence of her family and the caregivers at the Southwood Community Hospice. Jennifer Lillard's contribution to this chapter is dedicated to her memory.

SUICIDE AND THE ELDERLY

Patrick Arbore, MA

Arliss Thompson Willis, RN, MS

Between 20,000 and 30,000 Americans, 25% of whom are older adults, commit suicide every year. Nurses are often in the position to identify and assist those who may be at risk for suicide. This chapter describes the phenomenon of elderly suicide in terms of risk factors and research findings. Case studies are used to share the concerns of elderly clients at an urban suicide prevention agency.

Patrick Arbore is Director of the Geriatric Program of San Francisco Suicide Prevention, Inc. He has made significant contributions to the development and implementation of services to the elderly. His areas of particular emphasis include assisting families with their bereavement following the suicide of a family member.

Arliss Willis is Director of Medicare Risk Contract at the French Health Plan in San Francisco. Her experience in gerontologic nursing spans both academic and service settings. In her current position, she directs outpatient and home care services for the elderly.

Introduction

The elderly population has the highest rate of suicide of any age group (Gurland, Cross, 1983). This dictates that suicidology and suicide prevention cannot remain the exclusive domain of psychiatric mental health nursing. Nurses involved in broader aspects of community mental health, public health nursing, geriatric case management, hospice and bereavement care, and other related areas are often in the position to confront individuals who may be at risk of suicide.

We concur with Fitzpatrick (1983) when she states "Suicide is of concern to all health professionals and the study of suicide and suicide prevention have been truly interdisciplinary fields of endeavor." Thus, we have drawn from the literature of several disciplines—from nursing, psychology, medicine, social work, and gerontology—to develop the theme of this chapter.

Each year in the United States between 20,000 and 30,000 individuals will commit suicide. Of these reported suicides, at least 25% will be older adults (Bromberg, Cassel, 1983; Osgood, 1982; Shulman, 1978). Although the elderly currently represent only 11% of the population, they have the highest rate of suicide for any age group (Osgood, 1982). In absolute numbers, between 6000 and 10,000 Americans over the age of 60 take their own lives each year (Osgood, 1982; Bromberg, Cassel, 1983). Of the known suicides, it is generally accepted that the older male will be highly represented. Durkheim (1951) was the first to hypothesize that suicide rates increase with advancing age and that males were more at risk than females of the same age. White males over the age of 75 have a suicide rate (per 100,000 population) over seven times that of white females of the same age group (Gurland, Cross, 1983).

Not all authors agree that suicide rates among the elderly are so high. Stenback (1982) indicates that the United States has seen a decrease in suicide rates of the aged during the 1960s and 1970s. Kastenbaum (1985) clarifies this debate somewhat by taking gender differences into account. Regarding the overall suicide rate of 21.2 per 100,000 for persons in the 75 to 79 age group, there are 42.5 male suicides per 100,000 as compared with 7.5 for females. The statistics for the overall age group are very misleading.

According to Fitzpatrick (1983), suicide is the 10th leading cause of death among adults. She indicates, however, that suicide statistics are conservative estimates. If there are any doubts regarding a suicide—that is, an equivocal death—the coroner will most often indicate accidental death or death from natural causes. Among the elderly, a high incidence of physical illness provides a convenient cause of death whenever there is any doubt (Shulman, 1978).

In recent years, research has begun to focus on suicide and minority populations. Seiden (1981) found that nonwhite suicide rates tended to decline during older years. McIntosh and Santos (1981) also found suicide rates among nonwhites generally do not increase with age of the person as do suicide rates for whites. These authors indicate that the rate of suicides among nonwhites is greatest among those aged 20–30 and declines after age 30. Although available suicide figures for Chinese and Japanese–Americans are dated, the last published data show increases with age for Chinese, with peaks in the oldest age grouping (over 65 and over 75, respectively) (McIntosh, Santos, 1981). In a study conducted by Bourne (1973) of suicide among Chinese in San Francisco, data were collected over a 16-year period. One of his findings was that for both sexes the peak decade for suicide is between 55 and 65 years of age.

Among Blacks and Native Americans, however, suicide rates were extremely low for the aged (Bourne, 1973). Wylie (1971) reports on studies that suggest that American Blacks have a wider acceptance of the extended family, including persons of older generations. There is a certain respect and veneration of age in Black families that affects the place of the older person within the culture (Wylie, 1971).

In an 11-year period, from 1970 to 1980, a study was conducted on all elderly suicides in San Francisco (Arbore, Moy, 1984). Of the 617 suicides, 91.25% were committed by whites. Rates for nonwhites dramatically declined during this 11-year span, from a high of 62.44 in 1970 to 19.06 in 1980.

Although more knowledge must be gained regarding the degree of impact that suicide has on minority elderly, it is germane to notice some of the problems inherent in ethnic aging research. Bengtson (1979) addressed four problem areas:

1. The identification of problems, questions, and issues. The perspective of the researcher who may not be of the racial minority of the sample population may find the life circumstance of the subjects irrelevant to the issues.

2. The goals of the research may not benefit the members of the race from which the study subjects are drawn.

3. The methods of the research may not appropriately elicit the useful information for which the study was constructed.

4. The politics and accountability in research. Bengtson cautions that researchers frequently are "quite unprepared to negotiate for the right to carry out their studies, or to consider accountability beyond their own academic reference group" if they encounter the interest group "of the collectivity from which data are sought."

Research Theories

Alienation Theory

In terms of gerontological research, this is an exciting as well as a challenging time to investigate the world of the older adult. What are some of the theories that have motivated gerontological research? One such theory that has guided social gerontological research for the last 30 years is alienation theory. According to Shanas (1982), the alienation approach presupposes that elderly people who live alone or apart from family are, therefore, neglected by these relatives. This myth needs to be broken. Researchers who study older aging, Shanas argues, should begin by defining family as it relates to older people. According to Shanas (1982), the "family may include those persons somewhat distantly related by blood or marriage" (p. 67). She continues her definition of family to include "even more distant relatives as a need arises for information, services, or help from these relatives" (p. 67). The hidden implications that older individuals living in the same household with other relatives brings happiness and, conversely, that older individuals living in separate households are unhappy are entwined in the alienation myth. Shanas asserts that *household* or *family* be clearly defined.

Activity Theory

Another theoretical approach that has guided research in social gerontology for several decades is activity theory (Lee, 1985). In this theory, emotional adjustment of the elderly is positively related to their social involvement. Although a thorough review of activity theory is beyond the scope of this chapter, a few studies using this approach are worth mentioning. Lee describes a study conducted by Lemon et al that found that "only informal activity with friends was significantly related to a measure of life satisfaction." Lee refers to a number of studies that surprisingly suggest that emotional adjustment among the elderly is unrelated to the elders' interaction with relatives.

Another interesting study referred to by Lee (1985) draws the conclusion that an older person's self-image and emotional adjustment to potentially traumatic events can be heightened through the existence of even one very intimate friend or confidant. This study is particularly relevant to the nurse who encounters, for example, an elder who has been recently isolated through the death of a spouse. Allowing the grieving spouse the opportunity to confide in the nurse could have positive therapeutic repercussions. A 24-hour telephone line developed by a suicide prevention agency to provide emotional support and other services to the elderly is in keeping with this theory and is aptly called the Friendship Line for the Elderly.

Disengagement Theory

Another theory discussed by Lee (1985) as an alternative to activity theory is disengagement theory. Disengagement theory states that social involvement tends to decrease in later life. Although involvement in social networks among the elderly is crucial to both theories, Lee contends that neither theory is designed to predict or explain network involvement itself.

Exchange Theory

A fourth and final theory Lee (1985) offers as a more appropriate concept for aging research is the exchange theory. This theory "focuses analytic attention on the properties of specific relationships and kinds of relationships, variation in these properties, and variation in potential outcomes of social interaction for older persons" (p. 32).

If one accepts the premise that needs may increase as a person ages, exchange theory can be instrumental in understanding the deficiencies that can occur when formal or informal services are introduced to an elder. If, as Lee points out, the only reward an elder can offer a service provider is conformity, there may be an imbalance in terms of reciprocity. A result of this lack of balance or exchange in the relationship could result in the elder's withdrawal from the provider. See Chapter 2 for a more detailed discussion of social exchange theory.

Risk Factors

Keeping the theories related to aging research in mind, we will describe some of the risk factors endemic to elderly suicide.

Depression

Gurland and Cross (1983) reported on various studies that investigated important risk factors. In one study, researchers discovered that 94% of the suicide victims studied were mentally ill, and 68% had affective disorder or alcoholism. Another study discussed by these authors related factors associated with 30 elderly suicides. It was found that 87% were mentally ill, 63% had affective disorder, and the remainder suffered from a depressive illness in conjunction with terminal physical illness, alcoholism, or organic brain syndrome. What is meant by the term *mental illness*, ambiguous at best, needs refinement or clarification.

Because depression is more likely to lead to suicide in older than in younger patients according to Gurland and Cross (1983), a closer examination of this risk factor is warranted. It is suggested that most depressions related to elderly suicides had lasted less than a year; this short duration indicates the urgency of intervention to prevent suicide (Gurland, Cross, 1983). Psychiatric nurses' understanding of the link between depression and suicide is found in the work of Menninger, who is responsible for the anger-turned-inward hypothesis about suicide (Fitzpatrick, 1983).

Roose et al (1983) discuss a study where a group of depressed patients who committed suicide is compared with a demographically similar group of depressed patients who never attempted suicide. These researchers concluded that depressed patients who committed suicide were like the general population of depressed patients but more severely depressed in every way.

Although clinicians generally have little difficulty recognizing the severely depressed older patient, those elders with less severe forms of depression may be harder to detect (Okimoto et al 1983). Okimoto et al (1983) cite the following reasons why depression in the older patient is difficult to recognize:

1. The older depressed patient presents with vague, ill-defined somatic symptoms rather than with the psychologic and mood symptoms typical of a classic depressive syndrome.

2. The presence of medical disease complicates the diagnosis of depression in the older patient.

3. The attitude of the clinician toward aging may contribute to difficulties in recognizing depression in the elderly.

Fitzpatrick (1983) summarizes this discussion on depression by stating that "suicide is related to the depressed feeling state not necessarily to the psychiatric illness of depression. It is more accurate to say that even crazy people kill themselves rather than saying only crazy people kill themselves" (p. 23).

Bereavement

According to various authors (Bromberg, Cassel, 1983; Osgood, 1982; Shulman, 1978; Stenback, 1982) bereavement, a normal response to the death or loss of a deeply loved or important person or thing, is clearly a predisposing factor for depression and suicide. Stenback (1982) describes a study that compared 320 widowed suicide victims with the same number of widowed persons having died of other causes. In the older age groups, especially among males, deaths from suicide were particularly evidenced in the first year of bereavement.

Bromberg and Cassel (1983) state that 20% of widowers and widows manifest depressive syndromes in the year following the death of a spouse. It is suggested also that widowers experience more difficulty with this life transition. In addition, elderly widowed males generally are characterized by more unhappiness, mental disorders, high death rates, and high self-injury rates (Wenz, 1980). Because of a lack of supportive intervention networks, this transition to widowhood can be difficult.

According to the committee for the Study of Health Consequences of the Stress of Bereavement, the Institute of Medicine,* for some couples past middle age, feelings of attachment may intensify even when the death of one partner is imminent. The Committee points out that helping a spouse plan for the approaching death of the partner may arouse feelings of disloyalty.

Physical Illness

Gurland and Cross (1983) discuss other factors associated with elderly suicides, including physical illness and isolation. Many studies have shown a high incidence of serious physical illness in those individuals who attempt suicide in old age (Shulman, 1978). In a study commented on by Shulman (1978), which compared elderly suicides with an age-matched control group of accidental deaths, a clear excess of physical illness was found among the former group on postmortem examinations. Because of the preponderance of chronic physical ailments experienced by the elderly, Stenback (1982) cautions that a simultaneous estimation of the personal significance allocated to the illness be undertaken in suicides and attempted suicides.

Isolation

Social isolation and loneliness are frequently mentioned in the analysis of suicidal behavior among the elderly (Stenback, 1982). Recent isolates or those persons who have encountered a

---

*This project was launched at the Institute of Medicine. The Institute of Medicine, chartered in 1970 by the National Academy of Sciences, enlists distinguished members of appropriate professions in the examination of policy matters pertaining to the health of the public (Osterweis et al, 1984, p. ii).

very recent loss such as the death of a spouse are particularly vulnerable. Lifelong isolates appear adjusted to that state as long as they are well. Determining the type of isolation of an older adult seems to be more important than the isolation itself (Gurland, Cross, 1983).

Stenback (1982) reports on another study that described the reasons why 34% of 30 elderly suicide victims were living alone on the day of their suicide. In addition to marital break-up, other reasons given were the death or admission to the hospital of a friend or a relative. Stenback (1982) also found that the percentage of suicide victims living alone was as high as 29.7%. When those individuals aged 60 years and over were analyzed, it was found that 39% were living alone.

Shulman (1978) includes increasing age, unmarried marital status, living alone, poor physical health, psychosis, unemployed or retired work status, and lethality of method used in his list of risk factors based on studies of elders who have attempted to take their own lives.

Substance Abuse and Suicide

Case Study A

John G., a 74-year-old man, attempted suicide seven years ago through a combination of drugs and alcohol. Also, seven years ago John G. was divorced by his wife of many years. Although he survived that suicide attempt, John G. tried again 5 1/2 years later. This time he took an overdose of Tylenol followed by alcohol. He stated that prior to this second suicide attempt his son refused to see him because of the drinking. John G. said that he drinks one quart of vodka each day. John G. is dead. The cause of death was congestive heart failure and cirrhosis of the liver.

Case Study B

Eva D., a 78-year-old woman, begins each day by drinking a concoction of milk, egg, and whiskey. Although her refrigerator might be devoid of food, there is always a twelve pack of beer. When paramedics were called in to take her to the hospital, at least 25 prescription bottles were discovered. When asked if she used these medications, she responded that she took some of the pills from various bottles now and then. Some of the prescriptions were written over three years ago. Last year at this time, her companion of 27 years died. Eva D., terrified of nursing home confinement, was placed by her older daughter in a nursing home several hundred miles from the community where she had lived for 30 years.

Referring again to the study of elderly suicide in San Francisco, Arbore and Moy (1984) discovered that 35% of the 617 total elderly deaths were a result of an overdose of medication compounded in some cases by alcoholic beverages.

In both case studies, a loss was incurred either through divorce or death of an important person. The Committee for the Study of Health Consequences of the Stress of Bereavement, The Institute of Medicine (Osterweis et al, 1984) cites several studies that have relevance here. One small study found that 17% of their alcoholic subjects who committed suicide had experienced the death of someone close during the prior year. The central concern of other studies is that the loss of an affectional relationship can increase the risk of suicide for the alcoholic.

Until his death at age 74, John G. in Case Study A was among the growing ranks of elderly alcoholics in the United States. Although estimates vary, most authors tend to agree with Schuckit (1977) that alcohol problems in the elderly affect between 2% and 10% of the general elderly population (Brown, 1982; Lamy, 1984; Price, Andrews, 1982; Russell, 1984; Snyder, Way, 1979). Of these 2 to 3 million older alcoholics, those who are most affected are widowers, individuals with medical problems, and people who are in difficulty with the police (Schuckit, 1977).

Even the nonscientific literature cites the lonely older person as being vulnerable to alcohol dependency. Cowley (1980) writes, "If inner resources are lacking, old persons living alone may seek comfort and a kind of companionship in the bottle. I should judge from the gossip of various neighborhoods that the outer suburbs from Boston to San Diego are full of secretly alcoholic widows."

Brown and Chiang (1983, 1984) caution that estimates of elderly alcohol abuse are often tentative and imprecise. These authors suggest that older adults are more likely to abstain from alcohol than younger age groups. However, these authors agree with the contention of other investigators that alcohol abuse among the elderly is more extensive than most people realize.

The older alcoholic is invisible, except to his landlord and a few neighbors (Duckworth, Rosenblatt, 1976). Older alcoholics often tend to deny their drinking problem and thus hide their abuse from authorities (Brown, 1982). Medical personnel may often not diagnose alcoholism in their older patients because the symptoms elderly alcoholics present can be attributed to other degenerative diseases common in the aged or because those health care professionals are reluctant to label an elderly patient as an alcoholic (Snyder, Way, 1979). Although Snyder and Way (1979) state that the burden of identifying elderly alcoholics will fall heavily on physicians and social service personnel, it is very likely that nurses, often in a front-line position with the patient, will need to be educated not only about the identification of alcohol abuse but also about the most appropriate treatment plan.

In Case Study B, Eva D.'s physician of 25 years knew about but did not treat her alcohol dependency. At the time of her last hospitalization prior to her entry into a nursing home, Eva D.'s physician said that perhaps he "didn't handle her alcoholism well. She always bounced back before." During this hospitalization, she experienced nightmarish delusions and paranoia.

Several months after Eva D. was moved by her family to a nursing home, a call came from her on the Friendship Line for the Elderly. Although in a weakened condition, she had man-

aged, with the help of a long-time friend, to move back to her community. It did not seem surprising that her drinking had accelerated as she attempted to reestablish herself in the community where she had been living for over 30 years. Eva D. was hospitalized once more for problems related to her alcoholism. However, for the first time, she was enrolled in an alcohol rehabilitation program of a local hospital. She told the counselor from Suicide Prevention "I have it easier than most of the young people here because I only have one drug to fight. They have booze and other stuff." Although it is hoped that Eva will overcome her dependence on alcohol, we include her story to emphasize the need to offer alternatives to the older client who may suffer from alcoholism or other mental as well as physical health issues. Should she fail or not, Eva's enrollment in an alcohol rehabilitation program may open the minds of health care professionals to treatment programs that may positively affect the well-being of older adults.

Drug Use, Misuse, or Abuse

Case Study

> Interviewer: Have you taken your medication today?
>
> Alice: No. I'm not going to take my pills today.
>
> Interviewer: Why is that?
>
> Alice: I want to see what happens if I don't.
>
> Interviewer: Didn't your doctor tell you what will happen?
>
> Alice: He's never told me why I need to take them so I'm going to find out for myself.

Alice, a 70-year-old woman, is one of a growing number of adults over the age of 65 who consume 25% of all prescription drugs sold in the United States (Butler, 1975). Alice also is failing to comply with the instructions of her doctor regarding the taking of her medication. Alice is not unlike the typical respondent in a study referred to by Raffoul, Cooper, and Love (1981), where the most common type of inappropriate use of drugs was underuse, and none of the subjects reported receiving adequate information about the appropriate use of the medication. Alice is contributing to a problem of yet unknown proportions that deserves more attention and study—misuse of drugs among the elderly (Peterson, Whittington, Beer, 1979). Although not many studies exist that investigate the extent of this problem, a few are worth mentioning. La Rue, Dessonville, and Jarvik (1985) state that only a small percentage of older adults is seen in acute-care facilities for drug-related emergencies. Other studies discussed by these authors suggest that data collected from emergency rooms underestimate the extent of drug misuse among the elderly. In a survey reported by Moree (1985), a nurse reported that patients stop taking a medication if they are uninformed about the consequences of not taking the medication. Other respondents indicated that cost and confusion about the regimen resulted in noncompliance. Obviously, other studies must be initiated, coupled with education aimed at identifying older patients who may be seen in the emergency room and who may be misusing medications.

Caution must also be used when any medications are prescribed to an elderly patient. Although high usages of tranquilizers, sedatives, and hypnotics might reflect the greater anxiety, depression, and insomnia found in older adults, it may also point to the anxiety of doctors and other health personnel and to their impatience with elderly people (Butler, Lewis, 1977). Alice, for example, did not know why she was asked to take the tranquilizers prescribed by her doctor and was noncompliant as a result. According to Pascarelli and Fisher (1974), the elderly drug dependent person is more apt to be poor, isolated, and residing in an urban area. Pascarelli (1979) also suggests that older persons on Medicare and Medicaid have free access to different physicians and health care facilities, and can "shop around" for multiple prescriptions from a variety of sources.

Abuse is defined in one study reported by Pascarelli (1979) as the deliberate use of a drug, usually by self-administration in a manner inconsistent with or related to acceptable medical practice. The study netted the following results from nationwide sources such as hospital emergency rooms and medical examiners: Tranquilizers such as diazepam (Valium), chlordiazepoxide (Librium), and flurazepam (Dalmane) are the drugs of preference. Barbiturates are now second choice and secobarbital is used about one-third of the time. These data were gathered on persons 50 years of age and older. As mentioned earlier, caution is warranted when investigating emergency room statistics.

Antidepressant medications such as Elavil and Triavil are increasingly recognized as drugs of abuse that can produce euphoria (Pascarelli, 1979). These drugs rank 24th and 31st respectively in the top 40 DAWN II (Drug Abuse Warning Network) drugs of abuse (Drug Enforcement Administration, 1973–1974).

Combinations of drugs are used by all age groups, including the elderly; the most frequent combination is alcohol with tranquilizers or hypnotics (Pascarelli, 1979). Euphoria is enhanced by this combination, and the likelihood of an overdose is heightened (Pascarelli, 1979). Krupka and Vener (1979) suggest that multiple pathology of the aging leads to polypharmacy, which may lead to a greater number of problems, which are treated with an even greater number of drugs. Again, more care needs to be adopted on the part of health professionals, policy-makers, and others who work on behalf of the aging regarding drug interactions.

An important reason for monitoring treatment plans for older patients requiring multiple drugs is to be on the alert for adverse drug reactions. Patients who exhibit symptoms typically associated with old age (such as forgetfulness, weakness, confusion, anorexia, and anxiety), and who may be receiving psychotropic or hypnotic agents, may be victims of adverse drug reactions (Bressler, 1981). When the patient suffers from multiple pathology and receives multiple drugs, it is most difficult to predict patient response to a specific drug for a specific symptom (Lamy, 1980).

Daily drugs might be taken with a complex pattern of timing and dosage which even a young alert person would find difficult to maintain accurately (Atkinson, Gibson, Andrews (1977). Add to this an elder with poor eyesight or memory loss and confusion may occur regarding compliance. Even simple but differing instructions for taking more than one medication can result in misunderstanding and noncompliance (Atkinson, Gibson, Andrews, 1977).

Patterns are changing and will continue to change as the present day street narcotic users— many of whom use multiple drugs—grow older (Pascarelli, 1979). Schuckit (1977) writes that many addicts die young and as many as one-third of the survivors "mature out" of their addiction by age 50. He would agree, however, that older addicts exist. It can be suggested that the older opiate user will have unique treatment needs (Schuckit, 1977). In a study conducted by Pascarelli (1979), most of the drug abuse among his elderly sample involved the categories of depressants including alcohol. He reported that fewer problems occurred with the use of opiates.

Kastenbaum (1985) postulates that orientations toward self-destruction are becoming more common among the elderly. These orientations manifest as suicide ideation, suicide attempts, and a variety of behaviors that substantially increase the risk to one's life. Kastenbaum (1985) stresses the need to be alert to the ever-present danger of suicide and concludes by stating that "Greater awareness of suicidal thinking and self-injurious behaviors in later life can help us become more adept both as care-givers and researchers" (p. 636).

Summary

Although it is not our aim to promote a negative image of aging nor to suggest that all old people living alone are in a high-risk group, it is paramount to note that some older people contemplate and frequently complete the suicidal act.

Whether an older person's care comes primarily from the family as is suggested by Krout (1985) or from public or nonprofit organizations, the nurse must be aware of the danger signs that can signal a potentially suicidal elder. Nurses, especially those in the burgeoning role of geriatric case managers, must become knowledgeable regarding both the formal and informal support systems in the community that may aid an elder during stressful life transitions.

Research efforts designed to study suicide among the elderly must be supported and encouraged in order to understand the motivating factors behind this tragic act. Nurse researchers are in an ideal position to explore the area of suicide prevention.

Special considerations must be taken into account, however, in any study that attempts to investigate an elderly population. Not only does the 75-plus age population possess the highest suicide rate of any age group, but it is also the fastest growing segment of the U.S. population (Streib, 1983). Although many older individuals are healthy and living independent lives, many others are more likely to require numerous hospitalizations and extensive medical care. One study discussed by Streib (1983), which proposed to survey a random sample of the total noninstitutionalized population in the United States aged above 65, had a significant loss rate in the 75-plus age category because the subjects were too sick to be interviewed. Streib suggests that new methods and techniques be created in order to successfully study this older population.

Nurses can be very effective in studies focusing on the older adult since they are knowledgeable regarding the physical and mental functioning limitations in ill older persons. This is an asset since physical illness, isolation, and depression are critical risk factors in elderly suicide.

As Fitzpatrick (1983) instructs "Suicidal persons reach out to others asking for assistance.

Both knowledge and compassion will help us to more effectively help them" (p. 28).

Issues for Further Investigation

1. If, as Osgood (1982) discusses, 75% of elderly persons who kill themselves see a physician shortly before committing suicide, what are the factors that contribute to the perceived lack of intervention on the part of the health care professional?

2. At what point does an elder become suicidal? Does one risk factor carry more weight than others?

3. What steps need to be taken to strengthen the commitment of health care providers and others to an effective prevention strategy relative to elderly suicide?

4. How can nurses be more instrumental in reducing medication noncompliance in their patients? What could be the related impact on elderly suicide prevention?

5. Is a kin network as effective in diminishing elderly isolation and suicide as the introduction of an unrelated community worker or volunteer?

6. How can elderly suicide prevention training help a nurse intervene more successfully with a suicidal older patient?

References

Arbore P, Moy S (1984): Demographic study of suicide and the elderly in San Francisco from 1970 to 1980. Unpublished paper.*

*More information can be obtained by writing Patrick Arbore, San Francisco Suicide Prevention, 3940 Geary Blvd., San Francisco, CA 94118.

Atkinson L, Gibson IJM, Andrews J (1977): The difficulties of old people taking drugs. *Age and Aging,* 6: 144–150.

Bengtson VL (1979): Ethnicity and aging: Problems and issues in current social science inquiry. In: *Ethnicity and Aging: Theory, Research, and Policy,* Gelfand DE, Kutzik AJ (eds.). New York: Springer-Verlag.

Bourne PG (1973): Suicide among Chinese in San Francisco. *Am J Public Health,* 63(8): 744–750.

Bressler R (1981): Hazards of common drugs. *Drug Therapy,* 3: 135–139.

Bromberg S, Cassel CK (1983): Suicide in the elderly: The limits of paternalism. *J Am Geriatr Soc,* 31(11): 698–703.

Brown BB (1982): Professionals' perceptions of drug and alcohol abuse among the elderly. *Gerontologist,* 22:(6) 519–525.

Brown BB, Chiang C (1983–84): Drug and alcohol abuse among the elderly: Is being alone the key? *Int J Aging Hum Dev,* 18(1): 1–12.

Butler RN (1975): *Why Survive? Being Old in America.* New York: Harper & Row.

Butler RN, Lewis MI (1977): *Aging and Mental Health.* St. Louis: Mosby.

Cowley M (1980): *The View from 80.* New York: Penguin.

Drug Enforcement Administration (1973–1974): Drug abuse warning network phase II report, BNDD Contract No. 72-47. Washington, DC: Department of Justice.

Durkheim E (1951): *Suicide.* New York: Free Press.

Duckworth GL, Rosenblatt A (1976): Helping the elderly alcoholic. *Soc Casework,* 5: 296–301.

Fitzpatrick JJ (1983): Suicidology and suicide prevention: Historical perspectives from the nursing literature. *J Psychiatr Nurs,* 21(5): 20–28.

Gurland BJ, Cross PS (1983): Suicide among the elderly. In: *The Acting-Out Elderly,* Aronson MK, Gurland BJ (eds.). New York: Haworth.

Kastenbaum R (1985): Dying and death: A lifespan approach. In: *Handbook of the Psychology of Aging,* Birren JE, Schaie KW (eds.). New York: Von Nostrand Reinhold.

Krout JA (1985): Relationships between informal and formal organizational networks. In: *Social Support Networks and the Care of the Elderly,* Sauer WJ, Coward RT (eds.). New York: Springer-Verlag.

Krupka LR, Vener AM (1979): Hazards of drug use among the elderly. *Gerontologist, 19*(1): 101–105.

Lamy PR (1984): Alcohol misuse and abuse among the elderly. *Intell Clin Pharm, 18*: 649–651.

La Rue A, Dessonville C, Jarvik LF (1985): Aging and mental disorders. In: *Handbook of the Psychology of Aging*, Birren JE, Schaie KW (eds.). New York: Van Nostrand Reinhold.

Lee GR (1985): Theoretical perspectives on social networks. In: *Social Support Networks and the Care of the Elderly*, Sauer WJ, Coward RT (eds.). New York: Springer-Verlag.

McIntosh JL, Santos JF (1981): Suicide among minority elderly: A preliminary investigation. *Suicide Life Threat Behav, 11*(3): 151–166.

Moree NA (1985): Nurses speak out on patients and drug regimens. *Am J Nurs,* (1):51–54.

Okimoto JT, Barnes RF, Veith RC (1983): A simple screening test for depression in geriatric patients. *Geriatr Psychiatry, 2*(8): 51–55.

Osgood N (1982): Suicide in the elderly: Are we heeding the warnings? *Postgrad Med, 72*(2): 123–130.

Osterweis M, Solomon F, Green M (eds.) (1984): *Bereavement, Reactions, Consequences, and Care.* Washington, DC: National Academy Press.

Pascarelli EF (1979): An update on drug dependence in the elderly. *J Drug Issues, 9*(1): 47–54.

Pascarelli EF, Fischer W (1974): Drug dependency in the elderly. *Int J Aging Hum Dev, 5*(4): 347–356.

Petersen DM, Whittington FJ, Beer ET (1979): Drug use and misuse among the elderly. *J Drug Issues, 9*: 5–26.

Price JH, Andrews P (1982): Alcohol abuse in the elderly. *J Gerontol Nurs, 8*(1): 16–19.

Raffoul PR, Cooper JK, Love DW (1981): Drug misuse in older people. *Gerontologist, 21*(2): 146–150.

Roose SP et al (1983): Depression, delusions, and suicide. *Am J Psychiatry, 140*(9): 1159–1162.

Russell JF (1984): Alcohol and the elderly. *Alcohol Health Res World,* Spring, p. 18.

Schuckit MA (1977): Geriatric alcoholism and drug abuse. *Gerontologist, 17*(2): 168–174.

Seiden RH (1981): Mellowing with age: Factors influencing the nonwhite suicide rate. *Int J Aging Hum Dev, 13*(4): 265–284.

Shanas E (1982): Social myth as hypothesis: The case of the family relations of old people. In: *Adult Development and Aging*, Schaie KW, Geiwitz J (eds.). Boston: Little, Brown.

Shulman K (1978): Suicide and parasuicide in old age: A review. *Age and Aging, 7*: 201–209.

Snyder PK, Way A (1979): Alcoholism and the elderly. *Aging,* Jan/Feb: 97–100.

Stenback A (1982): Suicidal behavior in old age. In: *Adult Development and Aging*. Schaie KW, Geiwitz J (eds.). Boston: Little, Brown.

Streib GF (1983): The frail elderly: Research dilemmas and research opportunities. *Gerontologist, 23*(1): 40–44.

Wenz FV (1980): Aging and suicide: Maturation or cohort effect? *Int J Aging Hum Dev, 11*(4): 297–305.

Wylie FM (1971): Attitudes toward aging and the aged among Black Americans: Some historical perspectives. *Aging Hum Dev, 2*: 66–70.

29

ALCOHOLISM AND THE FAMILY

W. Carole Chenitz, RN, EdD

William Granfors, RN, BSN

Alcoholism is a chronic, progressive, and fatal disease that affects up to 10% of the population in the United States. The disease has profound impact on all family members and on the nurses that care for the family. This chapter describes the disease of alcoholism and its effect on the family. It also presents an overview of current theories and models for intervention, and describes one nurse-administered family program for alcoholics.

Carole Chenitz, Associate Chief of Nursing Service for Research at the Veterans Administration Medical Center in San Francisco, is recognized both for her clinical contributions to family treatment, care of the elderly, and substance abuse, and for her program of instruction for nurses on the utilization of grounded research theory methodology in their research. She is coauthor of From Practice to Grounded Theory.

William Granfors was formerly associated with Dr. Chenitz at the Veterans Administration Medical Center, and he now maintains a private practice for clients with substance abuse.

Introduction

Alcoholism has been called the "family disease" and with good reason. Each member of the alcoholic's family is affected by the disease, and in turn, the family affects the alcoholic. When alcoholism exists in the family, the entire family gets caught up in a complex interactional pattern that revolves around the drinking behavior and its sequelae. In this chapter, the disease of alcoholism and its effect on the family will be presented. An overview of current theories, treatments, and models for intervention with alcoholic families is presented. The relationship of nursing to alcoholic families and a nurse-administered family program for alcoholic families are described. We approach this chapter from the perspective of nurse clinicians who have been involved in the treatment of alcoholic families. This chapter draws heavily from this experience and from the extensive literature on alcoholism and alcoholic families.

The Disease Concept of Alcoholism

Alcoholism is a chronic, progressive, and fatal disease that affects between 3% and 10% of the population, depending on the definition of alcoholism that is used (Vaillant, 1983). According to the National Institute on Alcohol Abuse and Alcoholism, there may be as many as 10 million adults (7% of the adult population) and 3.3 million youths who are problem drinkers (Noble, 1979). Alcoholism is involved in a quarter of all admissions to general hospitals. Death can be directly related to alcoholism, as with cirrhosis of the liver, or indirectly related to alcoholism, as with car accidents, falls, fires, suicides, and homicides (Institute of Medicine, 1980). However, as a study by the Institute of Medicine points out, "These deaths are seldom ascribed to alcoholism, because of physician reluctance to

label alcoholics as such" (Institute of Medicine, 1980, p. 9).

There are many definitions of alcoholism. Based on the orientation of the person or provider, alcoholism is considered a disease or a social and psychologic problem. There is no specific etiology for alcoholism, which has increased the controversy about definition and therefore treatment. As Vaillant (1980) points out:

> Some people believe that if alcoholics are taught to regard alcoholism as a disease they will use the label as an excuse to drink or as a reason why they should not be held responsible for their own recovery. But the facts are that once patients understand that they have a "disease" they become more, not less responsible for self care (p. 19).

Alcoholism is incurable. Once the individual becomes an alcoholic there can be no return to "normal" drinking. As a chronic disease, alcoholism has remissions and exacerbations—that is, the disease may remain nonproblematic for a period of time, and a return of symptoms will precipitate a return of the drinking behavior. Daily management of the regimen can produce a state of recovery, which is a state of total abstinence from alcohol and other mind-altering drugs, with continuing improvement in the quality of the individual's life. (Abstinence is recommended because of cross-tolerance to other drugs; an alcoholic can stop alcohol use and become addicted to another mind-altering drug.) Recovery is impeded by denial and isolation. Denial is a defense mechanism against the reality that alcohol is causing a problem in the external or internal life of the individual. Denial of alcoholism and resistance to accepting the reality that alcohol is causing life problems plague the alcoholic and impede treatment and recovery. Isolation protects the denial as the alcoholic barricades himself or herself against any information that may threaten the distorted reality that alcohol is not a problem. The alcoholic isolates himself or herself from persons or situations as well as from internal feelings that may challenge the denial. Denial and isolation plague the alcoholic, prevent recovery, and often cause relapses into active alcoholism.

Denial and isolation enable the problematic drinking to continue and produce feelings of guilt, shame, loss of self-esteem, and loneliness. These feelings may confront the denial and thus are denied, rationalized, and projected onto others. Behavior that results from the problem-drinking and the response to the drinking are: loss of responsibility, dependence on others, lying about and making excuses for the drinking, and withdrawal and social isolation.

The Stages of Alcoholism

Jellinek (1960) first described the progression of alcoholism through four stages: the prealcoholic, the early alcoholic, the addicted alcoholic, and the chronic alcoholic. Forrest (1975) elaborated on the stages. Forrest identifies the first stage as the preproblematic, or experimental, social-drinking stage. In this stage, alcohol consumption is a social phenomenon that is established through peer pressure and wide acceptance of alcohol consumption. Controlled intoxication and socially acceptable intoxicated behavior characterize this stage. Most people never progress beyond this stage.

Stage two is called excessive drinking. Consumption is now more progressive, and there is more time and frequency spent on the act of drinking alcohol. Attending social events where drinking occurs and keeping company with people who drink now occupy the individual's time. The amount of alcohol consumed is not disclosed. Nondisclosure of alcohol consumption can take many forms, from hiding bottles to secretive drinking. Drinking that was once socially based is now motivated; the individual drinks to reduce tension and anxiety. Tolerance to alcohol increases with a growing, though unacknowledged, awareness of the increased alcohol consumption. This awareness is accompanied by feelings of guilt, which manifest as

denial about drinking. Blackouts or amnesic-like phenomena begin in this stage.

The third stage is called the addiction stage and is characterized by a loss of control over where and when drinking occurs, the accustomed pattern of drinking, and a loss of the ability to stop drinking once started. Drinking at this stage stops only when the individual passes out. The individual may then reawaken and resume the drinking. This "binge" can last from days to months. The individual drinks for the effect, and consumption of alcohol can take up most of his or her time. At this stage, memory loss, defensiveness and paranoia about the memory loss, loss of general intellect, and unstable behavior are common changes. The combined effect of the increased drinking and behavior changes affect both the job and the family. Work effectiveness, efficiency, and attendance begin to be compromised, and family relationships are affected. Parents begin to have serious disagreements, children disengage, and role boundaries deteriorate. The family as a unit disengages from social contacts and becomes enmeshed around the drinking behavior. Trust breaks down as the alcoholic lies about drinking. This leads to a negative self-concept in the alcoholic, who is at this time unable to stop. Blackouts become more common and suicidal impulses and attempts occur while the individual is drinking.

By stage four, the alcoholism is chronic, and life for the alcoholic is in shambles. Intoxication can last from months to years. Unlike the previous stage, in this stage tolerance for alcohol decreases. Physical problems such as encephalopathies, chronic malnutrition, liver disease, pancreatitis, and Korsakoff's syndrome are common. Family relationships have been severed either because the alcoholic left the family or the family asked the alcoholic to leave. The social network now includes other chronic alcoholics. This stage, if continued, ends in hospitalization or death.

We have reported here one version of the progression of alcoholism. These are not the only transitions and changes noted in alcoholics as the disease progresses. Because of the multiple factors involved in alcoholism and individual differences, there can be any number and combination of traits, and individuals can shift back and forth between behaviors that are characteristic of different stages. In fact, some alcoholics manifest few of the behavioral characteristics noted. These stages represent the mean and provide a sense of the progression experienced by many.

Diagnostic Criteria

There have been many attempts to establish a set of criteria to standardize the diagnosis of alcoholism. The most far-reaching attempt at defining diagnostic criteria is by the National Council on Alcoholism (NCA, 1972). They outline a two-track system that includes (1) physiologic and clinical criteria; and (2) behavioral, psychologic, and attitudinal criteria. In each track, a set of signs and symptoms is presented. These signs and symptoms can be used to analyze and differentiate a diagnostic picture (Estes et al, 1980). Once the diagnosis is made, an important emphasis in the initial phase of treatment is to assist the alcoholic and the family to deal with the disease and accompanying behaviors rather than beliefs about alcoholism and the etiology.

A major problem in the treatment of alcoholism is that the diagnosis is often never made known to the client in medical treatment. The treatment focus is on the medical problem, and the alcoholic denial is supported. Hence, diagnosis of alcoholism is a critical issue in the treatment of the disease.

Many treatments exist for alcoholism. The most standard form of treatment is individual, group, and family psychotherapy and the use of support groups such as Alcoholics Anonymous (AA). Psychotherapy is used to assist the alcoholic and family members identify, communicate, and cope more effectively with feelings and to foster new behavior in relation to the self and others. The support groups of AA provide rapid

identification, individual and group support, and a program for growth and change. Through participation in AA and active involvement in the 12 steps suggested as the means to recovery, there is an ongoing confrontation of denial and a decrease in personal and social isolation for the alcoholic.

Alcoholism and Families

Alcoholic families are families that have an alcoholic member, and the family is organized around the alcoholism. The organization of the family around the alcoholism affects all family members and the family's ability to function (Steinglass, 1971, 1980).

Alcoholism is a health problem for the alcoholic. The alcoholic's response to the health problem reverberates throughout the family. Vaillant (1980, p. 20) notes, "Outside of residence in a concentration camp, there are very few sustained human experiences that make one the recipient of as much sadism as does being a close family member of an alcoholic." The existence of alcoholism in the family affects family interactions and functioning and may threaten the survival of the family. Family unity for survival becomes a common goal for the family as a reaction to the threat posed by the alcoholism. Each member adjusts his or her behavior to fit the family goal, and the family as a whole continually adjusts to adapt to the alcoholic behavior.

Berenson describes two categories of family systems with alcoholism. The chief characteristic that differentiates these systems is the identification of alcohol as a problem in the system. In the first type, the "family agrees that alcohol is not a problem, or a minor problem" (Berenson, 1976, p. 290). In these families, alcoholism is acute to subacute and is secondary to other problems. Behavior in the family system has only slight changes when drinking occurs, and the amount and pattern of drinking is variable. In the second category, there is "agreement that alcoholism is a problem and there is intense conflict about it" (Berenson, 1976, p. 290). In these families, alcoholism is chronic and a primary problem that exacerbates other problems. The family's behavior changes are very common and intense, and the pattern of drinking remains variable.

Although the alcoholic has a health problem, the family also has a health problem in living with alcoholism. The family responds to alcoholism by denying it, trying to control it or eliminate it, and finally extruding the alcoholic either physically or functionally from the family.

Stages of Adjustment

Jackson (1954) described stages families go through in learning to adjust to alcoholism in an adult member of the family. The family first attempts to deny the problem. As the alcoholism progresses, there is recognition that the drinking is a problem, and the family then attempts to eliminate the problem by trying to keep the alcoholic from drinking. These attempts may be changes in family members' behavior or active control over the drinking, such as hiding the alcohol, removing alcohol from the house, or accompanying the alcoholic. When these attempts fail, disorganization follows. The family feels impotent and frustrated because their efforts to solve the problem have proven to be futile. Survival requires the family to reorganize in spite of the problem. The nonalcoholic spouse takes over more and more of the family functions, and the alcoholic's functions become divided among the spouse and children. The alcoholic at this stage is placed in the role of a child in the family and gradually loses more and more responsibility associated with their role in the family. Efforts to escape the problem through separation follow, and another reorganization then occurs. Jackson's (1954) stages have been refined and elaborated on as further studies of the alcoholic family have found variations in this pattern. As Kaufman (1984, p. 7) points out, "Most studies of alcoholic families have not addressed the changing relationship between stages of alcoholism and the family system operation."

Living with alcoholism in the family produces feelings of guilt, loss of self-esteem, shame, anger, frustration, hurt, and powerlessness in family members (Wegscheider, 1981). As one wife commented, "You're ashamed because you don't want anyone to know how you are living." She then went on to describe her anger and frustration, "There was nothing I could do for him, no matter what I did, it didn't work." Family members learn that their feelings must be denied for the sake of family unity. Denial requires that feelings cannot be acknowledged or shared with others. Members become isolated from each other and from their own feelings. Another wife of an alcoholic described her frustration, "I could never talk to him. When he was drunk, I couldn't talk because he wouldn't remember, and when he wasn't drinking I was afraid if I said anything, he would remember." Basic trust is shaken as promises are broken, responsibilities are not met, and intimacy is not permitted. The family sets up a rigid barrier to others, and social life becomes restricted. The family and its members withdraw into isolation and loneliness. The alcoholism in the family is a secret, and family members feel compelled to keep this secret. Family myths are created to maintain it. The basic myth is that the family will be destroyed if the secret is told. Paradoxically, it is the secret that destroys the family.

Steinglass (1980) reported a life history model of alcoholic families in interactional terms. Early in the drinking, families react to create enmeshed and chaotic systems, especially during periods of active drinking. Later, as the drinking progresses, the family adapts to exclude the drinker, or it may remain enmeshed and fused to the alcoholic with cycles of engagement and disengagement (Steinglass, 1980).

Wives of Alcoholics

Early interest in the effects of alcohol on family members focused on the wives of alcoholics.

Moos et al (1982) note that research in this area has been dominated by three perspectives: the personality perspective, the stress perspective, and the coping perspective. In the personality perspective, studies have tried to identify the personality traits of individuals who select and marry alcoholics or prealcoholics and foster their mates' alcohol abuse. In this view, spouses of alcoholics are considered to have negative personality characteristics that draw them to select and marry alcoholics. Studies within the stress perspective addressed the stress created by living with an alcoholic and have identified stress-related characteristics in spouses of alcoholics, such as depression, anxiety, poor health, and somatic complaints. Researchers adopting this view do not assume personality traits in the nonalcoholic spouse but focus attention on the functional differences between wives of recovered alcoholics and wives of nonalcoholics (Moos et al, 1982). Studies on the coping perspective focus on the ways spouses develop to cope with alcoholism in their mate and to create satisfactory lifestyles in spite of a disturbed marriage. Moos points out fundamental limitations in the methodology of these studies and notes that "Very few definite conclusions can be drawn from these studies" (Moos et al, 1982, p. 891). In his own research on alcoholic spouses, which compared spouses of relapsed alcoholics, recovered alcoholics, and matched community controls, Moos found that "Spouses of alcoholics are basically normal people who are trying to cope with disturbed marriages and behaviorally dysfunctional partners" (Moos et al, 1982, p. 905). In a later study of spouses, using the same type comparison groups, Moos and Moos (1984) found that families of recovered alcoholics when compared to community controls had fewer arguments, shared household tasks more, and showed higher agreement about their joint task performance but had a less active recreational orientation. Moos suggests that these findings are consistent with Jackson's (1954) stage of recovery and reorganization. Family functioning in the group of families of the re-

lapsed alcoholic was poorer than in either of the other groups (Moos, Moos, 1984).

Children of Alcoholics

Children of alcoholics respond to alcoholism in the family by developing characteristic, rigid behavior patterns that carry over into adult life. Children of alcoholics also become alcoholic at a higher rate than children from nonalcoholic families. The etiology remains unknown; however, emotional and behavioral responses of children of alcoholics have been described (Sloboda, 1974).

Children's specific patterns of reaction to living with alcoholism have been reported. These patterns are roles that the child assumes in the family that carry over into adult life (Black, 1982). These roles—the responsible one, the adjuster, the placater, and the acting-out child—have consequences on the future for these children. The responsible child takes over the work of a parent by caring for other children, setting rules, maintaining the house, and setting and achieving goals for themselves and others in the family. The adjuster remains detached from the family drama. These children make no effort to change or engage in the family and do not seem to experience any emotion over family crisis. The placater is the "sensitive" child and nurtures family members effectively. This child smooths over the situation and makes life easier for others in the family. The acting-out child is the stereotype of the child from a disturbed and chaotic family. The acting-out child is seen in child guidance clinics, school counseling programs, or law enforcement agencies. These children draw attention to themselves and their families in negative ways (Black, 1982).

Identification of the effects of alcohol on children in the family has recently emerged. Cermak and Brown (1982) analyzed group therapy sessions with adult children of alcoholics. Issues that emerged were control, trust, the identification and realization of personal needs, acceptance of responsibility for feelings and actions of others, and acceptance of one's feelings. They summarize, ". . . in terms of family structure, adult children of alcoholics share a history . . . there is exposure to a family system that is rigid, often chaotic and frequently rife with pressure to keep the obvious unnoticed" (Cermak, Brown, 1982, p. 385).

Enabling Alcoholism

Research has supported the idea that families play a role in maintaining alcoholism in the family member. Steinglass (1980) points out that the periodic symptomatic condition produced by active drinking acts as an adaptive or stabilizing mechanism for the family system. Sands et al (1971) identified a punitive mother–rebellious child interaction that emerged as a major theme during group psychotherapy with alcoholics and groups with spouses of alcoholics. In this interaction pattern, "the wife adopts the role of guardian of the home, a protector of the children and a watchdog in regard to the husband's drinking" (Sands et al, 1971, p. 475). At the same time, the alcoholic husband gives up the role of husband and father. However, Sands et al note that "when the drinking stops . . . the wife cannot or will not give his role back to him. In fact, she may undermine any effort he makes to resume his former role" (Sands et al, 1971, p. 476).

The process of maintaining the alcoholism is termed "enabling." Another term used to describe the family member's behavior in relation to alcoholism that may perpetuate the alcoholism is "coalcoholism." Both of these terms are used to describe behaviors that are well-intentioned but are nonproductive for the family member and assist in maintaining the alcoholism. The spouse of the alcoholic or the family member closest to the alcoholic, such as a parent, is considered a primary enabler, and other family members are considered enablers to some extent. The term *enabler* is used to describe how those closest to the alcoholic "become drawn into and affected by the very problem they would like to prevent. Thus a circular process is set up which can gather momentum of its own which is difficult to halt" (The Johnson Institute, 1982, p. 4). Enabling develops subtly and gradually over time and is characterized by behaviors that are aimed at doing the correct thing to help the alcoholic. Enabling behaviors are any attempts to protect the alcoholic from the full consequences of his or her behavior. Enabling may be making excuses for the drinking and the behavior, assuming responsibility for the alcoholic, and going along with the drinking. Specific examples of enabling behavior are calling in sick for the alcoholic when they have a hangover, lending money, making excuses to self and others for the drinking and behavior, restricting or eliminating family social life to protect the alcoholic from embarrassment, and trying to cover up the drinking (The Johnson Institute, 1980, 1982).

Family Treatment

Treatment of the family with an alcoholic member has included individual family therapy, spouse group therapy, and multiple family therapy (O'Farrell, Cutter, 1984; Anderson, Henderson, 1983; Sands, Hanson, 1982; Kaufman, Pattison, 1981; Davis, 1980; Steinglass, 1979; Shapiro, 1977). Each of these modalities has been found useful in treatment, mainly on an outpatient and long-term basis. Alcohol treatment and rehabilitation inpatient programs are a major form of treatment for alcoholism. The issue of family involvement has ranged from referral services to admitting the family into treatment with the alcoholic both on an inpatient basis and on an outpatient basis.

A goal in the treatment of the family is emotional detachment from the behavior of the alcoholic spouse. Once removed from the emotional engagement with the alcoholic, the spouse can begin to lead his or her own life. This includes a change in behavior in relation to the alcoholic

(Estes, 1974). A change in the system is made through a change in the nonalcoholic spouse. Emotional detachment allows the nonalcoholic spouse to assume responsibility for himself or herself and for the children but not for the behavior of the alcoholic. The overfunctioning member of the system is assisted to function more appropriately. This conversely allows the recovering alcoholic room in the family to resume previously neglected roles and responsibilities (Bowen, 1974).

Usher found that "because of the link between alcohol and specific family functions, the removal of alcohol in the initial phase of family therapy leaves the family vulnerable. They are exposed to their inadequacies and thus experience a threat previously concealed by the alcoholism" (Usher et al, 1982, pp. 928, 929). In the early stages of treatment, families may have mixed feelings about the treatment agency as well as about the treatment. Hope is remobilized, yet they may feel resentful of the support the alcoholic receives and of the possibility that the agency may accomplish what they have been unable to do for years (Jackson, 1954). During the early stage of treatment for alcoholism, the family needs support to deal with its ambivalence to treatment and the alcoholic.

An advantage of group counseling of alcoholics with their spouses is that identification with others in the group removes the pressure and blame from the alcoholic. In the group setting, the alcoholic is accepted as an individual with rights and feelings. This acceptance can be a motivating factor for the alcoholic to continue in treatment (Burton, 1962).

Nursing and Alcoholic Families

In 1980, the American Nurses' Association described nursing as "the diagnosis and treatment of human responses to actual or potential health problems." The unit of intervention for nurses can be the individual, family, group, or community. Nurses treat both the human response and the health problem. The focus of nursing intervention can be the health problem or the individual's response to the problem. The distinction of nursing from medicine and other health care disciplines is in the identification and treatment of the human response. Nursing and medicine may converge in the treatment of the health problem (ANA, 1980).

Nurses treat alcoholics in a variety of settings: hospitals, homes, clinics, psychiatric units and institutions, and alcohol treatment programs. The alcoholic family is also treated by nurses in schools, clinics, treatment programs, and health care institutions. Most often nurses treat alcoholics and their families for another health problem or for health maintenance.

Alcoholism is an encompassing health problem affecting the health not only of the alcoholic but of the family as well. There has been a growing recognition in society and in nursing that interventions with alcoholics and alcoholic families are needed and can be effective. The National Nurses' Society on Addictions (NNSA), a specialty organization in nursing, has identified five categories of nursing intervention in the treatment of alcoholism. The first category is identifying the problem with alcohol—that is, "systematically assess each patient in any setting for problems related to alcohol abuse and alcoholism. Each nurse should further identify the stage of progression of alcoholism based on the physical and psychological data obtained in the assessment" (NNSA, 1979, p. 7). In the second category of intervention, the nurse opens communications about the problem with alcohol with the patient, with the family or significant others, and with members of the health care team. The third category of intervention relates to the nurse as a health educator responsible for educating clients, families, and significant others about alcoholism. The fourth category asserts that "nurses in all settings should have a basic level of knowledge and skill to provide some alcoholism counseling" (NNSA, 1979). Finally, the nurse should have knowledge and information about available resources to refer clients and their families to appropriate treatment agencies (NNSA, 1979, p. 2).

Nurses are in a unique position to assist alcoholics and their families through the myriad of seeming contradictions to recovery and the development of coping styles and mechanisms that will promote a more healthy response to the disease of alcoholism. In order to do so, it is important to identify and understand factors that have influenced nurses' relationship with alcoholics. Naegle (1983) points out that several factors have influenced the character of nurse interaction with alcoholic clients. These are the nature of the disease of alcoholism and its increasing prominence as a health problem; social and professional attitudes toward alcoholism, which are marked by ambivalence and negativity; and problems associated with nursing's role development based on theory and practice. The result of these interacting factors is that nurses have not yet realized their potential as health care providers to alcoholic clients. Nurses reflect the larger society's ambivalent ideas and attitudes toward alcohol (Burkhalter, 1975). Throughout the ages, alcohol has been used as a social lubricant to assist in overcoming fears and to celebrate both large and small events. Alcohol is used in almost all social situations and in a wide range of places and occasions. Alcohol can be simultaneously viewed as a friend or foe. Although drinking alcohol is a cultural and social activity, there is a fine line between drinking alcohol and alcohol abuse. When an individual crosses the line into alcoholism, feelings, attitudes, and stereotypes about alcoholics and alcoholism are conjured up. Alcoholism has been termed the cancer of morals and dignity. In spite of growing awareness in society about the disease of alcoholism, the alcoholic has been and continues to be considered a moral reprobate, and many continue to stereotype alcoholics as people on skid row.

Nurses as part of society may, unbeknownst to themselves, reflect these attitudes. Health professionals generally view alcoholics negatively. The client's resistance to treatment and recurrent failure to attain goals for treatment set up an approach–avoidance conflict between the nurse and the client. It is difficult to invest a great deal of time and energy into a self-destructive individual. Relapse in alcoholism is common. The unspoken value that society places on alcoholism, which is reflected in the controversy over a definition and diagnostic criteria, is that this problem is not a "legitimate" medical problem. The client is seen as making a mindful choice to take the first drink and thereby restarting the binge and relapse.

Family members of alcoholics are also stereotyped and labeled. Family members can be seen as helpless victims or as willing accomplices, depending on the situation. Neither of these views is accurate, and neither is productive in assisting the family to make changes to cope effectively with the disease in a family member.

Nurses need to examine their feelings, attitudes, and beliefs about alcoholics and about working with this population. Knowledge of family systems and alcoholic family systems is needed. Nurses committed to this task are needed as role models and educators for other nurses and health professionals. These committed nurses can foster open communication and dialogue among colleagues and assist others to confront and break down myths, negative attitudes, and stereotypes. In terms of nursing's role with substance abusing clients, nurses in this specialty can advance and further develop the role of nursing with addicted clients.

The unique position of nurses in relation to the alcoholic client and the family is related to nursing's position in the health care system and nursing's image in society. First, nurses, as the largest single group of health professionals, engage with alcoholics and their families in a variety of health care contexts. Second, the image of nursing is as friendly, caring, and interested in helping. Attached to this stereotype of nursing and nurses is an inroad into the resistant, fearful, and unbalanced world of the alcoholic and the family. Although a number of counseling professions work with alcoholics, the image of nursing in society creates a nonthreatening, noninvasive, and safe role of the nurse to the client and family.

This role can be used to advantage to engage the alcoholic and/or the family. The family is entangled in a maze of maladaptive actions and reactions in response to the alcoholism. Although the family situation may be difficult, chaotic, painful, and almost unbearable for the family members, the situation is the family's best current balance at achieving unity and stability. Nurses, who have a caring image, availability, and visibility to families, are in an excellent position to enter into this system.

Nurses are able to assist alcoholic clients and their families with the social and psychologic recovery process balanced by a fund of physiologic and medical knowledge and a philosophy of care that addresses the complete needs of the individual and family. Nurses can incorporate knowledge of nutrition, positive health care practices, and instructions for prescribed medical treatment, and can develop programs to meet the needs of changing activities of daily living.

Nursing has claimed a holistic approach to health care with the goal of nursing to assist individuals and their families to attain, maintain, and regain their highest level of functioning. This philosophy and goal can be used with the alcoholic family to assist them in a step-by-step, task-oriented manner to develop coping skills to deal with the disease in the family. In this process, nurses need counseling skills and knowledge of alcoholism, the recovery process, families, and change. This knowledge combined with nursing's image in society and the profession's philosophy and goal enables nurses to engage and treat the alcoholic family effectively. The goal of treatment is to assist the family to develop ways to cope with the disease and a plan of action that takes into account the health

of each family member and the family as a whole. Nurses can assist families to develop this plan by providing information about positive health practices and to incorporate positive health practices into their daily lives.

Interventions with Alcoholic Families

The nurse's focus can be on the individual or on the family and on both the health problem of alcoholism or the response to the problem. Nursing interventions are aimed at engaging any of the alcoholic family members in treatment for the effects that alcoholism has had on them. Family members will resist the idea that they themselves need treatment. On alcohol inpatient units, it is common to find that families resist treatment because "he (alcoholic) is the problem and once he stops drinking we won't have a problem." Others resent the time and intrusion that treatment represents and are threatened by change.

The nurse can either treat the alcoholic or family, or encourage and refer them to treatment programs or the support groups of AA and Al Anon. Psychiatric or psychologic treatment is expensive and may not be readily available in the community. AA and Al Anon are free and readily available in most communities. Families can be referred to both or one of these, depending on the complexity and severity of the family problem and the present condition of the family.

Identification and diagnosis of the health problem of alcoholism is the first step in intervention. Communicating the diagnosis to the alcoholic and the family is the next step. At this juncture, it may be useful to call other members of the team together for a meeting with the alcoholic and the family for the purpose of communicating the diagnosis. Team members can support each other and take various approaches to deal with denial, anger, resentment, pain, and sadness that accompany a diagnosis of alcoholism. Often a nurse may not know if the client has been told this diagnosis in the past. The presence of alcoholism as a problem in the medical record does not indicate that the client and family have been told. The physician is a valuable member of the health team to have available for the initial meeting for diagnosis. The physical and medical problems of the alcoholic client that are related to alcoholism can be carefully outlined. The prognosis with continued drinking can be made.

Family members present in the initial interview for diagnosis can be very helpful in confronting the initial denial and anger. Families know the reality of the situation and more often than not believe that the alcoholic member needs help. Families can and will bring up specific incidents of drinking behavior to confront denial in this context. It is not uncommon for alcoholics in recovery to recall this type of interview as a precipitating event that led them to treatment. Often, this type of communication is not done formally or with the identified patient.

In other settings, the nurse will informally interact with the alcoholic client. One recovering alcoholic described an ICU nurse's interventions with her when she went to visit her family member who was terminal in the ICU as a result of alcoholism. The nurse asked her if she knew why her parent was in ICU. When the woman responded that she did, the nurse suggested that she may also have this problem. Angry and shocked, she was forced by this confrontation to recognize that she had a problem.

Violence is commonly reported by alcoholic families. In assessment, the nurse should ask specifically about violence in the family. Questions can be framed in a nonthreatening way, such as, "Many families with alcoholism report that they live with physical or verbal abuse. Has this been the case with your family?" Families with a history of violence are in physical danger, and the severity of this state must be communicated to them. These families should be referred to formal treatment programs or psychotherapy.

A Family Treatment Program

The philosophy of modern nursing espoused in the ANA Social Policy Statement and the roles and interventions for nurses presented by the National Nurses' Society for Addictions are consistent with the goal of alcohol treatment and rehabilitation. The following program description illustrates the implementation of nursing philosophy and roles to provide family treatment in an alcohol rehabilitation unit.

Family treatment has been an integral part of the inpatient alcohol rehabilitation unit at an urban Veterans Administration Medical Center since it opened eight years ago. In the early years of the unit, family treatment was provided by psychotherapists as an adjunct to primary treatment of the alcoholic in the program. Nursing input in family care was minimal. Over time, team members became increasingly aware of the visibility and importance of nurses on the unit both to clients and to families. There was also a growing recognition that nurses communicated easily and were motivated to work with families. Thus began the evolution to the current program for family treatment, which includes a nurse-coordinated and nurse-conducted family night.

Family involvement in treatment has three phases: family assessment, family program, and family referral, with individual family therapy.

Family Assessment

The program for family treatment begins with the client's assessment on entry into the unit. The configuration of a family system, identification of family members, and problems in the family are included in the assessment for each client. Family members are then referred by the client's coordinator to the family program.

Family Program

The family program is conducted in two segments one evening a week for two and a half hours. The first segment is family education; the second segment is a multifamily group.

Family Education   In family education, a series of four revolving classes is presented. The content for the classes was developed from a thematic analysis of family concerns during multifamily group meetings conducted over an 18-month period. The first class presents information on alcoholism and the recovery process. The majority of families entering this program have had limited knowledge of these concepts, and most often, they have had no involvement in treatment. In order for families to develop effective coping mechanisms during the recovery process, these basic concepts are presented.

The second class covers coalcoholism, or enabling. In this class, the focus is on how family members have coped with alcoholism and the effects of the disease on them. This information is critical because it provides a direction for change. Family members learn that by taking care of themselves they are taking care of the alcoholic, who needs to focus on his or her own recovery.

In the third class, specific information is presented about the support groups available to family and friends, such as Al-Anon, Al-Ateen, and Adult Children of Alcoholics. A major focus of this class is to encourage and support families to attend a meeting of these support groups while identifying common misgivings and beliefs about these groups.

In the fourth class, a film depicting the effects of alcoholism on child development is presented, followed by a discussion (Granfors, Chenitz, 1985).

These classes are conducted with only the family members and significant others present for several reasons. The alcoholic clients have been previously exposed to this material in other sections of the program. As noted earlier, families are new to treatment, and the tension level for them is high. When this material is presented in an educational format, anxiety levels drop, and families can more readily assimilate the in-

formation. Family members are able to ask questions and share information that they may not feel comfortable sharing with the alcoholic present, for fear of reprisal or embarrassment. As questions and concerns emerge, families are encouraged to share these with the alcoholic in a direct fashion. This educational component of the program also provides an opportunity for family members to identify and relate to each other, and it often generates questions and concerns that are carried over and addressed in the multifamily group (Granfors, Chenitz, 1985).

Multifamily Group   The multifamily group is the second part of the family program. The group begins after family education and a short break and lasts for 75 minutes. The alcoholic clients and their families are together for the group. This group provides an opportunity for alcoholic and family to examine and identify their responses to alcoholism, gain experience with new behaviors, and experience mutual support. A focus of these groups is communication of feelings, expectations, fears, and concerns. A major goal of the group is to provide a structure in which members can learn to identify, communicate, and tolerate the expression of emotions that can help them move past paralyzing pain and fear into new behaviors (Granfors, Chenitz, 1985).

The family program is coordinated, conducted, and supervised by nurses. Feedback to the team is provided in rounds the morning following the family program night. Family assessments are presented and recommendations for further treatment are made at this time.

Family Treatment

The third phase of treatment is short-term family treatment, usually one to three sessions. These are conducted by the client's coordinators, who are nurses, psychiatrists, social workers, and substance abuse fellows in psychiatry. The coordinator will conduct sessions for the family as problems are identified in the family program or the client's treatment. Referrals for ongoing treatment are made as needed for each family.

Treatment of the entire disease process and of the human responses to the disease of the affected individual and family is the highest form of health care delivery. When this can be implemented in an efficient, cost-effective manner, the program has viability and increased credibility. This program of family involvement in treatment is used to illustrate the role of nursing in family treatment.

Summary

In this chapter we have presented an overview of alcoholism; its effects on the family; family treatment; nursing's role; and a description of a nursing program for family treatment. Although much is known about alcoholic families and treatment is available for families, a central orientation of this chapter is on the critical nature of nursing's role in identifying, initiating, and in some cases, providing treatment for alcoholic families. The combination of nursing philosophy, knowledge, and image enhanced by knowledge of alcoholism and families creates a powerful force in the treatment of families affected by this disease. As one wife of an alcoholic noted, "I can't change him, all I can change is myself so that's what I am doing. Now I feel good about myself. Now I can hold my head up. I'm not ashamed anymore."

Issues for Further Investigation

1. Is there a relationship between the stages of alcoholism and family interactions and functioning?

2. What are the family functioning and family interaction patterns in families with an alcoholic member in late recovery, early recovery, and those not in recovery compared to "normal" (nonalcoholic) families?

3. Does the family exhibit different patterns of interaction when the alcoholic member is drinking than when the alcoholic is not drinking?

4. Does the family function differently when the alcoholic member is drinking than when the alcoholic is not drinking?

5. What is the incidence of alcoholism and drug addiction in children of alcoholics?

6. What is the incidence of recovery from alcoholism in alcoholic children of alcoholics when one or both parents entered recovery and when there was no recovery in the parent(s)?

7. Does a parent in recovery affect the experience of seeking help for alcohol and drug addiction for the addicted child? What is the experience of seeking help for an addiction among alcoholic children of recovered and nonrecovered parents?

References

American Nurses Association (1980): Nursing: A social policy statement. Kansas City, MO: ANA.

Anderson SC, Henderson DC (1983): Family therapy in the treatment of alcoholism. *Soc Work Health Care, 8*: 79–94.

Berenson D (1976): Alcohol and the family system. In: *Family Therapy: Theory and Practice,* Guerin PJ (ed.). New York: Gardner Press.

Black C (1982): *It Will Never Happen to Me.* Denver, CO: M.A.C. Printing and Publications.

Bowen M (1974): Alcoholism as viewed through family systems and family psychotherapy. *Ann NY Acad Sci, 42*: 115–122.

Burkhalter PK (1975): *Nursing Care of the Alcoholic and Drug Abuser.* New York: McGraw-Hill.

Burton G (1962): Group counseling for alcoholic husbands and their nonalcoholic wives. *J Marr Fam, 24*: 56–61.

Cermak TL, Brown S (1982): Interactional group therapy with adult children of alcoholics. *Int J Group Psychother, 32*: 375–389.

Davis DI (1980): The family in alcoholism. In: *Phenomenology and Treatment of Alcoholism*, Fann WE, Williams RL (eds.). New York: S.P. Medical and Scientific Books.

Estes N (1974): Counseling the wife of an alcoholic spouse. *Am J Nurs, 74*: 1251–1255.

Estes NJ, Smith-Dijulo KT, Heineman ME (1980): *Nursing Diagnosis of the Alcoholic Patient.* St. Louis: Mosby.

Forrest G (1975): *The Diagnosis and Treatment of Alcoholism.* Springfield, IL: Thomas.

Granfors W, Chenitz WC (April, 1985): Multifamily groups in an alcohol rehabilitation program. Paper presented at National Nurse's Society on Addiction, Washington, DC.

Institute of Medicine (1980): Report of a study: Alcoholism, alcohol abuse, and related problems, opportunities for research. Washington, DC: National Academy Press.

Jackson JK (1954): The adjustment of the family to the crisis of alcoholism. *Quarterly Journal on the Studies of Alcoholism, 15*: 562–586.

Jellinek EM (1960): *The Disease Concept of Alcoholism.* New Haven, CT: The Hillhouse Press.

Johnson Institute (1980): *Detachment: The Art of Letting Go While Living With an Alcoholic.* Minneapolis, MN: Johnson Institute.

Johnson Institute (1982): *The Family Enablers.* Minneapolis, MN: Johnson Institute.

Moos RH, Finney JW, Gable W (1982): The process of recovery from alcoholism. II. Comparing spouses of alcoholic patients and matched community controls. *J Stud Alcohol, 43*: 888–909.

Moos RH, Moos BS (1984): The process of recovery from alcoholism. III. Comparing functioning in families of alcoholics and matched control families. *J Stud Alcohol, 45*: 111–118.

Naegle M (1983): The nurse and the alcoholic. *J Psychosoc Nurs, 21*: 17–24.

National Council on Alcoholism, Criteria Committee (1972): Criteria for the diagnosis of alcoholism. *Am J Psychiatry, 129*: 41–49.

National Nurses Society on the Addictions (February 1, 1979): Position paper: The role of the nurse in alcoholism. Evanston, IL: NNSA.

Noble EP (ed.) (1979): The third special report to the Congress on alcohol and health, June, 1978. Technical Support Document. DHEW Publ. No. (ADM) 79-832. Washington, DC: US GPO.

Kaufman E (1984): Family system variables in alcoholism. *Alcoholism: Clin Exper Res, 8*: 4–8.

Kaufman E, Pattison EM (1981): Differential methods in family therapy in the treatment of alcoholism. *J Stud Alcohol, 42*: 951–971.

O'Farrell TJ, Cutter HS (1984): Behavioral marital therapy couples group for male alcoholics and their wives. *J Subst Abuse Treatment, 1*: 191–204.

Sands PM, Hanson PG (1982): Psychotherapeutic groups for alcoholics and relatives in an outpatient setting. *Int J Group Psychother, 21*: 1276–1278.

Sands PM, Hanson PG, Sheldon RB (1971): Recurring themes in group psychotherapy with alcoholics. *Psychiatr Quarterly, 41*: 474–482.

Shapiro RJ (1977): A family therapy approach to alcoholism. *J Marr Fam Counseling, 3*: 71–78.

Sloboda SB (1974): The children of alcoholics: A neglected problem. *Hosp Commun Psychiatry, 25*: 605–606.

Steinglass P (1980): A life history model of the alcoholic family. *Fam Process, 19*: 211–226.

Steinglass P, Weiner S, Mendelson J (1971): A systems approach to alcoholism. *Arch Gen Psychiatry, 24*: 401–408.

Steinglass P (1979): Family therapy with alcoholics: A review. In: *Family Therapy of Drug and Alcohol Abuse*, Kaufman E, Kaufman P (eds.). New York: Gardner Press.

Usher ML, Jay J, Glass BR (1982): Family therapy as a treatment modality for alcoholism. *J Stud Alcohol, 43*: 927–938.

Vaillant GE (1983): *The Natural History of Alcoholism.* Cambridge, MA: Harvard University Press.

Wegscheider S (1981): *Another Chance: Hope and Health for the Alcoholic Family.* Palo Alto, CA: Science and Behavior Books.

EPILOGUE

by Betty L. Highley

This closing gallery depicts a fractionated time slice of the family life cycle, as represented by a pre-birth interaction, a mid-life catastrophic illness, and an elderly couple faced with the long-term consequences of a stroke. The portrayal of older widowed women provides a final demographic statement.

Envision your idealized images of family life cycles in the 21st century and consider the implications those images convey for family nursing care through health and illness.

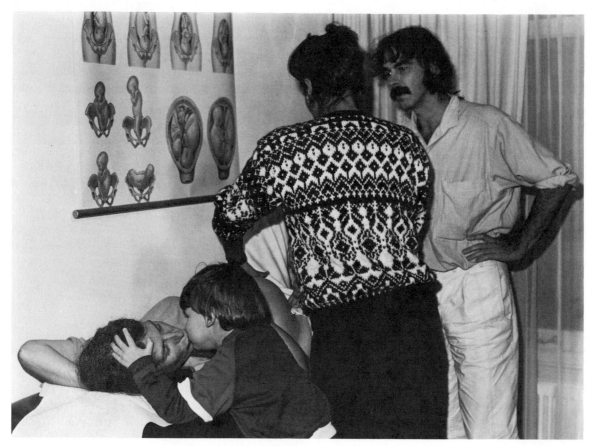

The photos in this gallery evolved from a photo study, sponsored by the European Region of World Health Organization, of nurses in Europe.

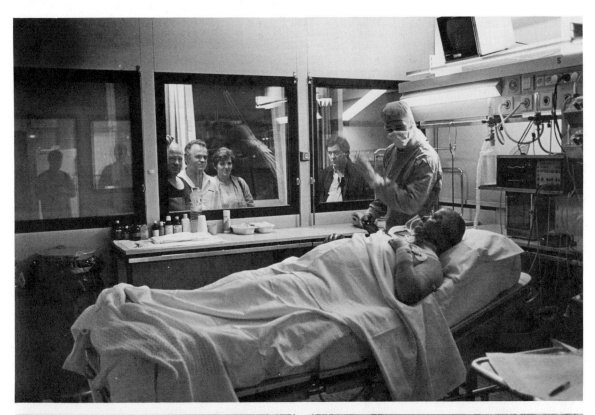

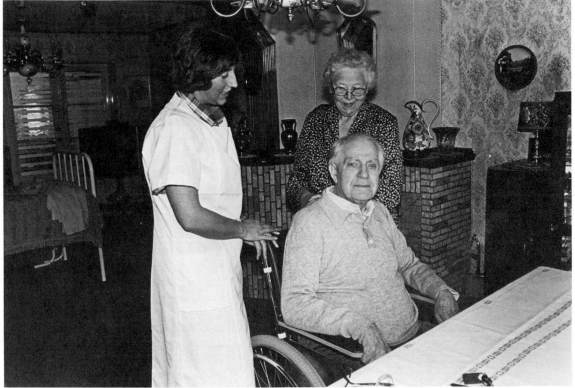

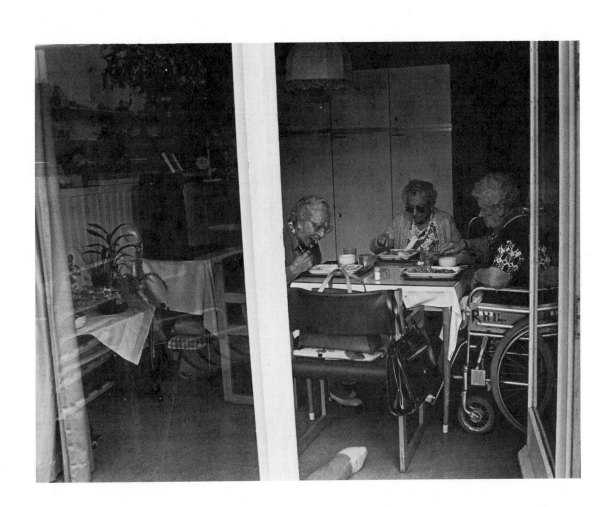

VISUAL MEDIA RESEARCH
REFERENCES

Books

Akeret R (1975): *Photoanalysis.* New York: Pocket Books.

Arbus D (1972): *diane arbus.* Millerton, NY: Aperture Monograph.

Becker H (1981): *Exploring Society Photographically.* Chicago: University of Chicago Press.

Bellak L, Baker SS (1981): *Reading Faces.* New York: Holt, Rinehart, Winston.

Bellman BL, Rosetto J (1977): *A Paradigm for Looking: Cross-Cultural Research with Visual Media.* Norwood, NJ: Ablex.

Berger J (1980): *About Looking.* New York: Pantheon.

Berger J (1972): *Ways of Seeing.* London: BBC and Penguin Books.

Callahan S (ed.) (1972): *The Photographs of Margaret Bourke-White.* New York Graphic Society.

Collier J Jr, Collier M (1986): *Visual Anthropology: Photography as a Research Method,* rev ed. Albuerque: University of New Mexico Press.

Cook T, Reichardt C (1979): *Qualitative and Quantitative Methods in Evaluation Research.* Beverly Hills: Sage.

Cunningham I (1977): *After Ninety.* Seattle: University of Washington Press.

Curtis E (1972): *In a Sacred Manner We Live.* New York: Weathervane Books.

(1970) *The Encyclopedia of Photography.* New York: Greystone Press.

Evans W (1971): *Walker Evans.* New York Graphic Society.

Fast J (1970): *Body Language.* New York: Pocket Books.

Featherstone D (1984): *Observations.* Carmel: The Friends of Photography.

Hattersley R (1971): *Discover Yourself Through Photography.* Dobbs Ferry, NY: Morgan & Morgan.

Heyman TT (1978): *Celebrating a Collection: The Work of Dorothea Lange.* Oakland, CA: The Oakland Museum.

Hirsch J (1981): *Family Photographs: Content, Meaning, and Effect.* New York: Oxford.

Johnson W (ed.) (1981): *W. Eugene Smith: Master of the Photographic Essay.* Millerton, NY: Aperture.

Jussim E (1974): *Visual Communication and the Graphic Arts.* New York: R. R. Bowker.

Krippendorff K (1980): *Content Analysis—An Introduction to its Methodology.* Beverly Hills: Sage.

Lange D (1967): *The American Country Woman.* Fort Worth, TX: The Amon Carter Museum of Western Art.

Lesy M (1980): *Time Frames: The Meaning of Family Pictures.* New York: Pantheon.

Life Library of Photography (1972): *Documentary Photography.* New York: Time-Life Books.

Lofland J (1970): *Analyzing Social Settings.* Belmont, CA: Wadsworth.

Mark ME (1981): *Falkland Road.* New York: Knopf.

Masayesva V, Younger E (eds.) (1983): *Hopi Photographers—Hopi Images.* Tucson: Sun Tracks and University of Arizona Press.

Mead M, Heyman K (1965): *Family.* New York: Macmillan.

Merton T (1956): *Silence in Heaven.* New York: Studio Publications.

Newhall B (1980): *Photography: Essays and Images.* New York Graphic Society.

Newhall B (1982): *The History of Photography.* New York: Museum of Modern Art.

Owens B (1978): *Documentary Photography: A Personal View.* New York: Addison House.

Owens B (1973): *Suburbia.* Straight Arrow Books.

Rothstein A (1986): *Documentary Photography.* Woburn, MA: Focal Press.

Rosenborg M (1980): *Patients: The Experience of Illness.* Philadelphia: Saunders.

Ruesch J, Kees W (1974): *Nonverbal Communication.* Berkeley, CA: University of California Press.

Simpson J (1976): *The American Family: A History in Photographs.* New York: Viking.

Smith EW, Smith A (1975): *Minimata.* New York: Holt, Rinehart, Winston.

Smith EW, Smith A (1972): *Master of the Photographic Essay.* New York: Aperture.

Sontag S (1977): *On Photography.* New York: Dell.

Steichen E (1955): *The Family of Man.* New York: Museum of Modern Art.

Sussman A (1973): *The Amateur Photographer's Handbook.* New York: Thomas Crowell.

Upton B, Upton J (1981): *Photography.* Boston: Little Brown.

Wagner J (1979): *Images of Information.* Beverly Hills: Sage.

Zakia R (1979): *Perception and Photography.* Rochester, NY: Light Impressions.

Zakia R (1980): *Perceptual Quotes for Photographers.* Rochester, NY: Light Impressions.

Articles

Bird G, Elwood PC (1983): The dietary intakes of subjects estimated from photographs compared with a weighed record. *Human Nutrition: Applied Nutrition, 37A:* 470–473.

Elwood PC, Bird G (1983): A photographic method of diet evaluation. *Human Nutrition: Applied Nutrition, 37A:* 474–477.

Grunsky O, Bonacich P (1984): Physical contact in the family. *J Marr Fam, 46(3).*

Higgins S, Highley B (1986): The camera as a tool: Photo interview of mothers of infants with congestive heart failure. *Children's Health Care,* Fall: 119–122.

Kalisch, P, Kalish B (1981): When nurses were national heroines: Images of nurses in American film. *Nursing Forum, 20(1):* 14–61.

Sedgwick R (1978): Photostudy as a diagnostic tool in working with families. *Current Perspectives in Psychiatric Nursing,* 60–69.

Woychik JP, Brickell C (1983): The instant camera as a therapy tool. *Social Work,* 316–318.

Ziller R, Smith D (1977): A phenomenological utilization of photography. *Psychology, 7:* 172–173.

INDEX

A

AA. *See* Alcoholics Anonymous
ABCX model of family stress, chronic illness studied using, 290–291
Abuse, 394–417
  attachment and loss theory and, 408–411
  causation theories for, 396–404
  child
    definition of, 395
    denial and, 410–411
    in modern families, 163
    crisis theory and, 407–408
    nursing interventions related to, 408
  definition of types of, 395–396
  denial of by victim, 410–411
  drug, and suicide in elderly, 468
  ecological model and, 398–399
  elder, definition of, 395
  emotional, definition of, 395
  exchange theory and, 402–403
  feminist model and, 403–404
  future directions in study of, 411–412
  future research issues and, 412
  grieving framework and, 408–411
  incidence of, 396
  individual psychopathology and, 396–397
  learned helplessness and, 404–406
  nursing interventions related to, 405–406
  Millor framework and, 399–400
  psychologic, definition of, 395
  rape-trauma syndrome and, 406–407
  response theories and, 404–410

social learning theory and, 400–402
  substance, and suicide in elderly, 466–467
  systems theory and, 397–398
  traumatic stress syndrome and, 406–407
    nursing interventions related to, 407
Acceleration model of day care, 231
ACCH. *See* Association for the Care of Children's Health
Activity theory, and suicide in elderly, 463–464
Adaptability, in systems approach to study of family, 21
Adolescent, chronically ill, 322–331
  effects on adolescent, 323–325
  effects on family unit, 326–327
  effects on grandparents, 326
  effects on parents, 325–326
  effects on siblings, 326
  factors affecting family responses, 327
  future research issues and, 330
  responses of adolescent to, 327–328
  responses of parents to, 328
  responses of siblings to, 328–329
Advocate, nurse as, for families experiencing chronic illness, 296–297
Affective disorders, 385–387
  and childhood relations of depressed adults, 386–387
  family risk of illness and, 386
  retrospectiove research and, 387
Alcoholic families, 475–478. *See also* Alcoholism

categories of, 475–476
children of alcoholics, 477–478
enabling alcoholism and, 478
interventions with, 481–482
stages of adjustment in, 476
treatment of, 478–479
  assessment and, 482
  education and, 483
  program for, 482–484
wives of alcoholics, 476–477
Alcoholics Anonymous (AA), 475
Alcoholism, 472–485. *See also* Alcoholic families
  cultural patterns
    in Irish catholic family, 133–137
    in Protestant family, 137–142
  diagnostic criteria for, 475
  disease concept of, 473
  family and, 475–478
    children and, 477–478
    enabling and, 478
    future research issues and, 484
    interventions with, 481–482
    nursing and, 479–481
    stages of adjustment to, 476
    wives and, 476–477
  family treatment program and, 478–479, 482–484
    assessment in, 482
    education in, 483
    multifamily group in, 483
    program of, 482–483
    treatment in, 483–484
  stages of, 474
  and suicide in elderly, 466–467
Alienation theory, and suicide in elderly, 463
Alzheimer's disease, 418–436
  behavioral manifestations of, 420

Alzheimer's disease *continued*
  biochemical changes in, 419–420
  caregiver burden and, 423–427
    instruments measuring, 425
    severity of illness and, 424
  causes of, 421
  dementia management and,
      427–428
  diagnosis of, 432–433
    criteria for, 432–433
    family members affected by,
      421–422
  family caregiver, case study of,
      428–429
  future research issues and, 434
  morphologic changes in, 419–420
  nursing implications and, 429–430
  and problems of families and
      caregivers, 422–423
  and quantification of dementia,
      430–431
  research implications and, 430–432
  significance of to family, 420–422
    family members as caregiver,
      420–422
Alzheimer's Disease and Related
    Disorders Association (ADRDA),
    428, 431–432
American Indians. *See* Native
    Americans
Antepartum stress, developmental
    framework in study of effects of,
    17
Antidepressants, and suicide in
    elderly, 468
Asians, and alternate family forms,
    79
Assessment
  caseload analysis and, 149–153
  Family Dynamics Measure for, 26
  of healthy families
    based on Barnhill's model, 5
    Family Assessment Guide for,
      87, 88–89
  and treatment of alcoholic families,
    482
Association for the Care of Children's
    Health (ACCH), 251, 257
Asthma, family relationships
    affecting, 7
Attachment
  abusive behavior in families and,
      408–411
  father-infant, chronic illness of
      infant affecting, 304–305
  mother-infant
    chronic illness of infant
        affecting, 303–304
    and limitations of developmental
        approach, 18

B

Baird, M., 68
Barbiturates, and suicide in elderly,
    468
Battering, of female partner. *See also*
    Abuse
  definition of, 395
Beavers, W., 80–81
Beavers systems model, research on
    healthy families and, 84–85
Berardo, F.M., 10
Bereaved family, 216–225. *See also*
    Bereavement; Death; Grief
  cancer and, 340
  clinical implications and, 222–223
  and consequences of grief, 221–222
  controversial issues and, 219–221
    replacement versus integration,
      219
    stages approach, 219–220
  future research issues and, 224
  nurse's role and, 222
  tasks of, 217–219
    extrafamilial role realignment,
      218
    increased solidarity, 218
    intrafamilial role realignment,
      217–218
    intrapsychic role reorganization,
      218
    object replacement, 218–219
    permission to grieve, 217
Bereavement. *See also* Bereaved
    family; Death; Grief
  abusive behavior in families and,
      408–411
  cancer and, 340
  clinical implications of, 222–223
  and consequences of grief, 221–222
  controversial issues in field of,
      219–220
    replacement versus integration,
      219
    stages approach, 219–220
  and death of cancer patient, as
      family crisis, 340
  future research issues and, 224
  and nurse's role, 223
  research implications and, 222–223
  as risk factor for suicide in elderly,
      465
Bertalanffy, L.V., 20–24
Blacks
  and alternate family forms, 79
  changes in family structure of,
      164–167
    economic issues affecting,
      165–166
    internal adaptation and, 166–167

and suicide in elderly, 462–463
Bonding, mother-infant. *See*
    Attachment, mother-infant
Bronfenbrenner, U., 24–26
Brown, J., 38–45
Burgess, A., 406, 407
Burr, W.R., 10, 11–14, 291

C

Calcium, intake of in American
    family diet, 102
Caloric intake, and nutritional risk
    factors, 104
Cancer, 332–343
  as end-stage illness
    as family problem, 438–440
    palliative care and, 437–460. *See
        also* Palliative care nursing
  impact of on family, 333–334
    clinical issues and, 341
    family support and, 341–342
    future research issues and, 342
    research issues and, 341
    staging models for, 334
  and nutritional risk factors,
      106–107
  psychosocial dimensions of, 333
  sociologic and psychologic crises
      precipitated by, 334–341
    bereavement, 340
    death, 340
    decline, 339
    diagnosis and, 335–336
    disclosure, 336
    ending treatment, 339
    family reorganization, 340–341
    home care stress, 339
    in prediagnostic phase, 335
    preparation for death, 339–340
    recurrence, 339
    role conflict, 338–339
    sexuality, 338
    stigma, 337
    suspicion, 335
    treatment decisions, 336–337
    uncertainty, 335
    uncertainty of chronic disease,
      337–338
Cardiac illness, 344–356. *See also*
    Coronary artery disease
  acute, 347–350
    and needs for specific
        information, 349–350
    patient-spouse differences and,
      348–349
    and preparation for discharge,
      350
    seeking care and, 348
    spousal distress and, 350

future research issues and, 353
prevention of, 345–347
  environmental manipulation
    and, 347
  lifestyle behaviors and, 345
  type A behavior and, 345–346
and promotion of family health,
  352–353
recovery from, 350–352
  family conflict and, 351
  spousal distress and, 351
  and spousal support of patient,
    352
Cardiac surgery, family response to,
  347–350. *See also* Cardiac illness,
  acute
Caregiver, mother as, 209
Caregiver burden, *See also* Family
  burden
  Alzheimer's disease and, 422–427
    Caregiver Burden Scale and,
      426–427
    case study of, 428–429
    description of, 423–427
    family support instrument and,
      426
    instruments measuring, 425
    as outcome variable, 423–427
    and problem behaviors of
      demented family member,
      422–423
    severity of illness affecting, 424
Caseload analysis, and health care
  financing and policy, 148–154
  case examples of, 150–153
  family assessment and, 149–150
  issues in, 149
Cerebrovascular disease, as end-
  stage illness
  as family problem, 438–440
  palliative care and, 437–460. *See
    also* Palliative care nursing
Change, in healthy family unit, 5
Chicago tradition, in family practice
  and research, 13
Child
  abused. *See* Child abuse of
    alcoholic, 477–478
  chronically ill, 300–321
    community support for family
      and, 315–316
    family triad affected during
      infancy, 305–306
    father-infant dyad affected
      during infancy, 303–305
    future research issues and, 316
    impact during infancy, 303–307
    influence of during early
      childhood, 307–310
    influence of during middle
      childhood, 310–311

mother-infant dyad affected
  during infancy, 303–305
newborn experience affected by,
  310–303
parental responses to birth of,
  301–303
peer relationships in school and,
  312–313
school and, 311–315
siblings affected by during early
  childhood, 308–309
day care for, 226–247. *See also* Day
  care
of depressed adult, 386–387
with diabetes mellitus, 358–371.
  See also Diabetes mellitus
disabled, day care programs for,
  240–241
hospitalized, 248–261
  basic principles for family
    centered care of, 257–258
  change of focus in family
    involvement in care of, 252
  changes in perception of
    hospitals and, 254–255
  changes in perception of role of
    family in care of, 254–255
  child life movement affecting
    family involvement in care
    of, 257
  consumer groups affecting
    family involvement in care
    of, 252–253
  current trends in family
    involvement in care of,
    256–257
  family adjustment and, 255–256
  family support and, 256
  future research issues in family
    involvement in care of, 259
  history of family involvement in
    care of, 249–251
  hospital design affecting family
    involvement in care of, 256
  parent programs affecting family
    involvement in care of,
    253–254
  parental housing and, 256–257
  parent's involvement in care of,
    248–261
  transition to family involvement
    in care of, 251–256
illnesses in, stressful family
  experiences and, 6–7
status in in modern family,
  163–164
  divorce affecting, 163–164
Child abuse
  definition of, 395
  denial and, 410–411
  in modern families, 163

Child day care, 226–247
  environment of, 236
  future of, 241–242
  future research issues and, 243
  health program in, 236–239
    health needs of infants and
      children, 237
    health needs of staff, 236–237
    infectious diseases and, 238–239
    injury control and, 237–238
    primary health care and, 239
  historical context of, 227–229
  models of, 230–232
    acceleration model, 231
    cognitive-play model, 231
    custodial model, 231
    deprivation-eduation model, 230
    empowerment model, 230–231
    infant programs, 231–232
    surrogate parenting model,
      231
  need for, 227
  political context of, 227–229
  regulation of in United States,
    229–230
  resources for, 246–247
  selection of program, 232–236
    minority families and, 234
    staff-child ratios and, 235–236
    supporting choice for, 232–234
    types available and, 234–235
  special needs and, 240–241
Child development. *See also*
  Developmental perspective
  chronic illness affecting, 300–321.
    See also Child, chronically ill
  diabetes mellitus affecting,
    360–361
  and healthy families, 80
Child life movement, 257
Child neglect. *See also* Child abuse
  definition of, 395
Child sexual abuse. *See also* Child
  abuse
  definition of, 395
Childbearing. *See also* Perinatal family
  changes in attitudes toward,
    163–164
  decision for, 200–201
  delayed, and alternate family form,
    78
  marital quality affected by, 187–198
    future research issues and, 196
    and intimacy as concept in
      childbearing literature, 193
    and intimate dyad, 188–189
    and marital dyad, 189–190
    and nurturance as concept in
      childbearing literature,
      193–194
    as outcome variable, 190–191

Childbearing *continued*
 as predictor of childbearing
   outcomes, 191–193
 and transitions in emerging
   families, 179–181
Childhood
 early, chronic illness influencing,
   307–310
 middle, chronic illness influencing,
   310–311
Childrearing
 changes in attitudes toward,
   163–164
 and transitions in emerging
   families, 179
Children In Hospitals, 252–253
Chinese, and suicide in elderly, 462
Chlordiazepoxide, and suicide in
   elderly, 468
Choline acetyltransferase (ChAT),
   reduction of in Alzheimer's
   disease, 419–420
Chronic obstructive lung disease, as
   end-stage illness
 as family problem, 438–440
 palliative care and, 437–460. *See
   also* Palliative care nursing
Circumplex model
 research on healthy familes and,
   83, 84
 in systems approach to study of
   family, 22
Clinic, as setting for family care,
   66–67
Cognitive-play model of child day
   care, 231
Cohesion, in systems approach to
   study of family, 21
Communication deviance, family and
   schizophrenia and, 382–383
 problems in research on, 383
Community
 and social support for families,
   113–123
 conceptual issues related to,
   115–117
 definition of terms and,
   114–115
 family as source of, 117–118
 measurement of, 117
 non-kin ties as source of,
   118–119
 sources of, 117–121
 and support for family with
   chronically ill child, 315–316
Conflict, diabetes as source for,
   361–362
Connectedness, in healthy family
   unit, 6
Contextualism, in study of
   developmental phenomena, 17

Contrived experiment, in ecological
   framework for study of family, 24
Coping, family, 293–295. *See also*
   Family coping
 as perspective for family practice
   and research, 26–27
Coping trajectory, in families coping
   with illness, 272–275
 multiple remissions affecting,
   274–275
 patient versus family, 273–274
Coronary artery disease. *See also*
   Cardiac disease
 dietary factors and, 107–108
Couples, healthy, and healthy
   families, 80–81
Crisis theory, abusive behavior in
   families and, 407–408
 nursing interventions related to,
   408
Cross-sectional approach, in
   developmental research, 17–18
Culture
 and alternate family forms, 79
 family centered care affected by,
   278
 family response to illness affected
   by, 124–145
 in American-Samoan family,
   129–133
 concepts in study of, 128–129
 and family health, 125–126
 and family structure, 126–127
 family studies of, 127–128
 and future research issues, 143
 in Irish-Catholic family, 133–137
 methods in study of, 128–129
 in middle-class Protestant family,
   137–142
 food decisions affected by, 96–99

D

Day care, *See* Child day care
Death. *See also* Bereaved family;
   Bereavement; Grief
 abusive behavior in families and,
   408–411
 of cancer patient
   as family crisis, 340
   preparation for as family crisis,
     339–340
 of child, developmental framework
   in study of effects of, 16
 palliative care and, 437–460. *See
   also* Palliative care nursing
 and time of death, 452–453
Dementia. *See also* Alzheimer's
   disease
 management of symptoms of,
   427–428

quantification of severity of,
   430–431
Depression. *See also* Affective
   disorders
 control of in palliative care
   nursing, 450
 as risk factor for suicide in elderly,
   464–465
Deprivation-eduation model of day
   care, 230
Developmental perspective. *See also*
   Child development; Family
   development
 on family practice and research,
   14–20
 assumptions of, 15–16
 constraints of, 18–19
 definition of stages in, 14–15
 epigenetic principle and, 14–15
 limitations of, 18–19
 methodology of, 17–18
 models for study of, 17–18
 orthogenetic principle and, 15
 problems addressed by, 16–17
 spirality principle and, 15
 strengths of, 19–20
Developmental stage, food decisions
   affected by, 93–95
Diabetes mellitus, 357–373
 current state of research on effects
   of, 364–368
 developmental stage of child and,
   360–361
 family orientation to care and,
   364–365
 future directions in health care
   and, 370–371
 future research directions and,
   368–369
 and future research issues, 371
 individual, care-cure orientation to
   care and, 364–365
 linear models in study of,
   366–368
 literature review of psychosocial
   implications of, 358–359
 and medical definitions of control
   and compliance, 365–366
 professional education programs
   and, 369–370
 significance of for families with
   adult with, 362–364
 significance of for families with
   children with, 359–360
 as source of family conflict,
   361–362
 systems models in study of,
   366–368
 teaching programs and, 366–368
Diagnosis, of life threatening disease,
   as family crisis, 335–336

Dialectical model, for study of developmental phenomena, 17–18
Diazepam, and suicide in elderly, 468
Diet. *See also* Nutrition
  compliance with, as source for conflict in families with diabetic children, 361–362
  problem areas in in American families, 100–108
    caloric intake, 104
    and cancer, 106–107
    and coronary artery disease, 107
    counseling guidelines and, 103
    dietary goals and, 100, 101
    disease influenced by, 105–108
    in elderly, 105
    and hypertension, 107
    in middle aged adults, 104
    nutrients, 100–104
    obesity, 104–105
    in young adults, 104
Disengagement theory, and suicide in elderly, 464
Distributive justice
  abusive behavior in families and, 402–403
  social exchange theory and, 27
Divorce
  singlehood and future of marriage affected by, 161–163
  status of child in family affected by, 163–164
Doherty W.J., 68
Double ABCX model
  chronic illness studied with, 292
  and stress and coping frameworks for family practice and research, 27
Drinking. *See* Alcoholism
Drugs, use, misuse, or abuse of in elderly, suicide and, 467–469
Duvall, E., 15, 178
Dyad
  family, 43
  father-infant, 204
    chronic illness of infant affecting, 304–305
    intimate, historical perspective of, 188–189
    marital
      in first pregnancy, 189–190
      in mid-life, 41
      overview of, 189
    mother-infant, 203–204
      chronic illness of infant affecting, 303–304
    parent-child, 41, 43
Dying. *See* Death

E

Ecological framework
  abusive behavior in families and, 398–399
  as theory for family practice and research, 24–26
    assumptions of, 24–25
    constraints of, 26
    limitations of, 26
    methodology of, 25–26
    problems addressed by, 25
    strengths of, 26
Economic issues
  Black family structure affected by, 165–166
  and health care financing policy, 146–155
    caseload analysis and, 148–153
    perspectives on family affecting, 147–148
    policy development and, 153–154
  nutritional care influenced by, 108–110
Ecosystem, in ecological framework for study of family, 24
Education
  and alcoholism, family treatment and, 483
  chronic illness in childhood affecting, 311–315
  and diabetes mellitus, 366–368
    programs for professionals, 369–370
Elder abuse. *See also* Abuse
  definition of, 395
Elder neglect. *See also* Abuse
  definition of, 395
Elderly
  and alternate family forms, 79
  diabetes mellitus in, 363–364
  nutritional risk factors in, 105
  suicide and, 461–471
    activity theory for, 463–464
    alienation theory for, 463
    bereavement and, 465
    depression and, 464–465
    disengagement theory for, 464
    drug use, misuse, or abuse and, 467–469
    exchange theory for, 464
    future research issues and, 470
    isolation and, 465–466
    physical illness and, 465
    research theories for, 463–464
    risk factors for, 464–466
    substance abuse and, 466–467
  and transitions in contracting families, 183

Emotion, expressed, research on in schizophrenic patients and families, 383–384
Empowerment model of day care, 230–231
Empty nest syndrome, 183
Entropy, and systems approach to study of family, 20
Environment
  change in as family transition, 176–177
  for emerging family, 181
  manipulation of, and cardiac disease prevention, 347
Epidemiology, social, and study of individual health and family, 4
Epigenetic principle, in developmental theories, 14–15
  limitations of, 18
Equifinality, and systems approach to study of family, 20–21
Equity theory. *See* Social exchange theory
Erikson, E.H., 14–20, 80
Ethnic variation, and alternate family forms, 79
Exchange theory. *See also* Social exchange theory
  abusive behavior in families and, 402–403
  and suicide in elderly, 464
Expressed emotion research, family and schizophrenia and, 383–384
  issues in, 384

F

Family
  abusive behavior in, 394–417. *See also* Abuse
  affective disorders and, 385–387. *See also* Affective disorders
  alcoholism affecting, 472–485. *See also* Alcoholism
  alterations in traditional patterns of, 78–79
  alternate forms of, 86–87
    nursing implications related to, 87–89
  Alzheimer's disease affecting, 418–436. *See also* Alzheimer's disease
  as basic unit of health, 4
  bereaved, 216–225. *See also* Bereaved family
  cancer affecting, 332–343. *See also* Cancer
  cardiac illness affecting, 344–356. *See also* Cardiac illness
  changes in

Family *continued*
　childbearing and, 163–164
　childrearing and, 163–164
　future research issues and, 169
　marriage and, 159–163
　sexual revolution affecting,
　　157–159
　chronic illness affecting, 287–299.
　　See also Illness, chronic
　chronically ill adolescent affecting,
　　322–331. *See also* Adolescent,
　　chronically ill
　chronically ill child affecting,
　　300–321. *See also* Child,
　　chronically ill
　cultural factors affecting response
　　to illness of, 124–145
　development of, 80–81
　　children, 80
　　couples, 80–81
　　parents, 80
　diabetes mellitus affecting,
　　357–373. *See also* Diabetes
　　mellitus
　emerging, transitions in, 179–181
　end-stage illness and, 438–440. *See
　　also* Palliative care nursing
　extended, and cultural patterns in
　　family health demonstrated by
　　Samoan family, 129–133
　functions of, 79
　future of, 167–168
　healthy, 5–6. *See also* Healthy
　　family
　　assessment of, 5–6, 87, 88–89
　day care for, 226–247. *See also*
　　child day care
　forms of, 77–91
　and future research, 90
　processes in, 77–91
　research on, 83–86
　in hospital, 262–283. *See also*
　　Hospital, family's experience
　　in
　hospitalized child affecting,
　　248–261. *See also* Child,
　　hospitalized
　individual health affected by, 4–5,
　　6
　models for study of, 4–5
　individual illness affecting, 5
　life cycle of, 81–83. *See also* Family
　　life cycle
　　transitions in, 173–186
　mental illness affecting, 374–393.
　　See also Mental illness
　nutritional needs of, 92–112. *See
　　also* Nutrition
　　factors affecting, 93–99
　　family health affected by, 99–100

　future directions for nutritional
　　care and, 108–110
　future research on, 110
　individual health affected by,
　　99–100
　problems areas and, 100–108
　perinatal, 199–215. *See also*
　　Childbearing; Perinatal family
　at risk, preventive care and, 69–70
　schizophrenia and, 382–385. *See
　　also* Schizophrenia
　social support for in the
　　community, 113–123
　　measurement of, 117
　　sources of, 117–121
　theoretical perspectives on, 9–36.
　　See also specific theory
　　coping framework, 26–27
　　current status of, 31–32
　　developmental perspective,
　　　14–20
　　ecological framework, 24–26
　　future directions for, 31–32
　　interactionist perspective,
　　　11–14
　　research issues in, 32
　　social exchange theory, 27–31
　　stress framework, 26–27
　　systems approach, 20–24
　transitions in, 173–186. *See also*
　　Family transitions
　as unit of care, 65–66
　violence in, 394–417. *See also*
　　Abuse
Family Assessment Guide, for
　healthy families, 87, 88–89
Family burden. *See also* Caregiver
　burden
　and mental illness in the family,
　　375–379
　correlates of, 377–379
　descriptive studies of, 378
　levels of, 377
　and research issues, 379
　treatment forms affecting,
　　376–377
Family centered care
　in families coping with illness,
　　269–272
　barriers to implementation of,
　　276–277
　clinical intervention guidelines
　　for, 275
　culture affecting, 278
　fallacies of, 270–271
　group support strategies and,
　　271–272
　implementation of, 276–277
　levels of intervention in,
　　269–270

　methodologic implications and,
　　277–278
　as tripartate construct, 277
　of hospitalized child, 248–261. *See
　　also* Child, hospitalized
　basic principles of, 257–258
Family coping, 293–295
　as perspective for family practice
　　and research, 26–27
　phases of, 294
　role of nurse in, 295–297
　　advococy and, 296–297
　　communication facilitation, 296
　　coordination of care and, 295
　　information and, 295–296
　　respite and, 297
Family development, transitions and,
　178–183
　in contracting families, 183
　in emerging families, 179–181
　in reconstituting families,
　　181–183
　in solidifying families, 181–183
Family Dynamics Measure, 26
Family ecology, 25–26
Family health and illness cycle, 5
Family Health Project, and cardiac
　disease prevention, 345
Family life cycle, 81–83
　stages of, 82
　food decisions affected by,
　　93–95
　transitions in, 173–186
　　in contracting families, 183
　　in emerging families, 179–181
　　environment changes, 176–177
　　family development and,
　　　178–184
　　future research issues and, 184
　　loved possessions changes,
　　　177–178
　　mental capacity changes, 177
　　personal relationship changes,
　　　175–176
　　physical capacity changes, 177
　　psychosocial, 175–178
　　in reconstituting families,
　　　181–183
　　role changes, 176
　　in solidifying families, 181–183
　　status changes, 176
Family nursing
　and family as unit of care, 65–66
　health care financing policy
　　affecting, 146–155
　　caseload analysis and, 148–154
　　future research issues in, 154
　　perspective on families affecting,
　　　147–148
　interventions in, 71–72

prevention and, 69–71
  primary, 69–70
  secondary, 70
  tertiary, 70
primary care and, 68–69
research needed in, 72
research summary of, 37–63
  design taxonomy for, 38
  discussion in, 43–44
  important citations in, 49–63
  methods in, 39
  results of, 39–43
settings for, 66–67
models for, 67–68
Family paradigm, chronic illness
  studied with, 292–293
Family stress theory, in study of
  chronic illness, 290–292. *See also*
  Stress
Family studies, cultural factors and,
  127–129
Family therapy, as level 5 of primary
  family care, 69
Family transitions, 173–186
  family development and, 178–183
    contracting families, 183
    emerging families, 179–180
    reconstituting families, 181–183
    solidifying families, 181–183
  future research issues and, 184
  psychosocial, 175–178
    environment changes, 176–177
    loved possessions chanages,
      177–178
    mental capacity changes, 177
    personal relationship changes,
      175–176
    physical capacity changes, 177
    role changes, 176
    status changes, 176
Family treatment programs
  alcoholism and, 478–479, 482–484
    assessment and, 482
    education and, 483
    multifamily group and, 483
    program for, 482–483
    treatment in, 483–484
  for families of mentally ill, 387–390
    implications for, 389–390
Father-infant dyad, 204
  chronic illness of infant affecting,
    304–305
Feedback, negative, in systems
  approach to study of family, 23
Feetham, S., 25, 38–39, 43–44
Feetham Family Functioning Survey
  (FFS), and family ecological
  systems perspective, 25
Female partner, battering of. *See also*
  Abuse
  definition of, 395

Feminist model, abusive behavior in
  families and, 403–404
FFS. *See* Feetham Family Functioning
  Survey (FFS)
First order changes, in family
  nursing, 70
Flurazepam, and suicide in elderly,
  468
Food. *See also* Nutrition
  factors affecting family decisions
    about, 93–99
    advertising, 95
    color, 98
    cost, 95–97
    developmental stage, 93–95
    external influences, 95
    internal influences, 98
    lifestyle, 97–98
    psychophysiologic responses to,
      98–99
    smell, 98
    sociocultural, 96–97

G

Gays. *See* Homosexual couples
Gelles, R.J., 10, 28, 29, 402
Grief. *See also* Bereaved family;
  Bereavement; Death
  abusive behavior in families and,
    408–411
  consequences of, 221–222
  controversial issues and, 219–220
    replacement versus integration,
      219
    stages approach, 219–220
  family tasks in process of, 217–219
    extrafamilial role realignment,
      218
    increased solidarity, 218
    intrapsychic role reorganization,
      218
    object replacement, 218–219
    permission to grieve, 217
    realignment of intrafamilial
      roles, 217–218
  future research issues and, 224
  process of in bereaved family,
    216–225
  research implications, 222–223

H

Hawthorne effect, in ecological
  framework for study of families,
  28
Health
  dietary factors in promotion of,
    99–100
  individual, family affecting, 4–5,
    6–7

Health care
  day care and, 236–239
  for diabetes mellitus, 370–371
    individual, care-cure orientation
      versus family orientation,
      364–365
  purpose of for families, 3–8
    and healthy family unit, 5–6
    individual health and, 4–5, 6–7
    individual illness and, 5
Health care financing policy, family
  nursing practice affected by,
  146–155
  caseload analysis and, 148–154
  caseload analysis affecting policy
    development, 153–154
  and elements of policy
    development, 148
  future research issues, 154
  perspective on families and,
    147–148
  policy and family relationships,
    147–148
Health program, for infants and
  children in day care, 236–239
Healthy family
  assessment of, 5–6
  Family Assessment Guide for
    study of, 87, 88–89
  forms of, 77–91
    alternate, 86–87
    alterations in, 78–79
    nursing implications and, 87–89
  processes in, 77–91
    and child development, 80
    and development of marital
      couple, 80–81
    and functions of family, 79
    and parental needs, 80
  research on, 83–86
    Beavers systems model in,
      84–85
    Circumplex model in, 83, 84
Heart disease, as end-stage illness
  as family problem, 438–440
  palliative care and, 437–360. *See
    also* Palliative care nursing
Hill, R., 10, 290–291
Hispanics, and alternate family
  forms, 79
Home, as setting for family care, 67
Home care, for cancer patient, stress
  of as family crisis, 339
Homeostasis, and systems approach
  to study of family, 20–21, 22
Homosexual couples. *See also*
  Lesbians
  AIDS and, 174
  childrearing decisions and, as
    transition in emerging family,
    179–181

Homosexual couples *continued*
  children raised by, as alternate
      family form, 78
Hospice care. *See also* Palliative care
    nursing
  introduction of, 440–441
Hospital
  design of, and family centered care
      for children, 256–257
  family's experience in, 262–283
    and barriers to family focused
        care, 276–277
    clinical intervention guidelines
        and, 275
    coping trajectory and, 272–275
    culture affecting, 278
    and fallacies of family centered
        services, 270–271
    and family care as tripartate
        construct, 277
    and family centered care,
        276–277
    and family intervention,
        269–272
    family needs and, 265–267
    family strengths and, 267–268
    future research issues and, 280
    and group support strategies,
        271–272
    and levels of family intervention,
        269–270
    method for study of, 264–265
    methodologic implications of,
        277–278
    and patient versus family coping
        trajectories, 273–274
    remissions affecting coping
        trajectory, 274–275
    research conclusions about,
        278–280
    role of stigma and, 268–269
  as setting for family care, 67
Hospitalization, of child, parents'
    involvement in, 248–261
  basic principles for, 257–258
  change of focus to, 252
  and changing perceptions of
      families, 254–255
  and changing perceptions of
      hospitals, 254–255
  and child life movement, 257
  and consumer groups as change
      force, 252–253
  current trends in, 256–257
  family adjustment and, 255–256
  family support and, 256
  and future research issues, 259
  history of, 249–251
  hospital design and, 256
  and parent programs as change
      force, 253–254

and parental housing, 256–257
  transition to, 251–256

I

Identity processes, in healthy family
    unit, 5
Idiographic approach, in
    developmental research, 17
Illness, family affected by, 4,
    262–283. *See also specific disease*
  cancer, 332–343
  cardiac disease, 344–356
  of child, hospitalization and,
      248–261. *See also* Child,
      hospitalized
  chronic, 287–299
    adaptation to uncertainty of in
        cancer, 337–338
    in adolescent family member,
        322–331. *See also*
        Adolescent, chronically ill
    assumptions about, 289–290
    in children, 300–321. *See also*
        Child, chronically ill
    family coping and, 293–295
    family frameworks used in study
        of, 290–293
    family paradigm in study of,
        292–293
    family stress theory in study of,
        290–292
    future research issues and, 298
    in infant, 303–307. *See also*
        Infant, chronically ill
    and nurse's role in family
        coping, 295–297
    palliative care and, 437–460. *See
        also* Palliative care nursing
    symbolic interactionism in study
        of, 12
    versus transition, 288–289
  and compliance with treatment,
      6–7
  as consequence of grief, 221
  diabetes mellitus, 357–373
  dietary patterns affecting, 105–108
  end-stage
    as family problem, 438–440
    palliative care and, 437–460. *See
        also* Palliative care nursing
  and family's experience in hospital,
      262–283. *See also* Hospital,
      family's experience in
  family's reaction to, 262–283
    and barriers to family focused
        care, 276–277
    and clinical intervention
        guidelines, 275
    and coping trajectory, 272–275
    and culture, 278

and fallacies of family centered
    services, 270–271
  and family care as tripartate
      construct, 277
  and family focused care,
      276–277
  and family intervention,
      269–272
  and family needs, 265–267
  and family strengths, 267–268
  and future research issues, 280
  and group support strategies,
      271–272
  and levels of family intervention,
      269–270
  method of study of, 264–265
  and methodologic implications,
      277–278
  and patient versus family coping
      trajectories, 273–274
  and remissions affecting coping
      trajectory, 274–275
  research conclusions about,
      278–280
  and role of stigma, 268–269
  individual, family affected by, 5
  mental, 374–393. *See also* Mental
      illness
  as risk factor for suicide in elderly,
      465
  stressful family experiences and,
      6–7
Indians, American. *See* Native
    Americans
Infant
  chronically ill, 303–307
    father-infant dyad affected by,
        303–305
    implications for nursing
        interventions and, 306–307
    mother-infant dyad affected by,
        303–305
  contribution of to perinatal family,
      204
  day care program for. *See also* Day
      care
  health program in, 237
  settings for, 231–232
  and father-infant dyad, 204
  as focal point of perinatal family
    postbirth, 208
    prebirth, 206–207
  and mother-infant dyad, 203–204
  sibling's response to, 204
  as unborn family member,
      202–203
Infectious disease, prevention and
    management of in day care
    programs, 238–239
Infertility, symbolic interactionism in
    study of, 12

Information processing, in healthy family unit, 5

Injury control, in day care programs, 237–238

Interactionist perspective, on family practice and research, 11–14
assumptions of, 11–12
constraints of, 13–14
limitations of, 13–14
methodology of, 12
problems addressed by, 12–13
strengths of, 14

Interventions
with alcoholic families, 481–482
and chronically ill infant, 306–307
clinical guidelines for, 275
fallacies of, 270–271
group support strategies and, 271–272
implementation of, 276–277
levels of, 269–270
crisis theory of abusive behavior and, 408
with families of mentally ill, 387–390
implications for family treatment, 389–390
learned helplessness theory of abusive behavior and, 405–406
nature of in family nursing, 71–72
and traumatic stress syndrome, 407

Intimacy, as concept in childbearing literature, 193

Irish family, cultural patterns in family health demonstrated by, alcohol use and, 133–137

Isolation, as risk factor for suicide in elderly, 465–466

Isomorphism, and systems approach to study of family, 21

J

Japanese Americans, and suicide in elderly, 462

L

Lesbians. *See also* Homosexual couples
parenthood and, 179–181

Learned helplessness, abusive behavior in families and, 404–406
nursing interventions related to, 405–406

Life cycle, of family. *See* Family life cycle

Lifestyle, food decisions affected by, 97–98

Linear approach, in study of diabetes mellitus, 366

LISREL VI, and systems approach to study of family, 23

Loss, abusive behavior in families and, 408–411

Lubricants, in control of constipation in palliative care nursing, 450

M

Macrosystem, in ecological framework for study of family, 24

Marriage
childbearing affecting quality of, 187–198
future research issues and, 196
and intimacy as concept in childbearing literature, 193
and intimate dyad, 188–189
and marital dyad, 189–190
and marital quality as outcome variable, 190–191
and marital quality as predictor of childbearing outcomes, 191–193
and nurturance as concept in childbearing literature, 193–194
singlehood affecting future of, 159–163
and transitions in emerging families, 179

McCubbin, H.I., 10, 23, 27, 291–292

Mead, G.H., 11–14

Mechanistic model, for study of developmental phenomena, 17

Memory impairment, in Alzheimer's disease, 420

Mental capacity, change in as family transition, 177

Mental illness, 374–393
affective disorders, 385–387
and childhood relations of depressed adults, 386–387
and retrospective research issues, 387
risk of illness and, 386
family attitudes to, 379–381
current research on, 380–381
family burden and, 375–379
correlates of, 377–379
descriptive studies of, 378
issues in research on, 379
levels of, 377
treatment forms affecting, 376–377
family needs and, research on, 381–382
family response to, 379–380

classic studies of, 380
family treatment programs for, 387–390
implications of, 389–390
future research issues and, 390
as risk factor for suicide in elderly, 464–465
schizophrenia, 382–385
and communication research problems, 383
and course of illness, 383–384
and expressed emotion research, 384
onset, 382–383
and risk of illness, 384–385
and risk research issues, 385
scope of, 375

Mesosystem, in ecological framework for study of family, 24

Mexican Americans, and alternate family forms, 79

Microsystem, in ecological framework for study of family, 24

Millor framework, abusive behavior in families and, 399–400
self-role definition and, 401

Minority families
and alternate family forms, 79
day care and, 234
and suicide in elderly, 462–463

Morphogenetic properties, in systems approach to study of family, 21

Morphostatic properties, in systems approach to study of family, 20–21

Mother
as essential caregiver, 209
working. *See also* Child day care

Mother-infant dyad, 203–204
chronic illness of infant affecting, 303–304

Myocardial infarction, family response to, 347–350. *See also* Cardiac illness, acute

N

National Council on Alcoholism, and diagnostic criteria for alcoholism, 475

Native Americans
and alternate family forms, 79
and suicide in elderly, 462–463

Needs, of families in hospital, 265–267

Negentropy, and systems approach to study of family, 20, 21
limitations and constraints and, 23

Neglect. *See also* Abuse
    child, definition of, 395
    elder, definition of, 395
Newborn, chronically ill, 301–303
    implications for nursing
        intervention and, 302–303
    parental response to birth of,
        301–302
Nomothetic approach, in
    developmental research, 17
Noncompliance, family affecting,
    6–7
Nuclear family, as assumption of
    developmental perspective, 15
Nurturance, as concept in
    childbearing literature, 193
Nutrients, problems with in
    American diet, 100–104. *See also*
    Nutrition
Nutrition, 92–112
    and dietary risk factors, 100–108
        calcium intake and, 102
        caloric intake and, 104
        cancer and, 106–107
        coronary artery disease and,
            107–108
        counseling guidelines and, 103
        dietary goals and, 101
        disease influenced by, 105–108
        in elderly, 105
        fat controlled diet and, 109
        hypertension and, 107
        iron intake and, 102
        magnesium intake and, 102
        in middle aged adults, 104
        nutrient intake and , 100–104
        obesity and, 104–105
        vitamin A intake and, 102–104
        vitamin C intake and, 102–104
        vitamin B_6 intake and, 102
        in young adults, 104
    and factors affecting family food
        habits, 93–99
        advertising, 95
        color of food, 98
        developmental stage, 93–95
        external influences, 95
        food cost, 95–96
        internal influences, 98
        lifefstyle, 97–98
        psychophysiologic responses,
            98–99
        smell of food, 98
        sociocultural factors, 96–97
    family health affected by,
        99–100
    and future directions for family
        care, 108–110
        economic conditions influencing,
            108–110
    future research issues and, 110

individual health affected by,
    99–100
in palliative care nursing, case
    study example of, 454
Nye, F.I., 10, 28–31

O

Obesity, and nutritional risk factors,
    104–105
Objective burden, and mental illness
    in the family, 376. *See also* Family
    burden
Oliveri, M.E., 292–293
Oral dysfunctions, control of in
    palliative care nursing, 452
Organismic model, for study of
    developmental phenomena, 17
Orthogenetic principle, in
    developmental theories, 15

P

Pain, control of in palliative care
    nursing, 445–449
    case study example of, 454
    intervention plans for, 447
    mild to moderate, 446
    severe chronic, 446–449
Palliative care nursing, 437–460
    case study illustrating, 453–457
    challenges of, 441–442
    clinical practice and,
        recommendations for care
        emerging from, 442–444
    and end-stage illness as family
        problem, 438–440
    essence of, 440–441
    future research issues and, 457
    research on, recommendations for
        care emerging from, 442–444
    symptom control and, 444–452
        anorexia, 451–452
        constipation, 449–450
        decubiti, 450–451
        depression, 450
        nausea, 449
        oral dysfunctions, 452
        pain, 445–449
        vomiting, 449
    and time of death, 452–453
Parenthood, changes in attitudes
    toward, 163–164
Parents
    developmental needs of, and
        healthy families, 80
    and hospitalized child, 248–261.
        See also Child, hospitalized
Parkes, C.M., 174, 175
Patterson, J., 10, 23, 27, 292
Peers, chronic illness during

childhood affecting relationships
    with, 312–313
Perinatal family, 199–215. *See also*
    Childbearing
    changing shape of, 210
    dynamics of, 204–210
        and infant as focal point
            (postbirth), 208
        and infant as focal point
            (prebirth), 206–207
        and mother as essential
            caregiver, 209
        and narrowing of social world,
            207–208
        postbirth, 208–210
        prebirth, 205–208
        and pregnant woman as
            centerpiece, 205–206
        and widening of social world,
            209–210
    and family as unit of care, 200
    future research issues and, 213
    and perinatal nursing, 210–212
    and postpartum changes and
        processes, 203–204
        father-infant interaction, 204
        maternal role attainment, 203
        mother-infant dyad, 203–204
        newborn's contribution, 204
        sibling response, 204
    and pregnancy experience,
        200–203
        childbearing decisionn, 200–201
        psychodynamics of pregnancy,
            201
        relationships during pregnancy,
            201–202
        unborn family member, 202–203
Perinatal nursing, nature of, 210–212
    case studies and, 211–212
    future directions and, 212
Physical capacity, change in as family
    transition, 177
    in contracting families, 183
Possessions, loved, changes in as
    family transition, 177–178
Pregnancy. *See also* Perinatal family
    and childbearing decision, 200–201
    and postpartum changes and
        processes, 203–204
        maternal role attainment, 203
        mother-infant dyad, 203–204
    and pregnant woman as
        centerpiece of perinatal family,
        205–206
    psychodynamics of, 201
    relationships during, 201–202
    and unborn family member,
        202–203
Premarital sex, modern family
    affected by, 157–159

Prevention, levels of applied to family care, 69–71
first-order changes and, 70–71
primary, 69–70
secondary, 70
second-order changes and, 70–71
tertiary, 70
Primary care
family involvement levels, 68–69
in day care programs, 239
Processes
developmental framework in study of, 16–17
symbolic interactionism in study of, 12
limitations and, 13–14
Psychopathology, in abusive families, 396–397
Psychosocial transitions, family life affected by, 175–178
environment changes, 176–177
loved possessions changes, 177–178
mental capacity changes, 177
personal relationship changes, 175–176
physical capacity changes, 177
role changes, 176
status changes, 176
Psychosomatic problems, family affecting, 7

R

Rape trauma syndrome, and abusive behavior in families, 406–407
nursing interventions related to, 407
Reality orientation, in management of symptoms of dementia, 427–428
Recommended Dietary Allowances (RDAs), and problem nutrients in American diet, 100
Reiss, D., 292–293
Relationships, changes in personal during pregnancy, 201–202
as family transition, 175–176
as family transition in contracting family, 183
as family transition in emerging family, 181
as family transition in solidifying or reconstituting family, 181–182
Research
on abusive behavior in families, future issues in, 412
on affective disorders in families, retrospective, 387

on alcoholism in families, future issues in, 484
on Alzheimer's disease affecting family
future issues in, 434
implications of, 430–432
on bereavement
future issues in, 224
implications of, 222–223
on cancer affecting family
future issues in, 342
issues in, 341
on cardiac disease affecting family, future issues in, 353
on childbearing decisions, future issues in, 196
on chronic illness affecting family, future issues in, 298
on chronically ill adolescent affecting family, future issues in, 330
on chronically ill child affecting family, future issues in, 316
on communication deviance, problems with, 383
on culture affecting family, future issues in, 243
developmental perspective for, 14–20
on diabetes mellitus affecting family
current state of, 364–368
future directions of, 368–368, 371
Double ABCX model and, 27, 292
ecological framework for, 24–26
on expressed emotion, 383–384
on family burden, future issues in, 379
on family changes, future issues in, 169
family coping perspective for, 26–27
on family experinece in hospitals
conclusions from, 278–280
future issues in, 280
on family life cycle, future issues in, 184
on family nursing
research needed in, 72
summary of, 37–63
on family reaction to illness
conclusions from, 278-280
future issues in, 280
on family transitions, future issues in, 184
on grief affecting familiy
future issues in, 224
implications of, 222–223
on health care financing affecting family practice, future issues

in, 154
on healthy families, 83–86
Beavers systems model for, 84–85
and Circumplex model, 83, 84
future issues in, 90
on hospitalized child, future issues in family centered care of, 259
idiographic approach to, 17
interactionist perspective for, 11–14
and mental illness affecting family
current, 380–381
future issues in, 390
issues in, 379
needs of family and, 381–382
retrospective, 386–387
on risk factors, 385
nomothetic approach for, 17
on nutritional needs of family, future issues in, 110
on palliative care nursing
future issues in, 457
recommendations for care from, 442–444
on perinatal family, future issues in, 213
social exchange theory for, 27–31
stress perspective for, 26–27
and suicide in the elderly
future issues in, 470
theories for, 463–464
summary of in family nursing, 37–63
design taxonomy for, 38
discussion, 43–44
methods, 39
results, 39–43
systems approach for, 4, 20–24
and theoretical perspectives on family, 32
Retrospective research, on families and affective disorders, 386–387
issues in, 387
Risk factors
affective disorders and, 386
nutritional, 100–108
caloric intake and, 104
cancer and, 106–107
coronary artery disease and, 107–108
disease affected by, 105-108
in elderly, 105
hypertension and, 107
in middle aged adults, 104
obesity and, 104–105
in young adults, 104
schizophrenia and, 384–385
issues in research on, 385
suicide in elderly and, 464–466
bereavement as, 465
depression as, 464–465

Risk factors *continued*
  isolation as, 465–466
    mental illness and, 465–466
    physical illness as, 465
Role
  change in as family transition, 176
    in contracting families, 183
    in emerging families, 181
  conflict in resulting from cancer, as
    family crisis, 338–339
  maternal, postpartum attainment
    of, 203
Role structuring, in healthy family
    unit, 5

S

Samoan family, cultural patterns in
    family health demonstrated by,
    129–133
Schizophrenia, 382–385
  and communication research
    problems, 383
  expressed emotion research and,
    384
  family affecting course of, 383–384
  and family treatment programs,
    387–390
  needs of families of, 381–382
  onset of, 382–383
  risk of illness in families and,
    384–385
  issues in research on, 385
School, chronic illness during
    childhood affecting, 311–315
Secobarbital, and suicide in elderly,
    468
Second order changes, family
    therapy for, 70
Senile dementia. *See* Alzheimer's
    disease
Separateness, in healthy family unit,
    6
Sex, premarital, modern family
    affected by, 157–159
Sexual abuse, child. *See also* Abuse
    definition of, 395
Sexual revolution, modern family
    affected by, 157–159
Sexuality, cancer affecting as family
    crisis, 338
Shame, and family attitudes to
    mental illness, 379
Sibling
  of hospitalized child, family
    adjustment and, 255–256
  response of to birth of additional
    child, 204
  response of to chronic illness of
    adolescent, 326, 328–329

response of to chronic illness
    during early childhood,
    308–309
Sibling behavior, individual illness
    affecting, 5
Single parents, as alternate family
    form, 78
Singlehood, future of marriage and,
    159–163
Social epidemiology. *See*
    Epidemiology, social
Social exchange theory. *See also*
    Exchange theory
  for family practice and research,
    27–31
    assumptions of, 28–29
    constraints of, 30
    limitations of, 30
    methodology of, 29–30
    problems addressed by, 29
    strengths of, 30–31
Social learning theory, abusive
    behavior in families and,
    400–402
Social network. *See also* Social
    support
    definition of, 115
Social rejection, and family attitudes
    to mental illness, 379
Social support
  conceptual issues related to,
    115–116
  definition of, 115
  measurement of, 117
  sources of, 117–121
    family, 117–118
    non kin ties, 118–119
Spanier, G. B., 188–189, 191–192
Spousal distress
  and acute cardiac disease, 350
  and recovery from myocardial
    infarction, 351
Status, change in as family transition,
    176
  in emerging families, 181
Stigma
  associated with cancer, as family
    crisis, 337
  role of in families coping with
    illness, 268–269
Straus, M., 397
Stress
  antepartum, developmental
    framework in study of effects
    of, 17
  and Double ABCX Model, 27
    chronic illness and, 292
  family
    and chronic illness, 290–292
    chronic illness studied using

ABC model of, 290–291
  and diabetes as source of family
    conflict, 361–362
  of home care of cancer patient, as
    family crisis, 339
  as perspective for family practice
    and research, 26–27
  spousal, individual illness
    affecting, 5
  as theoretical framework for study
    of family, 26–27
  traumatic syndrome, abusive
    behavior in families and,
    406–407
Stryker, S., 10
Subjective burden, and mental illness
    in the family, 376. *See also* Family
    burden
Substance abuse, and suicide in
    elderly, 466–467
Suicide, in elderly, 461–471
  activity theory for, 463–464
  alienation theory for, 463
  bereavement and, 465
  depression and, 464–465
  disengagement theory for, 464
  drug use, miscuse, or abuse
    and, 467–469
  exchange theory for, 464
  future research issues and, 470
  isolation and, 465–466
  physical illness and, 465
  research theories for, 463–464
  risk factors for, 464–466
  substance abuse and, 466–467
Surrogate parenting model of day
    care, 231
Symbolic interaction. *See*
    Interactionist perspective, on
    family practice and research
Systems approach
  abusive behavior in families and,
    397–398
  to family practice and research, 4,
    20–24
    assumptions of, 21–22
    constraints of, 23
    limitations of, 23
    methodology of, 23
    problems addressed by, 22–23
    strengths of, 23–24
  in study of diabetes mellitus,
    366–368

T

Therapy, family. *See* Family therapy
Tranquilizers, and suicide in elderly,
    468
Transition, versus chronic illness,

288–289
Traumatic stress syndrome, and
    abusive behavior in families,
    406–407
    nursing interventions related to,
    407
Triad, family, chronic illness of infant
    affecting, 305–306
Type A behavior, changing, and
    cardiac disease prevention,
    345–346

V

Violence
    crisis theory of response to, 407
    exchange or social control model in
        study of, 28
Vitamin A, intake of in American
    family diet, 102–104
Vitamin B$_6$, intake of in American
    family diet, 102

Vitamin C, intake of in American
    family diet, 102–104

W

Whall, A.L., 87
    assessment guide, 88–89